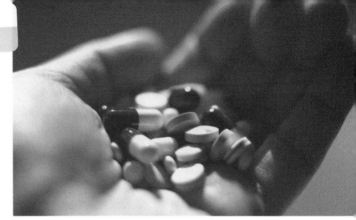

I dedicate this edition to my wife, Jeri, and children, Aaron and Meredith, who have shared in the journey of this book over the last 20+ years.

I wish to acknowledge David Brushwood, who coauthored with me the first three editions of this book and whose valuable contributions remain in this edition.

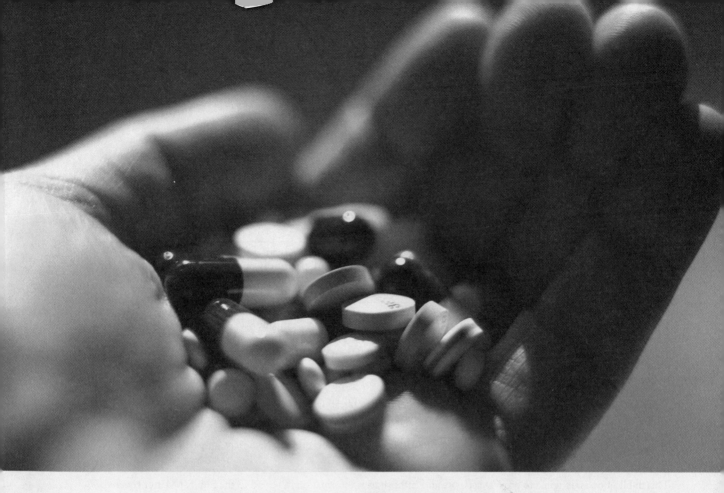

PHARMACY PRACTICE AND THE LAW

SEVENTH EDITION

Richard R. Abood, BS Pharm, JD
Professor of Pharmacy Practice
Thomas J. Long School of Pharmacy and Health Sciences
University of the Pacific
Stockton, California

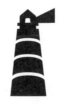

JONES & BARTLETT
LEARNING

World Headquarters
Jones & Bartlett Learning
5 Wall Street
Burlington, MA 01803
978-443-5000
info@jblearning.com
www.jblearning.com

Jones & Bartlett Learning books and products are available through most bookstores and online booksellers. To contact Jones & Bartlett Learning directly, call 800-832-0034, fax 978-443-8000, or visit our website, www.jblearning.com.

Substantial discounts on bulk quantities of Jones & Bartlett Learning publications are available to corporations, professional associations, and other qualified organizations. For details and specific discount information, contact the special sales department at Jones & Bartlett Learning via the above contact information or send an email to specialsales@jblearning.com.

Production Credits

Publisher: William Brottmiller
Senior Acquisitions Editor: Katey Birtcher
Associate Editor: Teresa Reilly
Editorial Assistant: Sean Fabery
Production Editor: Jessica Steele Newfell
Marketing Manager: Grace Richards
Manufacturing and Inventory Control Supervisor: Amy Bacus
Composition: diacriTech
Interior and Cover Design: Kristin E. Parker
Front Matter Opener Image: © Photos.com
Cover Images: (scales) © Pshenichka/ShutterStock, Inc.; (pharmacists working) © Dmitry Kalinovsky/ShutterStock, Inc.; (pharmacist consulting with customer) © Kzenon/ShutterStock, Inc.; (pills) © Stockbyte/Thinkstock
Printing and Binding: Edwards Brothers Malloy
Cover Printing: Edwards Brothers Malloy

To order this product, use ISBN: 978-1-284-02136-3

Library of Congress Cataloging-in-Publication Data
Abood, Richard R.
  Pharmacy practice and the law / by Richard R. Abood. — 7th ed.
       p. ; cm.
  Includes bibliographical references and index.
  ISBN 978-1-4496-8691-8 — ISBN 1-4496-8691-5
  I. Title.
  [DNLM: 1. Legislation, Pharmacy—United States. 2. Ethics, Pharmacy—United States. 3. Legislation, Drug—United States. 4. Liability, Legal—United States. QV 733 AA1]
  344.7304'16–dc23
                            2012032097

6048

Printed in the United States of America
16 15 14 13   10 9 8 7 6 5 4 3 2

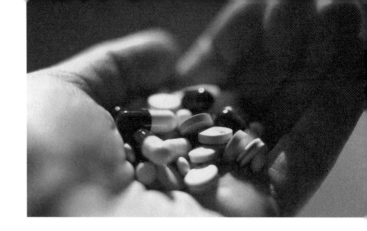

CONTENTS

the case and to generally cue the students as to what issues to think about as they read the case. As much as possible, the court's own language has been retained. By doing so, students learn that law is seldom "black and white" but rather requires a considerable measure of reasoning and analysis to reach a decision. Faculty should recognize that the questions raised in the overview are designed to stimulate discussion. A specific correct answer might not always exist; rather, there could be several answers to some of the questions. The notes following each case serve to address the questions arising from the case and to clarify certain points about the case.

The structure of all eight chapters remains essentially the same as that of the previous edition except, of course, for the updates. As in the *Sixth Edition*, this edition includes study scenarios and study questions after various chapter sections. The instructor can use these to lead class discussions. Additional study scenarios and study questions can be found in the Instructor Manual.

Chapter 1 provides an overview of law and the legal system. Chapters 2 and 3 cover the federal regulation of medications, with Chapter 2 describing the basic regulatory framework of food and drug law and Chapter 3 applying that framework to pharmacy practice.

Chapters 4 and 5 discuss relevant provisions of the federal Controlled Substances Act (CSA). Chapter 4 provides an overview of the framework of the CSA while Chapter 5 applies that framework more specifically to pharmacy practice.

The main focus of Chapter 6 is the significant influence of the federal government on the state-regulated practice of pharmacy and on business and financial issues related to the profession. From the standards established in the Omnibus Budget Reconciliation Act of 1990 (OBRA '90) to the Medicare and Medicaid laws and the federal antitrust laws, federal requirements for drugs have a profound effect on the professionals who dispense and monitor drugs. This chapter also discusses some very important recent developments involving privacy, electronic records, and pharmacy reimbursement.

Chapter 7 describes some of the basic principles of state regulation of pharmacy practice, including licensure and standards setting. Chapter 7 is intended to provide only a general overview of state law issues and contains a discussion of some important recent regulatory trends occurring among the states and discussions of the similarities and differences among state pharmacy practice acts.

Finally, Chapter 8 provides an overview of malpractice and product liability for order processing and pharmaceutical care activities, with specific tips on liability avoidance through risk management programs. Chapter 8 is important, not just to understand legal risk but also to understand the conflicting judicial opinions of the societal expectations of pharmacists, why those expectations exist, and whether they are changing. Courts mirror societal values and sometimes provide us with both flattering and unflattering perspectives of our profession.

Because the overall structure of the text remains the same, faculty who have used this text in the past should not have to make major adjustments in the way they use this new edition.

I am indebted to David Brushwood, for his friendship and for being my coauthor for the first three editions of this book, and also to those who have used this text in their classrooms and provided valuable suggestions.

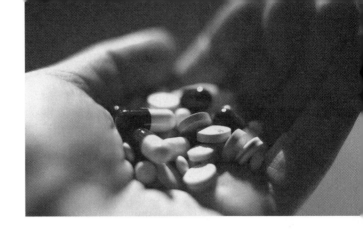

NEW TO THE *SEVENTH EDITION*

Several legal/regulatory developments directly affecting pharmacy practice or drug products have occurred since the publication of the *Sixth Edition* in 2010. This *Seventh Edition* attempts to include many of these recent developments relevant to the profession. A brief chapter-by-chapter description of those changes follows.

CHAPTER 1

Chapter 1 remains largely unchanged. Important legal terms have been accented with quotation marks so as to be more readily identifiable. A recent federal court decision where inmates sued the Food and Drug Administration (FDA) for allowing unapproved thiopental to be shipped into the country was added to the notes of *Heckler v. Chaney*.

CHAPTER 2

To the historical section was added a brief description of the Patient Protection and Affordable Care Act (PPACA, or ACA) and the FDA Safety and Innovation Act of 2012. Important provisions from each of these laws as they relate to pharmacy were added throughout Chapter 2 and in other chapters of the book.

Other changes in the chapter include new or updated discussions of the following topics:

- Whether the FDA can regulate electronic cigarettes as drug/device combination products
- Probiotics as nutraceuticals
- The FDA's enforcement emphasis on the Park Doctrine
- The FDA's reconsideration of the linear bar code requirement for labeling
- Risk evaluation and mitigation strategy (REMS) generally and REMS for extended-release and long-acting opioid drugs
- Litigation related to the legality of "pay for delay"
- Brand-name manufacturer use of a REMS requirement restricting drug distribution
- 505(b)(2) drugs
- FDA enforcement actions directed at unapproved drugs and revised compliance guidance
- FDA website where approved drug products can be identified
- Biosimilars under the Biologics Price Competition and Innovation Act
- FDA's Bad Ad Program

CHAPTER 3

Chapter 3 changes from the previous edition include new or updated discussions of these topics:

- State-standardized prescription labels
- A proposed class of drugs called "nonprescription under conditions of safe use"
- Emergency contraception product issues
- Conscientious objection and whether pharmacists can refuse to dispense prescriptions to which they are morally opposed
- FDA compliance guide related to MedGuides and REMS
- Proposed single-page consumer medication guides
- A drug information website for pharmacists
- Federal court decision analyzing whether compounding medications for animals constitutes manufacturing rather than compounding
- FDA's position on whether current bioequivalence standards are adequate for narrow therapeutic drugs
- The pedigree requirement under the Prescription Drug Marketing Act
- "Track and trace" requirements required by the FDA Amendments Act (FDAAA)

CHAPTER 4

Changes in Chapter 4 include new or updated discussions of the following items:

- "Herbal incense" and "bath salts" as schedule I substances
- Federal government policy related to state medical marijuana laws
- Carisoprodol as a schedule IV substance
- Reverse distributors included under the law as distributors
- The Drug Enforcement Administration's (DEA's) Distributor Initiative Program
- The DEA's interpretation of "constructive delivery"
- The Combat Methamphetamine Epidemic Act of 2005 and the Methamphetamine Production Prevention Act of 2008

CHAPTER 5

Changes in Chapter 5 include new or updated discussions of the following topics:

- Recent DEA actions as to whether a pharmacist can make changes to a written schedule II prescription
- Electronic refill records
- REMS for long-acting and extended-release opioid products
- REMS for transmucosal immediate release fentanyl products
- Electronic transmission prescription requirements
- Return of controlled substances to pharmacy by nonregistrants
- The Secure and Responsible Drug Disposal Act of 2010
- Central fill pharmacies
- Internet pharmacy prescriptions
- State electronic prescription monitoring programs
- Recent long-term care facility (LTCF) pharmacy issues including
  - LTCF nurses as agents of the prescriber
  - Dispensing from LTCF emergency kits

- Central recordkeeping requirements
- The filing of controlled substance prescriptions
- Disposal of controlled substances by a pharmacy
- Records of theft or loss
- Form 222 requirements
- Controlled substance ordering system (CSOS)

CHAPTER 6

Within the past few years there have been several significant changes or proposed changes in law related to electronic records, Medicare Part D, federal reimbursement determinations for prescriptions, and average wholesale prices. Perhaps there has never been a more uncertain financial climate for pharmacies.

Changes in Chapter 6 from the previous edition include new or updated discussions of these topics:

- Medicare Part D
  - Enrollment period
  - Beneficiary cost
  - Covered drugs
  - Electronic prescribing
  - Printed notice requirement
  - Fraud and abuse
  - Durable medical equipment accreditation exemption
- Average manufacturer price (AMP) regulation
- Centers for Medicare & Medicaid Services (CMS) proposed new benchmark to determine estimated acquisition cost
- U.S. Supreme Court decision on state Medicaid reimbursement cuts
- Fourteen-day dispensing cycle for long-term care facilities
- LTCF consultant pharmacist issues
- Flexible spending accounts

CHAPTER 7

Few changes were made to Chapter 7 in the *Seventh Edition*. The discussion of citizenship as a requirement for licensure was updated with a 2011 federal court decision. The continuing education section now includes a discussion of the National Association of Boards of Pharmacy's (NABP) collaborative effort with the Accreditation Council for Pharmacy Education (ACPE) called CPE Monitor where pharmacists and technicians can now be registered electronically. The discussion of state-standardized prescription labels was moved to Chapter 3.

CHAPTER 8

Chapter 8 remains largely unchanged; however, some important additions are included. The discussion under duty of care of whether a healthcare provider owes a duty to a third party was expanded by including summaries of two contrasting cases, one from Utah and one from Nevada. A subsection was added to the section on expanded view of pharmacist duty that discusses a compromise judicial position between no duty of care and a general duty of care. Correspondingly, the notes after the *Happel* case (see Case 8-1) were amended. The product liability section includes a recent state court opinion as to whether the learned intermediary doctrine is a defense when a manufacturer engages in direct-to-consumer advertising. The discussion of *Wyeth v. Levine* is expanded and supplemented with the U.S. Supreme Court's decision on the issue of whether the holding in *Levine* extends to generic drug manufacturers.

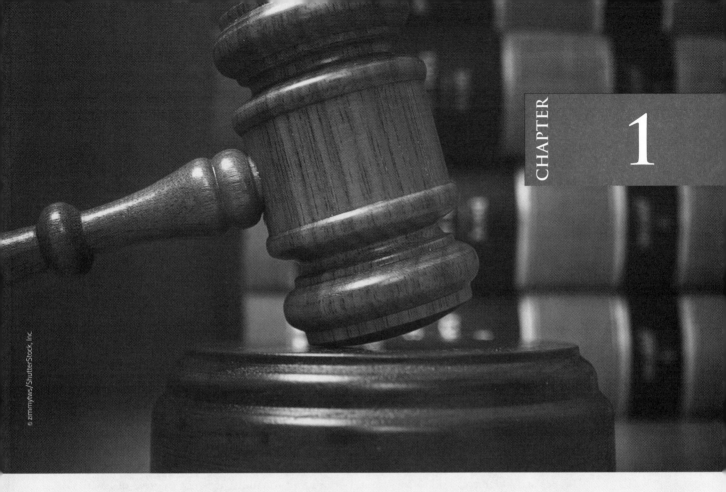

The Law and the Legal System

CHAPTER OBJECTIVES

Upon completing this chapter, the reader will be able to:

▸ Identify the reasons why society regulates medications, as well as the limitations of this regulation.

▸ Distinguish the sources and types of laws in the United States.

▸ Describe the federal and state legislative processes.

▸ Describe the structure and function of the U.S. judicial system.

▸ List the responsibilities of administrative agencies.

▸ Distinguish among criminal, civil, and administrative liability.

▸ Describe the relationship between federal and state law.

Pharmacy laws describe for pharmacists the basic requirements of day-to-day practice. Pharmacy laws also define the relationship pharmacists have with the public they serve. As health professionals, pharmacists are highly regulated because the slightest misstep in drug distribution or pharmaceutical care could cost a life. As custodians of the nation's drug supply, pharmacists are subjected to extensive regulation because the products pharmacists control are held to the most exacting standards of any consumer product. Pharmacists study the law because through the law society has described what is considered acceptable conduct for pharmacists, and pharmacists who fail to meet this level of acceptability will be held accountable for their failure.

In most pharmacy practice situations, the question of "What is legal?" can be addressed by answering the question "What is best for the patient?" Pharmacists may not always know the law, but they usually will know what is best for the patient, and this knowledge is ordinarily sufficient. However, sometimes things are more complicated than this simplistic approach would suggest. Pharmacy laws have been drafted to describe the best general approach to specific pharmacy practice situations. They provide guidance for pharmacists by establishing rules that reflect societal value choices. It is essential for pharmacists to know these rules and how to use them.

Although pharmacy laws can describe basic practice requirements, they cannot substitute for good professional judgment. Sports metaphors are not always valuable in describing professional responsibilities, but it may be useful to think of pharmacists as being on an athletic team that follows the rules of a game as they are interpreted and applied by referees or umpires. Pharmacy law provides the rules, whereas government agencies interpret and apply them. Within this framework, pharmacists are free to develop various strategies and exercise good judgment, just as athletes do. Some strategies and judgments lead to success and others lead to failure. It is not the role of law to dictate strategy and professional judgment. The law merely establishes the overall framework within which the strategy is developed. Following the law is necessary, but not sufficient, for professional success, just as following the rules is necessary, but not sufficient, for athletic success. To succeed in pharmacy, as in athletics, an effective strategy must be used together with good judgment, and it is up to pharmacists themselves to determine this, just as it is up to athletes to determine how they can succeed within the rules. Pharmacists who look to the law for an effective practice strategy and professional judgment will be disappointed because they will not find anything beyond the basic rules for behavior and appointed officials to enforce the rules.

THE NATURE AND ROLE OF LAW

Laws may generally be regarded as requirements for human conduct, applying to all persons within their jurisdiction, commanding what is right, prohibiting what is wrong, and imposing penalties for violations. The law, however, is much more than a collection of mandates and prohibitions. It is a framework through which people in a society resolve their disputes and problems in a way that does not involve force and consistently yields results that are acceptable to most of society. It is a socially prescribed process through which people declare their collective will and express their norms and values. This process of law accommodates the individual differences of every situation, but it recognizes as well the need to provide firm rules for people to follow. Therefore, the law attempts simultaneously to be flexible and also to maintain a reasonable degree of certainty. To achieve certainty, the law assumes the existence of a decision maker such as a legislature, an administrative agency, or a court that resolves disagreements by providing definitive, final answers reflective of society's expectations.

Answers in law are not often easily derived or black and white in nature. Many times an attorney's reply to a legal question is, "It depends." Many laws are necessarily vague and variable because they deal with human relationships. It is impossible for law-makers to foresee all the countless, ever-changing human relationships that may occur. Courts often can reach decisions in law only after considerable reasoning based on several factors that may include the following:

- Fundamental notions of fairness
- The custom or history involved
- The command of a political entity
- The best balance between conflicting societal interests

Recognizing the flexibility inherent in the law is important to understanding and critiquing how and why certain laws, regulations, or judicial decisions have been written.

REASONS TO REGULATE MEDICINAL DRUGS

The government regulates medicinal drugs very heavily because of the potential risks to users. The concept of government regulation to protect people from harming themselves through risky choices conjures up images of an overbearing, paternalistic bureaucracy that forces people to behave in prescribed ways. If it can be assumed that people tend to act in their own self-interest by making decisions that will increase their personal happiness (e.g., higher income, more free time, improved health status), why does the government need to make decisions for people? Why not simply allow people to look out for themselves? One possible answer is that the free market does not always act efficiently to promote happiness-maximizing behavior. Such market inefficiency, often referred to as "market failure," serves as justification for government regulation. The following four types of market failures are relevant to drug use:

1. Public goods
2. Externalities
3. Natural monopolies
4. Information asymmetry

Any legitimate government interference with a private choice to use medicinal drugs will be based on one or more of these identifiable market failures. In fact, government agencies should bear the burden of demonstrating that a market failure justifies interference with private choice. Government regulation need not occur in the absence of a specific reason to regulate.

Public goods are those necessary and beneficial commodities that private entities will not supply because there is no incentive for a private entity to provide them. National defense programs and lighthouses are classic examples of public goods; parks and intercity highways also fall within this category. Government must step in and regulate the market to provide these goods because an unregulated market will (probably) fail to provide them efficiently. Public goods in the drug industry include orphan drugs and vaccines. Orphan drugs are those drugs that are sufficiently safe and effective to be marketed, but the number of patients who need them is so small that it is not commercially feasible for a manufacturer to market them. Because the open market will not make these drugs available, government must step in to ensure their availability for those who need them. The need to regulate vaccines, on the other hand, stems from the fact that they benefit society as a whole by preventing epidemics, but because of acute reactions to them they are viewed as too risky by many individuals. If every individual made a rational decision not to accept the risk of vaccines because their benefit is to all of society rather than to the individual, there would be no benefit to anyone, and epidemics would be unpreventable. Prevention of epidemics is a public good, and government must regulate by requiring vaccinations. At the same time, the government must ensure the availability of vaccines. Because of mass product liability actions, most manufacturers stopped producing childhood vaccines in the 1980s, and the country faced a crisis when less than six months of vaccine stores remained. The federal government stepped in to provide liability protection for vaccine manufacturers, and manufacturers not only resumed production but also developed new vaccines safer than the older ones.

An externality, another type of market failure, exists when the production or consumption of a good affects someone who does not fully consent to the effect and when the costs of a good are not fully incorporated into the price a consumer pays for it. The parties who are directly involved in using the good may not consider the indirect impact of the production or consumption of the good for a party that is not involved in the use of that good. For example, people who purchase products manufactured in a factory that pollutes the air will probably not consider the costs associated with harm to the lungs of the people who live near the factory. In an unregulated market, where the manufacturer is not required to prevent air pollution, the purchase price of the product will not include the cost of the pollution. Because there is a market failure, government regulation is necessary. The overuse of antibiotics is an externality in drug therapy. A person who unnecessarily uses an antibiotic to treat a cold will probably not consider the cost to other people in terms of the increased resistance to the antibiotic within the general population. In part because of this externality, government must regulate the use of antibiotics by imposing a prescription requirement to ensure that unnecessary use by one person does not impose an indirect cost on other people.

A natural monopoly occurs when the fixed costs of providing a good are high relative to the variable costs, so the average cost declines over the time that the good is provided. Utilities that provide electricity, water, and natural gas are natural monopolies, for example, because the cost of establishing the infrastructure of supply lines vastly exceeds the cost of supplying the good once the infrastructure has been developed. Governments regulate these natural monopolies to promote efficiency. In drug therapy, the cost of demonstrating the safety and efficacy of a new drug is usually far greater than the cost of providing the new drug once it has been shown to be safe and effective. Government regulation ensures that there is an incentive to develop new drugs by initially providing an exclusive right to market them. After the period of exclusivity expires, regulation promotes efficiency by permitting competition by generic manufacturers.

Information asymmetry leads to market failures when the consumer is uninformed about the true value of a good. Some goods have characteristics that are obvious to a consumer before purchase (e.g., a chair, a tablet of paper). Consumers can evaluate other goods only after purchasing them (e.g., a used car, a meal at a restaurant). It is more difficult to evaluate medications because most consumers are unable to determine their value fully even after using them. Information about the benefits and detriments of medications does not flow freely within the lay public because it often is difficult for untrained individuals to understand these benefits and detriments. To minimize the possibility of market failure caused by information asymmetry, government regulation requires the provision of information and input by educated professionals into decisions about drug use. Without government regulation to promote the dissemination of information about drugs, patients and health care providers would find it more difficult to make good decisions about the benefits and detriments of drug therapy.

LIMITS OF THE LAW

Even though there may be good reasons for market regulations, there are limits on effective legal action. These limits originate not only in the constitutional parameters with which laws must harmonize but also in the human condition. Attempts to achieve overly broad objectives through the law will inevitably fail if they conflict with popular attitudes, habits, and ideals.

Human relationships, to the extent that they are well defined by society, are usually best left alone by legal institutions. In families, professions, and religious groups, for example, wholly internal disagreements are generally not amenable to legal resolution. Legal agencies lack the necessary expertise to deal with these problems, and the parties involved are not usually willing to abide by a legal pronouncement that fails to account for the peculiarities of a closely knit group. Excessively harsh enforcement of the law in the face of *de minimis* (very minor or trifling) violations counterproductively decreases respect for the law. No pharmacy can operate without occasional, very minor technical legal violations. If they have no real impact on the quality of drug therapy, such violations usually result only in warnings by law enforcers. This is not to say that the law will condone frequent or consistent minor violations. As a practical matter, however, there is little or nothing to be gained by pursuing occasional minor violations, obvious though they may be.

Avoidance of excessive punishment that does not "fit the crime" is usually a matter of enforcement discretion left to those who have legal authority at the "street level" to charge (or not charge) violators with infractions. However, in *Young v. Board of Pharmacy*, 462 P.2d 139 (N.M. 1969), the Supreme Court of New Mexico substituted its judgment for that of the enforcement authorities. The court reacted to what it believed was excessive punishment, ruling that charges made against a pharmacist were arbitrary, unlawful, and unsupported. The pharmacist had not kept accurate dispensing records and had been charged with "unprofessional conduct." The court acknowledged the deficiencies of the pharmacist's recordkeeping, but the court could not understand why accurate recordkeeping should be a test of a person's professional character. This ruling in favor of the pharmacist does not mean that sloppy recordkeeping is acceptable, only that it should not be punished oppressively.

The fact that individuals in a free society are permitted to act in ways that they deem best for themselves—as long as their actions do not interfere with another individual's right of action—also limits effective legal action. John Stuart Mill expressed this belief in his essay, "On Liberty," when he said, "The only purpose for which power can be rightfully exercised over any member of a civilized community, against his will, is to prevent harm to others" (1986, p. 16). The law does not always accede to the Mill principle. Drug abuse and the use of unsafe medications (e.g., Laetrile) are legally restricted, for example, either because of the potential harm to others or because of a belief that some individuals are incapable of knowing what is in their own best interests. However, under most circumstances, individuals are free to make decisions for themselves without legal intervention.

Slogans such as "You can't legislate morality" or its converse "There oughta be a law" oversimplify the role of the law in society. The law can influence behavior through its deterrent and educative role, but there are definite limits on that function. Society shapes the law, and the primary purpose of the legal system is to make the premises of society work.

© Stockbyte/Thinkstock

STUDY SCENARIOS AND QUESTIONS

1. You are a pharmacist talking to a patient. The patient remarks, "I really don't understand why the FDA has to approve every drug before it can be marketed. I have cancer, and there is a very promising drug in Europe that I can't get in the United States because of the FDA. Do you think that's fair?" Respond to this patient using market failures to justify your answer.

2. The patient continues, "I also don't understand why someone has to have a pharmacy degree and a license to practice pharmacy. Doesn't it make sense that anyone should be allowed to dispense medications? All that the law should require is that the dispenser be required to post his or her credentials. Then, let the patients decide if they want to go to a high school graduate or a PharmD." Respond to this patient using market failures to justify your answer. What are the advantages and disadvantages to society of licensure?

3. A female patient visits a pharmacy at night and needs a refill on her birth control prescription, which she has been taking for 2 years. She has no refills remaining, the physician is unavailable, and she is flying on a 6 a.m. flight with her husband for a 2-week trip out of the country. Assume there is no law allowing for emergency refills and the pharmacist refills the prescription anyway, violating both state and federal law. A state board of pharmacy inspector discovers what happened and files his report to the state board. You are on the state board and must decide what action to take. How could the board proceed as an administrative agency? How should the board proceed, and why?

SOURCES OF U.S. LAW

The U.S. government is a tripartite system consisting of the legislative, executive, and judicial branches. Each branch serves as a check to the power of the others, ensuring that no one branch can dominate and control the others. Most persons say that the legislative branch of government makes the laws, whereas the executive branch enforces the laws, and the judicial branch interprets them. In theory this may be correct; in practice, however, all three branches make law together with what can be considered a fourth branch of government—administrative agencies.

THE CONSTITUTION OF THE UNITED STATES

The supreme law of the United States is the Constitution. Any federal or state statute or regulation that conflicts with the Constitution is invalid. The Federal Convention ratified the basic Constitution in 1787, and the Bill of Rights (i.e., the first 10 amendments) was added in 1791. In addition to the Bill of Rights, there have been 16 amendments to the Constitution since it was enacted. The passage of so few amendments in such a short document is quite remarkable and illustrates the timeless manner in which the Constitution was written.

The Bill of Rights includes rights generally recognized by everyone such as freedom of speech, freedom of religion, freedom to be secure from unreasonable searches and seizures, protection against self-incrimination, and the right to due process. The Fourteenth Amendment, passed in 1870, applies the Bill of Rights to state governments.

LAW MADE BY LEGISLATURES: STATUTORY LAW

A legislature is an elected body of persons with the primary responsibility to enact laws, also called statutes. These statutes can be organized in a hierarchical order:

- Federal statutes
- State constitutions
- State legislation
- Ordinances

Article 1, section 1 of the U.S. Constitution provides that all legislative powers of the federal government shall be vested in a Congress, which shall be composed of a Senate and a House of Representatives. In addition to several specifically enumerated powers entrusted to Congress, article 1, section 8 provides that Congress shall have the power to make all laws "necessary and proper" for carrying out its responsibilities. Thus, Congress enacts laws that apply nationwide.

Each state has its own constitution, which is usually much more detailed than the U.S. Constitution. Just as the U.S. Constitution is the supreme law over the whole country, a state constitution is the supreme law of the state.

Under the Tenth Amendment to the U.S. Constitution, states have the power to legislate in all areas except those prohibited or given to Congress by the U.S. Constitution. As a result, state legislatures have extremely broad powers to pass laws to protect the health, safety, and welfare of the public.

Each state government has the authority to create political subdivisions, such as municipalities and counties, to which the state can delegate certain functions. These political entities can enact ordinances that are enforceable as laws.

LAW MADE BY ADMINISTRATIVE AGENCIES

A legislature may create administrative agencies to implement desired changes in policies or to administer a body of substantive law when the legislature itself cannot perform these functions. It is impossible, for example, for state legislatures to monitor the activities of pharmacists and pharmacies on a regular basis. Therefore, the legislatures have created state boards of pharmacy to administer and enforce state pharmacy practice acts. Although the legislature creates them, such agencies are housed in the executive branch of government.

Several administrative agencies affect pharmacists at both the federal and state levels. Federal agencies include the following:

- The Centers for Medicare & Medicaid Services (CMS), formerly the Health Care Financing Administration (HCFA), which is housed in the Department of Health and Human Services (DHHS), is responsible for reimbursement policies and procedures for pharmacies and other health care providers participating in the Medicare and Medicaid programs.
- The Food and Drug Administration (FDA), also housed in the DHHS, administers the federal Food, Drug, and Cosmetic Act (FDCA).
- The Federal Trade Commission (FTC), in administering the Federal Trade Commission Act, enforces unfair business practices and antitrust violations.
- The Drug Enforcement Administration (DEA) is under the jurisdiction of the U.S. Justice Department and administers the federal Controlled Substances Act.

Some state-level agencies of importance to pharmacists include the state board of pharmacy, which administers state pharmacy practice acts; the state department of health services; and state Medicaid agencies (usually under the department of health services), which determine state Medicaid policies and pharmacy reimbursement rates. Administrative agencies generally have considerable and broad authority, including the authority to perform legislative, judicial, and executive functions. Administrative agencies create law primarily through their authority to enact regulations and to render decisions at hearings.

Legislative Function

Administrative agencies accomplish their legislative function through the promulgation of regulations. Administrative regulations interpret and define statutes. For example, although the federal Food, Drug, and Cosmetic Act enacted by Congress requires compliance with "current good manufacturing practices," it is really the regulations promulgated by the FDA that precisely and extensively define these practices. Similarly, for example, several states mandate that pharmacists complete a certain number of continuing education units over a specified period of time. Regulations promulgated by state pharmacy boards provide the necessary details, such as the types of continuing education units that are acceptable, the records that must be furnished to the state pharmacy board, and the requirements that continuing education providers must meet.

Because administrative agencies have a greater level of expertise than does Congress or a state legislature, it makes good sense for such agencies to determine how legislative policy will be implemented on a day-to-day basis. Recognizing the technical expertise of agencies, courts generally presume the actions of an agency to be valid.

Most administrative agencies promulgate regulations pursuant to a process known as "notice and comment rulemaking." This process ensures that constituents whose interests are affected by the actions of the agency receive notice of any proposed regulation. Constituents then have an opportunity to comment on the proposed regulation. The agency considers all comments and may incorporate them into the regulation before its final promulgation. Although regulations are not statutes, they have the legal force of statutes and must be obeyed as such.

To be valid, a regulation must generally meet three legal tests. First, the regulation must be within the scope of the agency's authority. For example, a state board of pharmacy is charged with administering pharmacy practice laws. It generally would not, for example, have the authority to regulate such issues as pharmacy investment practices or wage standards for pharmacy personnel.

Second, and often directly related to the first test, the regulation must be based on a statute that gives the agency the authority to promulgate the regulation. Generally, it is not legal for agencies to create new substantive law unless there is a statute enabling the agency to regulate in that area. For example, a state board regulation authorizing licensed pharmacy technicians to assist pharmacists with dispensing functions is likely to be invalidated unless there is a statute that recognizes the status of pharmacy technicians. Some courts have interpreted enabling legislation quite liberally. In *Rite Aid of New Jersey, Inc. v. Board of Pharmacy*, 304 A.2d 754 (N.J. Super. 1973), the court upheld a regulation passed by the New Jersey Board of Pharmacy to require that pharmacies maintain patient-profile record systems. The board cited as the enabling law a state law requiring pharmacists to keep prescription records on file. Although the law made no mention of patient medication records, the court found that the regulation was valid because it furthered the objective of the state law requiring pharmacists to keep records to protect the public. The court stated that the legislature could not be expected to anticipate every possible problem when it wrote the law.

As another example, the North Carolina Board of Pharmacy proposed a regulation limiting the number of continuous hours a pharmacist may work to 12 hours and requiring pharmacists be given one 30-minute and one 15-minute break if working longer than 6 continuous hours. Chain drug stores argued against the proposed regulation and the Rule Review Commission (RRC), which must approve state agency regulations, vetoed the rule on the basis that the Board lacked statutory authority to regulate pharmacists' working conditions. The Board sued to force publication, but the trial court and state court of appeals, in a split decision, found for the RRC, concluding that the pharmacy board did not have the authority to regulate work conditions because it is a function of the North Carolina Department of Labor. The appellate court majority also concluded that setting limits on work hours and requiring breaks does not concern filling prescriptions. On appeal, the North Carolina Supreme Court reversed the court of appeals and sided with the dissenting appellate court judge that the Board did have the statutory authority to issue the regulation and that there is a relationship between continuous hours of work and accuracy in filling prescriptions (*North Carolina Board of Pharmacy v. Rules Review Com'n.*, 620 S.E. 2d 893 [App. Ct. N.C. 2005]; reversed 637 S.E.2d 515 (N.C. 2006)).

The third legal requirement for a regulation is that it must bear a reasonable relationship to the public health, safety, and welfare. Thus, regulations that specify a dress code for pharmacists or that require the front door of a pharmacy to face the north or south side of a street are likely to be invalid.

Judicial Function

An administrative agency exercises its judicial function through its enforcement activities. The decision to institute proceedings is discretionary with the agency. Hearings conducted by administrative agencies resemble civil or criminal court proceedings; evidence is presented, arguments made, and a decision rendered. The results favor either the agency or the regulated party, perhaps creating new substantive law by interpreting existing law. At one time, it was common to create new law through case-by-case enforcement (i.e., regulated parties discover that they have committed a violation only through an adjudicative proceeding), but notice and comment rulemaking has largely replaced that inefficient and unfair approach.

Agency decisions are usually subject to "judicial review" but only after the individual has availed him- or herself of every available administrative option, legally called "exhaustion of remedies." On judicial review, a court may examine the record of the administrative hearing. If the record shows that the agency's decision was based on "substantial evidence," the court often simply reviews the appropriateness of the decision in light of the evidence. If the court finds that the agency's decision was not based on substantial evidence, it may decide to hear the case *de novo*, meaning that the court will pay no heed to the hearing findings but instead will conduct an entirely new trial.

The *Federal Register* and *Code of Federal Regulations*

Administrative agencies exercise considerable authority over pharmaceutical distribution and pharmacy practice, and pharmacists must be aware of the proposed and final regulations that affect their professional lives. Congress has prescribed that federal agency regulations be recorded in a specific manner so the public will have notice. This notice occurs primarily through two sources:

1. The *Federal Register*
2. The *Code of Federal Regulations* (CFR)

These two publications can be found at many public libraries, university and law school libraries, county courthouse libraries, and several government websites, including the U.S. Government Printing Office website (http://www.gpoaccess.gov).

The *Federal Register* is a daily publication that lists various federal actions, including proposed regulations, final regulations, and various government notices. The CFR is an annually revised compilation of final regulations divided and indexed by subject matter. There are 50 titles (i.e., divided subject areas) in the CFR, and each title is further divided into chapters, subchapters, parts, subparts, and sections.

To pass a regulation that would add a labeling requirement for prescription drugs, for example, the FDA would first publish in the *Federal Register* the proposed regulation, a notice of the intent to enact this regulation, and its reasons for proposing the regulation. A number would be included to identify exactly where the regulation, if enacted, would be placed in the CFR. (All FDA regulations are contained in Title 21 of the CFR.)

The notice would invite public comment within a certain time frame. At the conclusion of the comment period, the FDA would review the comments, draft a final regulation, and publish this final regulation along with the agency's comments and the effective date in the *Federal Register*. Simultaneously this regulation would be inserted into its appropriate location within Title 21 of the CFR.

LAW MADE BY THE COURTS: COMMON LAW

When two or more parties cannot settle a dispute or controversy among themselves, they are likely to ask a court to settle the issue. The duty of the court is to apply the proper law to the facts before it and resolve the matter through judicial opinions (decisions). Whereas legislatures make law through statutes and administrative agencies make law through regulations and hearings, courts make law through judicial "opinions." The word *opinion* is potentially misleading. When a court issues an opinion, the rules of law stated within it are not merely a point of view, subject to debate but with no general applicability. Rather, these rules are enforceable as law; they are binding on lower courts within the same jurisdiction and are persuasive in other jurisdictions. Judicial opinions establish enforceable legal principles either by expanding the common law (i.e., a body of judge-made law with its roots in centuries of resolved disputes) or by interpreting statutes and regulations.

The subject matter considered by a court varies a great deal from one day to the next. Thus, a court that is resolving a controversy relating to drug use today may have been presiding over a divorce yesterday and may be facing a dispute over securities tomorrow. Given the vast differences in subject matter, it is remarkable that courts are consistently able to resolve conflicts in a way that makes contextual sense, and it is inevitable that a court's ruling will sometimes reflect a misunderstanding of the subject matter. There have been periodic calls for "science courts," in which experts in both law and science work to resolve legal controversies relating to drug risks and other complex scientific issues. To date, however, no coordinated effort toward that end has materialized, and the judiciary continues to lack scientific expertise.

The term "common law" refers to law developed from judicial opinions. Much of the common law in the United States is based on law developed in England during the 200 to 300 years that followed the Norman conquest of England in 1066. Because the English kings in this period wanted to establish a uniform set of national laws, judges recorded and followed court decisions made previously. The result was a body of legal rules, many of which courts are still following today.

The English colonists retained the common law legal system when they came to North America. Each state, except for Louisiana (whose law is based on French and Spanish law), then adopted common law into its system. Although many common law principles are uniformly applicable in all states, each state does have its own common law, and some common law principles differ from state to state. In some instances, common law principles have become so accepted and recognized that legislatures have codified them as statutes.

Stare Decisis

The essence of the common law system is the recording of judicial opinions and the reliance of courts on those previous opinions. This practice is called *stare decisis*, meaning "to abide by decided cases." In practice, a court's establishment of a certain rule of law based on a particular set of facts becomes a precedent that all lower courts in that jurisdiction must follow. *Stare decisis* serves two purposes:

1. Establishing continuity of decisions
2. Expediting judicial decision making

Stare decisis applies only to lower courts within the jurisdiction in which the precedent has been established. Thus, lower courts in one state need not follow a state supreme court ruling in another state. Similarly, a federal court of appeals in one circuit need not follow an opinion rendered in another circuit. Often, however, courts carefully consider opinions from other jurisdictions.

Stare decisis is not an inflexible principle. A court may vary from precedent primarily for two reasons. First, there may be factual distinctions between the case before the court and previous decisions on which the court relies. For example, a court may find that a pharmacist has a duty to warn patients of the drowsiness associated with an antihistamine drug but may later find that a pharmacist has no duty to warn patients of possible teratogenic effects associated with a sulfa drug. Lawyers commonly single out factual differences between cases in an attempt to convince a court that the present case is different from the precedent relied on by the other party in the lawsuit.

Second, courts may vary from a precedent because of changing times or circumstances since the precedent was established. A legal principle that was appropriate when the precedent was established may not be the best rule of law for society today. Thus, even if a court ruled in 1965 that pharmacists have no duty to warn a patient of adverse drug reactions, the court may be convinced to reverse that decision today, based in part on the different educational background of pharmacists in 1965 and today and the difference in societal expectations.

Relationship of Common Law to Statutory Law

Common law and statutory law merge when courts are required to interpret the meaning of statutes. It is virtually impossible for any legislature to write a law that is not ambiguous, vague, or confusing in some manner when applied to specific controversies. In fact, many statutes are deliberately written in very general language to provide flexibility. If a statute is too ambiguous or vague, however, courts may invalidate all or part of the statute as unconstitutional. For example, in an attempt to make it illegal to sell and possess devices for illicit drug use, some states in the late 1960s and early 1970s passed laws so broad and imprecise that even items like household teaspoons could have been considered illegal. In those states, the courts either invalidated all or parts of these laws. Courts do not commonly invalidate statutes unless they have no choice; they prefer to presume the constitutionality of a statute and make every attempt to interpret the statute in a way that results in a reasonable and fair application of the law to the facts of a case.

In numerous cases a court has had to interpret statutes and decide if the set of facts before it is subject to a particular law. What principles do courts apply when interpreting legislation? In conjunction with the rule of *stare decisis*, the most important approach that courts apply when interpreting statutes is to determine the legislative intent. In other words, the court attempts to put itself in the mind of the legislature and ask, "Did the legislature mean for the law to apply to the specific fact situation that the court is now considering?" Especially with respect to federal statutes, the court looks to legislative committee reports and any written legislative history to guide it in its interpretation. Often, the legislative history is of no assistance because the legislature never anticipated the type of situation that is the subject of litigation. In this event, the court looks to the overall intent and purpose of the legislation, asking, "Why did the legislature pass this law? What is the law attempting to accomplish? How does this particular situation apply to the law's purpose?"

A state may pass a law, for example, that requires pharmacies to offer counseling to patients but does not require the pharmacist to actually provide the service if the patient refuses it. In one pharmacy, a clerk informs all patients that they may receive counseling from the pharmacist but will have to wait 30 to 60 minutes. As a result, nearly all patients refuse the counseling. The state board charges the pharmacist with violating the statute, but the pharmacy contends that it has complied with the law. If this case goes to court, the pharmacy's actions may be ruled more an attempt to avoid the intent of the statute than an effort to accomplish the intent.

Although a determination of legislative intent generally prevails, courts often combine this analysis with other approaches to interpret a statute. One such other approach is to give the words in a statute their ordinary (commonly understood) meaning. Another is to support the position that best exemplifies current social policy. Yet another consideration that courts must heed is an individual's constitutional right of due process. In this context, due process means that a reasonable person would be expected to know that this law applies or does not apply to the particular activity in question. It is unfair to hold someone accountable for a law that the person could not know was applicable.

© Stockbyte/Thinkstock

STUDY SCENARIOS AND QUESTIONS

1. Assume the Board of Pharmacy passed a regulation prohibiting any pharmacy from accepting any third party plan whose dispensing fee is less than $2. You are the owner of a pharmacy that wants to accept a plan offering a fee of $1. On what basis might you challenge this regulation in court?

2. Assume the Board of Pharmacy passed a regulation that pharmacists may not wear facial jewelry (from piercing). You are a pharmacist who has a number of rings in your eyebrows, nose, and lips. On what basis might you challenge this regulation in court?

3. Apply the principle of *stare decisis* and precedent to the following related fictional cases:

1990 Case

Assume it is 1990 and a patient has been dispensed a prescription antihistamine. The pharmacist did not counsel or provide any warnings. The patient became drowsy while driving, had an accident, and was seriously injured. The patient sued the pharmacist for failing to warn him of the drowsiness. Assume no counseling statute or regulation is in effect in 1990.

There is a 1975 case decision in this same jurisdiction where the patient was dispensed Valium. The pharmacist did not counsel or provide any warnings. The patient took the drug and later while standing on a ladder fixing his roof, fell off the ladder and broke his back. The patient sued the pharmacist for failing to warn him that Valium could cause drowsiness and dizziness. The court found for the pharmacist and determined that the legal obligation a pharmacist owes a patient does not include warning the patient of a drug's dangers but to only fill the prescription correctly, exactly as written. During the trial:

- What arguments will the defendant pharmacist's lawyer make?
- What arguments will the plaintiff's lawyer make?

1998 Case

Now assume the plaintiff won the 1990 case and the court held that the pharmacist had a legal obligation to warn the patient of the drowsiness. In this 1998 case, the patient is dispensed an antibiotic. The pharmacist provided counseling and warnings but did not warn of myocardial infarction (MI), a relatively uncommon adverse effect. The patient suffered an MI and sued the pharmacist for failure to warn. Assume the state counseling statute or regulation is in effect.

- What arguments will the plaintiff's lawyer make?
- What arguments will the pharmacist's lawyer make?

2005 Case

Now assume a similar situation to the 1990 case occurred, except with the following differences: The patient taking the antihistamine ran her car into another car, injuring the occupants. The state counseling regulation or statute was in effect. The injured occupants of the other car are suing.

- What arguments will the plaintiff's lawyer make?
- What arguments will the pharmacist's lawyer make?

4. The state counseling regulation or statute is in effect. Your pharmacy is simply too busy to provide counseling personally and keep up with the volume so, being the tech wizard you are, you program computers to provide counseling to the patients. The computers are in a private area where a patient can simply enter the name of the drug and a pharmacist, who has been videotaped, comes on screen and provides all the required information. The board of pharmacy finds you have violated the counseling regulation. You contend otherwise and take your case to court representing yourself.
   - What would be critical to the court's analysis? In other words, how would you argue your case to the court? Conversely, what would the board argue? Assume the arguments applied to statutory analysis are the same for analysis of a regulation.

THE LEGISLATIVE PROCESS

FEDERAL LEVEL

At the federal level, the U.S. Congress, composed of the Senate and the House of Representatives, is the basis of legislative power. The Senate has 100 members; the House, 435 members. The primary function of the Congress is to enact statutes through vote of the full membership. Statutes are usually general in scope, establishing a framework within which the expressed intent of the law is to be achieved.

Ideas for bills originate from several sources, including lobbying groups, citizens, government officials, and the president. The sponsor of the bill, who must be a senator or representative, introduces the bill in Congress. After introduction, the bill moves to the particular congressional committee that has jurisdiction over that subject. The committee stage of a bill's life is by far the most important to its success or failure. The committee holds public hearings, conducts investigations, and works with the sponsor to ensure special interests are accommodated to the extent possible. Advocates and proponents of a bill concentrate their activities on the committee level because a bill cannot proceed to a vote by the Senate or House without the consent of a majority of the committee members.

If the committee votes favorably on the bill, it issues a report detailing the purpose of the bill, the reasons the committee approved it, any amendments, and the changes the bill would create in existing law. Often, individual committee members file supplemental opinions or views with the majority's report. Courts and administrative agencies may use the committee report to ascertain the legislative intent of the law.

After a bill has cleared the committee, the majority leadership places it on a calendar. This is a strategic step. If not impressed by a particular bill, the majority leadership may place it so late on the calendar that it will not come to a vote before Congress adjourns for the year. Once the bill is called for discussion in the Senate or House, it is usually extensively debated and amended.

After passage by one chamber, a bill goes to the other chamber's appropriate committee for further consideration. Again, hearings are held, and opponents and proponents do their best to influence committee members to vote for or against the bill. There are often differences between the version of a bill passed by the Senate and the version passed by the House. In this case, a conference committee rectifies the differences between the two. After the identical bill has been agreed on by both sides, it is signed by the president of the Senate and the Speaker of the House and sent to the president of the United States.

The bill becomes law on the signature of the president of the United States or if the president fails to return the bill to Congress within 10 days. If the president disapproves of the bill, the president may veto it; in this case, the president must return it with the reasons for disapproval to the chamber where the bill originated. Congress can override a presidential veto only by a two-thirds vote in favor of the bill. The president also can prevent a bill from becoming a law by means of a pocket veto, which occurs when the president fails to act on a bill within a 10-day period and Congress adjourns within that time period.

In addition to enacting statutes, Congress is responsible for overseeing the federal bureaucracy. Because Congress has a say in appointments to administrative agencies and appropriations for these agencies, congressional influence over substantive agency policy is significant. Congressional committee investigations, committee hearings, and statutorily required agency reports keep members of Congress informed of agency activities. They often are able, either individually or as members of a committee, to influence administrative agencies.

STATE LEVEL

Legislatures at the state level are modeled roughly after the U.S. Congress, although some differ from the federal body in one or more characteristics. For example, the Congress meets almost continuously, but some state legislatures meet in full session for only a few months of the year, usually every other year (with limited budget sessions during the off year).

State legislative committees differ from congressional committees at the federal level in that they are generally less prone to hold full hearings and do not usually issue fully informative committee reports on bills. Communication is sometimes poor on the state level, making it difficult for legislators to know the true nature of proposed bills, their status, and amendments. Thus, a statute's legislative history (i.e., early drafts, committee reports, relevant statements made on the floor), which usually plays a significant role in determining the meaning of a federal statute when a dispute arises, may be virtually nonexistent at the state level.

DISTINGUISHING CRIMINAL, CIVIL, AND ADMINISTRATIVE LAW

A pharmacist's wrongful act may subject the pharmacist to a criminal, civil, or administrative action, or perhaps all three at the same time. The government may initiate a "criminal action" if the pharmacist has violated a statute. For example, a pharmacist who sells a prescription-controlled substance without a prescription may be subject to a criminal action by the state or federal government. A person can only be charged with a crime if there is a statute prohibiting the conduct. The sanctions are usually a fine, a prison sentence, or both, depending on the severity of the crime and the penalties specified in the statute. The objectives of criminal statutes and prosecutions are to deter an undesirable activity as well as to punish and rehabilitate the wrongdoer.

A "civil action" is a lawsuit in which one private party sues another private party alleging an injury. If, for example, the pharmacist in the criminal case just discussed sold the controlled substance to a patient who was allergic to the drug and the pharmacist had knowledge of that allergy but simply forgot, the patient injured from ingesting the drug may sue the pharmacist for the injury. Civil actions may be based on common law, statutory law, or both. The objective of a civil action is to compensate the injured party for the damages caused by the wrongdoer.

An "administrative action" may occur when a pharmacist has violated a statute or regulation or has committed an act that, in the opinion of the agency, warrants an investigation. As discussed previously, such administrative actions are called "hearings." Depending on the statutes and the nature of the violation, they may lead to sanctions including:

- Warnings
- Fines
- License revocation
- License suspension
- Probation

The pharmacist in the situation discussed is likely to be subject to a state pharmacy board disciplinary hearing.

THE JUDICIAL PROCESS

THE FEDERAL COURT SYSTEM

Article 3 of the U.S. Constitution provides that there shall be a Supreme Court, and it authorizes Congress to establish additional federal courts as necessary (see **Figure 1-1**). At the trial court level, Congress has established district courts. Each state has at least one U.S. district court; more populated states have two or more. District courts have jurisdiction over controversies that involve the following:

- The U.S. Constitution or a federal law
- Ambassadors or consuls
- Admiralty and maritime issues
- The United States as a party
- A state as a party against another state
- A state as one party and a citizen of another state as the other party
- A citizen of one state against a citizen of a different state

There are 12 circuit courts of appeals, one for each judicial circuit and the District of Columbia. An appeal from a district court goes to the court of appeals in the circuit that

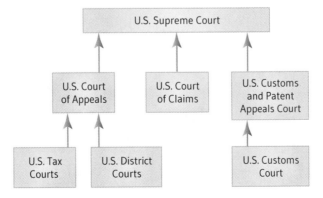

FIGURE 1-1 Federal court system.

includes both courts. Most cases before appellate courts are those on appeal from the district courts, but these courts can also directly review certain administrative agency decisions.

The U.S. Supreme Court has nine justices who hold lifetime appointments from the president, subject to Senate confirmation. As specified in the Constitution, the Supreme Court has "original" jurisdiction in all cases that affect ambassadors, other public ministers, and consuls as well as in all cases in which a state is a party. In most other cases, the Supreme Court has "appellate" jurisdiction. The Supreme Court primarily reviews cases from federal appellate courts, three-judge district court decisions, and final judgments from the highest court in a state when a federal question is involved. Although the Supreme Court is obligated to hear certain cases on appeal, most cases must be submitted through a "writ of certiorari," meaning, essentially, that the Court has the discretion to hear whichever cases it chooses by granting or denying certiorari.

The federal court system also includes special courts, such as tax courts for tax disputes, a customs court for issues involving imported goods, and a customs and patent appeals court that hears appeals from the customs court and from the patent and trademark office. A court of claims hears disputes lodged against the United States, although district courts also may have jurisdiction.

THE STATE COURT SYSTEM

Although each state has its own court system, there are many similarities among the states (see **Figure 1–2**). Every state has one highest review court, usually called the state supreme court. Many of the more densely populated states, such as California, Florida, and New York, have intermediate appellate courts. Below the appellate courts, all states have trial courts with very broad jurisdiction; these may be called county courts, superior courts, district courts, or circuit courts, depending on the state. In addition, most states have limited jurisdiction trial courts, such as probate courts, juvenile courts, and family courts. Below the trial courts are courts with very limited jurisdiction, such as police courts, traffic courts, small claims courts, and justice of the peace courts. Disputes in these courts often involve relatively small amounts of money or minor statutory violations. No record of the proceedings is kept, and the individuals involved often represent themselves.

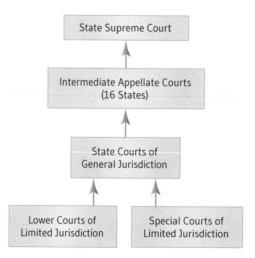

FIGURE 1-2 Typical state judicial court system.

CIVIL COURT PROCEDURES

Controversies are resolved in court through an adversarial process. Each attorney has the obligation to present the best legal arguments possible on behalf of a client while also attempting to refute the other party's arguments. The intent of the adversarial process is to bring out all possible legal arguments and rationale that are relevant to the issue so an impartial judge or jury may apply the best ones.

Every party in a court case must follow specific procedures as prescribed by statutes and court rules. The procedures differ somewhat, depending on the following:

- Whether the action commences in a federal court or a state court
- Whether the action is civil or criminal

Many of the procedures in the following hypothetical civil action are generally applicable to criminal actions as well:

> Gail Bond has delivered a baby with birth defects. During the pregnancy, her physician prescribed a benzodiazepine drug for her. Sally Walker, a pharmacist and owner of Walker Pharmacy, dispensed the drug. Bond believes the drug caused her baby's birth defects and sues Walker for not warning her that this could happen.

Selection of a Court

To start this lawsuit, Bond's attorney must first file the case in the proper court. An action can be filed in a court only if that court has jurisdiction over both the subject matter of the dispute and the parties involved. Occasionally, the jurisdiction issue is so complicated that the parties must spend considerable time and money to resolve it before the case can proceed. In this hypothetical case, there are no jurisdictional problems, and the case is filed in a state trial court. Filing in federal court would not likely be an option because both Bond and Walker are citizens of the same state and there is no federal law in question.

The Parties

The person who brings the lawsuit is called the "plaintiff." The person against whom the lawsuit is brought is called the "defendant." The plaintiff's name appears first in the name of the case. Thus, the title of the hypothetical case would be *Bond v. Walker Pharmacy*.

A party bringing a lawsuit must prove "standing"; that is, the plaintiff must show that the challenged conduct has caused the plaintiff injury and that the plaintiff's interest is a legally protectable interest. In *Bond v. Walker Pharmacy*, there would be no dispute that Bond has standing. If Bond did not wish to bring a lawsuit against the pharmacist but a friend of hers did—who believed that such a suit was necessary to establish the social policy that pharmacists must warn of these types of dangers—the friend would likely not have standing to bring the lawsuit because Walker's conduct did not harm the friend. Similarly, courts have maintained that pharmacists do not have standing to sue a state on behalf of Medicaid patients who may be denied quality services because of state policy. The Medicaid patients must bring the lawsuit.

Statute of Limitations

Bond cannot wait too long before filing a lawsuit against Walker. All states have "statutes of limitations" requiring that lawsuits be brought within a certain period of time after the injury. The period of time in which the suit must be brought usually depends on the nature of the lawsuit and the state in which the suit is brought. In most states, the statute of limitations is 2 years for this type of case.

The Complaint, Summons, and Answer

To initiate the lawsuit, the plaintiff, Bond (herself or through her attorney), would file a "complaint" that contains all the material facts of her case and the remedy requested with the clerk of the court. The clerk of the court would then issue a document called a "summons," and the sheriff of the county or a deputy would likely serve the summons, together with a copy of the complaint, to the defendant. The summons would command Walker to file an "answer" to Bond's complaint within a specific period of time, usually about 30 days. Walker's answer may admit or deny any of Bond's allegations. If Walker fails to submit an answer within the required time period, however, the court would probably issue a "default judgment" in favor of Bond. A defendant must never ignore a summons and should notify the insurance company or an attorney the instant a complaint is received.

Often called the "pleadings" of the case, the complaint and answer serve two purposes:

1. They provide the defendant with the constitutional due process right of notice.
2. They constitute the basis on which the trial is built.

No facts or legal issues not stated in the pleadings may be admitted in court, unless the court allows amendments to the pleadings. Thus, the complaint and answer must be drafted very thoroughly and carefully.

Discovery

Contrary to widespread public beliefs, surprise evidence and witnesses are unusual during a trial (civil or criminal). Nearly all courts allow the parties to use the pretrial process called "discovery." Each party must give the other party all the facts, evidence, and names of witnesses on which that party relies. Each lawyer generally questions the key witnesses who will testify for the opposing party. This questioning takes place in a "deposition," a procedure in which the opposing party's lawyer interrogates a witness in the presence of the other party's lawyer outside of a courtroom. A court-approved stenographer records the deposition. There are three major purposes for a deposition:

1. It allows the attorneys to know in advance what the witnesses will say at trial.
2. If a witness cannot appear at trial, the deposition may be admitted to serve as the witness's testimony.
3. The deposition can be used to impeach the credibility of a witness whose testimony on the witness stand deviates from that in the deposition.

If it is not practical or necessary to depose a witness, the lawyers may use an "interrogatory." An interrogatory requires the witness to respond in writing under oath to written questions.

Pretrial Motions

At the pleadings stage, either party may file various "motions" with the court. For example, Walker might file motions of objection against Bond's complaint, pointing to errors in the complaint or in the procedure process or asserting that there are no legal grounds for a lawsuit. If the court grants the motions, either the case would be dismissed or the court would allow Bond to correct the errors.

Jury Selection and Role

The parties must decide whether to have a jury trial or to allow the judge to decide the case. If they want a jury, the clerk of the court requires a number of potential jurors to appear at the courthouse. The attorneys then question each potential juror through a process known as *voir dire* examination to determine if they want that person on the jury. Ultimately, they accept the required number of jurors, and the trial proceeds.

The jury's role is to determine all questions of fact presented at the trial. In the hypothetical case, the jury would have to decide, for example, if Walker provided the warnings. The judge's roles are to determine the law involved in the case (e.g., does the pharmacist have a legal duty to warn patients of these types of drug dangers?) and to instruct the jury as to what law to apply to the facts. If there is no jury, the judge both determines the facts and applies the proper law.

Witnesses

As discussed earlier, the witnesses for both sides are generally identified and depositions taken before the trial. As an additional precaution to ensure a witness's presence, either party's attorney may choose to subpoena one or more witnesses. A "subpoena" is an order to appear in court at a specified time and place. Failure to appear in court can result in a contempt of court citation. Subpoenas serve valuable functions, even for a party's own witnesses. If a subpoenaed witness cannot appear in court, the trial may be postponed. A subpoena may also ease the conscience of a witness who must testify against a friend or relative because an order to appear may reduce the witness's sense of betraying the party.

When certain factual subject matter is beyond the scope of knowledge of jurors, "expert witnesses" are used to explain the technical facts to a jury and to render professional opinions. For example, in *Bond v. Walker Pharmacy*, pharmacists could be called as expert witnesses to testify about pharmacists' functions when they dispense prescriptions. The expert witnesses would be allowed to render opinions as to whether a reasonable pharmacist has a duty to warn patients of a drug's side effects, particularly its potential teratogenicity. The jury would then have to decide whether it agreed with the expert witness's assessment of the case.

The Trial

Before or during the trial, either side may ask the judge to decide the case without trying the facts. This is called a motion for "summary judgment." One party attempts to convince the judge that the other party's claim or defense has no merit even if all the facts are correct. For example, in *Bond v. Walker Pharmacy*, Walker might make a motion for a summary judgment. By doing so she concedes that the facts are not in dispute and she did not warn Bond but that it does not matter because she has no legal duty to do so and thus there is no substance to Bond's claim.

Assuming summary judgment is denied before the trial, at the trial, each party usually makes an opening statement. The plaintiff's attorney begins by highlighting the issues involved and the reasons that the jury should ultimately decide in the plaintiff's favor. The witnesses for the plaintiff are then sworn, examined (i.e., questioned under oath) by the plaintiff's attorney, and cross-examined by the defense attorney. After all the plaintiff's witnesses have testified and all of the plaintiff's evidence has been introduced, the focus of the trial shifts to the defendant. At this point, the defendant's attorney may make a motion for a "directed verdict," on the basis that the plaintiff did not introduce sufficient evidence to justify the complaint. If granted, the defendant wins; if not, the defense then presents its witnesses and evidence. After the presentation of the defendant's case, the plaintiff also may make a motion for a directed verdict on the ground that a defense has not been established.

At any time during the trial, either side may voice "objections" to certain testimony or evidence. The judge must decide whether to overrule or to sustain each objection.

Timely objections are crucial. A party that fails to object to evidence or testimony at the proper time cannot later issue an objection. A failure to object to evidence properly can be devastating to a party's case at the trial level because objections can sometimes block the introduction of damaging evidence. The failure to object also can be damaging on appeal because the appellate court cannot consider if the introduction of evidence was proper unless objections had been raised at trial.

In the absence of a directed verdict, each side provides its closing arguments and summation to the jury. The judge then instructs the jury as to what law to apply to the determined facts. For example, assume the judge instructs the jury that the law states that a pharmacist only has a duty to warn patients of those adverse effects highly probable to occur. After being instructed, the jury would retire to another room and deliberate the probability of teratogenicity occurring with a benzodiazepine drug and if it is a risk of which a reasonable pharmacist would warn. Any time before or during the trial and before the jury reaches its verdict, the parties can agree to settle the case. Settlements are common and encouraged by the court. Assuming a settlement is not reached, the jury would then return with the verdict.

The Verdict

The jury's verdict may not end the controversy. If the jury has clearly reached the wrong verdict, the losing party may ask the judge to rule contrary to the jury, called a "judgment notwithstanding the verdict." Alternatively, if an egregious error was made during the trial (e.g., a juror talking to a witness outside the courtroom and then influencing other jurors with information thus obtained), the losing party may ask for a "mistrial" and have the verdict thrown out. If the verdict is final, the disgruntled party may appeal the case to a higher court.

The Appeal

In most cases, the dissatisfied party has a right to "appeal" the decision of the trial court. The party bringing the appeal is known as the "appellant," whereas the party defending the appeal is known as the "appellee." The appellant's name appears first. Thus, if Walker lost in the hypothetical *Bond v. Walker Pharmacy* at the trial level and appealed, the case would become *Walker Pharmacy v. Bond* at the appellate level. Notice of the intent to appeal must usually be filed within a 30-day period after the trial court's decision. The appeal documents usually include a transcript of the trial court proceedings for review by the appellate court judges.

To succeed on appeal, the appellant must convince the appellate court that the trial court committed an "error of law" that was material to the decision in the case. Generally only questions of law are considered on appeal because the appellate court, which usually consists of three judges, does not second-guess the trial court on questions of fact. Every time a judge rules on an objection or instruction to the jury, this ruling creates a question of law on which a party may base an appeal. The appellant's attorney attempts to convince the appellate court of the trial court's legal errors and the significance of the errors by means of a written legal document called a "brief." The brief not only provides the reason for the appeal but also specifies the alleged errors of law committed by the trial court and cites the legal principles and cases that support the appellant's arguments. The appellee's attorney also files a brief with the court, refuting the appellant's claim and citing legal principles and cases in the appellee's favor. If Walker lost at the trial level, her lawyer's brief might contend that the judge improperly allowed certain testimony by a witness or improperly instructed the jury as to the law in that jurisdiction; the attorney would cite previous cases in support of these contentions.

At the appellate hearing, the attorneys for each party present their oral arguments and answer questions from the judges. Presumably, the judges will have read the briefs and be quite familiar with the case. After hearing oral arguments, the court is likely to move on to hear other cases; it may not render a judgment for weeks or months.

Although attorneys can file various motions for rehearing, the judgment of an appellate court is usually final. The losing party has the option to file an appeal to the highest state court, however, if the appeal had been to an intermediate court. After the highest state court hears the appeal, there is likely to be no further review, unless one of the parties has raised a constitutional or federal law issue that may entitle the case to be reviewed by the U.S. Supreme Court.

CRIMINAL COURT PROCEDURES

Some important differences exist between criminal and civil court procedures. As is true of civil cases, criminal procedures vary somewhat depending upon the statutes and court rules in a particular jurisdiction. Nonetheless some general observations can be made. A defendant can be charged with a crime in different ways but most often either by an "indictment" or by "arrest." An indictment is issued by a "grand jury," called such because it normally has more jurors than an ordinary trial jury. The grand jury hears evidence presented by the government to determine if a trial should be held. If enough evidence ("probable cause") exists, the grand jury will issue an indictment leading to an arrest and trial.

Alternatively, the government may directly arrest an individual for a crime. In this case it must afford the defendant a preliminary hearing before a judge to determine if probable cause exists for the arrest. If probable cause exists, the defendant will face an arraignment, where in front of a judge the defendant will be given the right to enter a plea of guilty or not guilty. In most jurisdictions the defendant also has the right to plead *nolo contendere* ("I do not wish to contend"). Although this is a guilty plea, it might not bind the defendant in other proceedings, such as an administrative hearing or civil case.

Defendants in a criminal trial have considerable rights that the government must not violate, ranging from the right to not self-incriminate to the legality of the arrest. This provides the defendant the opportunity to make various types of pretrial motions to challenge nearly every aspect of the government's case. Also, the defendant may wish to negotiate a "plea bargain." In a plea bargain the defendant agrees to plead guilty to a lesser offense instead of risking the results of a jury trial and being found guilty of a greater offense. Plea bargains benefit the government by saving considerable expense and resources.

The burden of proof in a criminal trial is much higher than in a civil trial. In a civil trial the plaintiff must establish proof by a "preponderance of the evidence." In a criminal trial the government must prove its case "beyond a reasonable doubt." Thus, evidence that would result in a victory for a plaintiff in a civil trial might not be near enough evidence to convict a defendant in a criminal trial.

CASE CITATION AND ANALYSIS

Trial court opinions at the state level are not usually reported (published). Most state and federal appellate opinions and many federal trial court opinions are reported, however. These are the opinions that courts use as precedents. When a case is reported, it is titled with the names of the parties involved and a citation to indicate which court decided the case and where its record can be found. For example, the case citation *United States v. Guardian Chemical Corporation*, 410 F.2d 157 (2nd Cir. 1969), means that this is a Court of Appeals for the Second Circuit decision issued in 1969 and can be found in volume 410 of the second Federal Reporter series, starting on page 157. All case citations containing F., F.2d, or F.3d are federal courts of appeal opinions. Any case citation containing F. Supp. is a federal district court opinion, and any case citation containing U.S. or S. Ct. is a U.S. Supreme Court opinion. Citations containing the abbreviation of a state (e.g., 145 N.M. 322) or the abbreviation of a region of the country (e.g., 323 P.2d 445) are state court opinions. Regional reporter abbreviations include P. (Pacific), N.W. (Northwestern) N.E. (Northeastern) A. (Atlantic), S.E. (Southeastern) and So. (Southern).

Studying actual court cases is an excellent method of learning law and is used by nearly all law schools and in many undergraduate and graduate programs. Any law librarian can help a person find published cases.

© Stockbyte/Thinkstock

STUDY SCENARIO AND QUESTIONS

1. A patient, Molly, contends that Bill, a pharmacist for DrugEm Pharmacy, dispensed the wrong drug to her and that she suffered serious injury as a result. Bill denies this claim and believes that Molly somehow transferred the wrong drug to the container at her home. Molly plans to sue Bill and DrugEm Pharmacy jointly as codefendants.
   - Is this a civil and/or criminal case, and why?
   - Can the patient sue in either federal or state court, and why?
   - How would Bill know he is being sued?
   - Could Bill ask for a summary judgment at the beginning of the trial, and, if so, would the judge grant it?
   - Could Bill ask for a directed verdict at the beginning of the trial, and, if so, would the judge grant it?
        During the trial, Molly introduced a surprise witness who testified she saw the tablets in the vial when Bill dispensed them to Molly and that they were the wrong tablets Molly contended she received.
   - What process might prevent Molly from introducing this surprise witness, and why might it prevent a surprise witness?
   - Assume the jury concluded that Bill dispensed the wrong drug and found for Molly. Can Bill appeal, and, if so, on what basis?

FEDERAL VERSUS STATE LAW

The practice of pharmacy and the distribution of drug products are subject to both federal and state regulation. As a general rule, a state has the authority to regulate in any area that Congress has regulated, as long as there is no conflict between state and federal law. If a conflict exists, federal law always prevails over state law under the Supremacy Clause of the Constitution. This principle of federal law also is known as the "preemption doctrine."

Most conflicts occur when state law is less strict than federal law and compliance with a state law could lead to the violation of federal law. For example, federal law provides that a pharmacist can refill prescriptions for some controlled substances only five times within a 6-month period. If a state were to pass a law permitting 10 refills, that law would directly conflict with federal law and, if legally challenged, would be preempted. A pharmacist who complies with state law by dispensing a sixth refill during the fourth month would be in violation of federal law. On the other hand, if a state passed a law allowing no refills of the controlled substances that are refillable under federal law, this stricter law would not conflict with federal law. A pharmacist who complies with state law by refusing all refills would not be in violation of federal law.

FEDERAL AUTHORITY TO REGULATE

The U.S. Congress and federal administrative agencies derive their authority to regulate drug distribution from the Interstate Commerce Clause of the Constitution. The courts have liberally interpreted this clause on several occasions to give Congress considerable power to regulate commerce among the states. Technically, the federal government regulates drug distribution through the Interstate Commerce Clause and reserves for the states the authority to regulate the practice of pharmacy. In actuality, however, regulation of drug distribution often results in professional regulation as well.

The reach of the federal government's authority under the Interstate Commerce Clause was put to the test in a landmark Supreme Court case, *United States v. Sullivan*, 332 U.S. 689 (1948). In *Sullivan*, a community pharmacist contended that the Federal Food, Drug and Cosmetic Act did not apply to transactions between his pharmacy and his customers because these were entirely intrastate transactions. The facts of the case showed that a pharmaceutical manufacturer in Chicago, Illinois, shipped properly labeled bottles of sulfathiazole tablets to an Atlanta, Georgia, wholesaler. The label stated that the drug was to be sold by prescription only. Sullivan, a pharmacist in Columbus, Georgia, purchased the drug from the wholesaler and proceeded to sell the drug without prescription and without the labeling required under the Food, Drug, and Cosmetic Act. Finding against the pharmacist, the Court held that the Act extends to even these intrastate transactions because its intent is to protect the public and that intent would be subverted by a narrow definition of interstate commerce.

STATE AUTHORITY TO REGULATE

State government receives the authority to regulate pharmacy practice and the distribution of drugs through the Tenth Amendment of the Constitution, which, as noted earlier, gives the states all powers not delegated to the federal government or prohibited by the Constitution. States also have the authority to regulate drugs and the professions through the common law concept of "police powers," which allow the state to enact laws promoting the health, safety, and welfare of its people. State laws are considered valid as long as they do not conflict with the U.S. Constitution or federal laws, and as long as they bear a reasonable relationship to the protection of the public health, safety, and welfare. For example, if a state passed a law that all over-the-counter drugs must be sold only in licensed pharmacies, opponents could challenge this law on the ground that the law does not bear a reasonable relationship to the protection of the public health, safety, and welfare.

© Stockbyte/Thinkstock

STUDY SCENARIOS AND QUESTIONS

1. Makeit Laboratories in New Jersey shipped one of its prescription drugs to a wholesaler in Sacramento, California, which sold it to a pharmacy in Stockton, California. The pharmacy in Stockton sold it to a Stockton patient without a prescription. The FDA charged the pharmacy with violating federal law

pursuant to the Federal Food, Drug, and Cosmetic Act (FDCA). The defendant pharmacy argued that the FDCA does not apply to this situation.
- On what basis would the defendant argue this?
- What would the court likely decide, and why?
- Does the FDA have jurisdiction to charge the pharmacy, or is this a state law issue?

2. A state passed a law that a pharmacist could refill a schedule II prescription two times when the patient requires continual use of the medication. Federal law states that a schedule II prescription may not be refilled. If you were a pharmacist in that state, which law would you follow, and why?

BIBLIOGRAPHY

Adverse Drug Events: The Magnitude of Health Risks Is Uncertain Because of Limited Incidence Data. Publication No. GAO/HEHS-00-21. Washington, DC: U.S. General Accounting Office; January 2000.

Feinberg, J., and H. Gross. *Law in Philosophical Perspective.* Encino, CA: Dickenson Publishing Co., 1977.

Fuller, L. L. *Anatomy of the Law.* New York: The New American Library, 1968.

Fuller, L. L. The case of the speluncean explorers. *Harvard Law Review* 62 (1949): 616.

Levi, E. H. *An Introduction to Legal Reasoning.* Chicago: University of Chicago Press, 1948.

Mill, J. S. *On Liberty.* New York: Prometheus Books, 1986.

CASE STUDIES

CASE 1-1   *People v. Stuart*, 302 P.2d 5 (Cal. 1956)

Issue

Whether a pharmacist should be held criminally liable for having inadvertently made a mistake in dispensing a medication to a patient.

Overview

In criminal law, the state takes action against an individual who has committed an act so unacceptable that all of society is offended by it. Theft and assault are examples of crimes that harm all of society, not just their immediate victims. Reprehensible crimes such as these threaten to degrade the moral fiber of an entire society. Reaction to them is not left only to their immediate victims. Society collectively reacts to crime because everyone is harmed by them.

After a crime has been committed, a prosecutor representing either a locality, the state, or the entire country files charges against the perpetrator. If found guilty, a convicted criminal will usually serve time in jail. Criminal law isolates a criminal who might otherwise continue to act unacceptably and harm others. It deters unacceptable conduct by others who prefer not to face the same consequences as the criminal who has been made an example. Criminal law also provides vengeance for a society that feels the need to strike back at a person who has broken well-established rules of conduct.

In the case presented here, a pharmacist has been charged with both manslaughter (a relatively serious crime) and misbranding (a relatively minor crime). As you read this case, ask yourself what the purpose of criminal law is and if that purpose is being met by this prosecution. Also ask yourself what the consequences might be if pharmacists were to be held criminally liable for an error in order processing. If any pharmacist who makes a mistake in filling a prescription is a criminal, how many pharmacists are criminals at some point during their decades–long careers?

The court opinion began by describing the facts of the case:

Defendant was charged by information with manslaughter (Pen. Code, § 192) and the violation of section 380 of the Penal Code. He was convicted of both offenses by the court sitting without a jury. His motions for a new trial and for dismissal (Pen. Code, § 1385) were denied, sentence was suspended, and he was placed on probation for 2 years. He appeals from the judgment of conviction and the order denying his motion for a new trial.

Defendant was licensed as a pharmacist by this state in 1946 and has practiced here since that time. He holds a BS degree in chemistry from Long Island University and a BS degree in pharmacy from Columbia University. In April 1954, he was employed as a pharmacist by the Ethical Drug Company in Los Angeles.

On July 16, 1954, he filled a prescription for Irvin Sills. It had been written by Dr. D. M. Goldstein for Sills' 8-day-old child. It called for "sodium phenobarbital, grains eight. Sodium citrate, drams three. Simple Syrup, ounces two. Aqua peppermint, ounces one. Aqua distillate QS, ounces four." Defendant assembled the necessary drugs to fill the prescription. He knew that the simple syrup called for was unavailable and therefore used syrup of orange. The ingredients were incompatible, and the syrup of orange precipitated out the phenobarbital. Defendant then telephoned Dr. Goldstein to ask if he could use some other flavoring. Dr. Goldstein told him that since it was midnight, if he could not find any simple syrup "it would be just as well to use another substance, elixir Mesopin, P.B." Defendant spoke to a clerk and learned that there was simple syrup behind the counter. He mixed the prescription with this syrup, put a label on the bottle according to the prescription, and gave it to Sills. Sills went home, put a teaspoonful of the prescription in the baby's milk and gave it to the baby. The baby died a few hours later.

Defendant stipulated [admitted] that there was nitrite in the prescription bottle and that "the cause of death was methemoglobinemia caused by the ingestion of nitrite." When he compounded the prescription, there was a bottle containing sodium nitrite on the shelf near a bottle labeled sodium citrate. He testified that at no time during his employment at the Ethical Drug Company had he filled any prescription calling for sodium nitrite and that he had taken the prescribed three drams of sodium citrate from the bottle so labeled.

On August 11, 1954, another pharmacist employed by the Ethical Drug Company filled a prescription identical with the Sills' prescription. He obtained the sodium citrate from the bottle used by defendant. The prescription was given to an infant. The infant became ill but recovered. In the opinion of Dr. Goldstein, it was suffering from methemoglobinemia. An analysis of this prescription by a University of Southern California chemist disclosed that it contained 5.4 grams of sodium nitrite per 100 cc's and 4.5 grams of sodium citrate per 100 cc's.

An analysis made by the staff of the head toxicologist for the Los Angeles County coroner of contents of the bottle given to Sills disclosed that it contained 1.33 drams of sodium citrate and 1.23 of sodium nitrite. An analysis made by Biochemical Procedures, Incorporated, a laboratory, of a sample of the contents of the bottle labeled sodium citrate disclosed that it contained 38.9 milligrams of nitrite per gram of material. Charles Covet, one of the owners of the Ethical Drug Company, testified that on the 17th or 18th of October, 1954, he emptied the contents of sodium citrate bottle, washed the bottle but not its cap, and put in new sodium citrate. A subsequent analysis of rinsings from the cap gave strong positive tests for nitrite. Covet also testified that when he purchased an interest in the company in April 1950, the bottle labeled sodium citrate was part of the inventory, that no one had put additional sodium citrate into the bottle from that time until he refilled it after the death of the Sills child; he had never seen any other supply of sodium citrate in the store.

There was testimony that at first glance sodium citrate and sodium nitrite are identical in appearance, that in form either may consist of small colorless crystals or white crystalline powder, that the granulation of the crystals may vary with the manufacturer, and that there may be a slight difference in color between the two. The substance from the bottle labeled sodium citrate was exhibited to the court, but no attempt was made to compare it with unadulterated sodium citrate or sodium nitrite. A chemist with Biochemical Procedures, Incorporated, testified that the mixture did not appear to be homogeneous but that from visual observation alone he could not identify the crystals as one substance or the other. Defendant testified that he had no occasion before July 16th to examine or fill any prescription from the sodium citrate bottle.

No evidence whatever was introduced that would justify an inference that defendant knew or should have known that the bottle labeled sodium citrate contained sodium nitrite. On the contrary, the undisputed evidence shows conclusively that defendant was morally entirely innocent and that only because of a reasonable mistake or unavoidable accident was the prescription filled with a substance containing sodium nitrite.

The court then reviewed the necessary elements of criminal misconduct, noting particularly that "intent" is a necessary element of virtually any crime. In other words, one cannot usually be held criminally liable for that which one unintentionally did.

Section 20 of the Penal Code makes the union act and intent or criminal negligence an invariable element of every crime unless it is excluded expressly or by necessary implication. Moreover, section 26 of the Penal Code lists among the persons incapable of committing crimes "[persons] who committed the act or made the omission charged under an ignorance or mistake of fact, which disproves any criminal intent" and "[persons] who committed the act or made the omission charged through misfortune or by accident, when it appears that there was no evil design, intention, or culpable negligence." The question is thus presented if a person can be convicted of manslaughter or a violation of section 380 of the Penal Code in the absence of any evidence of criminal intent or criminal negligence.

The answer to this question as it relates to the conviction of manslaughter depends on if the defendant committed an "unlawful act" within the meaning of section 192 of the Penal Code when he filled the prescription. The attorney general contends that even if he had no criminal intent and was not criminally negligent, the defendant violated section 26280 of the Health and Safety Code and therefore committed an unlawful act within the meaning of section 192 of the Penal Code.

The court described the elements of the crime of manslaughter, noting that there are two types of conduct that may lead to conviction of this crime; one type is voluntary, based on killing in the "heat of passion," whereas the other type is involuntary, based on killing during the commission of an unlawful act.

Manslaughter is the unlawful killing of a human being, without malice. It is of two kinds:

1. Voluntary—upon a sudden quarrel or heat of passion.
2. Involuntary—in the commission of an unlawful act, not amounting to felony; or in the commission of a lawful act that might produce death, in an unlawful manner, or without due caution and circumspection; provided that this subdivision shall not apply to acts committed in the driving of a vehicle. . . .

The court considered if the misbranding violation by the defendant pharmacist was an unlawful act sufficient to form the basis of an involuntary manslaughter charge.

Section 26280 of the Health and Safety Code provides: "The manufacture, production, preparation, compounding, packing, selling, offering for sale, advertising or keeping for sale within the State of California of any drug or device which is adulterated or misbranded is prohibited." In view of the analysis of the contents of the prescription bottle and the bottle labeled sodium citrate and defendant's stipulation, there can be no doubt that he prepared, compounded, and sold an adulterated and misbranded drug.

Because of the great danger to the public health and safety that the preparation, compounding, or sale of adulterated or misbranded drugs entails, the public interest in demanding that those who prepare, compound, or sell drugs make certain that they are not adulterated or misbranded, and the belief that although an occasional nonculpable offender may be punished, it is necessary to incur that risk by imposing strict liability to prevent the escape of great numbers of culpable offenders, public welfare statutes like section 26280 are not ordinarily governed by section 20 of the Penal Code and therefore call for the sanctions imposed even though the prohibited acts were committed without criminal intent or criminal negligence.

So-called "strict liability," or liability without fault, may apply to some activities of pharmacists and lead to minor criminal liability for acts such as misbranding because this is the best way to protect the public health. However, misbranding violations do not fit within the realm of unlawful acts that may form the basis of an involuntary manslaughter charge.

It does not follow, however, that such acts, committed without criminal intent or criminal negligence, are unlawful acts within the meaning of section 192 of the Penal Code for it is that this section is governed by section 20 of the Penal Code.

It follows, therefore, that only if defendant had intentionally or through criminal negligence prepared, compounded, or sold an adulterated or misbranded drug would his violation of section 26280 of the Health and Safety Code be an unlawful act within the meaning of section 192 of the Penal Code. When, as in this case, the defendant did not know, and could not reasonably be expected to know, that the sodium citrate bottle contained nitrite, those conditions are not met and there is therefore lacking the culpability necessary to make the act an unlawful act within the meaning of section 192.

The judgment and order are reversed.

Notes on *People v. Stuart*

1. Criminal prosecutions of health care providers based on harm caused by inadvertent errors have been rare in American law. This is, of course, contrasted with prosecutions for flagrant disregard of professional responsibilities, such as the sale of prescription narcotic medications without a prescription. Controlled substance diversion is frequently prosecuted as a criminal violation, and pharmacists should be aware that they cannot expect to commit such illegal acts and be free of legal consequences. The difference between these two types of conduct, of course, is that although one is volitional, the other is not. As the *People v. Stuart* case suggests, there is no point in punishing people for things they nonvolitionally do because only volitional conduct can be controlled. To criminally punish a pharmacist for merely making a mistake would be to criminalize the human condition of fallibility. All pharmacists would be criminals because all pharmacists make mistakes. As this case illustrates, such a result would be absurd and it is not the law. Nonetheless, in 2007 an Ohio hospital pharmacist was indicted for involuntary manslaughter for failing to check an IV erroneously compounded by a technician that caused the death of a 2-year-old girl. The pharmacist ultimately

pleaded no contest in 2009 and was sentence to 6 months in jail, 6 months of house arrest, 3 years probation, a $5,000 fine, and 400 hours of community service. The technician was not charged.

2. The effect of criminal liability for honest error would probably be to cause pharmacists to be extremely cautious and risk averse in their practice. Those prescriptions or medication orders that presented a potential risk to the patient might be avoided by pharmacists simply because the possibility of criminal liability would exist if an error were to occur; better to play it safe when prison or a stiff fine is a possibility. Caution of this kind could prevent patients from receiving necessary medications in extreme circumstances of need simply because their prescribed medication posed a risk of harm (that to them was acceptable but to the pharmacist might seem unreasonable). The threat of criminal liability might cause pharmacists to focus their attention on risks to themselves rather than on risks to patients. The threat might also chill pharmacists from documenting errors, a critical component to any pharmacy continuous quality improvement program.

3. In this case, the court ruled that "intent" is a necessary element of a serious criminal violation such as manslaughter; however, intent is hard to see in a person. It exists primarily in the mind of an individual and only perhaps for a fleeting period of time. One may intend to do harm to another, but that intent will never be known to anyone unless some act accompanies it. Thus, the law usually requires for criminal liability that there be both an intent to do harm and some act in furtherance of that intent. Fortunately, we are not criminals simply for thinking occasional bad thoughts about harm to others. As the court notes, there are some minor crimes (such as the misbranding and adulteration in this case) that are so-called strict liability or no-fault crimes. These crimes require no proof of intent because there is a strong social purpose in deterring them, and it would be virtually impossible to prove them if proof of intent were required.

CASE 1-2   *Cohen v. Missouri Board of Pharmacy*, 967 S.W.2d 243 (Mo. App. 1998)

Issue

Whether the Missouri Board of Pharmacy exceeded the scope of its statutory authority by imposing a penalty against a pharmacist.

Overview

This case explored the limits of the authority of a state board of pharmacy to discipline a pharmacist for obviously inappropriate conduct. There was no question that the pharmacist described in this case violated the law, but the board of pharmacy did not follow the rules it was given by the legislature. Boards of pharmacy are created by the legislature, and they are limited by the authority the legislature gives them. In most states, a pharmacy act describes how the board of pharmacy will function and the limits of what it can do. Simply because a pharmacist has committed a violation of the law does not mean the board of pharmacy can do anything it pleases to discipline the pharmacist. In most states, specific penalties are prescribed for specific violations. The board of pharmacy may punish pharmacists only in the ways it is authorized to use under the enabling legislation.

As you read this case excerpt, ask yourself if the board of pharmacy should be given wider latitude in determining the discipline it may use for a pharmacist who has violated the law. Are the rules so difficult to understand that pharmacies will inevitably violate them, or are they possible to understand and easily applied? To what extent should "legal technicalities" be permitted to stand in the way of disciplinary action that is clearly warranted?

The court opinion began by describing the facts of the case:

> Sylvan H. Cohen has been a registered pharmacist in Missouri since 1965. In August of 1976, he was convicted in the United States District Court, on a plea of guilty, of one felony count of "devising and intending to devise a scheme to defraud and obtain money and property by false pretenses" from Venture Stores, Inc. As a result, on July 24, 1978, his pharmacist license was suspended for 1 year by the Missouri Board of Pharmacy (the "Board"). Although the record does not reflect the date, the Board at some point filed another complaint against the appellant based upon a charge related to his addiction to Demerol. On April 18, 1988, based upon this complaint and pursuant to a "Joint Stipulation of Facts, Waiver of Hearings Before the Administrative Hearing Commission and the State Board of Pharmacy, and Consent Order," the Board suspended the appellant's license for 1 year, to be followed by 5 years of probation.

> On April 27, 1993, while on probation, an inspection of the appellant's pharmacy by the Bureau of Narcotics and Dangerous Drugs revealed 24 dispensing infractions in violation of CSR 220-2.110(1). On April 20, 1994, the appellant's 5-year probation expired. On June 28, 1994, the Board filed a "Complaint in Violation of Disciplinary Order," which alleged that 24 dispensing infractions violated the terms of the appellant's probation. On August 5, 1994, the Board conducted a "Violation of Disciplinary Order Hearing" to determine whether discipline should be imposed based upon these violations of probation. On September 20, 1994, the Board issued its "Findings of Fact, Conclusions of Law and Disciplinary Order," which provided that the appellant's probation was to be "extended" for 1 year beginning on October 20, 1994.

> In August of 1995, while on probation, the appellant suffered a relapse of his chemical dependency. As a result, on October 18, 1995, the Board filed a "Complaint in Violation of Disciplinary Order," alleging that appellant violated the terms of his probation imposed by the Board's 1994 disciplinary order and was subject to further discipline. The complaint reflected that a staff pharmacist reported that the appellant had diverted approximately 400 hydrocodone/acetaminophen tablets from the pharmacy. After this violation was reported, the appellant self-reported that he had suffered a relapse of his chemical dependency. The complaint also reflected that, after being confronted by an employee concerning missing drugs, the appellant wrestled with the employee, and that, at the time, he possessed two concealed weapons. As to this complaint, on January 30, 1996, the appellant and the Board entered into a "Joint Stipulation of Facts, Waiver of Hearings Before the Administrative Hearing Commission and the State of Pharmacy, and Consent Order," wherein appellant stipulated that all of the facts alleged in the October 18, 1995, complaint were true.

> On February 1, 1996, the Board held a hearing on the violations of the appellant's probation as alleged in the Board's October 18, 1995, complaint to determine whether his probation should be revoked, and what discipline, if any, should be imposed. At the hearing, the appellant again admitted to the allegations in the complaint and explained his illness and progress to the Board. On February 22, 1996, the Board issued its "Findings of Fact, and Conclusions of Law and Disciplinary Order," revoking the appellant's license for a violation of his probation imposed by the Board's 1994 disciplinary order.

> It is undisputed that the February 22, 1996, order, revoking the appellant's pharmacist license based upon alleged violations by the appellant of the September 20, 1994, probation order, extended his original 1988 5-year probation for another year. The alleged violations of the 1994 probation order, professional misconduct and inaccurate controlled substance recordkeeping, were set forth in the Board's "Complaint in Violation of Disciplinary Order."

The court then described the contention by the pharmacist that he was being disciplined in a way the pharmacy act did not permit. Specifically, his license was being revoked because he had violated conditions of a probation that was longer than the statute permitted by the board of pharmacy to extend a probationary period.

The appellant claims that the Board lacked the authority to revoke his license for a violation of the 1994 probation order because the order was void. Because we agree with the appellant that, if the probation order was void, the 1996 order revoking the appellant's license based on a violation and revocation of the same would be void as well, then the issue we must decide is whether the Board had the authority to enter its 1994 probation order.

The appellant's claim that the Board's September 20, 1994, probation order was void is premised upon his assertion that the Board's authority to enter the order was based on a violation and revocation of the appellant's 5-year probation ordered in the Board's April 20, 1988, disciplinary order, and that its authority to enter the 1994 probation order for a violation of the 5-year probation had expired on April 20, 1994, prior to the entry of the 1994 order. The record reflects that the 1988 disciplinary order imposed a 1-year suspension of the appellant's license to be followed by a 5-year probation, the maximum allowed. As such, the appellant's 5-year probation would have expired on April 20, 1994. Thus, the appellant contends that because his 5-year probation had already expired at the time of his revocation and entry of the September 20, 1994, probation order, the Board lacked authority to enter a disciplinary order based on a violation and revocation of his 5-year probation, rendering the 1994 order void.

Based upon the 1988 complaint, the appellant entered into a "Joint Stipulation of Facts, Waiver of Hearings Before the Administrative Hearing Commission and the State Board of Pharmacy, and Consent Order." As a result, on April 20, 1988, pursuant to § 338.050.3, the Board suspended the appellant's license for 1 year, which was to be followed by a 5-year probation. Unlike the 1988 disciplinary order, which was entered in accordance with § 338.055 authority and procedures, the 1994 probation order and the 1996 order revoking the appellant's license were entered based upon violations and revocations of the 1988 and 1994 probation orders, respectively, which resulted from the original 1988 complaint. Thus, the issue becomes whether the Board had the authority to enter its 1994 and 1996 disciplinary orders based upon violations of the 1988 and 1994 probation orders, which sprang from the original 1988 complaint.

In assessing the persuasiveness of the pharmacist's argument, the court noted the well-recognized principle that administrative agencies may exercise only the powers given them in their enabling statutes. The court then applied that fundamental concept to the facts of the case.

A key principle of administrative law "is that administrative agencies—legislative creations—possess only those powers expressly conferred or necessarily implied by statute." In this regard, the authority which allows the Board to take disciplinary action against a pharmacist licensed in Missouri and the procedures by which such must be done are contained in § 338.055. As such, it is clear that for each complaint filed pursuant to § 338.055, on which the administrative hearing commission (AHC) finds that the grounds for disciplinary -action are met, the Board has the authority to: (1) censure the person named in the complaint; (2) impose up to 5 years probation on him or her; (3) suspend his or her license for up to 3 years; or (4) revoke his or her license. In this regard, the 1988 order, which was entered as a result of a § 338.055 complaint, imposed the maximum 5-year term of probation. Although § 338.055.3 expressly authorizes the Board to impose up to 5 years of probation for a substantiated complaint filed pursuant to § 338.055.2, it does not expressly authorize it to discipline a licensee based upon an alleged violation of such probation. In the absence of express statutory authority to discipline a licensee based upon an alleged violation of such probation, the issue is whether the Board has the inherent authority to do so.

Logically, the Board would be limited to those dispositions provided for in § 338.055.3, which would include extending the term of the probation which was violated. However, even assuming the Board has the authority in the case of a probation revocation to impose discipline on a licensee pursuant to § 338.055, including extending the term of probation, the question arises as to whether the Board could extend a term of probation beyond the maximum term of 5 years provided for in § 338.055.3. The answer to this question is significant to the case at bar because, if we assume the Board did not have the authority to extend the appellant's probation beyond the 5-year term originally ordered in the 1988 disciplinary order, the 1994 probation order extending the appellant's probation for another year would be void, which, as discussed, would render the 1996 order revoking the appellant's license, based upon a violation of the 1994 probation order, void as well. Thus, we must decide whether the Board had the authority in 1994 to extend by 1 year the appellant's 5-year probation ordered in 1988, which had expired prior to the entry of the 1994 probation order, for an alleged violation of that probation.

Because the Board was prohibited by § 338.055.3 from extending the appellant's probation beyond the original 5 years, we find it had no authority to enter its 1994 order extending the appellant's probation for one more year. Thus, the 1994 order was void.

Having decided that the board of pharmacy was without authority to extend the probation beyond the 5 years authorized by the statute and having decided also that the license revocation was void for having been based on the violation of an unauthorized probation, the court then took care to describe the narrowness of its ruling.

In holding as we do, we do not decide whether the Board, after revoking the appellant's probation, could have ordered him censured, or his license suspended or revoked as provided in § 338.055.3, rather than extending his probation beyond the maximum term of 5 years. We also do not decide whether the Board could have sought to discipline the appellant pursuant to a new § 338.055 complaint based on the alleged violations of probation, rather than revoking and extending his probation. We only decide that in revoking the appellant's 5-year probation ordered pursuant to § 338.055, the Board was prohibited by § 338.055.3 from extending his probation for another year.

The judgment of the circuit court affirming the order of the Missouri Board of Pharmacy revoking the appellant's pharmacist license is reversed, and the cause is remanded to the circuit court for it to order the Board to reinstate the appellant's pharmacist license in accordance with this opinion.

Notes on *Cohen v. Missouri Board of Pharmacy*

1. All citizens have a right to know what the rules are before they engage in activity that may expose them to government punishment. It is not fair, thus it is a denial of due process, for a governmental agency to "make up the rules as it goes." In this case, it is a stretch to suggest that the pharmacist was unfairly treated by the board of pharmacy because he obviously knew he was violating the law and that punishment was a very real possibility. However, the protections of the law extend to those who deserve them, as well as to those who do not. The obvious culpability of this pharmacist was irrelevant to the core issue in the case; the board of pharmacy had exceeded the scope of its statutory authority.

2. At first blush, it may appear that this pharmacist was let off on a trivial technicality. Although he may have been the beneficiary of a technicality, it is important to note that the law is full of similar technicalities, all of them designed to

protect citizens from arbitrary government action. Society's interest in removing incompetent pharmacists from practice is a compelling reason to "let it slide" if a board of pharmacy fails to adhere to the letter of the law. However, even more compelling is the interest in protecting citizens from arbitrary government action. The state board of pharmacy may only discipline pharmacists because it is authorized to do so by the legislature through its enabling legislation, and in this case that authority was clearly exceeded.

3. It is interesting to note that the court provided a not-too-subtle primer on appropriate administrative enforcement for the board of pharmacy. Just to make sure there were no misunderstandings of the meaning of this legal opinion, the court specified that it would have been fully acceptable for the board of pharmacy to have used one of the other enforcement mechanisms available to it under the statute. Boards of pharmacy have undoubtedly heeded this advice.

| CASE 1-3 | *Malan v. Huesemann*, 942 S.W.2d 424 (Mo. App. 1997) |

Issue

Whether a pharmacist's admission of errors in a state board of pharmacy administrative action may be admitted into evidence in a subsequent malpractice case to show a propensity of the pharmacist to commit errors.

Overview

This case is a lawsuit within a lawsuit. The primary case was a malpractice lawsuit brought by a patient against a pharmacist who had allegedly dispensed to her an incorrect medication. The judge in that lawsuit ruled that evidence from a previous board of pharmacy disciplinary action could be used in the malpractice case. The pharmacist then filed an action against the judge who issued that ruling, seeking to have the ruling set aside by the appellate court on review.

As you read this case, reflect on the differing purposes of administrative actions brought by the board of pharmacy against a licensee and of malpractice cases brought by patients against their pharmacist. In the former, the purpose is to protect the public in the future, whereas in the latter the purpose is to award compensation for a problem of the past. Might admissions made in one type of action be inappropriate for consideration in the other type of action on the basis of the difference in character of the two proceedings? On the other hand, why should a person who has made an admission in one legal proceeding not be forced to live with that admission in another, albeit different, proceeding? How might practical matters, such as the availability of funding to support litigation, the relatively slight punishment one expects, and the confidentiality of a disciplinary action, influence pharmacists to admit to charges that they would prefer to contest?

The court opinion began by describing the facts of the case:

> Mary Malan is a registered pharmacist, practicing in Clinton, Missouri. In September 1990, the Missouri Board of Pharmacy seized Ms. Malan's bulk chemicals because it believed that her process of compounding drugs from them was illegal. On October 19, 1990, the Board also informed Ms. Malan that it was not renewing her pharmacy permit. Ms. Malan petitioned the Administrative Hearing Commission (AHC) for relief. The AHC subsequently ordered the Board to reinstate Ms. Malan's permit.
>
> On February 4, 1991, the Board filed a 16-count Expedited Complaint against Ms. Malan with the AHC, alleging that she had compounded drugs from bulk chemicals and had made dispensing errors or illegal substitutions that endangered the health

of her customers. The Board requested an expedited hearing and asked the AHC to immediately suspend Ms. Malan's license until a full hearing could be held to determine whether cause existed to discipline her.

The AHC held a hearing on March 20, 1991. In its order, the AHC denied the Board's request to suspend Ms. Malan's license and dismissed the Board's complaint. It found that most of Ms. Malan's compounding was not illegal, and in those instances that may have been illegal there was no clear and present danger to public health or safety because Ms. Malan testified that she had stopped this compounding. The AHC also noted that the Board's seizure of her bulk chemicals was done without authority and the Board's 5-month delay between the seizure and filing the complaint indicated there was not a present danger.

Regarding the alleged dispensing errors, the AHC found that Ms. Malan had a low error rating and the instances were mere mistakes. Although there was evidence of one serious incident, the AHC did not believe this warranted suspension of her license. The AHC did state, however, that it would have been willing to restrict her from dispensing anything other than acceptable commercial products if the Board had requested this relief.

Thereafter, the Board refiled its complaint with the AHC, seeking a full hearing. Before a hearing was held, however, the parties settled the dispute by entering into a "Joint Stipulation of Facts, Waiver of Hearings Before the Administrative Hearing Commission and State Board of Pharmacy, and Consent Order with Joint Proposed Findings of Fact and Conclusions of Law" on October 10, 1991. Ms. Malan suggests in this Court that she entered into the settlement because defense of the Board's prior unsuccessful actions against her had taken all of her funds. In any event, the Joint Stipulation stated in numerous places it was solely for the purposes of settlement that Ms. Malan did not contest the Board's allegations. The Joint Proposed Findings of Fact similarly recited that, on specified occasions, Ms. Malan agreed, again for settlement purposes only, that she had filled prescriptions by compounding bulk chemicals and had substituted drugs other than those prescribed.

Pursuant to the terms of the settlement, Ms. Malan's pharmacist's license and pharmacy permit were placed on probation for 5 years beginning on November 6, 1991.

On May 12, 1995, the Pharmacy Board issued a Complaint of Violation of Disciplinary Order against Ms. Malan alleging she had incorrectly filled prescriptions and made improper substitutions. This second Board complaint was not filed with the AHC, however. Instead, on August 4, 1995, Ms. Malan and the Board again entered into a settlement in the form of a Joint Stipulation extending Ms. Malan's probation. The Findings of Fact in this Joint Stipulation stated that Ms. Malan agreed, again solely for the purposes of settlement and not as an admission of liability, that she incorrectly filled prescriptions and substituted drugs for a person designated as "Patient I." The Joint Stipulation also recounted incidents involving other patients.

The Executive Director of the Board executed a Consent Order, purporting to find that the facts the Board had itself alleged, and which were stipulated to by Ms. Malan for purposes of settlement only, were true and that Ms. Malan was subject to discipline. No hearing was held on this order and neither it nor the Joint Stipulation on which it was based were ever filed with the AHC. The AHC issued no order at all in regard to the 1995 complaint.

After this lengthy description of the protracted problems between the pharmacist and the board of pharmacy, the court then described the lawsuit that served as the basis of the action brought by the patient against the pharmacist.

Also on May 12, 1995, Lois Ruth Kalberloh, the person identified as "Patient I" in the 1995 Joint Stipulation, filed a Petition against Ms. Malan alleging pharmaceutical malpractice. Ms. Kalberloh alleged that Ms. Malan filled Ms. Kalberloh's prescription for Eldepryl with the drug Prednisone. In her amended Petition, Ms. Kalberloh made a claim for punitive damages, alleging that Ms. Malan had repeatedly demonstrated willful, wanton, and malicious conduct in her practice as a pharmacist. As support, Ms. Kalberloh included as exhibits copies of the 1991 and 1995 Joint Stipulations between Ms. Malan and the Board. She sought to read portions of these stipulations to the jury.

Punitive damages are awarded when a defendant is determined to have acted with willful disregard of the interests of the plaintiff. The only way in which the plaintiff in this case could claim willful disregard would be if there was a pattern of pharmacy errors and if this pattern showed willful, wanton, and malicious conduct toward the public. To show such a pattern, the plaintiff sought to introduce evidence of the pharmacist's admissions of other errors made within the administrative action.

Judge Raymond T. Huesemann ruled that portions of the settlement agreements dealing with misfilling of other prescriptions were admissible and could be read to the jury, and that the fact they are settlements went only to their weight, not to their admissibility.

We hold that the court below erred in ruling that Ms. Kalberloh could read or introduce portions of the joint stipulations during the trial of her suit against Ms. Malan. Each explicitly states that it is being entered into solely for the purposes of settling the dispute, and not as any admission of liability by Ms. Malan. Each forms a part of a settlement between Ms. Malan and the Board of Pharmacy. As such, it is not admissible in evidence nor may the jury be informed about the fact of the prior settlements.

The court reviewed the policy of courts toward settlements generally, noting that out-of-court settlements are favored under the law because there is no purpose in using judicial resources when no real controversy exists. Courts are usually quite happy to let parties iron out their own disagreements, without resort to litigation.

In order to further the public policy favoring the settlement of disputes, it is well established that settlement offers are not admissible in a subsequent trial. This is because settlement negotiations "should be encouraged and a party making an offer of settlement should not be penalized by revealing the offer to the jury if the negotiations fail to materialize."

The danger of admitting evidence of settlements is that the trier of fact may believe that the fact that a settlement was attempted is some indication of the merits of the case. As a result, "if offers of settlement were admitted in evidence, they would have the natural tendency with the jury to denigrate the position at trial. No one would make offers if the risk of their being before the jury were a necessary corollary of the offer."

The desire to encourage settlements is fully applicable to settlement of administrative actions. This policy rationale supporting exclusion of evidence of settlements fully applies here. Ms. Malan had twice successfully defended against actions taken by the Board. The third action involved similar issues, and she nowhere admitted that her conduct had been improper. For practical reasons, however, she claims, she desired to settle, as did the Board. In any event, the settlements stated repeatedly that the facts stated therein were admitted solely for purposes of settlement. To now admit the stipulations contained in the settlement in this civil action would clearly be contrary to the intent of the settling parties, and would discourage further settlements in future cases, in derogation of the policy favoring settlements. For these reasons, no evidence of the settlement agreements may be admitted below.

Notes on *Malan v. Huesemann*

1. The court in this case was quite clearly considering the public policy implications of its actions. Although every case has as its main purpose the settlement of a dispute between two or more parties, the ruling of any case has the potential to set precedent that will extend beyond the confines of the parties to the case. The court recognized that had it ruled in favor of admitting into evidence in a malpractice case the admissions from an administrative case, there would be a deterrent to the settlement of administrative cases in the future. Why should a person admit error in an administrative hearing if the admissions are going to come back to haunt that person in a later malpractice case? The best approach might be to refuse to admit everything and force the administrative agency to prove its case, then continue with the denials in any subsequent malpractice case. The obvious problem with this result would be that administrative actions would continue long after they could have been settled, expending scarce resources and wasting the time of all involved. The court considered that a bad policy for the public and ruled in a way that would avoid such a problematic result.

2. In a pharmacist malpractice case such as this one, based on an alleged misfill of a prescription with one drug instead of another, the plaintiff is obligated to prove the facts alleged. Although evidence of past errors is irrelevant to prove a present error, evidence of past errors may be relevant to prove carelessness, sloppiness, and recklessness. Should these undesirable characteristics be proven for a pharmacist, a finding of willful disregard with attendant punitive damages may be supported. Of course, the plaintiff may be able to prove such facts and receive punitive damages, but this case stands for the principle that the plaintiff will not be permitted to use admissions from an administrative hearing as proof. Other means of developing evidence must be used to support an award of punitive damages.

3. The difficulties that can occur for a pharmacist who is noticed by the board of pharmacy are quite evident in this case. Most pharmacists hope to complete their entire career of years of pharmacy practice without at any time ever coming to the attention of the board of pharmacy. Because this pharmacist had attracted so much attention from the board of pharmacy, she had apparently expended significant financial resources in defending charges against her. It just seemed best to admit her mistakes and get on with her life. Although the board of pharmacy could revoke a license, the penalty in this case was evidently much less severe. However, the penalties of a malpractice case, especially punitive damages that usually are not paid for by insurance, are more significant and worth defending.

CASE 1-4	*Heckler v. Chaney*, 470 U.S. 821 (1984)

Issue

Whether an administrative agency has the discretion to decide not to enforce rules it is authorized to enforce, even though there is a possibility that the law would permit such an enforcement.

Overview

This case attracted national attention when it was appealed to the Supreme Court of the United States, but the attention was because of the controversial subject matter and not the important legal question it addressed. It was a dark case brought by condemned prisoners who contended that the drugs used for the execution of people in circumstances such as theirs were not approved by the FDA for this purpose and therefore were unlawful when used for execution by lethal injection. The prisoners sought a ruling to that effect by the FDA, but the FDA refused to even consider the issue.

As a general matter, administrative agencies have considerable discretion to choose when to enforce their rules and when not to enforce them. Rarely does an agency enforce every possible violation of the rules it is authorized to enforce. Rather, the agency prioritizes violations and enforces the rules against only those violations that are considered to be important enough to warrant agency attention. The FDA certainly functions in this way, with many trivial violations being ignored by the agency. In this case, the court was asked to force the FDA to take action against state governments that the prisoners believed were violating the FDCA.

The court opinion began by describing the facts of the case:

> Respondents have been sentenced to death by lethal injection of drugs under the laws of the States of Oklahoma and Texas. Those States, and several others, have recently adopted this method for carrying out the capital sentence. Respondents first petitioned the FDA, claiming that the drugs used by the States for this purpose, although approved by the FDA for the medical purposes stated on their labels, were not approved for use in human executions. They alleged that the drugs had not been tested for the purpose for which they were to be used, and that, given that the drugs would likely be administered by untrained personnel, it was also likely that the drugs would not induce the quick and painless death intended. They urged that use of these drugs for human execution was the "unapproved use of an approved drug" and constituted a violation of the Act's prohibitions against "misbranding." They also suggested that the FDCA's requirements for approval of "new drugs" applied, since these drugs were now being used for a new purpose. Accordingly, respondents claimed that the FDA was required to approve the drugs as "safe and effective" for human execution before they could be distributed in interstate commerce. They therefore requested the FDA to take various investigatory and enforcement actions to prevent these perceived violations; they requested the FDA to affix warnings to the labels of all the drugs stating that they were unapproved and unsafe for human execution, to send statements to the drug manufacturers and prison administrators stating that the drugs should not be so used, and to adopt procedures for seizing the drugs from state prisons and to recommend the prosecution of all those in the chain of distribution who knowingly distribute or purchase the drugs with intent to use them for human execution.

> The FDA Commissioner responded, refusing to take the requested actions. The Commissioner first detailed his disagreement with respondents' understanding of the scope of FDA jurisdiction over the unapproved use of approved drugs for human execution, concluding that FDA jurisdiction in the area was generally unclear but in any event should not be exercised to interfere with this particular aspect of state criminal justice systems.

Although the court could have spent significant time addressing the social issues surrounding capital punishment and the Constitutional prohibition against cruel and unusual punishment, the case instead was decided on the basis of principles of administrative law.

> For us, this case turns on the important question of the extent to which determinations by the FDA not to exercise its enforcement authority over the use of drugs in

interstate commerce may be judicially reviewed. This Court has recognized on several occasions over many years that an agency's decision not to prosecute or enforce, whether through civil or criminal process, is a decision generally committed to an agency's absolute discretion. This recognition of the existence of discretion is attributable in no small part to the general unsuitability for judicial review of agency decisions to refuse enforcement.

The court explained that it is unusual for there to be judicial interference with a decision of an administrative agency because agencies usually have expertise that courts do not have, and the availability of this expertise is a sound basis for judicial deference to administrative authority.

The reasons for this general unsuitability are many. First, an agency decision not to enforce often involves a complicated balancing of a number of factors which are peculiarly within its expertise. Thus, the agency must not only assess whether a violation has occurred, but whether agency resources are best spent on this violation or another, whether the agency is likely to succeed if it acts, whether the particular enforcement action requested best fits the agency's overall policies, and, indeed, whether the agency has enough resources to undertake the action at all. An agency generally cannot act against each technical violation of the statute it is charged with enforcing. The agency is far better equipped than the courts to deal with the many variables involved in the proper ordering of its priorities. Similar concerns animate the principles of administrative law that courts generally will defer to an agency's construction of the statute it is charged with implementing, and to the procedures it adopts for implementing that statute.

In addition to these administrative concerns, we note that when an agency refuses to act, it generally does not exercise its coercive power over an individual's liberty or property rights, and thus does not infringe upon areas that courts often are called upon to protect. Similarly, when an agency does act to enforce, that action itself provides a focus for judicial review, in as much as the agency must have exercised its power in some manner. The action at least can be reviewed to determine whether the agency exceeded its statutory powers. Finally, we recognize that an agency's refusal to institute proceedings shares to some extent the characteristics of the decision of a prosecutor in the Executive Branch not to indict—a decision which has long been regarded as the special province of the Executive Branch, inasmuch as it is the Executive who is charged by the Constitution to "take Care that the Laws be faithfully executed."

The court considered the argument of the petitioners that despite general deference to agency decisions, some enforcement actions were specifically mandated by the statute and thus were not discretionary.

To enforce the various substantive prohibitions contained in the FDCA, the Act provides for injunctions, 21 U.S.C. § 332, criminal sanctions, §§ 333 and 335, and seizure of any offending food, drug, or cosmetic article, § 334. The Act's general provision for enforcement, § 372, provides only that "[the] Secretary is authorized to conduct examinations and investigations." The section on criminal sanctions states baldly that any person who violates the Act's substantive prohibitions "shall be imprisoned or fined." Respondents argue that this statement mandates criminal prosecution of every violator of the Act but they adduce no indication in case law or legislative history that such was Congress' intention in using this language, which is commonly found in the criminal provisions of the United States Code. We are unwilling to attribute such a sweeping meaning to this language, particularly since the Act charges the Secretary only with recommending prosecution; any criminal prosecutions must be instituted by the Attorney General. The Act's enforcement provisions thus commit complete discretion to the Secretary to decide how and when they should be exercised.

Notes on *Heckler v. Chaney*

1. Government agencies usually are criticized for what they do, not for what they fail to do. However, in this case, the FDA was accused of having failed to do its duty to protect individuals for whom approved drugs were used (although admittedly a distinct and small class of individuals). The Supreme Court did not agree with the approach taken by the agency; it merely said that if the agency chose to take this approach, it was within its rights to do so. As a general matter, courts are highly deferential to administrative decisions.

2. The substantive claim in this case, that the FDA may forbid uses of medications in ways that fall outside their product labeling, has consistently been a losing argument. Product labeling is a guideline as to appropriate use, but it does not define the universe of appropriate use. So-called "off-label" uses, when physicians prescribe and pharmacists dispense in ways that are not fully supported by the product labeling, have generally been held not to violate the FDCA. Although the FDCA regulates drug distribution, it does not regulate professional practice. Even had the FDA exercised its discretion to consider the complaint by the prisoners, their claim would probably have failed on its merits.

3. In a 2012 case, *Beaty v. Food and Drug Admin.*, 2012 WL 102108 (D.D.C. March 27, 2012), plaintiff death row inmates sued the FDA, contending that the agency violated the FDCA by improperly allowing shipments of thiopental from foreign manufacturers for the purpose of being used in lethal injections. The court found for the plaintiffs, noting that the FDCA mandates the FDA to require registration of foreign drug manufacturers and to refuse entry to any drug that appears to be misbranded or unapproved. The court distinguished *Beaty* from *Heckler* by noting that *Heckler* centered on the FDA's discretion to decline to pursue enforcement actions contained in administrative rules. *Beaty*, however, deals with the agency's failure to carry out a statutory mandate. The court considered the FDA's failure to enforce the statute as arbitrary and capricious because it enforced this statute in other instances.

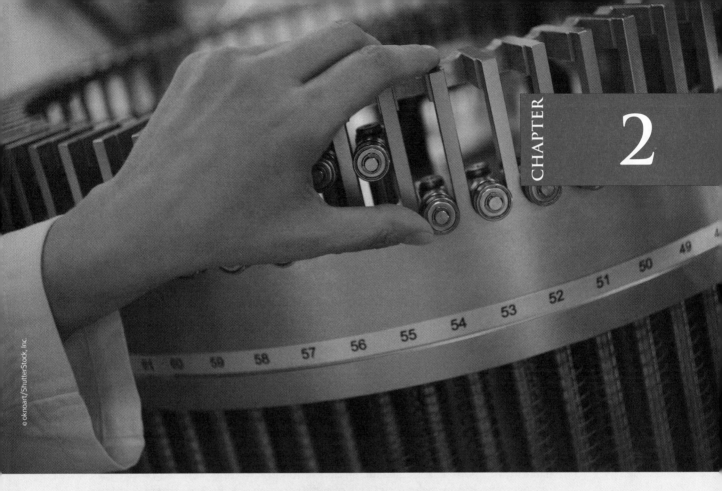

CHAPTER 2

FEDERAL REGULATION OF MEDICATIONS: DEVELOPMENT, PRODUCTION, AND MARKETING

CHAPTER OBJECTIVES

Upon completing this chapter, the reader will be able to:

▸ Identify the significant historical events that have shaped the current federal Food, Drug, and Cosmetic Act (FDCA).

▸ Distinguish among the definitions of food, drug, dietary supplement, cosmetic, device, label, and labeling.

▸ Recognize the prohibited acts, penalties, and enforcement mechanisms in the FDCA.

▸ Identify the situations that may cause a drug to be adulterated or misbranded.

▸ Differentiate FDCA requirements for prescription drugs from those for over-the-counter drugs.

▸ Understand the issues and procedures pertaining to new drug approval.

▸ Describe the legal requirements for manufacturers that advertise prescription drugs to health care professionals and consumers.

The federal Food, Drug, and Cosmetic Act (FDCA) (21 U.S.C. § 301 et seq., 52 Stat. 1040 (1938)) provides for the comprehensive regulation of all drugs introduced into interstate commerce. The intent of the law is to protect consumers from adulterated or misbranded foods, drugs, cosmetics, or devices. Under the act, no new drug may be marketed and sold unless it has been proved both safe and effective for its intended use and approved by the federal Food and Drug Administration (FDA).

This chapter discusses relevant history, definitions, and provisions of the FDCA related to the development, production, and marketing of products, from the discovery of a new concept by a scientist to the delivery of a therapeutically appropriate product to a pharmacy. In many sections, the reader will note that the applicable law is either cited or summarized first, followed by an explanation of the law from the perspective of the author.

HISTORICAL OVERVIEW OF THE FEDERAL FOOD, DRUG, AND COSMETIC ACT

In order to protect public health, governments of nearly every civilization have sought to protect the public from adulterated food products. More modern laws in the United States in the 1800s against the adulteration of foods and drugs were led by two factors: one, advances in analytical chemistry and microscope technology, and two, studies showing the impact of adulterated foods and drugs on human life. One such study in 1850 showed that average life expectancy actually decreased by as many as 7 years over certain periods of time in Boston and New York in part because of adulterated drugs and foods. (See Hyman, 2002, Chapter 2.)

Our present-day food and drug regulatory system in the United States, represented by the FDCA, has been shaped by several important amendments and events and warrants a brief historical discussion at this point. The purpose of this historical overview is to provide the reader a general background of the act. Many of the amendments and events chronicled here are discussed in greater detail later.

PURE FOOD AND DRUG ACT OF 1906

At the turn of the century, investigative reports revealed widespread food and drug adulteration problems. Most notably, the 1906 novel, *The Jungle*, by Upton Sinclair, described atrocious adulteration problems in the meat industry. Concern for the risks to public health and safety associated with unsanitary and poorly labeled foods and drugs prompted Congress in 1906 to pass the Pure Food and Drug Act (34 Stat. 768). The law prohibited the adulteration and misbranding of foods and drugs in interstate commerce. It fell short of providing the protection that Congress intended, however, because a 1911 U.S. Supreme Court decision, *United States v. Johnson*, 221 U.S. 488, held that the misbranding provision in the law did not prevent false or misleading efficacy claims. In *Johnson*, the manufacturer claimed on the label that the drug was effective against cancer, knowing that this representation was false. The Court ruled that the misbranding provision in the law prevented false statements only as to the drug's identity (i.e., strength, quality, purity). Some manufacturers, fearing a violation of the labeling provision, simply omitted information from the label because the act did not require the label to list the ingredients, include directions for use, or provide warnings. Moreover, the act failed to regulate cosmetics or devices.

The *Johnson* decision prompted Congress to amend the Pure Food and Drug Act in 1912 to prohibit false and fraudulent efficacy claims. Even with this amendment, however, the act failed to achieve its purpose. The amendment was difficult to enforce because it required the government to prove fraudulent intent on the part of one who made false statements on the label. By pleading ignorance, violators could escape enforcement.

Despite public awareness that the 1906 law was inadequate, there was no new legislation until 1938. By that time, pressure for a new law had been building for many years. A catalyst for the new law was the sulfanilamide elixir tragedy of 1937. Sulfanilamide was one of the first of the "miracle" anti-infective sulfa drugs marketed. A manufacturer who sought to produce the drug in an elixir form seized upon diethylene glycol as the best solvent. (Diethylene glycol is used today as an industrial solvent and for other industrial uses.) No toxicity tests had been done, despite the fact that little was known about the use of diethylene glycol in humans. The solvent proved to be a deadly poison, and 107 deaths were ultimately at+tributed to this elixir. The 1906 law had not granted the FDA the authority to ban unsafe drugs, so the FDA had to remove the product on the basis of a technical misbranding violation—that an elixir must contain alcohol, and the product did not.

FOOD, DRUG, AND COSMETIC ACT OF 1938

The FDCA of 1938 (21 U.S.C. § 301 et seq. 52 Stat. 1040), with amendments, forms the nucleus of today's law. All the amendments and laws described subsequently in this section are amendments to the 1938 act. It provided that no new drug could be marketed until proven safe for use under the conditions described on the label and approved by the FDA. The law also expanded the definitions of misbranding and adulteration used in the earlier act, requiring that labels must contain adequate directions for use and warnings about the habit-forming properties of certain drugs. The 1938 law applies to cosmetics and devices as well. Significantly, however, the act exempted drugs marketed before 1938 from the requirement that new drugs be proven safe before being marketed.

In 1941, the FDCA was amended to allow the FDA to require batch certification of the safety and efficacy of insulin to ensure uniform potency. Because of concern over the quality of penicillin production, the FDCA was amended to allow the FDA to require batch certification of the safety and efficacy of penicillin in 1945. Subsequent amendments extended the certification requirement to other antibiotic drugs or any derivative of an antibiotic drug. (In 1997, the Food and Drug Administration Modernization Act eliminated the batch certification requirement for insulin and antibiotics.)

In 1948, the extent of the FDCA's jurisdiction was challenged in *United States v. Sullivan*, 332 U.S. 689. The defendant pharmacist contended that federal law did not apply to his acts because his acts only affected intrastate transactions. The U.S. Supreme Court, however, declared that the jurisdiction of the act extends to transactions between the pharmacist and the patient. Therefore, the FDCA applies to drugs held for sale in a pharmacy.

DURHAM-HUMPHREY AMENDMENT OF 1951

The 1938 FDCA required all drugs to be labeled with "adequate directions for use." When the act was passed, however, many drugs on the market were not safe for use except under medical supervision. These drugs could not meet the "adequate directions for use" requirement. The Durham-Humphrey Amendment (also often referred to as the Prescription Drug Amendment) was enacted in 1951 (65 Stat. 648) to solve this problem. The amendment established two classes of drugs, prescription and over the counter, and provided that the labels of prescription drugs need not contain "adequate directions for use" so long as they contain the legend, "Caution: Federal law prohibits dispensing without a prescription." When dispensed by a pharmacist, inclusion on the label of directions from the prescriber satisfies the "adequate directions for use" requirement. In addition to establishing the two classes of drugs, the amendment also authorizes oral prescriptions and refills of prescription drugs.

FOOD ADDITIVES AMENDMENT OF 1958

After several years of hearings, Congress amended the FDCA to require that components added to food products must receive premarket approval for safety (P.L. 85-929). The law also contains an anticancer provision, commonly known as the Delaney Clause, which prohibits the approval of any food additive that might cause cancer.

COLOR ADDITIVE AMENDMENTS OF 1960

In 1960, Congress amended the FDCA to require manufacturers to establish the safety of color additives in foods, drugs, and cosmetics. Under the Color Additive Amendments, the FDA can approve a color for one use but not for others (e.g., external use only). The amendments also contain a Delaney Clause, similar to the one contained in the Food Additives Amendment.

KEFAUVER-HARRIS AMENDMENT OF 1962

In the late 1950s, a popular sedative, thalidomide, was being marketed in Europe. The William S. Merrell Company distributed the drug experimentally in the United States in 1960, but the FDA withheld final approval of the new drug application (NDA) pending additional safety information. In 1961, it was confirmed that the drug had caused a birth defect, phocomelia (seal limbs), in thousands of infants. Because the FDA had refused to allow the marketing of thalidomide in the United States, the number of birth defects caused by the drug in this country was low. Nonetheless, the worldwide disaster caused Congress to enact the Kefauver-Harris Amendment to the FDCA.

This amendment, also called the Drug Efficacy Amendment (76 Stat. 780), strengthened the new drug approval process by requiring that drugs be proved not only safe but also effective. The efficacy requirement was made retroactive to all drugs marketed between 1938 and 1962. The amendment also:

- Transferred jurisdiction of prescription drug advertising from the Federal Trade Commission (FTC) to the FDA
- Established the Good Manufacturing Practices (GMP) requirements
- Added more extensive controls for clinical investigations by requiring the informed consent of research subjects and reporting of adverse drug reactions

MEDICAL DEVICE AMENDMENTS OF 1976

Under the 1938 Act, the FDA had no authority to review medical devices for safety and efficacy before marketing. As a result, the agency resorted to classifying devices as drugs when it deemed appropriate and necessary. Prompted by public safety concerns with certain devices such as the Dalkon Shield, an intrauterine device, Congress amended the FDCA in 1976 to provide for more extensive regulation and administrative authority regarding the safety and efficacy of medical devices. The Medical Device Amendments (P.L. 94-295; 90 Stat. 539) require

- Classification of devices according to their function
- Premarket approval
- Establishment of performance standards
- Conformance with GMP regulations
- Adherence to record and reporting requirements

ORPHAN DRUG ACT OF 1983

For years, pharmaceutical manufacturers had urged Congress to recognize that the NDA process was too expensive to warrant the development and marketing of drugs for diseases that affect relatively few people. In fact, the FDA acknowledged that between 1973 and 1983 only 10 products were approved for the treatment of rare diseases. In response, Congress passed the Orphan Drug Act (P.L. 97-414) in 1983 to provide tax and exclusive licensing incentives for manufacturers to develop and market drugs or biologicals for the treatment of "rare diseases or conditions" (defined as those affecting fewer than 200,000 Americans). Between the act's passage and the year 2000, the FDA approved about 172 orphan drugs and biological products, and 700 additional orphan-designated products were being developed.

DRUG PRICE COMPETITION AND PATENT TERM RESTORATION ACT OF 1984

Also called the Waxman-Hatch Amendment, the Drug Price Competition and Patent Term Restoration Act (P.L. 98-417) was enacted in 1984 to streamline the generic drug approval process while giving patent extensions, in certain cases, to innovator drugs. The intent of the law is to make generic drugs more readily available to the public and, at the same time, provide incentives for manufacturers to develop new drugs. The law is the result of intense lobbying and negotiating between generic drug manufacturers and the manufacturers of innovator drugs.

PRESCRIPTION DRUG MARKETING ACT OF 1987

Congress enacted the Prescription Drug Marketing Act (P.L. 100-293) in 1987 in response to growing alarm that a secondary or diversionary distribution system for prescription drugs was threatening the public health and safety and creating an unfair form of competition. This law establishes sales restrictions and recordkeeping requirements for prescription drug samples. It also prohibits hospitals and other health care entities from reselling their pharmaceutical purchases to other businesses and requires the state licensing of drug wholesalers.

SAFE MEDICAL DEVICES ACT OF 1990

This act further strengthened the Medical Devices Amendment Act of 1976, giving the FDA additional authority especially related to postmarketing requirements and premarket notification and approval, while expediting the premarket device approval process.

THE GENERIC DRUG ENFORCEMENT ACT OF 1992

This act warrants discussion to highlight a scandal that occurred when some FDA staff accepted bribes from generic drug industry personnel in order to facilitate the approval process of certain generic drug products. These individuals were convicted and the scandal prompted Congress to pass this law authorizing the FDA to ban individuals or firms from participating in the drug approval process if convicted of related felonies. The law also imposes severe civil penalties for any false statements, bribes, failures to disclose material facts, and other related offenses.

PRESCRIPTION DRUG USER FEE ACT OF 1992 (PDUFA)

Although the FDA was called on to review an ever-increasing number of drugs for approval, it found Congress unwilling to expand its budget. Instead, the administration and Congress took the approach that private industry should shoulder part of the costs for new drug approval rather than the taxpayers. Thus, Congress passed the Prescription Drug User Fee Act (PDUFA), which requires manufacturers seeking NDAs to pay fees for applications and supplements when the FDA must review clinical studies (P.L. 102-571). The fees provide the FDA with the resources to hire more reviewers to assess these clinical studies and hopefully speed up the NDA reviews. PDUFA must be reauthorized every 5 years.

NUTRITION LABELING AND EDUCATION ACT OF 1990 (NLEA)

Capitalizing on increased consumer interest in health and nutrition, the 1980s witnessed many food companies promoting their food products with nutritional claims. Congress enacted the Nutrition Labeling and Education Act (NLEA) (P.L. 101-535) to encourage this trend. The NLEA mandates nutrition labeling on food products and authorizes health claims on product labeling, as long as they are made in compliance with FDA regulations.

DIETARY SUPPLEMENT HEALTH AND EDUCATION ACT OF 1994 (DSHEA)

Dietary supplement manufacturers felt that the NLEA left too much authority with the FDA and unduly restricted the promotion of dietary supplements. As a result, Congress was persuaded to pass the Dietary Supplement Health and Education Act (DSHEA) (P.L. 103-417) to define dietary supplements and permit manufacturers to make certain claims that otherwise would have been illegal under the FDCA. The DSHEA in essence forced the FDA to regulate dietary supplements more as foods than as drugs.

FOOD AND DRUG ADMINISTRATION MODERNIZATION ACT OF 1997 (FDAMA)

FDA critics—which included drug manufacturers, Congress, and consumer groups— believed that the FDA was not efficiently administering its statutory responsibilities and that the FDCA itself produced too burdensome a regulatory system for drug approval. The Food and Drug Administration Modernization Act of 1997 (FDAMA) was passed primarily to streamline regulatory procedures to ensure the expedited availability of safe and effective drugs and devices.

Building on the Prescription Drug User Fee Act, FDAMA increases the FDA's public accountability, requires an FDA mission statement to define the scope of its responsibilities, and requires the agency to publish a compliance plan in consultation with industry representatives, scientific experts, health care professionals, and consumers. The intent is to eliminate backlogs in the approval process and ensure the timely review of applications. In particular, the FDAMA creates a fast-track approval process for drugs intended for serious or life-threatening diseases, establishes a databank of information on clinical trials, authorizes scientific panels to review clinical investigations, and expands the rights of manufacturers to disseminate unlabeled use information.

The FDAMA also expands the FDA's authority over over-the-counter (OTC) drugs and establishes ingredient-labeling requirements for inactive ingredients. States are preempted from establishing labeling requirements for OTC drugs and cosmetics when federal requirements exist. The law also affects the regulation of medical devices in part by mandating priority review for breakthrough technologies in medical devices and allowing the FDA to contract with outside scientific experts for review of medical device applications.

FOOD AND DRUG ADMINISTRATION AMENDMENTS ACT OF 2007 (FDAAA)

Congress passed the Food and Drug Administration Amendments Act in September of 2007 (P.L. No. 110-85) reauthorizing and amending many drug and medical device provisions that were set to expire, while providing the FDA with new funding and significantly more authority over drug safety. The FDAAA allows the FDA broader use of the fees generated from PDUFA, while substantially increasing the fees. In response to postmarket problems with certain drug products, such as Vioxx, which had to be removed from the market because of safety concerns, the law provides the FDA with significantly enhanced responsibilities and authority to regulate drug safety, including to: mandate labeling changes related to safety; require clinical trial data reporting and registries; require postmarket clinical studies to assess risks; and require companies to implement risk evaluation and mitigation strategies (REMS) when necessary. These features and others of the FDAAA will be described in greater detail later in this chapter.

PATIENT PROTECTION AND AFFORDABLE CARE ACT OF 2010 (PPACA/ACA)

The Patient Protection and Affordable Care Act (PPACA or ACA) (P.L. No. 111-148), enacted in March 2010, provided sweeping changes throughout the entire health care system. The U.S. Supreme Court has ruled that most of the provisions in the act are constitutional (*National Federation of Independent Business v. Sebelius*, 132 S.Ct. 2566 (June 28, 2012)). Although the ACA added health care law far beyond the FDCA, it bears mentioning in this historical section because it did add provisions to the FDCA and directly and indirectly affected other law related to pharmacy practice.

FDA SAFETY AND INNOVATION ACT OF 2012 (FDASIA)

The primary purpose of the FDA Safety and Innovation Act (P.L. No. 112-144) is to reauthorize PDUFA, which was to sunset in September 2012. The law allows the FDA to continue to collect user fees from manufacturers seeking NDAs or medical device approvals, but also adds new user fees for generic drugs and biosimilars. The law also contains several other provisions directed at reducing drug counterfeiting, blocking the import of adulterated products, detecting and reducing drug shortages, and enhancing the exchange of prescription drug diversion information across state lines. Additionally, the law enables the FDA to inspect foreign drug manufacturers more regularly and requires the agency to target problematic manufacturing sites, whether in the United States or not. Congress anticipates that the law will help bring critical drugs and medical devices to market faster and enhance the availability of generic drugs.

RATIONALE FOR FEDERAL DRUG REGULATION

The primary goal of the Pure Food and Drug Act of 1906 and the succeeding drug-related legislation was the protection of the public welfare. Few can deny that the public should be protected or that government should play a role in the protective effort. Nonetheless, there is a legitimate concern by some that government may go too far in protecting people from the consequences of their own risky choices.

The development of federal drug regulation shows a pattern of increasing government intrusion into the decisions of the people who use drugs. The 1906 law was an example of "indirect regulation." Its purpose was to help people make their own decisions by providing accurate and useful information through appropriate labeling. The 1938 act reinforced the indirect regulation by expanding the labeling requirements, but it also introduced an important piece of "direct regulation" by keeping off the market those drugs that have not met government safety standards. This type of regulation is direct because it makes decisions for people rather than helping them to make decisions for themselves. The 1951 and 1962 amendments increased direct regulation by mandating prescriptions for certain drugs and requiring proof of efficacy as well as safety for drug approval. At present, most of the drugs available cannot be used unless the government has certified them as safe and effective and another person (an authorized prescriber) has decided to permit their use.

Against this background of increasingly paternalistic drug laws, modern-day consumers have developed an independence regarding therapeutic choices and have matured in their ability to make sophisticated decisions for themselves. It is perhaps no coincidence that the Omnibus Budget Reconciliation Act of 1990 (OBRA '90) (P.L. 101-508), one of the later major federal drug laws, focuses on informed decisions by patients rather than on decisions by government or health care providers on behalf of patients. It also is perhaps no coincidence that the past 20 years or so have witnessed an unprecedented number of drugs switched from prescription status to OTC status. This may signal the beginning of a trend away from direct regulation and back toward indirect regulation, empowering patients to participate actively in health care decisions rather than passively accepting therapies decided on by others.

THE FOOD AND DRUG ADMINISTRATION (FDA)

Because primary enforcement of the FDCA is vested in the FDA, it is important to know a little about the agency. The FDA is a component of the Department of Health and Human Services (DHHS), and actual authority for administering the FDCA is really vested with the secretary of DHHS. In fact, until 1988 the secretary appointed the commissioner of the FDA. The act now directs the president to appoint the commissioner with the confirmation of the Senate; however, the commissioner still remains accountable to the secretary. In reality, the secretary has delegated most of the secretary's authority to the commissioner, who in turn has delegated the majority of authority to various FDA directors. The FDA's website can be accessed at http://www.fda.gov.

The agency is structured around the concept of the national headquarters providing policy and decision making, together with an extensive field force of professionals throughout the country to provide additional decision making and regulatory enforcement. At the headquarters level, five centers share the authority for scientific and regulatory evaluations and interpretations:

- Center for Biologics Evaluation and Research
- Center for Food Safety and Applied Nutrition
- Center for Drug Evaluation and Research
- Center for Veterinary Medicine
- Center for Devices and Radiological Health

Each center has a director and several managers. The field is divided into six geographic regions with 20 district offices. The district offices provide inspections and work cooperatively with state and local agencies and provide source information to headquarters.

Because the FDA is an administrative agency, it has rulemaking authority (Section 707 of the FDCA). In fact, the FDA prefers to regulate by regulation if at all possible. But, the agency also may pursue a less formal avenue by publishing guidance documents. The purpose of guidance documents is to clarify laws or regulations, to explain how compliance with the laws or regulations may be achieved, and to outline review and enforcement approaches. The FDA has issued several guidance documents, some of which will be referred to in this book. Guidance documents are not legally binding, nor legally enforceable. Nonetheless, these guides represent the agency's best thinking upon a particular subject and should be followed.

Although the FDA is staffed with considerable scientific expertise, it also regularly relies on advice from outside experts in the form of standing advisory committees. Most members of these committees are physicians, but they also include nurses, pharmacists, statisticians, epidemiologists, and other professionals. Members are recruited through the *Federal Register*, and often are nominated by professional organizations and professional schools. The secretary of DHHS makes the final selection of members from the list of nominees. Committee size ranges from 9 to 15 members. Although the FDA is not obligated to follow a committee recommendation, it often does.

DEFINING AND DISTINGUISHING DRUGS FROM FOODS, DIETARY SUPPLEMENTS, DEVICES, AND COSMETICS

THE LAW

Section 201 of the FDCA (21 U.S.C. § 321) provides definitions for the important terms used in the act. Understanding these definitions is critical to understanding the FDCA.

> (f) The term "food" means (1) articles used for food or drink for man or other animals, (2) chewing gum, and (3) articles used for components of any such article. (§ 201(f); 21 U.S.C. § 321(f))

> (g) (1) The term "drug" means (A) articles recognized in the official United States Pharmacopoeia, official Homeopathic Pharmacopoeia of the United States, or official National Formulary, or any supplement to any of them; and (B) articles intended for

use in the diagnosis, cure, mitigation, treatment, or prevention of disease in man or other animals; and (C) articles (other than food) intended to affect the structure or any function of the body of man or other animals; and (D) articles intended for use as a component of any articles specified in clause (A), (B), or (C).

(2) The term "counterfeit drug" means a drug which, or the container or labeling of which, without authorization, bears the trademark, trade name, or other identifying mark, imprint, or device, or any likeness thereof, of a drug manufacturer, processor, packer, or distributor other than the person or persons who in fact manufactured, processed, packed, or distributed such drug and which thereby falsely purports or is represented to be the product of, or to have been packed or distributed by, such other drug manufacturer, processor, packer, or distributor. (§ 201(g); 21 U.S.C. § 321(g))

(h) The term "device" . . . means an instrument, apparatus, implement, machine, contrivance, implant, in vitro reagent, or other similar or related article, including any component, part, or accessory, which is

> (1) recognized in the official National Formulary, or the United States Pharmacopoeia, or any supplement to them,

> (2) intended for use in the diagnosis of disease or other conditions, or in the cure, mitigation, treatment, or prevention of disease, in man or other animals, or

> (3) intended to affect the structure or any function of the body of man or other animals, and which does not achieve any of its principal intended purposes through chemical action within or on the body of man or other animals and which is not dependent upon being metabolized for the achievement of any of its principal intended purposes. (§ 201(h); 21 U.S.C. § 321(h))

(i) The term "cosmetic" means (1) articles intended to be rubbed, poured, sprinkled, or sprayed on, introduced into, or otherwise applied to the human body or any part thereof for cleansing, beautifying, promoting attractiveness, or altering the appearance, and (2) articles intended for use as a component of any such articles; except that such term shall not include soap. (§ 201(i); 21 U.S.C. § 321(i))

EXPLANATION OF THE LAW

Ask people about their perception of a drug and they will likely respond that it is a chemical entity for introduction into the body in one manner or another to improve one's health. The legal definition of drug (see preceding subsection g), however, in the FDCA leaves little doubt that Congress intended the term "drug" to have a much broader meaning than that, broader even than any scientific or medical definition. Note that subsection g uses the term "articles" to describe a drug. Articles can include chemical and nonchemical entities, and in fact most anything. Part B of the drug definition addresses products intended for use with diseases, whereas part C recognizes that even products not intended for use with diseases may still be drugs if they make a structure or function claim. For example, a product claimed by a manufacturer to prevent pregnancy may not be a drug under part B (because pregnancy is not a disease) but may be a drug under part C (because preventing pregnancy means that the product intends to affect the function of the body).

The FDA has used the drug definition to its advantage on several occasions by adjudicating an article to be a drug and then removing it from the market for failing to meet the premarket approval required of new drugs. Establishing that an article is a drug, as opposed to say a food, dietary supplement, or cosmetic, provides the agency with considerably more authority over the article.

The crucial issue in the determination of whether a product is a drug centers on whether the supplier made a therapeutic or health claim, or a structure/function claim. In other words, was the article intended to diagnose, cure, mitigate, treat, or prevent a disease, or (for articles other than food) was it intended to affect the body structure or function? The fact that a supplier, even in good faith, does not believe that its product is a drug or does not want its product to be a drug has little relevance. If therapeutic or structure/function claims are made, an article is a drug, no matter what disclaimers may be included in the labeling. Thus, a supplier cannot mitigate a therapeutic or structure/function claim for a product by proclaiming that the product is not a drug. For example, assume that a company that manufactures alfalfa pellets for animals decides to produce alfalfa tablets for humans, claiming that the tablets will cure ulcers and other gastrointestinal disorders. The label specifically notes that the tablets are not drugs. On the basis of the therapeutic claims, however, a court is likely to consider the product a drug, even though the manufacturer says it is not, and even though alfalfa by itself is certainly not a drug.

As a distinction, it is the supplier's intended use of the product that is important, not the purchaser's intended use. The mere use of an article for therapeutic purposes by purchasers, where the supplier does not intend the product to be used therapeutically or makes no therapeutic claims, does not usually make the product a drug. Health food stores and pharmacies have hundreds of examples of these types of products on their shelves. Similarly, although some hardware stores sell dimethyl sulfoxide (DMSO) as an industrial solvent and some purchasers apply it externally to reduce joint pain, this use does not make it a drug.

In contrast, some products that contain ingredients normally considered drugs might not be classified as drugs. For example, in the case of *Action on Smoking and Health v. Harris*, 655 F.2d 236 (D.C. Cir. 1980), a public interest group sought to have cigarettes declared drugs on the ground that they contain nicotine. The FDA, however, determined that the drug definition applies only to those brands of cigarettes about which a vendor makes therapeutic claims, and the court supported the FDA's position. Changing its position in the 1990s, the FDA asserted that nicotine is a drug and that cigarettes and smokeless tobacco are drug-delivery devices. The agency found that tobacco products are intended to satisfy addiction, stimulation and tranquilization, and weight control. As a result, the FDA, issued a regulation in 1996 intended to reduce tobacco consumption among children and adolescents (61 Fed. Reg. 44397). Tobacco manufacturers, retailers, and advertisers challenged the FDA, arguing that the agency lacks authority to regulate tobacco products. In a 5 to 4 decision, the U.S. Supreme Court agreed with the plaintiffs, finding that Congress intended to exclude tobacco from the FDA's jurisdiction (*Food and Drug Admin. v. Brown & Williamson Tobacco Corp.*, 529 U.S. 120 (2000)). The Supreme Court decision played a role in stimulating Congress to enact legislation in June 2009, known as the Family Smoking Prevention and Tobacco Act (P.L. No. 111-31), granting the FDA authority to regulate tobacco products. The FDA may now regulate the contents of tobacco products, require disclosure of product contents, prohibit certain additives, require more effective warnings, and strictly control or prohibit marketing and sales campaigns, especially those directed at children. Between 2008 and 2010, the FDA determined that electronic cigarettes were unapproved drug/device combination products. Manufacturers of these products challenged the FDA's assertion. The U.S. Court of Appeals for the D.C. Circuit found for the manufacturers on the basis that the agency can regulate the products under the 2009 Tobacco Act and that they are not drugs or devices unless marketed for therapeutic purposes (*Sottera, Inc. v. Food & Drug Administration*, 627 F.3d 891 (D.C. Cir. 2010)).

Although courts interpret the definition of the term "drug" broadly and often defer to the expertise of the FDA, the agency does not always prevail, even in nontobacco cases. In *National Nutritional Foods Association v. Mathews*, 557 F.2d 325 (2nd Cir. 1977), the FDA was unsuccessful in its attempt to classify vitamins A and D in high dosages as drugs on the basis of a lack of nutritional value and potential toxicity. The court held that nutritional value and toxicity were not relevant to the statutory definition of a drug.

A court will admit evidence of therapeutic intent from sources other than the labeling of the product. Thus, therapeutic claims that the manufacturer made while advertising on radio or television, or in newspapers or brochures, will be considered evidence that a product is a drug. Moreover, the fact that a product is being marketed as an injection, capsule, or tablet may add evidence of therapeutic intent, despite the absence of therapeutic language in the labeling.

FOODS VERSUS DRUGS

The distinction between food and drug has become an important issue, especially in view of the proliferation and popularity of natural products, dietary supplements, and other "health food" type products. As you likely surmised from the previous discussion, almost any food might be considered a drug if a therapeutic or health claim is made for it under part B of the drug definition. Part C of the drug definition, however, specifically excludes foods. This then raises the question: How is food defined for the purpose of part C? Stated another way, is it the intent of part C to exclude all substances normally defined as foods, regardless of their intended use? Reading the definition of food under subsection f is hardly helpful.

This issue was partially answered in the case of *Nutrilab, Inc., et al. v. Schweiker*, 713 F.2d 335 (7th Cir. 1983) (discussed in the case studies section of this chapter), in which the court considered whether a weight-reduction product known as a starch blocker is a food or drug. The plaintiffs argued the product was a food because it was derived from kidney beans. The court disagreed, finding for the FDA on the basis that the product neither fit the statutory definition of food nor the commonsense definition of food, in that people use food primarily for taste, aroma, or nutritive value. Most likely Congress intended to exclude foods when consumed in their ordinary manner from part C because all foods when ingested affect the structure or function of the body in some manner merely because of metabolism. Thus, unless excluded, all foods would become drugs by virtue of part C. Congress did not likely intend to exclude foods that are not intended or consumed for their ordinary purpose.

The FDCA has created at least two special categories of foods, including "special dietary foods" and "medical foods." Without this legal recognition, the FDA would likely regard articles falling into these categories as drugs.

Special Dietary Foods

Under the FDCA, special dietary foods include, but are not limited to those supplying a special dietary need that exists by reason of a physical, physiological, pathological, or other condition, including but not limited to the condition of disease, convalescence, pregnancy, lactation, infancy, allergic hypersensitivity to food, underweight, overweight, or the need to control the intake of sodium (21 U.S.C. § 411(3)(A)). Examples of products in this category include infant formulas, artificial sweeteners, and caloric supplements.

Medical Foods

Medical foods include foods formulated for oral use under the supervision of a physician and that are intended for the specific dietary management of a disease or condition for which distinctive nutritional requirements are established by medical evaluation

(21 U.S.C.A § 360ee). Examples of medical foods include foods formulated without the amino acid phenylalanine for phenylketonuria, and folic acid, B_6, B_{12} combination products for hyperhomocysteinemia.

Nutraceuticals and Functional Foods

Some believe that the FDA should recognize additional classifications of food products called "nutraceuticals" and "functional foods." The vague and broad category of nutraceuticals would include foods that provide health or medical benefits, including the prevention and treatment of disease. Advocates of this product classification contend that the current system deters the development of a substantial number of beneficial food-related products because the FDA could regard the products as drugs.

Another category of product some would like distinguished by law is one called "functional foods." These include foods or nutraceuticals that have been fortified or enhanced, often with a dietary supplement, such as drinks with ginseng or kava kava added and foods fortified with calcium. Probiotics are yet another example of products that would likely fall into this category. Probiotics are defined as live microorganisms that when administered in adequate amounts produce healthy results. Currently, the law does not recognize any category of articles as nutraceuticals or functional foods, and Congress has apparently not felt the need to do so. (Some nutraceuticals or functional foods can be defined as dietary supplements, as discussed later.)

Health Claims for Foods

Occasionally food manufacturers make health claims for their products, causing considerable controversy with the FDA. One such controversy arose in the 1980s when studies at the time indicated that the ingestion of psyllium might lower cholesterol levels. Cereal manufacturers whose products contained fibrous psyllium thus proclaimed the value of their products in reducing cholesterol levels. The FDA believed that these claims made the products drugs and warned the cereal manufacturers. OTC drug manufacturers who produced psyllium laxatives also were concerned but for a different reason; their products were regulated as drugs and because of this, they could not promote their products as effective for lowering cholesterol without being charged for misbranding. Thus, they felt the cereal manufacturers had an unfair advantage if the FDA allowed them to label their products with the health claim.

The FDA continued to struggle with this issue for years, as evidenced by the case of *United States v. Undetermined Quantities of an Article of Drug Labeled as Exachol*, 716 F. Supp. 787 (S.D.N.Y. 1989). In this case, the manufacturer of a product called Exachol distributed literature proclaiming that the product was useful in the prevention and treatment of coronary disease. As a result, the FDA brought legal action against the company, contending that the product, composed of lecithin, phosphatidyl ethanolamine, phosphatidylcholine, and several other natural products, was a drug on the basis of the therapeutic claims. The manufacturer then argued that the product was a special dietary food, not a drug. The court found that the FDA permitted some foods to be labeled with appropriate health-related messages. The court noted that the FDA was still trying to determine what types of health-related messages would be appropriate and, while doing so, had allowed manufacturers of other products (e.g., Kellogg's All-Bran, fish oils) to continue making health claims. Thus, concluded the court, it would be inconsistent for the agency to single out Exachol as a drug while failing to take action against other such products.

This confusion over what health claims would be appropriate for food products and whether they could escape being branded as drugs by sliding into the special dietary food category prompted Congress to enact the Nutrition Labeling and Education Act of 1990 (NLEA) (P.L. 101–535) that amends section 403 of the FDCA. In part, the amendment for the first time allowed food labeling to contain a health or disease-prevention claim, but only if the FDA had promulgated a regulation approving the claim and establishing the conditions under which the claim can be used. The FDAMA has since modified the NLEA to permit health claims without the requirement that the FDA must issue a regulation, as long as there is "significant scientific agreement," as determined by the FDA. Pursuant to this law, the FDA issued regulations for food products in 1993 (58 Fed. Reg. 2478, January 6, 1993; 21 C.F.R. part 101) and for dietary supplements in 1994 (59 Fed. Reg. 395, January 4, 1994; 21 C.F.R. parts 20 and 101). Under the regulations, the FDA will authorize a health claim for a food or dietary supplement only if the supplier submits a petition containing considerable information and evidence supporting the claim.

Even when FDA regulation authorizes a health claim, food manufacturers may still wander over the food/drug line if they exceed the strict limits and restrictions of that regulation. For example, the FDA issued a regulation (21 C.F.R. 101.81) authorizing a health claim associating soluble fiber from whole grain oats with a reduced risk of coronary heart disease. Pursuant to the regulation the manufacturer may also include a statement that the reduced risk of coronary heart disease occurs by lowering blood total and LDL cholesterol. General Mills labeled its Cheerios Toasted Whole Grain Oat Cereal with the claims: "you can Lower Your Cholesterol 4% in 6 weeks" and "Did you know that in just 6 weeks Cheerios can reduce bad cholesterol by an average of 4%?"

The FDA issued a warning letter to General Mills in May 2009, contending that these claims indicate that Cheerios is intended for use in lowering cholesterol, and therefore preventing and treating the disease of hypercholesterolemia, thus making Cheerios an unapproved new drug (http://www.fda.gov/ICECI/EnforcementActions/WarningLetters/ucm162943.htm). The FDA has taken the position that the claims are separate, stand-alone claims from the permissible health claim that General Mills also did include on the box; and, even if the claims were part of the permissible claim, they would not qualify because the regulation does not allow attributing any degree of risk reduction for coronary heart disease.

DIETARY SUPPLEMENTS VERSUS DRUGS

The NLEA was not popular among suppliers and consumers of dietary supplements, who feared that the law unduly empowered the FDA to restrict the dietary supplement industry. It is important to recognize that at that time, even though dietary supplements were commonly known by the public by that term and commonly marketed, the law did not recognize dietary supplements as a separate legal class of products. After intense lobbying, Congress reacted by passing the Dietary Supplement Health and Education Act of 1994 (DSHEA) (P.L. 103–417), further amending the FDCA by legally creating the category of dietary supplements and significantly altering the FDA's authority to regulate dietary supplements. The NLEA and its regulations remain in effect to the extent that they are not specifically contradicted by DSHEA.

Essentially, DSHEA mandates that the FDA regulate dietary supplements more as a special type of food than as drugs. The FDA cannot require premarket approval of dietary supplements as they do for drugs. Thus, the manufacturer is responsible for determining if its product is safe and that its claims about the product are substantiated by adequate evidence. Moreover, except for new dietary supplements, the manufacturer does not have to provide the FDA with the evidence upon which it relies to substantiate the product's safety and efficacy. DSHEA generally prohibits the FDA from regulating dietary supplements as food additives as well. Since food additives require premarket approval by the FDA, Congress wanted to ensure that the FDA did not attempt a back-door approach at requiring premarket approval. Stripped of premarket approval authority means that the agency must prove that a dietary supplement is unsafe before it can remove the product from the market. Under DSHEA, a dietary supplement is defined as a product that is intended for ingestion, is intended to supplement the diet, and contains any one or more of the following:

- A vitamin
- A mineral
- An herb or other botanical
- An amino acid
- A dietary substance for use by humans to supplement the diet by increasing the total dietary intake
- A concentrate, metabolite, constituent, extract, or combination of the previous (§ 201(ff); 21 U.S.C. § 321(ff))

Nutritional Support (Structure/Function) Statements

DSHEA allows dietary supplement suppliers to make four types of nutritional support statements without fear that the statements would cause the FDA to consider the product to be a drug. These are:

1. Statements that the product will benefit a classical nutrient deficiency disease as long as it also discloses the prevalence of the disease in the United States
2. Statements that describe the role of the dietary supplement in affecting the structure or function of the body
3. Statements that characterize the documented mechanism by which a nutrient or dietary supplement acts to maintain structure or function
4. Statements describing the general well-being from consumption of a nutrient or dietary ingredient (e.g., "energizer," "relaxant," "muscle enhancement")

DSHEA thus exempts dietary supplements from part C of the drug definition by permitting structure/function claims. For example, a seller could promote that its cranberry tablets increase the acidity of the urine and help to maintain a healthy urinary tract. If, however, the seller made the claim that its product prevents urinary tract infections, this assertion could make the product a drug under part B of the drug definition. Similarly, a seller could not claim a product helps avoid diarrhea associated with antibiotic use but could state that it "helps maintain healthy intestinal flora." In an attempt to clarify the dividing line between acceptable structure/function claims and disease claims, the FDA enacted a regulation on January 6, 2000 (65 Fed. Reg. 1000; 21 C.F.R. part 101).

To make any of these four nutritional support statements, the seller must have substantiation that they are truthful and not misleading, and the label of the product must contain the disclaimer, "This statement has not been evaluated by the Food and Drug Administration. This product is not intended to diagnose, treat, cure, or prevent any disease." Also, the manufacturer must notify the FDA within 30 days if it makes one of the permitted statements.

Health or Disease Claims

Despite the fact that DSHEA greatly restricts the FDA's premarket authority over dietary supplements and exempts dietary supplements from part C of the drug definition, as discussed the law does not allow manufacturers to make unapproved health (disease) claims that fall under part B of the drug definition. DSHEA does allow manufacturers to make limited health claims for dietary substances that describe the relationship between a food substance and a disease, such as "folic acid may reduce the risk of neural tube birth defects" and "calcium may reduce the risk of osteoporosis." In order to make these claims, however, the manufacturer must receive FDA approval for the health claim as judged by the "significant scientific agreement" standard. By 1999 the FDA had approved only about 11 health claims for foods and dietary supplements, including the claims for folic acid and calcium.

Because the FDA had approved so few health claims, frustrated dietary supplement manufacturers challenged the legality of the FDA's premarket approval requirement for health claims and the legality of the FDA's procedure for determining "significant scientific agreement" in a 1999 U.S. Court of Appeals decision, *Pearson v. Shalala*, 164 F.3d 650 (1999). In *Pearson*, four dietary supplement manufacturers, who had their health claims rejected by the FDA, successfully argued that requiring premarket approval of health claims violates the First Amendment, and that the FDA lacks sufficient criteria for explaining why a health claim does not meet the "significant scientific agreement" standard. The court agreed with the plaintiffs and felt that complete suppression of health claims, unless they are false or misleading, is too restrictive, when disclaimers (e.g., "the evidence is inconclusive that antioxidant vitamins will reduce the risk of certain kinds of cancer") on the label would accomplish the FDA's objective. The court of appeals ordered the case remanded back to the district court, whose decision it reversed, with instructions that the FDA articulate clear standards as to what constitutes "significant scientific agreement." The FDA declined to appeal *Pearson* to the Supreme Court.

The *Pearson* decision ultimately produced a profound change in how the FDA evaluated health claims. The agency now essentially allows two types of health claims, unqualified and qualified. Unqualified health claims are allowed if authorized by the agency pursuant to the significant scientific agreement test. Qualified health claims (pursuant to *Pearson*) may be made when the claim does not meet the significant scientific agreement test and the claim would be misleading without the qualification. Qualified claims will be allowed when there is more evidence for the claim than against it. (See 65 Fed. Reg. 59,855 (Oct. 6, 2000).) The qualified claim must be truthful and not misleading and appropriately indicate the level of scientific support; for example, "Scientific evidence suggests but does not prove" or "Some evidence shows the nutrient may be beneficial, but there is insufficient scientific evidence to prove the effect." The agency continues to aggressively police manufacturers who make unapproved health claims that it regards as false or misleading.

Dietary Supplements Containing Drugs

On occasion a dietary supplement may contain a drug, raising the issue of whether the product is actually a drug and not a dietary supplement. The FDCA excludes from the definition of dietary supplement any article that was approved as a new drug, unless prior to the approval it was marketed as a dietary supplement or food (21 U.S.C. §321(ff)(3)(B)). In the case of *Pharmanex, Inc. v. Shalala*, 35 F. Supp. 1341 (2001 WL 741419 (D.Utah)), Pharmanex challenged the FDA's decision that its product, Cholestin, which contained red yeast rice, was a drug and not a dietary supplement. Traditional red yeast rice has been eaten by the Chinese for centuries and is regarded by the Chinese as a health food. On this basis, the manufacturer argued Cholestin is a dietary supplement. The court, however, agreed with the FDA's determination. The FDA established that Cholestin contained significant amounts of lovastatin, a cholesterol-lowering drug approved by the FDA in 1987. The FDA further proved that Pharmanex carefully manufactured the production of Cholestin to contain high levels of lovastatin not found in traditional red yeast rice. In effect, the agency proved the company was marketing lovastatin, not traditional red yeast rice. Pharmanex retorted that, nonetheless, lovastatin was present in some foods marketed in the United States long before it was approved by the FDA, and therefore it must be considered a dietary supplement. The court, however, agreed with the FDA's interpretation that traditional red yeast rice does not contain lovastatin, and that lovastatin itself was not marketed as a dietary supplement, food, or food component prior to 1987.

Safety Issues and Ephedra Products

Because dietary supplements are regulated much as foods rather than drugs, the FDA can only remove a dietary supplement from the market on the basis of public safety if the agency can prove the product is adulterated (21 U.S.C. § 331(a), (b), (c), (k)). DSHEA provides that a dietary supplement is adulterated if it presents a "significant or unreasonable risk of illness or injury under the conditions of use recommended or suggested in the labeling; and, if no conditions of use are recommended or suggested, then under ordinary conditions of use" (21 U.S.C. §342(f)(1)).

Pursuant to its application and interpretation of the law, the FDA issued a final regulation in 2004 banning all ephedrine alkaloid dietary supplement (EDS) products (69 Fed. Reg. 6788 (Feb. 11, 2004)). (*Note:* Ephedrine alkaloids [ephedra] is an extract of the ma huang plant and has been used as a natural medicinal agent in China for centuries. It should be distinguished from OTC drug products with structurally related active ingredients.) This final regulation was the culmination of a long investigative process beginning in the early 1990s when the FDA began receiving adverse event reports suggesting injury and illness associated with the use of EDS products. The administrative record reflecting the regulatory process contains over 133,000 pages of scientific data, expert reviews, comments, and other materials. In addition, the FDA commissioned expert reviews of the scientific evidence and assessed the findings of these expert reviews. After all this review, the FDA concluded that, although EDS is promoted to achieve weight loss, enhance athletic performance, and increase energy, its effects are temporary, modest, and generally do not improve health. In contrast, the agency found that EDS increases the risk of serious adverse events including heart attacks, strokes, and death.

The passage of the regulation was hastened after highly publicized accounts that EDS use led to the death of some high profile athletes, such as Korey Stringer of the Minnesota Vikings and Steve Bechler of the Baltimore Orioles. Accounts such as these prompted Congress to issue a resolution that the FDA should immediately remove EDS from the market. Shortly after the enactment of the regulation, however, an EDS manufacturer sued the FDA in federal court in Utah, contending that the regulation was invalid (*Nutraceutical Corp. v. Crawford*, 364 F.Supp.2d 1310 (April 12, 2005)). The court ruled for the plaintiff and invalidated the regulation on the basis that the FDA improperly applied a risk-benefit analysis and failed to provide sufficient evidence that EDS poses a significant risk in the dose recommended by the plaintiff. The FDA appealed, resulting in the court of appeals finding for the FDA, reversing the district court's decision and reinstating the regulation banning EDS products (*Nutraceutical Corp. v. Von Eschenbach*, 459 F.3d 1033 (10th Cir. 2006)). In a lawsuit against the FDA by another EDS manufacturer (*NVE, Inc. v. Department of Health and Human Services*, 463 F.3d 182 (3rd Cir. 2006)), the court also sided with the FDA, ruling that plaintiffs could not present additional evidence about EDS, but rather are limited to review of the FDA's administrative record.

The Dietary Supplement and Nonprescription Drug Consumer Protection Act

The EDS situation prompted Congress to enact serious adverse event reporting requirements for dietary supplement manufacturers in December of 2006 in a law entitled the Dietary Supplement and Nonprescription Drug Consumer Protection Act (P.L. 109–462). This law adds two parallel mandatory serious adverse events reporting systems: one for nonprescription drugs and the other for dietary supplements. Manufacturers, packers, or distributors whose name appears on the label must submit to the Secretary of Health and Human Services (through the MedWatch program described later) any report of a serious adverse event within 15 business days. They also must submit any subsequent medical information received within 1 year of the initial reported event. Product labeling must include either the supplier's domestic address or a continuously operating toll-free telephone number so consumers can report serious adverse events. Suppliers also must maintain records related to each report for 6 years and allow inspection of the records. The FDA published a draft guidance in October 2007 to assist the dietary supplement industry in complying with the law (72 Fed. Reg. 58313–01).

Criticisms of DSHEA

DSHEA has proved thus far to be an extremely controversial law. Critics have three major concerns about DSHEA. First, they fear that the law allows the marketing of unsafe dietary supplements and contend that it prevents the FDA from acting aggressively enough to protect the public. Second, critics are concerned over a lack of consumer information about the dangers of taking many dietary supplements with certain OTC and prescription medications. Most dietary supplement labeling does not warn users of these potential adverse effects. Third, critics argue that dietary supplements lack quality standards for strength and purity because manufacturers are not required to register themselves or their products with the FDA prior to marketing them, and no manufacturing standards exist for dietary supplements. Quality assays of some dietary supplements have shown that strengths vary from those on the label and even vary from pill to pill in the same bottle. Some products were found not to contain the active ingredient, and some contained ingredients other than those stated on the label.

In response to these concerns over quality standards, the FDA issued a final rule in June 2007 (72 Fed. Reg. 34752 (June 25, 2007)) requiring that dietary supplement manufacturers comply with current good manufacturing practices (CGMP) in such a manner that the products will not be adulterated or misbranded. The regulations also require manufacturers to evaluate the identity, purity, quality, strength, and composition of their products. Dietary supplements containing contaminants or lacking the ingredient they represent would be adulterated or misbranded.

Implications of DSHEA for Pharmacists

In light of the decreased government regulation over dietary supplements since DSHEA, pharmacists have an important role in providing accurate product information to patients and assisting them with product selection. If possible, pharmacists should steer patients to products conforming to United States Pharmacopeia (USP) or National Formulary (NF) standards, or at least products in which manufacturers can attest to quality and uniformity standards.

Pharmacists should not promote dietary supplements on the basis of unapproved health or disease claims because this could violate the FDCA. However, pharmacists should not hesitate to counsel, educate, and provide advice to patients about the use of a supplement product for a disease, especially when asked by the patient. DSHEA permits pharmacists to display certain publications, such as articles, book chapters, books, and abstracts of peer-reviewed scientific publications, used in conjunction with the sale of dietary supplements. To conform to the law, however, these publications must be reprinted in their entirety; must not be false or misleading; must be presented with other publications, if available, about the product so as to present a balanced view; must be physically separate from the actual product; and must not have appended to them any information by sticker or other method.

DRUGS VERSUS DEVICES

Before the passage of the Medical Device Amendment (MDA) of 1976, the FDA lacked the authority to approve devices for safety and efficacy prior to their commercial distribution. This inadequacy forced the FDA to declare that certain devices were drugs, which often resulted in litigation. For example, in *United States v. Article of Drug Bacto Unidisk*, 394 U.S. 784 (1969), the FDA successfully established that antibiotic sensitivity disks fall under the drug definition. In another case, *United States v. Article of Drug Ova II*, 414 F. Supp. 660 (D.N.J. 1975), the FDA failed to prove that a home pregnancy testing kit is a drug. The court determined that because pregnancy is not a disease, the kit is not a diagnostic test for a disease. The MDA differentiates devices from drugs by stating that a device does not achieve any of its principal intended purposes through chemical action and is not dependent on being metabolized for the achievement of any of its principal intended purposes. The term "device" does include in vitro diagnostic products used to aid in the diagnosis of disease or verification of pregnancy.

When a device is used in conjunction with a drug, the legal distinction becomes less clear. The FDA has stated that many factors may determine whether a product is a device or a drug:

- Is the product intended to deliver drugs to the patient, but is not prefilled by the manufacturer (e.g., an empty implantable infusion pump)?
- Is the drug component included solely to make the product safer (e.g., a surgical drape impregnated with antimicrobial agents)?
- Is the drug component intended to have a therapeutic effect (e.g., an intrauterine contraceptive device that releases a hormone)?

The manufacturer of a drug delivery device must establish that the device and the drug will not have deleterious effects on one another. Although problems of classification still occur, the 1976 device amendment has greatly clarified the distinction between drugs and devices, and has given the FDA significantly more enforcement authority over devices. The MDA's comprehensive device classification system is discussed later in this chapter.

DRUGS VERSUS COSMETICS

A cosmetic may become a drug if its manufacturer promotes it for a therapeutic purpose, despite the product chemistry. In *United States v. An Article . . . Consisting of 216 Cartoned Bottles, More or Less*, "Sudden Change," 409 F.2d 734 (2nd Cir. 1969), the manufacturer distributed a lotion composed of bovine albumin and distilled water. When applied to the skin and allowed to dry, the lotion left a film that tightened the skin, thus temporarily masking imperfections and making the skin look smoother. The manufacturer's advertisements claimed that the lotion would "lift out puffs" or give a "facelift without surgery." The court refused to apply to these claims the standard of what a reasonable consumer would believe, but rather applied the standard of what an "ignorant, unthinking, and credulous" consumer would believe. On the basis of this standard and the manufacturer's claims, the court found that the lotion was a drug but would cease to be a drug once the claims were discontinued.

On the other hand, in *United States v. An Article of Drugs . . . 47 Shipping Cartons, More or Less . . .* "Helene Curtis Magic Secret," 331 F. Supp. 912 (D. Md. 1971), the court concluded that such claims as being a "pure protein" and causing an "astringent sensation" would not persuade even ignorant, unthinking, and credulous consumers that the product would alter their appearance. Therefore, this product was not held to be a drug.

Labels and Labeling

The FDCA differentiates the definition of label from that of labeling:

> (k) The term "label" means a display of written, printed, or graphic matter upon the immediate container of any article; and a requirement made by or under authority of this Act that any word, statement, or other information appearing on the label shall not be considered to be complied with unless such word, statement, or other information also appears on the outside container or wrapper, if any there be, of the retail package of such article, or is easily legible through the outside container or wrapper. (§ 201(k); 21 U.S.C. § 321(k))

> (m) The term "labeling" means all labels and other written, printed, or graphic matter (1) upon any article or any of its containers or wrappers, or (2) accompanying such article. (§ 201(m); 21 U.S.C. § 321(m))

The term "label," as the definition indicates, refers to information required on the container or wrapper. The term labeling has a far broader application. Although the term labeling includes the label, it also applies to the information "accompanying" the drug, such as the package insert. The legal interpretation of the word accompanying can be important in establishing whether misbranding has occurred. If the literature is deemed to accompany the product, it is labeling. If it is deemed not to accompany the product, it is advertising. The line between labeling and advertising is not always a clear one, leading to controversies.

In *United States v. Guardian Chemical Corporation*, 410 F.2d 157 (2nd Cir. 1969), the manufacturer discovered that its product, sold for the purpose of cleansing dairy apparatus, also was effective in treating kidney and bladder stones. Ultimately, the company prepared and distributed brochures to the medical profession to promote the product, now named Renacidin, for these purposes. The FDA contended that Renacidin was a drug and that the bottles and the brochures were misbranded because they did not contain the label and labeling information required by law. The court agreed with the FDA, holding that printed pamphlets or brochures need not be shipped with the article to constitute labeling. They may be sent either before or after the article and still "accompany" it as long as the distribution of the drug and the brochures are part of an "integrated distribution program" to sell the product.

In general, courts have held that information is labeling if the written materials are part of an integrated distribution program, have a common origin and destination, and explain the drug. The distinction between labeling and advertising for prescription drugs may not be that important today because each is subject to regulation by the FDA and must contain all the information approved by the FDA, as discussed later in this chapter.

OFFICIAL COMPENDIA

Part A of the drug definition recognizes particular compendia as legal sources of drug standards. One of these compendia, the *USP*, is published by the United States Pharmacopeial Convention (USPC), an independent, private organization jointly founded in 1820 by physicians and pharmacists of the time, who were concerned that various medicinal ingredients and preparations under the same names differed considerably in potency, quality, and composition. To set uniform standards for these products, the USPC elected scientific experts to publish the *USP*. It has continued to establish standards ever since.

Although the USPC is a private organization, independent of the FDA, the FDA actively participates in the development and modification of the standards contained in the *USP*'s monographs, which establish the approved titles, definitions, descriptions, and standards for identity, quality, strength, purity, packaging, stability, and labeling for a drug. The USPC publishes the monographs of many of the drugs marketed in the United States. Before 1980, the *USP* contained monographs of active ingredients, and the NF contained monographs of inactive ingredients. In 1980, the two books were combined into one compendium, commonly referred to as the *USP/NF*, which now serves as the official compendium for drug standards in the United States.

The other official compendium stated under the FDCA is the *Homeopathic Pharmacopoeia of the United States (HPUS)*, which has been in continuous publication since 1897. The *HPUS* defines homeopathy as the "art and science of healing the sick by using substances capable of causing the same symptoms, syndromes, and conditions when administered to healthy people" (http://www.homeopathicdoctor.com). The standards for the homeopathy products contained in the *HPUS* are established by the Homeopathic Pharmacopoeia Convention of the United States (HPCUS). This is a private, nonprofit organization of scientific experts in homeopathy. Because of the recent resurgence of homeopathy and a resultant need for continuous updates, HPCUS has republished the *HPUS* since 1988 as the *HPUS Revision Service*, a loose-leaf binder publication that allows for continual revisions without the need to reprint an entirely new volume.

Under the FDCA, a drug recognized in the *USP/NF* or *HPUS* must meet all compendium standards or it will be considered misbranded or adulterated. Similarly, a drug is considered misbranded or adulterated if it is not recognized in the *USP/NF* or *HPUS*, yet purports to be so recognized.

© Stockbyte/Thinkstock

STUDY SCENARIOS AND QUESTIONS

1. A company manufactures and markets capsules filled with pulverized sheep bone. It promotes the product as a treatment for anemia and various blood disorders. Explain whether this product is a drug or a dietary supplement.
2. Assume for question 1 that the company promoted the product with the claim that it "restores healthy blood" instead. Explain whether this would change your answer to question 1.

Questions 3 through 7 relate to the following hypothetical situation:

Sue is a pharmacist who loves to travel internationally, studying the use of natural products in other societies and cultures. On one of her trips to a rain forest in Africa she noticed that a few natives of one of the tribes chewed a certain wild root known as acumana to help them sleep. She chewed the root and indeed felt it helped her sleep. While investigating this root she was surprised to find that although the root was not uncommon, its medicinal effects, if any, were scarcely mentioned in any literature. Sue brought the root back to the United States and found it grew readily under greenhouse conditions. Sue formed a company that produced and bottled tablets made from the dehydrated and pulverized root. She heavily marketed the product, which she labeled with the name Acuxen, across the country as an "aid in relaxation and sleep." The FDA is investigating Sue's company to determine if she is marketing a drug or dietary supplement.

3. Based on the facts in this case, is Acuxen most likely a food, drug, or dietary supplement, and why? (To answer this question you must consider both the composition of Acuxen and the indication.)
4. If Sue made the root product as a topical patch, why might your answer be different than the previous one?
5. Assuming the product in question 3 is a dietary supplement based on composition and it is a structure/function claim, on what legal basis could the FDA still challenge the product?
6. Explain why your answer in question 3 might change if Sue labeled Acuxen for use in insomnia? Assuming this is a health or disease claim, would it matter whether the claim was made on the label or in pamphlets attached to the product?
7. Assume that, before purchasing Acuxen, a patient in a pharmacy asked the pharmacist about the product and that the pharmacist remarked that in his opinion the product seemed to be effective for insomnia and also in preventing some types of dementia. Has the pharmacist violated the FDCA?
8. The *Exachol* decision was issued prior to DSHEA. How might the decision be different today?
9. Differentiate between the disclaimer required for a structure/function claim on a dietary supplement product label and a health claim pursuant to the *Pearson* decision.

PROHIBITED ACTS, PENALTIES, AND ENFORCEMENT

PROHIBITED ACTS: THE LAW

Section 301 of the FDCA in part prohibits the following acts:

(a) The introduction or delivery for introduction into interstate commerce of any food, drug, device, or cosmetic that is adulterated or misbranded.

(b) The adulteration or misbranding of any food, drug, device, or cosmetic in interstate commerce.

(c) The receipt in interstate commerce of any food, drug, device, or cosmetic that is adulterated or misbranded, and the delivery or proffered delivery thereof for pay or otherwise.

(d) The introduction or delivery for introduction into interstate commerce of any article in violation of section 404 or 505.

(e) The refusal to permit access to or copying of any record as required . . . or the failure to establish or maintain any record, or make any report, required . . . or the refusal to permit access to or verification or copying of any such required record.

(f) The refusal to permit entry or inspection as authorized by section 704.

(g) The manufacture within any Territory of any food, drug, device, or cosmetic that is adulterated or misbranded.

(i) (3) The doing of any act which causes a drug to be a counterfeit drug, or the sale or dispensing, or the holding for sale or dispensing, of a counterfeit drug.

(k) The alteration, mutilation, destruction, obliteration, or removal of the whole or any part of the labeling of, or the doing of any other act with respect to, a food, drug, device, or cosmetic, if such act is done while such article is held for sale (whether or not the first sale) after shipment in interstate commerce and results in such article being adulterated or misbranded.

(v) The introduction or delivery for introduction into interstate commerce of a dietary supplement that is unsafe under section 413 of this title. (§ 301; 21 U.S.C. § 331)

Section 303(a)(1) then provides that any violator of section 301 shall be imprisoned for not more than 1 year, fined not more than $1,000, or both. Under section 301(a)(2), if the violator commits a second offense of the act or commits a violation with the intent to defraud or mislead, the violator could be imprisoned for up to 3 years and/or fined up to $10,000. (See *United States v. Hiland* in the case studies at the end of this chapter.) Section 303 also singles out several violations that warrant much more severe penalties, such as violations of the Prescription Drug Marketing Act.

EXPLANATION OF THE LAW

The FDCA establishes two major offenses—adulteration and misbranding—which are explained later in this chapter. Nearly every violation of the FDCA constitutes one or both of these offenses. The violations are of a strict liability nature. In other words, the commission of any of the listed offenses violates the FDCA, regardless of the person's intentions or knowledge. Under section 301(c), for example, a pharmacist who unknowingly and innocently receives an adulterated or misbranded drug and subsequently sells it to a consumer has violated the act. Section 303(c) of the act, however, provides that a pharmacist who sells the drug in good faith will not be subject to any penalties if on request the pharmacist furnishes the FDA with information about the source of supply.

Although section 301 is mostly self-explanatory, certain sections warrant more attention by pharmacists. Section 301(i)(3) makes it illegal for a pharmacist to make, dispense, or hold for dispensing a counterfeit drug. The definition of counterfeit drug in section 201(g) suggests that a pharmacist may violate section 301(i)(3) if the pharmacist dispenses a placebo or dispenses a particular drug and labels it as another drug.

Pharmacists who repackage or relabel drugs, either prescription or OTC drugs, must pay particular attention to section 301(k). If the new label does not conform to FDA specifications in all particulars, the pharmacist may be charged with misbranding. Pharmacists should ensure that the label of the repackaged drug contains the identical information that the manufacturer's label contains.

ENFORCEMENT

The FDA has the authority to enforce the FDCA in several ways. Under section 302, the FDA can bring an injunctive action against the violator to cause it to cease its illegal activity. Under section 303, the FDA can institute criminal proceedings against violators, resulting in fines, imprisonment, or both. Section 304 allows the FDA to seize any adulterated or misbranded food, drug, or cosmetic in interstate commerce. Because of the strict liability nature of section 302 and the realization that minor violations of the act should not be subject to criminal prosecution or seizure actions, Congress added section 309, which allows the FDA to send a warning letter to the violator as a first step when such an action would adequately serve the public interest.

CORPORATE OFFICER LIABILITY

The U.S. Supreme Court has held that corporate officers can be convicted when other corporate employees violate the FDCA. In *United States v. Dotterweich*, 320 U.S. 277 (1943), the president of a repackaging and relabeling company was convicted of adulteration and misbranding even though there was no evidence that he knew of the wrongful acts. The Court's rationale was that it is better to place the burden on those in a position to discover the violations than on an innocent and helpless public.

In *United States v. Park*, 421 U.S. 658 (1975), the president of a nationwide grocery chain was charged with holding food products under unsanitary conditions. He contended that he delegated the responsibility for sanitation to employees and could not be expected to oversee all corporate operations personally. The Court acknowledged that a defendant's "powerlessness" to prevent or correct the violation may be raised as a defense, but the burden falls on the defendant to prove this. Finding the defendant liable under the FDCA, the Court stated that the act imposes a duty not only to seek out and correct violations, but also to implement procedures to ensure that violations will not occur. This requirement on corporate officers may be demanding and onerous, stated the Court, but no more so than the public has a right to expect in light of the effect on the public health and well-being.

These two decisions are collectively known as the "Park Doctrine" and establish that corporate officials can be personally prosecuted without proof they acted intentionally or with negligence and even if they had no knowledge of the offense. After years of dormancy, the FDA announced that it will increase enforcement of the Park Doctrine against corporate officers and in 2011 published criteria that it will consider in such prosecutions (http://www.fda.gov/ICECI/ComplianceManuals/Regulatory-ProceduresManual/ucm176738.htm). The agency is frustrated that large fines against manufacturers for marketing violations, such as fines of $1.4 billion against Eli Lilly, $2.3 billion against Pfizer in 2009, and $3 billion against GlaxoSmithKline in 2012, have not seemed to deter violations of the FDCA. The FDA hopes that imposing personal liability will change the corporate culture.

PRODUCT RECALLS

One method of removing adulterated or misbranded products in interstate commerce is by means of recall. Prior to the passage of the FDAAA in 2007 the FDA did not have the statutory authority to order a product recall but rather had to request a company to recall a product as an alternative to injunctive action or seizure. Now the FDA can order a recall, or alternately, a manufacturer may initiate a product recall without FDA involvement. In either event, the FDA has the authority to prescribe the procedures to which the recall must conform.

Drug recalls are divided into three classes:

1. Class I recalls are issued when there is a reasonable probability that the product will cause serious, adverse health consequences or death.
2. Class II recalls occur when the product may cause temporary or medically reversible adverse health consequences, but the probability of serious adverse consequences is remote.
3. Class III recalls apply to products that are not likely to cause adverse health consequences.

The manufacturer is responsible for notifying sellers of the recall. In turn, sellers are responsible for contacting consumers, if necessary. Manufacturer recall notices may be delivered by means of letter, telegram, telephone, sales representatives, and so forth.

Guidelines issued by the FDA require that written notices for class I, class II, and some class III recalls be sent by first-class mail with the envelope and letterhead conspicuously marked, preferably in red, URGENT: DRUG RECALL. Many pharmacy publications also provide current lists of recalled products.

A pharmacist is responsible for knowing which drug products have been recalled. Furnishing a recalled product may violate the FDCA because the product is likely adulterated or misbranded, and a pharmacist might have difficulty asserting a good-faith defense. The pharmacist might also be subject to civil liability in the event of patient injury.

ADULTERATION

ADULTERATION: THE LAW

Section 501 of the FDCA in part provides that a drug or device shall be deemed to be adulterated:

> (a)(1) If it consists in whole or in part of any filthy, putrid, or decomposed substance; or (2)(A) if it has been prepared, packed, or held under insanitary conditions whereby it may have been contaminated with filth, or whereby it may have been rendered injurious to health; or (B) if it is a drug and the methods used in, or the facilities or controls used for, its manufacture, processing, packing, or holding do not conform to or are not operated or administered in conformity with current good manufacturing practice . . .; or (3) if its container is composed, in whole or in part, of any poisonous or deleterious substance which may render the contents injurious to health; or (4) if (A) it bears or contains, for purposes of coloring only, a color additive which is unsafe . . .

> (b) If it purports to be or is represented as a drug the name of which is recognized in an official compendium, and its strength differs from, or its quality or purity falls below, the standards set forth in such compendium. ***No drug defined in an official compendium shall be deemed to be adulterated under this paragraph because it differs from the standard of strength, quality, or purity therefore set forth in such compendium, if its difference in strength, quality, or purity from such standards is plainly stated on its label.***

> (c) If it is not subject to the provisions of paragraph (b) of this section and its strength differs from, or its purity or quality falls below, that which it purports or is represented to possess.

> (d) If it is a drug and any substance has been (1) mixed or packed therewith so as to reduce its quality or strength or (2) substituted wholly or in part therefore. (§ 501; 21 U.S.C. § 351)

EXPLANATION OF ADULTERATION

Most of the adulteration provisions apply to manufacturers. A pharmacy may be deemed a manufacturer if it repackages or compounds medications for sale under certain conditions, however.

A drug may be adulterated under the act, even if it is pure, because a drug is deemed adulterated if it is

- Prepared, packed, or held in conditions where it may have been contaminated
- Exposed to a container that may have contaminated it
- Manufactured under conditions that do not conform to current GMP

These provisions in the law are intended to regulate the facility and the means of production rather than the product itself. There are two reasons for this approach. First, it is much easier for the FDA to inspect a relatively few manufacturing plants than the thousands of drug products that these plants produce. Second, the health and safety risk to the public is much lower if the FDA can prevent adulteration rather than wait and remove an adulterated product from the market.

The law also provides that a drug is adulterated if it contains an unsafe color additive. Moreover, a drug that is subject to compendia standards is deemed adulterated if its strength, quality, or purity differs from those standards, unless the variations are stated on the label. If the drug is not subject to compendia standards, it is deemed adulterated if its strength, quality, or purity differs from those stated on the label. On the basis of this provision, a drug could be simultaneously adulterated and misbranded.

Current Good Manufacturing Practice (CGMP)

Section 501(a)(2)(B) specifically declares that a drug is adulterated unless it is manufactured in accordance with "current good manufacturing practice." CGMP is a set of regulations that establishes minimum requirements for the methods, facilities, or controls used in the manufacture, processing, packaging, or holding of a drug product (21 C.F.R. §§ 211.1–211.208). The intent of the CGMP regulations is to ensure that the drug is safe and meets the quality and purity requirements. The CGMP applies to manufacturers, not pharmacies, unless the pharmacies engage in activities in which they may be deemed manufacturers.

Manufacturers must be registered with the FDA and are normally inspected by the FDA for compliance with CGMP once every 2 years. The inspections are designed to

- Confirm that the production and control procedures result in the proper identity, strength, quality, and purity of the drugs
- Identify deficiencies
- Ensure correction of the deficiencies

Noncompliance with the CGMP could result in litigation against the company and a declaration that the drugs are adulterated. Drugs under the CGMP are selected for analysis on the basis of their medical importance, market share, number of similar products in the marketplace, and the previous compliance record of their manufacturer. The FDA looks for various defects, such as subpotency, particulates, lack of content uniformity, and dissolution failures. When unacceptable deviations are substantiated by further testing, the manufacturer is asked to investigate the problem and, if necessary, recall the drug voluntarily. If the manufacturer does not correct the problem, the FDA may seize the product.

Product Tampering

In response to the intentional contamination of Tylenol capsules on retailers' shelves in 1982, Congress passed the Federal Anti-Tampering Act (18 U.S.C. § 1365), making it a federal offense to tamper with consumer products. Tampering is defined in the act as improper interference with the product for the purpose of making objectionable or unauthorized changes. The act gave regulatory authority to the Federal Bureau of Investigation, the U.S. Department of Agriculture, and the FDA.

The FDA promulgated regulations in 1982 (21 C.F.R. § 211.132) requiring that certain OTC drugs, cosmetics, and devices be manufactured in tamper-resistant packaging. Violation of this regulation may be deemed adulteration, misbranding, or both.

A tamper-resistant package is defined as "one having an indicator or barrier to entry which, if breached or missing, can reasonably be expected to provide visible evidence to consumers that tampering has occurred." The regulations require tamper-resistant packaging, not tamper-proof packaging, because technology does not exist to eliminate the risk of tampering completely.

MISBRANDING

MISBRANDING: THE LAW

Section 502 of the FDCA provides that a drug or device shall be deemed to be misbranded:

(a) If its labeling is false or misleading in any particular. Health care economic information provided to a formulary committee, or other similar entity, in the course of the committee or the entity carrying out its responsibilities for the selection of drugs for managed care or other similar organizations, shall not be considered to be false or misleading under this paragraph if the health care economic information directly relates to an indication approved . . . for such drug and is based on competent and reliable scientific evidence. Information that is relevant to the substantiation of the health care economic information presented pursuant to this paragraph shall be made available to the Secretary upon request. In this paragraph, the term "health care economic information" means any analysis that identifies, measures, or compares the economic consequences, including the costs of the represented health outcomes, of the use of a drug to the use of another drug, to another health care intervention, or to no intervention.

(b) If in a package form unless it bears a label containing (1) the name and place of business of the manufacturer, packer, or distributor; and (2) an accurate statement of the quantity of the contents in terms of weight, measure, or numerical count. . . .

(c) If any word, statement, or other information required is not prominently placed on the label, with such conspicuousness and in such terms as to render it likely to be read and understood by the ordinary individual under customary conditions of purchase and use.

(e)(1)(A) If it is a drug, unless its label bears, to the exclusion of any other nonproprietary name (except the applicable systematic chemical name or the chemical formula) (i) the established name (as defined in subparagraph (3)) of the drug, if there is such a name; (ii) the established name and quantity or, if determined to be appropriate by the Secretary, the proportion of each active ingredient, including the quantity, kind, and proportion of any alcohol, and also including whether active or not the established name and quantity or if determined to be appropriate by the Secretary, the proportion of any bromides, ether, chloroform, acetanilide, acetophenetidin, amidopyrine, antipyrine, atropine, hyoscine, hyoscyamine, arsenic, digitalis, digitalis glucosides, mercury, ouabain, strophanthin, strychnine, thyroid, or any derivative or preparation of any such substances, contained therein, except that the requirement for stating the quantity of the active ingredients, other than the quantity of those specifically named in this subclause, shall not apply to nonprescription drugs not intended for human use; and (iii) the established name of each inactive ingredient listed in alphabetical order on the outside container of the retail package and, if determined to be appropriate by the Secretary, on the immediate container, as prescribed in regulation promulgated by the Secretary, except that nothing in this subclause shall be deemed to require that any trade secret be divulged, and except that the requirements of this subclause with respect to alphabetical order shall apply only to nonprescription drugs that are not also cosmetics and that this subclause shall not apply to nonprescription drugs not intended for human use.

(3) As used in paragraph (1) the term "established name" means (A) the applicable official name, or (B) if there is no such name and the drug is an article recognized in an official compendium, then the official title in the compendium or (C) if neither clause (A) nor clause (B) of this paragraph applies, then the common or usual name.

(f) Unless its labeling bears (1) adequate directions for use; and (2) such adequate warnings against use in those pathological conditions or by children where its use may be dangerous to health, or against unsafe dosage or methods or duration of administration or application, in such manner and form, as are necessary for the protection of users, except that where any requirement of clause (1) of this paragraph, as applied to any drug or device, is not necessary for the protection of the public health, the Secretary shall promulgate regulations exempting such drug or device from such requirement.

(g) If it purports to be a drug the name of which is recognized in an official compendium, unless it is packaged and labeled as prescribed therein.

(h) If it has been found to be a drug liable to deterioration, unless it is packaged in such form and manner, and its label bears a statement of such precautions.

(i)(1) If it is a drug and its container is so made, formed, or filled as to be misleading; or (2) if it is an imitation of another drug; or (3) if it is offered for sale under the name of another drug.

(j) If it is dangerous to health when used in the dosage or manner, or with the frequency or duration prescribed, recommended, or suggested in the labeling, thereof.

(m) If it is a color additive the intended use of which is for the purpose of coloring only, unless its packaging and labeling are in conformity with applicable packaging and labeling requirements.

(n) Unless the manufacturer, packer or distributor includes in all advertisements and other descriptive printed matter a true statement of (1) the established name printed prominently and in type at least half as large as that used for any trade or brand name, (2) the formula showing quantitatively each ingredient of the drug and (3) such other information in brief summary relating to side effects, contraindications, and effectiveness.

(p) If it is a drug and its packaging or labeling is in violation of an applicable regulation of the Poison Prevention Packaging Act of 1970. (§ 502; 21 U.S.C. § 352)

As noted previously, failure to manufacture certain OTC products in a tamper-resistant package also is misbranding.

EXPLANATION OF MISBRANDING

Whereas adulteration deals with a drug's strength, purity, and quality, misbranding focuses on representations made by the manufacturer on the label or labeling. The FDA must approve, as part of the premarket approval process, the exact wording of a drug's label and labeling. The agency often has used the misbranding provisions of the act to prevent manufacturers from marketing products in violation of the law.

False or Misleading Labeling

That a label shall not be false or misleading under section 502(a) is self-explanatory. The FDAMA added the provision regarding health care economic information. Before the FDAMA, the subject of drug manufacturers supplying pharmacoeconomic information to health care decision makers had been controversial. Because the FDA does not approve pharmacoeconomic data as part of the drug's labeling, the question was whether a manufacturer that provided this information would be guilty of misbranding. Now, under the law, health care economic information provided to formulary decision makers is permissible as long as the information is accurate and reliable.

Habit-Forming Drugs

Before the FDAMA, section 502 contained a provision stating that the labeling of any drug containing a substance found to be habit-forming must contain a warning to this effect. The FDAMA deleted this provision, thus making whether to include the warning discretionary with the manufacturer. Manufacturers are still required to adequately describe the habit-forming characteristics of the drug in the "Drug Abuse and Dependence" section of the package insert.

Established Names of Drugs

Section 502(e) obviously contains a significant amount of information. The important points to note from this section are that the law requires the listing of any active ingredient for both prescription and nonprescription drugs and the quantity of each active ingredient (unless the nonprescription drug is not for human use). Section 502(e) also requires that in most situations the labeling contain a list of the established name of each inactive ingredient in alphabetical order for both prescription drugs and nonprescription drugs (unless the nonprescription drug is also a cosmetic or not for human use). Before the FDAMA, the listing of inactive ingredients was not required.

Adequate Directions for Use

Section 502(f) states that the labeling must contain "adequate directions for use," and "adequate warnings against use" by children and others for whom use may be dangerous. "Adequate directions for use" in the regulations means "directions under which the layperson can use a drug safely and for the purposes for which it is intended" (21 C.F.R. § 201.5). The regulation continues by stating that the directions for use may be deemed inadequate unless the labeling contains statements of all conditions, purposes, or uses for which the drug is intended and for which the drug is commonly used. As the court held in *Alberty Food Products Co. v. United States*, 185 F.2d 321 (9th Cir. 1950), merely stating the proper way to take a drug is not adequate. The labeling must be complete enough to inform the consumer that the drug should be used for the consumer's particular ailment.

In addition to the statements of all conditions, purposes, or uses, "adequate" labeling of a drug must include

- The quantity or dosage for each intended use and for persons of different ages and physical conditions
- The frequency of administration or application
- The duration of administration or application
- The time of administration or application (in relation to meals, onset of symptoms, or other factors)
- The route or method of administration or application
- The preparation necessary for use (e.g., shaking, dilution)

Adequate Information for Use

Some drugs cannot be labeled adequately to protect the consumer and meet the "adequate directions for use" requirement of section 502(f). The FDA classifies these drugs as prescription drugs, which makes them exempt from the requirements of section 502(f). Prescription drugs must contain "adequate information for use" rather than adequate directions for use (21 C.F.R. § 201.100(c)(1)). Thus, the labeling must include such information as

- The drug's indications
- Side effects
- Dosages
- Routes, methods, frequency, and duration of administration
- Contraindications
- Other warnings and precautions that enable a practitioner to administer, prescribe, or dispense the drug safely

Prescription drug labeling is directed to the practitioner, not the patient. Nonetheless, the FDA has increasingly been concerned that patients receive understandable information about their prescription drug medication, as evidenced by the Medication Guide program.

Imitation Drugs

Section 502(i)(2) of the FDCA provides that it is misbranding if a drug is an imitation of another drug. The FDA has invoked this section against drugs sold as imitations of controlled substances. In *United States v. Articles of Drug* (Midwest Pharmaceuticals), 825 F.2d 1238 (8th Cir. 1987), for example, Midwest distributed and promoted a drug containing caffeine, ephedrine, and phenylpropanolamine. Advertisements for the drug contained pictures of capsules and tablets that looked exactly like various well-known amphetamine-type controlled substances. The advertisements contained no information about the drug's ingredients, but they described the drug using various street names, such as 20/20, White Mole, and Mini-White. Finding for the FDA, the court held that a product is an imitation if it is

- Identical in shape, size, and color
- Similar or virtually identical in gross appearance
- Similar in effect to controlled substances

Batch Certification

Before the FDAMA, section 502 had required batch certifications for insulin and antibiotics. Early insulin preparation techniques were often crude, resulting in problems of product purity and potency. Similarly, early antibiotic preparations relied on fermentation, extraction, and purification techniques that at the time were inconsistent, resulting in variability of stability and potency. Therefore, Congress gave the FDA the authority to require that batches of insulin and antibiotics be certified by the agency before their marketing. Because antibiotics and insulin products today no longer exhibit the problems they presented in earlier years, the FDA no longer has the statutory authority to require batch certification for either insulin or antibiotics.

NONPRESCRIPTION DRUG LABELING

Nonprescription drugs, or OTC drugs, are those that are safe and effective for self-medication by consumers. Pursuant to regulations finalized in 1999 with the intent to make OTC drug labeling more "user friendly," the label of a nonprescription drug must contain in part the following information (see 64 Fed. Reg. 13254; 21 C.F.R. part 201 subparts A and C):

- A statement of the identity of the product, including the established name of the drug, if any, followed by an accurate statement of the general pharmacological category of the drug or principal intended action(s) (e.g., Suphedrin, pseudoephedrine hydrochloride, nasal decongestant)
- The name and address of the manufacturer, packer, or distributor
- The net quantity of the contents of the package
- Cautions and warnings needed to protect the consumer
- Adequate directions for use (as discussed previously)
- A "Drug Facts" panel containing the following information in the following order (21 C.F.R. § 201.66):
  - Active ingredient(s) (including dosage unit and quantity per dosage unit)
  - Purpose (general pharmacological category or principal intended action)
  - Use(s) (indications)
  - Warnings (including the following subheadings in bold type)
    - "For external use only" (for topical products) or "For rectal (or vaginal) use only" for products intended for these uses
    - Do not use (listing of all contraindications)
    - Ask a doctor before use if you have (listing of all conditions and situations when the product should not be used)
    - Ask a doctor or pharmacist before use if you are (listing of all drug–drug and drug–food interactions)
    - When using this product (listing of possible side effects and substances or activities to avoid)
    - Stop use and ask a doctor if (listing of signs of toxicity and other reactions requiring immediate discontinuation)
    - "If pregnant or breast feeding" warning
    - "Keep out of reach of children" and accidental overdose/ingestion warning
  - Directions
  - Other information (as required by the monograph, by regulation, or in the approved labeling)
  - Inactive ingredients (listed in alphabetical order)
  - Questions? or Questions and Comments (followed by a telephone number)

Regulations (21 C.F.R. § 201.5) further require adequate directions for use to contain:

- The normal dose for each intended use and the doses for individuals of different ages and different physical conditions
- The frequency and duration of administration or application
- The administration or application in relation to meals, onset of symptoms, or other time factors
- The route or method of administration or application
- Any required preparation for use

The regulations provide that OTC drug labels must be easy to read and easy to understand, as well as be of a minimum size type. These format requirements are designed to make it easier for consumers to select the appropriate product and help them use the product more effectively.

Pharmacists who repackage or relabel OTC drugs for resale must comply with the same labeling requirements as manufacturers.

Professional OTC Labeling

For some OTC drug products, manufacturers publish additional labeling specifically for the health care professional, not the consumer. Called "professional labeling," it is intended to provide information for conditions not appropriate for lay diagnosis or treatment. The FDA does not allow this information on the labeling of the marketed OTC product because it does not contain "adequate directions for use." The concept of professional labeling arose in 1973 when panels of experts reviewing OTC drugs for safety and efficacy recommended additional labeling for such situations as pediatric dosing and the use of antacids for ulcer therapy. For example, the allowed OTC labeling indications for antacids include "heartburn," "sour stomach," "acid indigestion," and so forth. The professional labeling includes indications for "the symptomatic relief of hyperacidity associated with the diagnosis of peptic ulcer, gastritis . . ." (21 C.F.R. part 331).

The FDA's position is that the information contained in professional labeling can be safely used only under the supervision of the licensed prescriber. Therefore, a pharmacist should not provide a patient with professional information even if the manufacturer has mailed this information to the pharmacist, unless the patient requests it. Of course, the pharmacist may provide the labeling to the prescriber. Although a pharmacist may recommend an OTC drug to a patient for a condition or a dosage not listed on the label, doing so may increase the pharmacist's risk of civil liability in the event of patient injury.

Drugs That Are Both OTC and Prescription

The issue of adequate directions for use labeling also explains why some drugs are both OTC and prescription. With these drugs, the FDA has made the determination that the drug can be labeled with adequate directions for use for some indications but not others. For example, meclizine is sold OTC for the indications of nausea, vomiting, and dizziness associated with motion sickness. The drug is sold by prescription with the added indication of being possibly effective for vertigo associated with diseases affecting the vestibular system. It also explains why some drugs, such as ibuprofen, are OTC at one strength and prescription at other strengths. The 200-mg OTC ibuprofen carries the indication for mild to moderate pain, whereas the higher strengths prescription ibuprofen add indications of rheumatoid arthritis and osteoarthritis. (A drug can be both OTC and prescription, depending upon how it is switched from prescription to OTC status.)

PRESCRIPTION DRUG LABELS AND LABELING

As noted earlier, prescription drugs are labeled for the health care professional, not the patient.

The Commercial Container Label

The applicable regulations are somewhat detailed and, in general, require the following information on the commercial label (21 C.F.R. §§ 201.1 201.55 and 201.100):

- The name and address of the manufacturer, packer, or distributor
- The established name of the drug product
- Ingredient information, including the quantity and proportion of each active ingredient
- Names of inactive ingredients (with certain exceptions) if not for oral use
- A statement of identity (generic and proprietary names)

- The quantity in terms of weight or measure (e.g., 100 mg)
- The net quantity of the container (e.g., 100 tablets)
- A statement of the recommended or usual dosage or reference to the package insert
- The symbol "Rx Only" or the legend (e.g., "Caution: Federal law prohibits dispensing without prescription.")
- The route of administration, if it is not for oral use
- An identifying lot or control number
- A statement directed to the pharmacist specifying the type of container to be used in dispensing the drug (e.g., "Dispense in tight, light-resistant container as defined in the National Formulary.")
- The expiration date, unless exempted (*Note:* When an expiration date is stated only in month and year, the expiration date is the last day of the month.)

If the container is too small or unable to accommodate a label with space for all the information and is packaged within an outer container, the recommended dosage, route of administration, inactive ingredients, and statement regarding type of container may be contained in other labeling on or within the package. Moreover, the "Rx Only" statement may be placed only on the outer container and the lot number may be printed on the crimp of the dispensing tube.

Unit Dose Labeling

Unit dose packaging is when a single dosage unit of a drug is prepackaged and prelabeled for direct administration. Many hospitals, skilled nursing facilities, and other institutions commonly use unit dose systems because they reduce errors and diversion and permit the return of unused sealed doses. It would not be practical to require the label of a unit dose package to contain the same information as a commercial container because of the package size. Thus, the regulations require a label on the unit dose container to include (see Compliance Policy Guide (7132b.10)):

- The established name of the drug
- The quantity of the active ingredient in each dosage unit
- The expiration date
- The lot or control number
- The name or place of business of the manufacturer, packer, or distributor
- Any statements required by a compendia if an official drug, or for unofficial drugs, any pertinent statement regarding special characteristics

The Package Insert

The package insert is a pamphlet that must accompany the drug product and contains the essential scientific and medical information needed for safe and effective use of the drug by health care professionals. It cannot be promotional in nature, false, or misleading. FDA regulations specify not only the contents and format of the prescription drug's label but also the package insert and other labeling (21 C.F.R. §§ 201.56, 201.57, and 201.100).

Health care professionals had not found the package insert very useful, and many did not use it as their primary source of drug information. They found that the format and content of the insert made it difficult to read and difficult to distinguish important information and warnings from information clutter and "legalese." In 2000, after evaluating extensive information and feedback from health care professionals regarding how the content and format of the package insert could be improved to enhance safer and more effective use of prescription drugs, the FDA proposed a regulation to make major revisions in the package insert (see 65 Fed. Reg. 81082, Dec. 22, 2000, and 66 Fed. Reg. 17375-01, March 23, 2001). The FDA made the regulation final in January 2006 (see 71 Fed. Reg. 3922-01; 21 C.F.R. parts 201, 314, and 601).

The new package insert is designed to reduce preventable adverse drug events by making information about the drug more easily accessible, more memorable, and less complex. The insert reorganizes critical information so health care professionals can find the information they need quickly. This is accomplished by including a "Highlights" section at the beginning, which summarizes the most important information about the product, including Boxed Warnings, Indications and Usage, and Dosage and Administration. The Highlights section will also refer the reader to the appropriate section of the Full Prescribing Information. To ensure health care professionals have the most up-to-date information, manufacturers must include a list of all substantive changes made within the past year.

In order to help health care professionals find critical information more quickly, a Table of Contents has been added. The Full Prescribing Information is reorganized to give more prominence to the most important and most commonly referenced information. In addition, a Patient Counseling Information section has been added, designed as the FDA has stated: "to help doctors advise their patients about important uses and limitations of medications." It is also hoped that this section will serve as a guide for discussions about potential risks and how to manage those risks. Any FDA-approved patient information is included immediately after the Patient Counseling section.

Unfortunately for health care professionals, the new package insert requirements apply only to drugs whose new drug applications were submitted after June 30, 2006, and will be phased in gradually for drugs approved 5 years prior to June 30, 2006. The FDA hopes manufacturers of other drug products will comply voluntarily. Health care professionals do have access to a recent e-Health initiative from the FDA called "DailyMed," which is an online information clearinghouse through the National Library of Medicine. Accessible at http://dailymed.nlm.nih.gov/dailymed/about.cfm, its objective is to provide the most up-to-date medication information to consumers and health care professionals. Ultimately, the same information on DailyMed will be provided on a website called Facts@FDA, which will offer one-stop access for information about all FDA-regulated products.

Black Box Warnings

When the use of a drug may lead to death or serious injury, the FDA may require the warning of the special problem in the package insert to be placed within a prominently displayed box, also known as a black box warning (21 C.F.R. §201.57(c)(1)). The FDA considers a decision to require a boxed warning to be a dramatic step, and only about 450 prescription drugs contain a black box warning. Despite the prominence of the boxed warning in the insert and the seriousness of the warning, the FDA and most professional organizations agree that they are usually ineffective. Reports indicate that many prescribers are either unaware of the warnings or simply do not heed them. Many drugs (e.g., Propulsid, Duract) may not have needed to be withdrawn from the market if health care professionals simply observed and managed the risks contained in the boxed warning. The FDA is hoping that the new revisions to the package insert will improve the effectiveness of the boxed warnings. If not, the FDA will likely require other risk management strategies for high-risk drugs.

Pregnancy Warnings

The labeling regulations also require that the package insert contain information about use of the drug during pregnancy, unless the drug is not absorbed systemically and not known to harm the fetus (21 C.F.R. §201.57(c)(9)). There are five categories of risk in pregnancy into which a drug might be placed:

- Category A: Adequate and well-controlled studies in pregnant women have not demonstrated a risk to the fetus. The labeling for drugs in this category also must contain a notice that because studies cannot rule out the possibility of harm, however, the drug should be used during pregnancy "only if clearly needed."
- Category B: Animal studies have failed to demonstrate a risk to the fetus and there are no adequate well-controlled studies in pregnant women. As with Category A, a statement must be included providing that the drug should be used during pregnancy "only if clearly needed."
- Category C: Either animal studies have shown an adverse effect on the fetus or there are no animal reproductive studies, and there are no adequate well-controlled studies in pregnant women. A statement must be included that the drug should be used during pregnancy "only if the potential benefit justifies the potential risk to the fetus."
- Category D: Positive evidence of fetal risk exists based upon data from investigational or marketing experience or studies in humans; however, potential benefits from the drug may be acceptable despite potential risks (e.g., in life-threatening or serious disease situations for which a safer drug cannot be used). A statement must be included in the Warnings and Precautions section that the drug can cause fetal harm, and that the patient should be apprised of the risk if pregnant.
- Category X: Studies in animals or humans have demonstrated fetal risk, and that risk in pregnant women clearly outweighs any benefit. The Contraindications section must state that the drug "may cause fetal harm when administered to a pregnant woman." A statement must also be included that the patient should be apprised of the potential hazard to the fetus if used while pregnant. Accutane and Thalidomide are examples of drugs that fall into this category.

In May of 2008 the FDA published a proposed regulation to amend the pregnancy labeling requirements (73 Fed. Reg. 30831). If enacted, the regulation would require that prescription drug labeling include a summary of the risks of using the drug during pregnancy and lactation, require that the labeling include relevant clinical information to help health care providers make prescribing and counseling decisions, and eliminate the current A, B, C, D, and X categories. Pharmacy organizations are generally supportive of the proposed new regulation because it will require that labeling contain more comprehensive information about the benefits and risks of medication use during pregnancy and lactation than current labeling. On the other hand, the organizations would prefer that some form of the category labeling also be retained as a quick reference guide for practitioners.

NATIONAL DRUG CODE NUMBER

Drug products are identified and reported using a unique, 11-digit, 3-segment number (e.g., 55555-4444-22) called the National Drug Code (NDC) (21 C.F.R. §§ 201.2 and 207.35). Under the original system, the NDC number contained nine characters, either as numbers or letters. In the 1970s, however, it was changed to a 10-digit number, and the original 9-character codes previously assigned to products received a leading zero. Today, under the code system assigned to new products, the code is an 11-digit number. The first segment of the code is assigned by the FDA and identifies the manufacturer or distributor. The second segment of the code number identifies a specific strength, dosage form, and formulation for a particular firm. The third segment identifies package size and type of drug.

The presence of the NDC number on the label or labeling does not indicate that a drug has received an approved NDA. The FDA assigns the number simply for identification purposes. It has proved invaluable for facilitating the processing of third-party prescription drug claims and for distributing products among manufacturers, wholesalers, and pharmacies.

In 2004 the FDA enacted a regulation requiring that certain human drug and biological labeling include a linear bar code that contains at a minimum the NDC number. The intent of this requirement is to help reduce the number of medication errors by enabling health care professionals to scan the bar code to verify that the right drug, dosage, and route of administration are provided to the patient (69 Fed. Reg. 9120-01, February 26, 2004). Since the regulation was enacted, advances in alternative technologies have occurred and many products have presented unique bar coding problems. As a result, the agency has announced it will reassess the regulation (76 Fed. Reg. 66235, October 2011).

© Stockbyte/Thinkstock

STUDY SCENARIOS AND QUESTIONS

1. A pharmacist received a bottle of cephalosporin capsules. Unknown to the pharmacist, the tablets also contained small amounts of penicillin. The pharmacist dispensed the capsules to a patient who is allergic to penicillin and who then suffered an anaphylactic shock. Explain whether the drug is misbranded and/or adulterated. Explain whether the pharmacist has violated the FDCA, and if so, whether the pharmacist might face sanction by the FDA.

2. A hospital pharmacy received ampules of a commonly stocked drug contained in a pink solution. The drug has always been in a clear solution previously. The pharmacist dispensed the drug for IV administration. The drug was contaminated and injured the patient. Explain the difference between this situation and the one in question 1 as related to the pharmacist involved.

3. A pharmacist received a prescription for a brand-name drug and legally substituted a generic drug. The pharmacist labeled the dispensed generic drug with the brand-name drug. Explain whether the pharmacist has violated the FDCA.

4. A pharmacist received a call from a physician who ordered ibuprofen 600 mg for a patient but instructed the pharmacist to label the drug as oxycodone. Explain whether the pharmacist would violate the FDCA if he or she complies, and whether this situation differs from question 3.

5. A patient hands a pharmacist a prescription for Spondicin 20 mg, a prescription-only drug. As the patient is waiting for the prescription to be filled, the patient notices that Spondicin 10 mg is available over the counter and asks the pharmacist how it can be that one strength is prescription only and the other is OTC. What should the pharmacist say? Would the pharmacist violate the FDCA by telling the patient to use the OTC drug for the prescribed indication in the prescribed dose when that indication or dosage is not contained in the OTC drug's labeling?

6. A pharmaceutical manufacturer issued a Class I recall for one of its prescription drug products. How might a pharmacist learn of this recall? Explain whether a pharmacist would violate the FDCA if he or she dispensed the drug after the recall notice. If it is a violation, explain whether it would be a defense if the pharmacist did not know of the recall.

NEW DRUG APPROVAL

The FDCA provides that no person shall introduce into interstate commerce any "new drug," unless that drug has an approved application by the FDA (Section 505; 21 U.S.C. § 355(a)). If the drug is not a generic of a currently marketed drug, this means that drug manufacturers must apply for and receive FDA approval of a new drug application (NDA), an extremely expensive and lengthy process.

Some of the extensive information that the applicant must provide to the FDA as part of the application includes (Section 505(b)):

- Full reports of investigations showing the drug's safety and efficacy
- The drug's components and composition
- The methods, facilities, and controls used in manufacturing, processing, and packaging the drug
- Samples of the drug and its components
- The proposed labeling of the drug

Regarding the safety of the drug, applicants must submit adequate information to demonstrate the drug's safety for use under the conditions prescribed, recommended, or suggested in the proposed labeling (Section 505(d)). With respect to efficacy, the law stipulates that the applicant must submit "substantial evidence that the drug will have the effect it purports or is represented to have under the conditions or use prescribed, recommended, or suggested in the proposed labeling." Substantial evidence is defined as the findings of adequate and well-controlled investigations by experts qualified by scientific training and experience to evaluate the drug's effectiveness (Section 505(d)).

DEFINING "NEW DRUG"

The FDA must approve every "new drug" prior to marketing, so the question becomes, what is a "new drug"? Section 201(p) of the FDCA defines a "new drug" as a drug that is not generally recognized by qualified experts as safe and effective for use under the conditions recommended in the drug's labeling. The definition also provides that, even if the drug is so recognized, it must also have been used to a "material extent or for a material time under the conditions recommended in the labeling." Importantly, a drug marketed before 1938 is exempt from proving either safety or efficacy, provided that it is marketed in accordance with the labeling requirements as then existed.

As will be discussed, some drugs have been marketed for several years without FDA approval. If the FDA ultimately decides that these drugs must now be approved, the new drug definition seems to suggest that a manufacturer should be able to demonstrate that its product is not new and be able to market the drug without going through the NDA process. If the manufacturer can demonstrate that its product is generally recognized by experts as safe and effective (commonly termed GRASE) and has been used to a material extent and for a material time, the drug should not be new. In actuality this does not happen (except in some instances with OTC drugs). The FDA will not GRASE a product, but rather requires the drug manufacturer to prove safety and efficacy through the NDA process. The manufacturer has no choice but to comply because the courts will not second guess the agency's decision.

An example of this situation occurred with levothyroxine products. Levothyroxine products had been lawfully marketed for over 40 years without FDA approval until problems surfaced in the 1990s regarding bioavailability and bioequivalence. The FDA thus ordered that all levothyroxine products must have an approved NDA by August 2003. Abbott attempted to convince the FDA that its product, Synthroid, was not a new drug because it had been used safely and effectively for so many years. The FDA rejected the GRASE approach, however, and required Abbott to apply for and ultimately receive an approved NDA.

APPROVED DRUGS AS NEW DRUGS

Although typically one thinks of a new drug as some novel and as yet unapproved chemical entity, an approved drug may become a new drug if

- The drug contains a new substance (e.g., active ingredient, excipient, carrier, coating).
- There is a new combination of approved drugs.
- The proportion of ingredients in combination is changed.
- There is a new intended use for the drug.
- The dosage, method, or duration of administration or application is changed (21 C.F.R. § 310.3(h)).

It is not always obvious when an approved drug will become a new drug. In *United States v. Baxter Healthcare Corporation*, 901 F.2d 1401 (7th Cir. 1990), the court considered whether reconstituting, repackaging, freezing, and distributing approved antibiotic drugs make them new drugs. Baxter owned a compounding center that performed these functions on antibiotic powders and concentrates to prepare them for immediate use by health care providers. Baxter argued that it simply prepared the drugs according to the label instructions exactly as a physician or pharmacist would and, thus, the drugs could not be new drugs. Giving great deference to the judgment of the FDA, however, the court found that the reconstitution did indeed make the drugs new drugs because the procedure raised concerns about the safety and efficacy of the final product. To support its conclusion, the court referred to the statute and regulations that require a full description of the methods, facilities, and controls used in manufacturing, processing, and packaging with the submission of an NDA.

THE ROAD TO AN APPROVED NEW DRUG APPLICATION

In seeking approval for an NDA, an applicant must submit evidence (pursuant to § 505(d)) that the drug is safe and effective. This evidence must be obtained through animal and clinical (human) studies. Section 505(a), however, forbids the shipment of any new drug unless the drug has an approved NDA. This seemingly contradictory situation is avoided by section 505(i), which allows the FDA to exempt a drug from the NDA requirement for the pursuit of clinical investigations. To receive this exemption, the manufacturer must apply for a "Notice of Claimed Investigational Exemption for a New Drug," commonly called an Investigational New Drug (IND) Application. If approved, the manufacturer may then conduct clinical studies of its investigational new drug. Application of an IND follows extensive preclinical investigation by the applicant, where through laboratory experimentation and animal testing the applicant has determined that the drug has potential merit and would be reasonably safe to test in humans.

Investigational New Drug Application

The law requires a sponsor seeking an IND application to submit a substantial amount of information, including:

- The name of the drug
- Its composition

- Methods of manufacture and quality control
- Information from preclinical (animal) investigations regarding pharmacological, pharmacokinetic, and toxicological evaluations

The application must also include information about the experience and qualifications of the clinical investigators, as well as a complete outline of the proposed clinical trials. The primary purpose of the approval process for an IND is to protect the safety of the humans who will participate in the clinical trials. Secondarily, the process is intended to ensure that the clinical studies are designed properly so as to prevent problems during the NDA review.

If the FDA does not reject the IND request within 30 days of submission, human clinical testing may begin. The testing proceeds through three phases. In phase 1, which involves a small number of subjects, investigators examine the drug's toxicity, metabolism, bioavailability, elimination, and other pharmacological actions. Doses of the drug are initially low, then gradually increased. The purpose of phase 1 is to detect adverse effects, not to determine efficacy.

If the drug passes phase 1, it moves to phase 2, where it is tested on a limited number of patients who actually have the disease for which the drug is an intended treatment. The purpose of phase 2 is to determine the efficacy of the drug and the dosages at which the efficacy occurs. Investigators also continue to conduct pharmacological testing to determine further the drug's safety.

If the drug's safety and efficacy appear promising, the study proceeds to phase 3, where the drug is tested for safety and efficacy in hundreds or even thousands of patients. These tests often occur in actual clinical settings, such as physicians' offices and hospitals that have contracted with the manufacturer to conduct the studies. Usually, the studies are double-blinded and compared with a control group that receives a placebo.

The FDA may terminate the testing of an IND at any time if studies show that the drug is too toxic under the agency's benefit/risk ratio criteria. The FDA's determination is final and not subject to appeal or judicial review. If the phase 3 study results are favorable, the drug's sponsor may submit an NDA to the FDA. Only about 1 in 10 drugs demonstrates enough merit to make it this far in the process, however.

Public Registry of Clinical Trials

The FDAAA amended the FDCA to require that NDA sponsors must publish summary information about any post phase 1 clinical trial on a public registry. This public disclosure requirement allows health care providers, as well as the general public, to track the safety and efficacy data generated in the study. Prior to the FDAAA, sponsors only had to post clinical study information for drugs intended to treat serious or life-threatening diseases.

Informed Consent

In all three IND clinical phases, the FDCA (section 505(i)) requires the investigators to secure the informed consent of the patient or a representative for the administration of an experimental drug. This requires that potential participants know the risks, possible benefits, and alternative courses of treatment. In addition, if the study is to take place in an institutional setting, the local institutional review board (IRB) must approve the study. An IRB is a committee designated by the institution charged with reviewing any research projects involving human subjects.

The patient's consent must be in writing in phases 1 and 2. In phase 3, patient consent may be oral if the physician decides it is necessary or it is preferable to written consent, and this decision is recorded in the patient's medical record. Patient consent may not be necessary when it is not feasible to obtain the consent of the patient or a representative, or when, in the professional judgment of the physician, informed consent is not in the best interest of the patient.

The New Drug Application

As a compilation of all information obtained during the IND process, an NDA contains a complete evaluation of the drug's safety and efficacy. There may be 100,000 to 200,000 pages of summary and raw data. This information includes, in part, details of drug chemistry, preclinical studies, manufacturing processes, clinical studies, labeling, and packaging. In all, an NDA has five to six technical sections, each to be reviewed by an expert in that scientific discipline.

By statute, the FDA has 180 days in which to act on a completed NDA, but significant delays are common (§ 505(c)(1)). Manufacturers will rarely launch a legal challenge against the FDA to expedite action, preferring cooperation and realizing that lengthy litigation would be self-defeating. The potential importance of the drug usually dictates the length of approval time. Proof of the drug's safety and efficacy, the proposed manufacturing process, and benefit/risk ratio generally determine whether the FDA will approve an NDA. If the FDA proposes to disapprove an NDA, it will notify the applicant and provide the applicant with an opportunity for a hearing. Although the applicant may judicially contest the FDA's determination to refuse to approve an NDA, no applicant has ever succeeded in court.

The Prescription Drug User Fee Act of 1992 (PDUFA) is generally credited as having reduced the FDA review time for NDAs from a median approval time of 23 months before the act to 15 months for 1995. The law, by requiring substantial user fees from product sponsors, accomplishes this purpose in two ways: First, the fees allow the FDA to hire hundreds of extra reviewers. Second, the high fees discourage sponsors from submitting applications until they have a high probability of success, reducing the review effort required.

FDA Drug Rating and Classification System

Since 1974, the FDA has used a priority classification system that rates new drugs by chemical type and therapeutic potential. The rating assigned to a drug determines how rapidly it will proceed through the NDA process. Usually, FDA reviewers assign a rating when the IND request is made, but the rating may be changed during the subsequent approval process. The rating of an approved drug often is important because physicians and pharmacists may consider it when evaluating new drug therapies and making drug formulary decisions.

In the FDA classification system, a number indicates the drug's chemical type; a letter indicates its therapeutic potential. For chemical type, the six designations are:

1. The active moiety is a new molecular entity.
2. The active moiety is in a new salt or ester form.
3. The dosage form or formulation is new.
4. The product is a new combination of compounds.
5. The drug product is essentially a duplicate of another drug product.
6. The drug is a product previously marketed by the same firm (used primarily for new indications).

These types are not mutually exclusive because a new formulation (type 3) or a new combination (type 4) also may contain a new molecular entity (type 1) or a new salt (type 2).

For therapeutic potential, the FDA uses the letters P for priority or S for standard (replacing the A, B, and C letter ratings used before 1992). A rating of P indicates that the drug may represent a therapeutic advance for one or more of these reasons:

- No other effective drugs are available.
- It is more effective or safe than drugs currently used.
- It has important advantages, such as greater convenience, reduced side effects, or improved tolerance or usefulness in special populations.

An S rating means that the drug may have therapeutic properties similar to those of drugs already on the market and offers at best only minor improvements over existing drug therapies.

Supplemental New Drug Applications

After the approval of an NDA, a manufacturer may not usually make any changes in the drug or its production, even the most minor ones, unless it submits for approval a supplemental NDA (21 C.F.R. § 314.70). Depending on the type of change intended, a supplemental NDA falls into one of three procedural categories. For changes in any part of the production, ranging from the synthesis of the drug, to the manufacturing processes of the drug, to most of the labeling of the drug, a "prior approval" supplement is required, whereby the agency must approve the change before the sponsor can implement it. For certain types of labeling changes such as those that strengthen warnings or dosage and administration information, or for certain changes in manufacturing methods, facilities, and controls, a "change being effected (CBE)" supplement may be allowed. The CBE supplement allows the sponsor to implement the change before the FDA approves it. For labeling changes, however, the regulation requires that the change must reflect "newly acquired information" that strengthens a contraindication, warning, precaution or adverse reaction; and then only if there is sufficient evidence of a causal association (21 C.F.R. 201.57). The final category of supplemental NDA allows very minor changes, such as editorial changes in labeling or changes in container size to merely be reported in the annual report that the sponsor must file to the FDA.

Supplemental NDAs requiring preapproval usually have a lower priority than do original NDAs and, thus, may take years to be approved. A manufacturer may, however, ask the FDA to expedite its review "if a delay in making the change described in it would impose an extraordinary hardship on the applicant."

Postmarketing Surveillance

Once the new drug application has been approved, the manufacturer may legally distribute the drug in interstate commerce. Section 505(k) of the FDCA, however, requires that the manufacturer maintain and establish postmarketing records and reports. Under this provision, the manufacturer must submit to the FDA reports of any serious adverse drug reactions (21 C.F.R. § 314.80) and any new information relating to the drug's safety and efficacy (21 C.F.R. § 314.81), including information about current clinical studies, the quantity of drug distributed, labeling, and advertising. This postmarketing surveillance is necessary for two reasons. First, an investigational drug is tested in a relatively small number of patients compared with the number of patients who may use the drug after it is marketed; second, long-term adverse effects may not be discoverable before approval. As a result of postmarketing information, the FDA may withdraw its approval of an NDA and, in fact, has done so on some occasions.

Phase IV Studies

Manufacturers engage in postmarket clinical studies, known as phase IV studies, for a variety of reasons, including to determine new uses or abuses for a drug, or to obtain additional safety or efficacy data for labeled indications. Historically the FDA has lacked clear statutory authority to require phase IV testing, even when safety controversies arise about a drug. FDAMA gave the FDA that authority for "fast-track" drug approval (as discussed later in this text), but it was not until the FDAAA that Congress granted the agency authority to require phase IV testing for any prescription drug. Now the FDA can require a phase IV study to assess serious risks when adverse event reporting or active surveillance would not be sufficient.

Risk Evaluation and Mitigation Strategy (REMS)

The FDAAA granted the FDA yet another important safety tool called "risk evaluation and mitigation strategy" (REMS), whereby the FDA can require a drug product sponsor to establish special procedures directed at patient safety. The intent of REMS is to manage known or potential serious risks of the product. The FDA can require a sponsor to include a REMS in a pending NDA or mandate a REMS postmarket when the FDA believes it necessary to ensure that the benefits of the drug outweigh its risks. A REMS will require the manufacturer to submit periodic postmarket assessments of whether the drug's risks are being adequately managed.

A REMS can require a variety of procedures including distribution of Medication Guides, a patient package insert, a communication plan aimed at health care professionals, or elements to assure safe use (commonly known as ETASU). If the drug has a particularly high potential for harm, the REMS may require that the health care providers have special training or experience, that the drug may be dispensed only in specified settings, and/or that the patient enroll in a registry and agree to testing and monitoring. For example, in March 2008 the FDA issued a notice requiring that the manufacturers of 25 high-risk drugs, including abarelix, alosetron, clozapine, fentanyl citrate, and thalidomide, must submit REMS plans (73 Fed. Reg. 16313). Certain drugs such as isotretinoin had REMS in place prior to the FDAAA. (*Note:* Although Accutane [brand of isotretinoin] was removed from the market in 2009 by its manufacturer, some generic versions of isotretinoin continue to be marketed.)

In July 2012, the FDA approved a REMS for extended-release and long-acting (ER/LA) opioid drugs (information at http://www.fda.gov/Drugs/DrugSafety/InformationbyDrugClass/ucm309742.htm#Q7). The central component of the REMS is an education program for prescribers made available by the ER/LA sponsors. It was expected that the FDA would make the education program mandatory for prescribers, but the FDA declined to do so at this time. (A "blueprint" outlining the core messages that should be conveyed to prescribers in an education program is available for downloading at http://www.fda.gov/Drugs/DrugSafety/InformationbyDrugClass/ucm163647.htm).

The FDA has also developed a REMS for transmucosal immediate-release fentanyl (TIRF) products. The FDA has published tables of all drug products with currently approved individual REMS, currently approved single shared system REMS, and released REMS at http://www.fda.gov/Drugs/DrugSafety/PostmarketDrugSafetyInformationforPatientsandProviders/ucm111350.htm. Providers and patients can use the tables to determine the REMS requirements for each listed product.

Postmarket Labeling

Surprisingly, prior to the FDAAA, the FDA did not have the authority to require manufacturers to include additional safety information or warnings in its labeling after the drug had been marketed. Generally manufacturers complied with the FDA's requests to edit the labeling, however, on occasion the changes were not effected until months after the FDA's requests and only after extensive negotiations occurred. The FDAAA provided the agency the authority to compel safety-related labeling changes when the FDA becomes aware of a serious drug risk that it believes should be included in the labeling.

Postmarket Drug Safety Information for Patients and Providers

An important feature of the FDAAA required that the FDA develop and maintain a consolidated and easily searchable website for patients and providers, including patient and professional labeling, recent safety information, information about implemented REMS, drug safety guidance documents and regulations, and drug-specific summary analyses of adverse drug reaction reports. Pharmacists should find the website a valuable resource for drug information, and it is accessible at http://www.fda.gov/cder/drugSafety.htm.

Another important safety provision the FDAAA established is known as the Sentinel Initiative. This is a proactive surveillance system designed to detect early signs of medication risk and safety problems. Under the Sentinel Initiative, the FDA is developing a new electronic system that will enable it to query a broad array of information data sources to identify possible postmarket adverse events. The FDA has partnered with CMS to analyze Medicare Part D claims data and also will partner with the Veterans Administration and an array of private health care organizations to analyze their data.

Acknowledging the importance of communicating risk to health care providers, patients, and consumers about all FDA-regulated products, the FDA published a risk communication strategic plan in September 2009, which is accessible from its homepage. This plan outlines the efforts that the agency will take to release communications and mentions pharmacists as a targeted group to receive this information.

DRUG EFFICACY STUDY IMPLEMENTATION

The FDA initiated the Drug Efficacy Study Implementation (DESI) program in 1968 in response to the 1962 Kefauver-Harris Amendment requiring that drugs be effective as well as safe. The FDA applied the efficacy requirement retroactively to all drugs marketed after 1938 (pioneer drugs as well as generic drugs). Until the efficacy requirement was added, the FDA had established an informal policy of allowing many post-1938 generics to be marketed as not new drugs to facilitate generic competition. The FDA considered these generics as "generally recognized" as safe if the pioneer drug had a safe marketing history. Under DESI, however, the FDA changed its policy and regarded generic drugs as new drugs, and required generic manufacturers to prove efficacy. Several drug manufacturers balked at having to establish efficacy for their currently marketed drug products and contested the legality of the government action. However, in three 1973 decisions (*Ciba Corporation v. Weinberger*, 412 U.S. 640; *Weinberger v. Bentex Pharmaceuticals, Inc.*, 412 U.S. 645; and *USV Pharmaceutical Corporation v. Weinberger*, 412 U.S. 655), the U.S. Supreme Court upheld the retroactive efficacy requirement for drugs as well as the FDA's authority to determine whether a drug is a new drug.

Making proof of efficacy retroactive to innovator and generic drugs burdened the FDA with the responsibility for evaluating the efficacy of the several thousand drugs that had been approved between 1938 and 1962. To obtain some assistance with this overwhelming project, the FDA commissioned the National Academy of Sciences National Research Council to study the drugs and submit its recommendations. The National Academy divided the task among 30 panels of experts within specific drug categories. Each drug was to be classified into one of six categories:

1. Effective
2. Probably effective (additional evidence required)
3. Possibly effective (little evidence submitted)
4. Ineffective (no acceptable evidence)
5. Effective, but . . . (effective but better, safer, or more conveniently administered drugs are available)
6. Ineffective as a fixed combination

To further lighten its burden, rather than requiring NDAs for generic drugs, the FDA created a new form of NDA, called an abbreviated new drug application (ANDA). Under an ANDA, proof of safety and efficacy was not required but rather only proof of bioequivalence and proof of acceptable manufacturing methods and controls. Because the agency became swamped with ANDA proposals, it began allowing manufacturers of generic drugs to continue to market their products pending the approval of their ANDAs. This practice prompted a lawsuit, *Hoffman LaRoche, Inc. v. Weinberger*, 425 F. Supp. 890 (D.D.C. 1975), in which a U.S. district court held that the FDA could not allow drugs to be marketed unless their ANDAs or NDAs had been approved.

The court ruling frustrated certain generic manufacturers who faced substantial economic losses if they could no longer market their products. Some of these manufacturers ignored the ruling and continued to market their generic drugs, prompting the FDA to seize some of their products. The manufacturers then sued the FDA. In *United States v. Articles of Drug . . . Lannett Co.*, 585 F.2d 575 (3rd Cir. 1978), and *Premo Pharmaceutical Laboratories, Inc. v. United States*, 629 F.2d 795 (2nd Cir. 1980), the generic manufacturers raised a very interesting argument, contending that because the active ingredients in the parent drugs had already been approved as safe and effective, their generic drugs were not new drugs. Therefore, they advanced, the FDA had no statutory authority to withhold the approval of generic drugs. The FDA countered that new drug status is warranted for generic drugs because their safety and efficacy cannot be determined until such questions as the methods of manufacture and proof of bioequivalence are answered. Federal courts reached contrary decisions on this issue until the U.S. Supreme Court finally determined in *United States v. Generix Drug Corporation*, 103 S. Ct. 1298 (1983), that a generic drug is a new drug, thus subject to FDA approval.

"PAPER" NEW DRUG APPLICATIONS

Although the FDA would accept ANDAs for generic drug equivalents marketed between 1938 and 1962, it did not accept ANDAs for generic equivalents marketed after 1962. The FDA held the position that it lacked statutory authority to do so. Recognizing the inconsistency of allowing ANDAs for pre-1962 generic drugs but requiring NDAs for post-1962 generic drugs, the FDA compromised by implementing its "paper" NDA policy in the late 1970s. Under this policy, a generic drug manufacturer would not have to duplicate the actual research establishing the safety and efficacy of the innovator drug, as a full NDA would require. Rather, the generic drug manufacturer could submit evidence of its drug's safety and efficacy on the basis of the published scientific data generated from the innovator manufacturer's studies. Needless to say, innovator drug manufacturers were not pleased with this policy and judicially challenged the practice of "paper" NDAs in *Burroughs Wellcome Co. v. Schweiker*, 649 F.2d 221 (4th Cir. 1981), but the FDA prevailed. Nonetheless, the policy helped only a small number of post-1962 generic drugs because there was seldom enough published literature to support the manufacturer's claims of safety and efficacy for the drug. Clearly, a legislative solution was needed, and that solution came in the form of an amendment to the FDCA in 1984 called the Drug Price Competition and Patent Term Restoration Act (PTRA), as discussed next.

DRUG PRICE COMPETITION AND PATENT TERM RESTORATION ACT (PTRA) OF 1984

Essentially, the PTRA (Hatch-Waxman amendment) (P.L. 98-417) statutorily created the ANDA, which had been the FDA's policy for pre-1962 generic drugs. As discussed previously an ANDA allows a sponsor to streamline the approval process because it does not have to conduct clinical studies to establish safety and efficacy. Rather, the sponsor needs only to submit sufficient information to demonstrate that the generic contains the same active ingredient, route of administration, dosage form and strength as the pioneer drug; is bioequivalent to the pioneer drug; and has acceptable manufacturing methods and control procedures. The FDCA establishes a presumption that if the products are bioequivalent then the generic drug is as safe and effective as the innovator drug.

Bioequivalence must usually be established through evidence obtained from human clinical trials establishing either that the generic drug's extent of absorption (maximum concentration, Cmax) and rate of absorption (area under the curve, AUC) at the site of action are not significantly different from those of the pioneer drug or that the extent of absorption is the same and the rate of absorption is intentionally different, as long as the difference is not essential to attaining effective drug concentrations in the body and is considered medically insignificant for the drug. The different rate of absorption must be reflected in the drug's labeling. A company is not required to conduct clinical trials to establish bioequivalence if the FDA can conclude bioequivalence from other studies or other facts submitted by the company.

The significant statutory concession for generic drug manufacturers was not without two important concessions for innovator drug manufacturers. First, the law allows the FDA to grant innovator drugs patent-term extensions. The innovator drug manufacturers lobbied hard for patent extensions because their products normally receive patents long before the products are ultimately approved for marketing. As a result, often only a few of the 20 years granted for patent protection remain after the drug is marketed. It is during this time of patent protection that innovator manufacturers generally must recover the costs incurred during the IND/NDA phase. Patent extensions are available only if the patent has not expired. The second benefit the law provides is market exclusivity for an innovator manufacturer that develops a new chemical entity or a new use for a previously approved drug. Market exclusivity works independently of the drug's patent status. In general, for new chemical entities approved under an NDA, the market exclusivity provision prevents a generic drug application from being submitted for 5 years from the date of approval of the drug. For a new use for a previously approved drug, the act grants 3 years exclusivity against an ANDA.

In order to ultimately obtain approval for an ANDA, the generic manufacturer must make a patent certification. The law provides four types of certification a generic applicant can make relevant to the patent of the reference drug:

(I) That the NDA holder did not file information on the patent to the FDA
(II) That the patent already had expired
(III) The date that the patent will expire
(IV) That the patent is invalid or will not be infringed by the manufacture, use, or sale of the generic applicant's drug

If the applicant submits a paragraph I or II certification, the FDA will approve the ANDA provided all other requirements of the application are met. If a paragraph III certification is filed, the approval will likely be effective on the patent expiration date. If, however, a paragraph IV certification is filed, the process gets considerably more complicated. The applicant must notify the patent owner and NDA holder, citing the factual and legal bases for why the applicant believes the patent is invalid. If the patent owner sues the generic applicant, the FDA is automatically enjoined from approving the ANDA for 30 months, unless a court issues a final ruling that the patent is invalid prior to expiration of 30 months. To encourage generic manufacturers to challenge patents, since to do so is very costly, the law awards 180 days of marketing exclusivity to the first generic applicant to file an ANDA containing a paragraph IV certification. Of course, the generic applicant must obtain a favorable court decision on the patent issue to obtain this exclusivity.

Controversies for Health Care Practitioners

The PTRA created two controversies for health care practitioners. First, the law allows a generic drug to statistically vary in its rate and extent of absorption by 620 percent from the parent and still be considered as bioequivalent. This led to the position that if a patient used generic X 1 month, which was 120 percent, and generic Y the next month, which was 220 percent, there could be a 40 percent blood level difference between the two products, resulting in adverse clinical outcomes for the patient. The FDA countered this concern in public announcements by clarifying the statistical procedure involved. It further provided that in analyzing data on generic drugs approved between October 1984 and September 1986, the average difference in absorption between generic and pioneer products was only 63.5 percent, which should not produce clinical differences in patients. Nonetheless, the controversy continues for some drug products.

The second controversy created by the act centered on whether a generic drug product could be prescribed and dispensed for an indication that the innovator drug product has been granted exclusivity. For example, can a pharmacist legally substitute a generic propranolol prescribed for postmyocardial infarction when the innovator brand propranolol has marketing exclusivity for that indication? The general answer to this question is yes because this is really the use of an approved drug (the generic drug) for an off-label indication.

A separate but related issue is whether the FDA can legally approve an ANDA for a new generic drug product even though the labeling of the generic product will not include one or more of the indications appearing on the labeling of the innovator drug product because of the exclusivity provisions. (The law provides that the labeling of the generic drug must be the same as the innovator drug. This creates a dilemma, however, because if the innovator drug has exclusivity over certain indications, those indications could not be included in the generic drug's labeling.) The federal court in *Bristol-Myers Squibb Co. v. Shalala*, 91 F.3d 1493 (D.C. Cir. 1996) held that the FDA indeed could still approve the ANDA for a new generic drug, despite the fact that the manufacturer held exclusivity rights for 3 years to an indication approved by supplemental application and that this indication is not included on the generic's labeling. Bristol-Myers argued that the statute, § 355(j)(2)(A)(v), requires that the generic label be "the same" as that of the innovator and because it cannot be the same, the ANDA must be rejected. The court, however, agreed with the government's analysis that the manufacturer's interpretation is at variance with other provisions in the law and legislative intent, that being that the new generic drug be safe and effective for each indication appearing on the label. The fact that the label does not list every indication listed on the pioneer's label is irrelevant. Even more persuasive to the court, however, was the fact that if Bristol-Myers's interpretation prevailed, a new generic drug product would be precluded from the market for 3 years every time a manufacturer added a supplemental indication. Theoretically, then, the manufacturer of an innovator drug product could strategically file supplemental indications over several years, precluding any generic competition.

Drug Manufacturer Controversies

The PTRA has created some very controversial practices by drug manufacturers. Some of these practices have existed since the act's passage, but in the past few years have they captured the attention of Congress and the public because several blockbuster drug patents either have recently expired or will soon do so. One such practice involves an innovator manufacturer producing a generic version of its brand-name product, called an "authorized generic," just as its patent is about to expire or be successfully challenged by a generic competitor. The FDA takes the position that the innovator may do this without an ANDA, because the generic and brand-name drug products are the same and thus approved under the NDA. This means that the innovator manufacturer can produce the generic and compete directly with a generic manufacturer who filed a successful paragraph IV ANDA. The generic manufacturer no longer derives as much value from the 180-day market exclusivity, and the innovator manufacturer retains some market share it otherwise would have lost.

Another controversy involves the 30-month stay in ANDA approval when the patent holder sues the generic company for patent infringement. Critics contend that many innovator manufacturers sue to obtain the 30-month exclusivity, even though they have very weak legal arguments on their side and no chance of ultimately prevailing. Some manufacturers have piggybacked lawsuits to allow for additional 30-month exclusivity periods, although recent legislation has limited this practice. To make matters even more difficult for generic manufacturers attempting to invalidate patents, innovator manufacturers commonly file secondary patents after the initial patent, covering such things as manufacturing processes, methods of use, and even new tablet coatings. These secondary patents can add to the legal complexities facing generic companies.

Some innovator manufacturers engage in a related practice, often called product hopping. When a product nears its patent expiration, a manufacturer may make some type of product change, such as extended release or a different salt, and secure an additional patent. The manufacturer will then extensively market the new product, encouraging patients to switch from the old product to the new product, thereby reducing the market for generic versions of the old drug.

Yet another practice and one under investigation by the FTC, Justice Department, and Congress involves the innovator company paying the generic manufacturer not to market its generic—a practice sometimes called exclusion payments or pay-for-delay agreements. Recall that a generic company filing a successful paragraph IV ANDA enjoys a 180-day exclusivity period. To prevent this from occurring, some innovator manufacturers have entered into patent settlement agreements with generic companies.

The settlement agreement includes payment to the generic manufacturer for all litigation costs plus a significant sum, usually more than the generic manufacturer would make marketing the drug for the 180-day period. The innovator manufacturer still profits significantly by retaining marketing exclusivity for an additional 180 days. In 2011, the U.S. Supreme Court denied a writ of certiorari and let stand a federal court of appeals ruling that a pay-for-delay agreement between Bayer and Teva involving Cipro did not violate the antitrust laws (*Louisiana Wholesale Drug Co., Inc. v. Bayer AG*, 131 S.Ct. 1606 (2011)). The federal court of appeals found that the settlement agreement did not exceed the scope of the Cipro patent and thus did not cause cognizable injury (*Arkansas Carpenters Health and Welfare Fund v. Bayer AG*, 604 F.3d 98 (C.A.2 (N.Y. 2010))). Conflicting courts of appeal decisions on this issue, however, will likely require a Supreme Court determination.

Finally, some generic manufacturers have contended that some brand-name manufacturers have refused to provide them samples of the brand-name drug that they need for use in clinical trials testing for bioequivalence. They allege the brand-name companies with products subject to REMS are distorting a REMS provision that restricts distributing drugs that are dangerous or subject to abuse.

SECTION 505(B)(2) NDAS

The PTRA not only statutorily created the ANDA but also established what is known as a 505(b)(2) application, replacing the old paper NDA. A manufacturer might choose this route of application for a drug product, which is similar to the reference product but contains significant changes. The 505(b)(2) application is intended to encourage sponsors to develop improved generics that could not be approved under an ANDA because of the significant changes. Under this application, the sponsor is allowed to rely, at least in part, on safety and efficacy data furnished by another applicant—even unpublished data that are not legally protected—thus reducing the number of clinical trials required. Depending on the extent of the changes from the reference product, the manufacturer could be granted 3 to 5 years of market exclusivity. The 505(b)(2) application has received considerable notoriety in recent years as manufacturers have used it to receive approval for new indications of established drugs by relying on safety reports in a previous NDA. Some generic manufacturers have used the 505(b)(2) application process to obtain market approval when their generic drug does not qualify for ANDA submission because the dosage form or route of administration varies from the pioneer drug.

OVER-THE-COUNTER (OTC) DRUG REVIEW

The 1962 efficacy requirement retroactively applied not only to prescription drugs for which NDAs had been approved, but also to OTC drugs. As a result, after 10 years of attention to prescription drugs under the DESI review, in 1972 the FDA began reviewing OTC drugs marketed between 1938 and 1962. Although the FDA examined the efficacy of each prescription drug on a case-by-case basis in the DESI review, the agency initiated a different system to review OTC drugs. This system, which continues today for post-1962 OTC products, evaluates OTC products on the basis of therapeutic category, rather than individually, and classifies products through rule making rather than on a case-by-case basis. The agency took this approach for several reasons. First, there were between 100,000 and 500,000 OTC drug products on the market, many of which did not have approved NDAs; reviewing each of these products would overwhelm the FDA's resources. Second, litigation to remove unsafe or ineffective individual OTC products would be prohibitively time-consuming and expensive. Third, nearly all the OTC drugs were prepared from only about 200 active ingredients.

Under the procedures for classifying OTC drugs as safe and effective (21 C.F.R. part 330), the FDA appoints advisory review panels of qualified experts to consider the drugs by class (e.g., analgesics, antacids) and to make recommendations to the agency. The FDA then publishes the panels' recommendations in the *Federal Register*, requesting public comment. After receiving public comments, the agency publishes a proposed rule in the *Federal Register*. Then, the agency publishes a monograph, identifying which active ingredients are generally recognized as safe and effective and, thus, may be marketed. The monograph further specifies the labeling. Products that do not contain approved active ingredients or labeling must be removed and, if possible, reformulated and relabeled. Alternately, the manufacturer of a product that does not conform to the criteria in the monograph may withdraw the product and follow the NDA procedures or petition to amend the monograph. New OTC drug products that conform to the published monograph requirements may be marketed without FDA approval.

The final monograph on a reviewed ingredient specifies in which of three categories the ingredient is placed:

1. Category I includes ingredients generally recognized as safe, effective, and not misbranded.
2. Category II includes those ingredients that are not generally recognized as safe and effective or that are misbranded.
3. Category III includes ingredients for which data available are insufficient to permit classification.

Since the implementation of the OTC drug review, the FDA has allowed by regulation the continued marketing of drugs placed in category III until evidence was sufficient to place them in categories I or II. Otherwise, the FDA feared, drug manufacturers would not submit their products for review, and the FDA would be forced to bring new drug litigation against each product. In *Cutler v. Kennedy*, 475 F. Supp. 838 (D.D.C. 1979), however, a group of consumers contested the FDA's policy and demanded that the FDA remove all category III products from the market. The court agreed with the plaintiffs that an FDA regulation allowing these OTC drugs to be marketed pending the agency's determination of safety and efficacy was an affront to the FDCA's premarketing procedures. Although the court concluded that the FDA did not have the authority to continue this practice, the court disagreed with the plaintiff's claim that the FDA must seek out and remove category III drugs from the market, finding that there was no statutory ultimatum for this action. In effect, the *Cutler* decision caused the FDA to revise its regulations but continue informally to do what it had been doing by regulation.

MARKETED UNAPPROVED DRUGS

Based upon the preceding discussions, one might be led to believe that except for some drugs marketed prior to 1938, all marketed drugs today have been approved by the FDA. For various reasons, however, this is not the case. In fact, in a compliance policy guide (CPG) published in June 2006 and revised in September 2011, the FDA estimated that there are as many as several thousand prescription and OTC drug products marketed illegally without required FDA approval (http://www.fda.gov/ICECI/ComplianceManuals/CompliancePolicyGuidanceManual/ucm074382.htm). The 2006 CPG signifies the beginning of what the agency terms its "Unapproved Drugs Initiative" and describes the FDA's enforcement intentions toward these unapproved products. The FDA stated that since the initiative started it has removed more than a thousand unapproved drugs from the market (76 Fed. Reg. 58398, 2011). In 2011, the agency launched major enforcement actions against hundreds of marketed unapproved cough, cold, and allergy drug products (76 Fed. Reg. 11794, March 3, 2011). In July 2012, based upon reports of medication errors causing serious adverse events, the FDA announced that it was taking enforcement action against companies manufacturing or distributing "unapproved" single-ingredient, immediate release oxycodone products (77 Fed. Reg. 40069).

As explained in the CPG, there are many reasons why unapproved drug products exist on the market:

1. Recall in the DESI discussion that until DESI was instituted in 1968, the FDA had a policy of allowing many post-1938 generics to be marketed as not "new drugs" if the pioneer or innovator drug had a safe marketing history.
2. During that same time period, the FDA allowed some drugs to be marketed that were not identical or similar to other marketed drugs, either on the basis that the FDA felt that they were not new drugs or simply because the agency did not take action against them.
3. Some drugs are still being marketed pending a final determination of their efficacy under DESI reviews. (Technically these drugs should not be considered illegally marketed because the FDA has allowed the products to be marketed pending DESI review.)
4. Some products that have been determined to lack evidence of efficacy after DESI review have yet to be removed from market.
5. Some similar drugs to the products pending DESI review, which have never submitted applications for review, remain on the market.
6. Many drugs are being marketed claiming to be grandfathered as pre-1938 drugs, yet have changed labeling or composition, thus voiding their exemption status.
7. Some drug manufacturers simply market their product without approval, hoping to get away with it for as long as possible.
8. There are illegally marketed OTC drugs either because monographs do not allow their ingredients or because they were never subject to the OTC review.

In the CPG, the agency explains that these illegally marketed drugs remain on the market because first they have to be identified (no easy process), and then to remove each product requires a considerable amount of scarce FDA resources and time to comply with legal procedures. As a result, the FDA prioritizes enforcement, with highest priority going to drugs that present safety risks, those that lack evidence of effectiveness, and those that involve health fraud. Despite the FDA's attempts to remove unapproved drugs through the initiative, new unapproved drugs have constantly appeared on the market since the issuance of the 2006 CPG. Relying on the FDA's slow enforcement procedures and scarce resources, unscrupulous manufacturers have attempted to capitalize on profits before the FDA can force their products off the market. As a result, the 2011 revised CPG announced that any unapproved drugs introduced onto the market after September 19, 2011, are subject to immediate enforcement action, without prior notice and without regard to the enforcement priorities established in the CPG.

The FDA will more likely take enforcement action against unapproved identical or similar products when one manufacturer obtains NDA approval for its product. The agency stated it will generally allow a 1-year grace period from the date of NDA approval before it will initiate enforcement action against the unapproved products of the same type. The 1-year grace period, however, is dependent upon various factors and will be determined on a case-by-case basis. Pharmacists should exercise professional judgment when dispensing drugs of a particular type where one is approved and the others are not.

From a risk management perspective, it might generally be wise to dispense the approved product. Approved drug products can be identified at the Drugs@FDA website (http://www.accessdata.fda.gov/scripts/cder/drugsatfda/index.cfm).

DRUGS INTENDED TO TREAT SERIOUS AND LIFE-THREATENING DISEASES

Over the years, the new drug approval process and the FDA have been criticized for denying or impeding access to new drugs for people with serious and life-threatening diseases for which no other treatment exists. In *United States v. Rutherford*, 442 U.S. 544 (1979), reported in the case studies section, terminally ill patients unsuccessfully sued the FDA in an attempt to obtain an unapproved drug for cancer treatment. The FDA continually faces the dilemma of expediting patient access to drugs intended to treat these conditions, while protecting patients against unsafe, ineffective, or even fraudulent products.

The FDA has not been unsympathetic to the plight of those with life-threatening diseases. In recent years, it has modified its policy by enacting regulations with respect to both patient treatment with investigational drugs and drug approval for potentially life-saving drugs. These regulations were essentially codified and replaced by the FDAMA, as discussed here.

PATIENT TREATMENT WITH INVESTIGATIONAL DRUGS (§ 561)

The FDA had long held the position that investigational drugs must be used only for experimentation, not treatment. That position changed, however, as the incidence of acquired immune deficiency syndrome (AIDS) skyrocketed in the United States and researchers began to develop new drugs that showed promise for treating this and other serious diseases. The FDAMA modified the FDCA to state that an investigational drug may be provided for widespread access outside controlled clinical trials to treat patients with serious or immediately life-threatening diseases for which no comparable or satisfactory alternative therapy is available. The FDA will approve the investigational drug for treatment only if:

1. It is to be used for a serious or immediately life-threatening disease or condition.
2. There is no comparable or satisfactory alternative therapy available.
3. The drug is under investigation for the disease or condition.
4. The sponsor is actively pursuing marketing approval of the drug.
5. In the case of serious diseases, there is sufficient evidence of safety and effectiveness for the use.
6. In the case of immediately life-threatening diseases, there is a reasonable basis to conclude that the drug may be effective and would not expose patients to unreasonable and significant risk.

INDIVIDUAL PATIENT ACCESS TO INVESTIGATIONAL DRUGS FOR SERIOUS DISEASES (PARALLEL TRACK POLICY) (§ 561)

With respect to investigational drugs, the FDAMA also provides that an individual patient acting through a physician may request an investigational drug from the manufacturer if the physician determines that the patient has no comparable or satisfactory alternative therapy and that the risk to the patient from the drug is no greater than the risk from the disease or condition. To qualify, the FDA must determine that there is sufficient evidence of safety and effectiveness to support its use and that use of the drug will not interfere with clinical investigations in support of marketing approval. The sponsor also must submit to the FDA a protocol describing the use of the drug.

FDA policy has restricted the medical treatment with an IND to those drugs in phase 3 of the NDA process. A public interest group, formed on behalf of terminally ill patients, sued to enjoin the FDA from enforcing this policy and thus allow terminally ill, mentally competent adults, acting on a prescriber's advice, to obtain IND drugs that have reached phase 2 (*Abigail Alliance for Better Access to Developmental Drugs and Washington Legal Foundation v. Eschenbach*, 445 F.3d 470 (C.A.D.C. 2006)). A three-judge panel of the District of Columbia Court of Appeals reversed and remanded the district court's decision, finding for the plaintiffs. The justices concluded that terminally ill, mentally competent adults have a protected liberty interest under the Due Process Clause of the Constitution to IND drugs in phase 2 when there are no alternative approved treatment options available. The court relied heavily on the U.S. Supreme Court decision of *Cruzan v. Director, Missouri Department of Health*, 497 U.S. 261 (1990), holding that an individual has a due process right to refuse life-sustaining medical treatment. The court could find no substantial difference between the due process right in *Cruzan* and the one plaintiffs sought in this case because both involve the right of the individual to the "possession and control of his own person . . ." (p. 484).

On December 11, 2006, without mentioning the *Abigail* decision, the FDA announced a proposed regulation to make experimental drugs more widely available to seriously ill patients with no other treatment options (http://www.fda.gov/NewsEvents/Newsroom/PressAnnouncements/2006/ucm108798.htm). Under the proposed regulation, access to experimental drugs even in phase 1 would be available to individual patients, as well as small patient groups and larger populations. The proposed regulation was amended and became final in August 2009 (74 Fed. Reg. 40900), together with the announcement of a new FDA website for patients and health care professionals (http://www.fda.gov/Drugs/DevelopmentApprovalProcess/HowDrugsareDevelopedandApproved/ApprovalApplications/InvestigationalNewDrugINDApplication/ucm172492.htm). The final regulation expands and clarifies the treatment use of experimental drugs and was accompanied by another final regulation clarifying and establishing the criteria for drug manufacturers to charge patients for investigational drugs (74 Fed. Reg. 40872).

FDA's final regulation might be particularly favorable for patients in need of investigational drugs since the full D.C. court of appeals issued an 8 to 2 decision in August 2007 reversing the decision of the three-judge panel in *Abigail* (495 F.3d 695, C.A.D.C). The majority noted that it was reluctant to create new constitutional rights and that a right to experimental drugs is not a fundamental right deeply rooted in the nation's history and tradition. The court felt that this was an action better left to Congress. The majority also distinguished *Cruzan*, stating that the decision in that case was predicated on a common-law rule that forced medical treatment is battery and that there is a long tradition of protecting the patient's decision to refuse unwanted medical treatment. The plaintiffs appealed to the U.S. Supreme Court, but the Court declined to consider the case thus allowing the court of appeal's decision to stand (128 S.Ct. 1069 (January 14, 2008)).

Expedited Approval of Drugs Intended to Treat Life-Threatening Illnesses ("Fast Track Approval") (§ 506)

Motivated primarily by the AIDS epidemic, the FDA enacted regulations in 1988 and 1992 (21 C.F.R. § 312.80–312.88, modified by § 314.50) to expedite the development, evaluation, and marketing of new drugs intended to treat serious or life-threatening illnesses. The substance of these regulations has been codified by the FDAMA, which generally provides that at the request of a new drug's sponsor, the FDA will expedite the review of the drug if (1) it is intended for the treatment of a serious or life-threatening condition and demonstrates the potential to address unmet medical needs for the condition, and (2) the product has an effect on a clinical endpoint or on a surrogate endpoint reasonably likely to predict clinical benefit. Approval will be conditioned on the completion of postmarketing, or phase 4, clinical studies to verify and describe the drug's clinical benefit. The drug's sponsor must submit all promotional materials for FDA approval at least 30 days before dissemination. The FDA may use expedited procedures to remove the drug if phase 4 studies do not confirm the drug's safety and effectiveness.

BIOLOGICS

Biologics or biologicals are products derived from living organisms, and include viruses, therapeutic serums, toxins, antitoxins, vaccines, blood and blood components, and derivatives applicable to the prevention, treatment, or cure of a disease or condition of humans (42 U.S.C. § 262(i)). Biological products have had a history of government regulation since 1902 (4 years prior to the first federal drug law) and today are regulated under both the Public Health Service Act (PHSA) and the FDCA. Although biological products require premarket approval by the FDA and are subject to the FDCA requirements like new drug products, unlike drugs, biologicals are licensed under the PHSA. The FDA will approve a license upon demonstration that the product is safe, pure, and potent, and that the facility meets required standards. If a biological product contains a drug, it will be classified as either a biological or a drug depending upon the product's primary mode of action.

Unlike with drugs, the law has not recognized generic biological products until the passage of the ACA in 2010. The health care reform law contains a subtitle called the Biologics Price Competition and Innovation Act (BPCIA) intended to create a regulatory framework to facilitate the approval of generic biologics, also called biosimilars or follow-on biologics. The BPCIA grants the FDA the authority to determine whether a biosimilar is therapeutically equivalent to a reference biologic and thus can be substituted in the same manner as generic drug products. The notion of allowing generic versions of biologics has been (and still is) controversial because some contend that current science may not be adequate to ensure that a biosimilar is as safe and effective as the reference biologic. This is because the manufacturing process for many biologics is very complex and involves numerous steps. Often, it is not even known which of the components are the active ingredient(s), and efficacy may be a sum of the parts rather than a particular component. In February 2012, the FDA released three draft guidance documents in an effort to initiate the process of determining what factors must be considered in the biosimilar approval process. The BPCIA grants a 12-year marketing exclusivity period to the reference product.

MEDWATCH VOLUNTARY REPORTING PROGRAM

The FDA maintains a voluntary reporting system called MedWatch that allows health care professionals to report any serious adverse events, potential and actual product use errors, and product quality problems related to drugs, biologics, medical devices, special nutritional products, and cosmetics directly to the agency. An official reporting form (FDA 3500) can be accessed and completed online at http://www.fda.gov/downloads/Safety/MedWatch/HowToReport/DownloadForms/UCM082725.pdf. Pharmacists submit the largest number of adverse drug reaction reports and also are urged to report any problem with a drug product, including improper labeling, the presence of foreign or particulate matter, imperfectly manufactured dosage forms, abnormal color or taste, and questionable stability. The FDA emphasizes that it is the moral obligation of health care professionals to furnish the agency with information about suspected adverse events, product quality problems, and product errors. The agency encourages practitioners to submit reports, pointing out that a report is not a legal claim, nor an acknowledgment that there is an adverse event, problem, or error. The identities of the practitioners and the patients are confidential.

In addition to reports related to drugs, biologics, and devices, the FDA requests practitioners to submit reports of clinically significant toxicity that may be related to the ingestion of substantial quantities of nutrients or food components in dietary supplements, including vitamins and minerals. It also seeks reports of severe and well-documented nonmicrobiological reactions associated with food and food additives.

The MedWatch program not only provides for reporting but also provides a wealth of safety information on products, accessible from its website at http://www.fda.gov/medwatch.

PHARMACY REQUIREMENT TO PROVIDE PATIENTS WITH MEDWATCH NUMBER

Although the MedWatch program was intended initially for reporting by health care professionals, the scope has been broadened by the FDAAA to include patient reporting. The FDAAA requires the FDA to implement a dormant 2004 regulation mandating that pharmacies must provide patients with notification of a toll-free number so they can report adverse events (73 Fed. Reg. 402, Ja. 3, 2008). As of July 1, 2009, pharmacies must provide patients with the statement: "Call your doctor for medical advice about side effects. You may report side effects to the FDA at 1-800-FDA-1088" (which is the MedWatch number). Notification to patients must be distributed to patients with each new and refill prescription and may occur by any of the following means:

- On a sticker attached to the container or package
- On a preprinted vial cap
- On a separate sheet of paper
- In patient medication information distributed by the pharmacy
- In a MedGuide

MEDICAL DEVICES

Before 1976, the adulteration and misbranding provisions of the FDCA did not provide the FDA with enough authority to protect the public adequately in the face of a proliferation of quack products and the advances in sophisticated device technologies. As a result, Congress enacted the Medical Device Act of 1976 (P.L. No. 94-295), amending the FDCA to establish a comprehensive system of device regulation that includes device classification, premarket testing, and standards of performance. Devices marketed before the act, called "preamendment devices," were permitted to remain on the market pending classification or other type of action by the FDA.

Pursuant to the device amendments, the FDA must classify all devices marketed after 1976 into one of three classes:

1. Class I devices require the least regulation because they pose the least potential harm to users; therefore, "general controls" are adequate to ensure safety and effectiveness. General controls require that device manufacturers register their facility and list their products with the FDA, provide premarket notification in some cases, maintain records and reports, and adhere to good manufacturing practices. These devices include needles, scissors, examination gloves, stethoscopes, and toothbrushes.

2. Class II devices are those for which general controls alone are insufficient to ensure safety and effectiveness. These products must meet specific performance standards established by the FDA before the FDA will permit marketing. Such products include insulin syringes, infusion pumps, thermometers, diagnostic reagents, tampons, and electric heating pads.

3. Class III devices must have premarket approval because they are life–supporting or life–sustaining or they present a potential unreasonable risk of illness or injury. Class III devices include pacemakers, soft contact lenses, and replacement heart valves. Any devices not marketed before 1976 initially fall into class III, unless the FDA determines that they are substantially equivalent to a class I or II device.

Like certain drugs, certain devices may be available by prescription only. Under the law, these are devices that have a potential for harm or require collateral measures to ensure their proper use. Examples of restricted devices include diaphragms and contact lenses.

Custom devices ordered by health care professionals to meet the special needs of individual patients, such as orthopedic footwear, are generally exempt from some requirements such as registration, performance standards, and premarket approval. Other general control requirements do apply, however, such as conforming to good manufacturing practices and the adulteration and misbranding provisions.

The FDA can reclassify devices on the basis of new information of safety and efficacy, and has reclassified hundreds of devices from class III to class II and from class II to class I. If a manufacturer's petition for reclassification is approved, the reclassification applies to the generic type of device, not just the specific device in question. Thus, the reclassification will benefit not only the particular manufacturer but also its competitors.

Medical device firms must report to the FDA any death or serious injury that may be related to their products. If the FDA determines that a device presents an unreasonable risk of substantial harm, it may require the manufacturer to notify all health care professionals or to recall the product. If this action is insufficient, the FDA may require the manufacturer to (1) repair the device, (2) replace the device, or (3) refund the purchase price of the device. Alternately, the FDA can seize medical devices, enjoin shipment, and withdraw marketing approval to protect the public.

In 1990, Congress amended the FDCA device provisions by enacting a law that requires device-user facilities and distributors to report to the Secretary of Health and

Human Services any death, serious injury, or serious illness that may be related to the product (Safe Medical Devices Act of 1990). A device-user facility is defined as "a hospital, ambulatory surgical facility, nursing home, or outpatient treatment facility that is not a physician's office." Before this law, only manufacturers were required to report adverse incidents. This law was modified and expanded in 1992 (P.L. 102-300). Subsequently, the FDAMA has removed the requirement that distributors must submit adverse event reports to the FDA or to device manufacturers. Distributors must, however, maintain records of adverse events.

COSMETICS

Sections 601 to 603 of the FDCA and 21 C.F.R. parts 700 to 740 regulate cosmetics. Cosmetics do not have the same stringent legal requirements that drugs and devices have. Premarket approval from the FDA is not necessary for a cosmetic, although manufacturers must substantiate the safety of their cosmetic product and each of its ingredients. Moreover, the manufacturer of a cosmetic does not have to conform to current good manufacturing practices or even register with the FDA; registration is voluntary. The FDA may, however, remove a cosmetic from the market if it is misbranded, adulterated, or determined to be a health hazard.

A cosmetic must be labeled with a list of its ingredients in descending order of predominance. Fragrances or flavors may simply be listed as "fragrances" or "flavors." The ingredients must be placed on the outside of the package or container so the consumer can read them at the point of purchase. This information is especially important to consumers with allergies to certain ingredients.

Some cosmetics must have specified warning statements. For example, cosmetics in self-pressurized containers must contain the warning: "Intentional misuse by deliberately concentrating and inhaling contents can be harmful or fatal."

A cosmetic may be misbranded if its labeling is false, misleads the consumer, or lacks the required information, or if the label information is not clear enough to be read and understood by an ordinary consumer. In addition, the product may be deemed misbranded if the container is made or filled so as to be misleading or if the packaging and labeling do not conform to the requirements of the Poison Prevention Packaging Act. If substantiation of the product's safety is not available, the principal display panel must contain: "Warning—The safety of this product has not been determined," or the product will be deemed misbranded.

A cosmetic is adulterated if

- It contains any poisonous or deleterious substances that may injure users.
- It contains any filthy, putrid, or decomposed substance.
- It was prepared under unsanitary conditions.
- The container contains a substance that may contaminate the contents.
- It contains an unsafe color additive but is not a hair dye.

Hair dyes that contain coal tar are exempt from the adulteration and color additive provisions of the law, even though coal tar is an irritant to many users. The product with coal tar must have a warning label, stating

Caution—this product contains certain ingredients that may cause skin irritation on certain individuals, and a preliminary test according to accompanying directions should first be made. This product must not be used for dyeing the eyelashes or eyebrows; to do so may cause blindness.

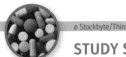
© Stockbyte/Thinkstock

STUDY SCENARIOS AND QUESTIONS

1. A drug manufacturer wishes to market its approved drug for use in a disease for which it has not been approved (off-label use). Explain whether marketing the drug for this use would make it a new drug.

2. A patient who has been prescribed a newly marketed drug complains to you, the pharmacist, about the high price of the drug. The patient remarks that it cannot cost more than a few cents to make such a little tablet. "Who is making all the profit?" the patient queries. How would you address the patient's concerns?

3. A pharmacist who is a member of a managed care formulary evaluation committee is evaluating whether to include on the formulary a newly marketed drug. The drug is more expensive than other drugs in its class and is rated by the FDA as type 5 and S. If you were the pharmacist, explain why you would or would not include the drug on the formulary.

4. As a pharmacist, you inform a patient that the patient's copay will be $15 less if the patient gets the generic drug rather than the brand prescribed. The patient is concerned about quality and asks you whether generic drugs are as safe and effective as brand-name drugs. How would you explain this to the patient?

5. A patient asks you, a pharmacist, whether OTC drugs are evaluated the same as prescription drugs for safety and efficacy. Provide an explanation to this patient.

6. Mentadine is an IND drug in phase 3. One of your terminally ill patients asks you if it is legally possible for her to get this drug. Respond to the patient's inquiry.

7. A patient is prescribed a brand-name drug. The patient asks if generics are available. Your research shows generics are available but unapproved by the FDA. You tell the patient this and the patient asks how it is legally possible that unapproved drugs can be sold and whether they are safe. Respond to the patient's inquiry.

8. A physician calls you, a pharmacist, and tells you she suspects that a drug is causing a certain adverse reaction in some of her patients. She asks you if you have noticed anything similar and you report you have. She asks you if the adverse reaction should be reported, and if so, how and to whom?

9. A physician asks you, a pharmacist, what the difference is between class I, II, and III devices, and whether devices have to be approved by the FDA prior to marketing. Respond to the physician's inquiry.

DRUG ADVERTISING AND PROMOTION

Product advertising and promotion is essential in order to inform and educate the public about new and existing products, and at the same time is critical to the commercial success of the products, and drug products are no exception. Because drugs are more dangerous than most products, however, and in the case of prescription drugs often require evaluation beyond the expertise of the consumer, the federal government has chosen to regulate the advertising and promotional activities of drug products more strictly than typical products. Of particular regulatory concern are communications promoting drugs for "off-label use," false and misleading claims, unsupported product comparisons, and overstatements of efficacy or understatements of risk. Congress has made two federal agencies responsible for the regulation of drug advertising. The FDA regulates prescription drug advertising under the FDCA (15 U.S.C. § 352(n)), whereas the FTC (usually in collaboration with the FDA) regulates nonprescription drug advertising under the Federal Trade Commission Act (15 U.S.C. § 45). Another federal law, the Lanham Trademark Act (15 U.S.C. § 1125), allows private parties a cause of action against false and misleading advertising. At the state level, most pharmacy practice acts prohibit pharmacists from false, misleading, or deceptive advertising.

THE FIRST AMENDMENT TO THE U.S. CONSTITUTION

Any government regulation of advertising and promotion creates legal controversy in light of the U.S. Constitution's First Amendment guarantee of free speech. The U.S. Supreme Court has held that commercial speech (e.g., promotional activities by product sellers) falls under the First Amendment, but has also recognized the need for government regulation of commercial activities, even when that regulation may have an incidental effect on speech in certain cases. Thus, government regulation must always walk the tightrope between protecting the public and violating free speech rights.

The Supreme Court has articulated the application of the First Amendment to commercial speech in the case of *Central Hudson Gas v. Public Service Commission*, 447 U.S. 557 (1980). When evaluating the governmental regulation of commercial speech, four factors must be considered:

1. The speech must not be misleading or related to an unlawful activity.
2. The government interest in the regulation must be substantial.
3. The regulation must directly advance the government interest asserted.
4. The restriction of speech cannot be more extensive than necessary to serve that interest.

There is no question that the FDA should be able to regulate drug product promotional activities under *Central Hudson*, but the issue becomes which activities, in what manner, and to what extent. For example, government regulation of company-sponsored educational symposia and company distribution of off-label use materials have faced First Amendment challenges. Any future governmental attempts to regulate activities such as direct-to-consumer advertising and Internet drug promotion must also pass the test under the First Amendment.

PRESCRIPTION DRUG ADVERTISING: MANUFACTURER TO PROFESSIONALS

Pharmaceutical manufacturers promote their products to health care professionals in several ways. Their methods range from advertising in professional journals to person-to-person contact through sales representatives. More controversial methods involve the sponsorship of medical symposia and the presentation of gifts and trips to health care professionals.

Applicable Statute and Regulations

Section 502(n) of the FDCA, enacted in 1962, provides that a drug shall be deemed misbranded unless the manufacturer includes in all advertisements and other descriptive printed matter issued a "true statement" of

- The established name of the drug
- The formula, showing quantitatively each ingredient
- A "brief summary" of other information relating to side effects, contraindications, and effectiveness, required by regulation

Pursuant to this statute, the FDA has issued detailed regulations (21 C.F.R. parts 200 and 201). The regulations mandate both the substance of the information that must be included (or not included) in the advertising and the manner in which it is presented (e.g., relative size of type, order of information).

The "true statement" requirement generally applies to all advertising, with certain exceptions. It does not apply to reminder advertising. "Reminder advertisements are those which call attention to the name of the drug product but do not include indications or dosage recommendations for use of the drug product" (21 C.F.R. § 202.1(e)(2)(i)). In addition to reminder advertisements, the regulations also exempt advertisements of bulk sale drugs (i.e., drugs intended to be processed, manufactured, or repackaged) and advertisements of prescription compounding drugs (i.e., drugs intended for use in compounding by pharmacists), as long as no safety or effectiveness claims are made.

A manufacturer has not met the true statement requirement if the advertising

- Is false or misleading
- Does not present a "fair balance" between side effects and contraindications information and effectiveness information
- Fails to reveal material facts

Fair balance essentially requires that the same scope, depth, and detail of information be presented for side effects and contraindications as for effectiveness.

The regulations list several examples of information in advertisements that are false, lacking in fair balance, or misleading (21 C.F.R. § 202.1(e)(6) and (7)). For example, an advertisement may not contain any representation or suggestion regarding a drug's effectiveness or lack of side effects that has not been approved for use in the labeling, nor may an advertisement suggest that a particular drug is safer or more effective than another when this has not been demonstrated by substantial evidence. As another example, an advertisement is false, lacking in fair balance, or misleading if it contains favorable information from a study inadequate in its design, scope, or conduct.

Under the regulations, advertising includes advertisements in journals and other periodicals, advertisements in the broadcast media, and telephone communications. Brochures, booklets, mailing pieces, bulletins, calendars, price lists, references (e.g., the *Physicians' Desk Reference*), and other such information disseminated by the manufacturer for use by health care professionals are considered labeling. Advertising and labeling must meet the same general standards; however, advertising need only contain a "brief summary" of the risks, whereas labeling must include the entire package insert.

The regulations somewhat modify the "true statement" requirements for advertising in broadcast media, such as radio and television. Because the brief summary requirement is really not that brief, manufacturers struggled to include all the required information in a short broadcast ad. As a result, prescription drug advertising in broadcast media need only include information about "major risks" instead of a full "brief summary," provided that the manufacturer makes "adequate provision for the dissemination of the approved package labeling." This alternative is called the "adequate provision" requirement, and is further described later in this text in the section discussing direct-to-consumer advertising.

Journal Advertising

Even a casual reader of medical journals cannot help but notice that many journal pages are devoted to pharmaceutical advertising. In 1991, the federal Office of the Inspector General (OIG) conducted a much publicized study to assess the accuracy, truthfulness, educational value, and quality of prescription drug advertisements in leading medical journals. Among other findings, the researchers concluded that most advertisements potentially violated FDA regulations and, if relied on, would lead to improper prescribing. The study confirmed and quantified what the FDA had suspected; in fact, the FDA had begun to step up its scrutiny and enforcement of prescription drug advertising before the study. Today the agency actively scrutinizes advertisements, and when necessary takes enforcement actions ranging from warning letters to lawsuits to requiring companies to run remedial advertisements and send corrective letters to health care professionals.

Industry-Supported Educational Programs Distinguished from Promotional Programs

For several years, pharmaceutical manufacturers have sponsored and funded educational programs (usually for continuing education credit [CE]) for health care professionals. In pharmacy, this sponsorship often is important in the production of high-quality educational programs at a reasonable registration fee for the pharmacist attendees. Concerns arise, however, when industry-supported programs are really product promotional activities disguised as educational programs.

A congressional investigation raised concerns about the objectivity of some manufacturer-sponsored educational programs and the inducements that some manufacturers were offering health care providers to attend (e.g., fees, free vacations). As a result of the congressional investigation, the FDA published a Draft Policy Statement on Industry-Supported Scientific and Educational Activities on November 27, 1992 (57 Fed. Reg. 56412-01), maintaining the agency's traditional position that scientific and educational activities performed by or on behalf of drug manufacturers are subject to regulation under the FDCA. This policy statement was substantially modified and published as the Final Guidance on Industry-Supported Scientific and Educational Activities on December 3, 1997 (62 Fed. Reg. 64074).

The guidance attempts to distinguish between activities supported by companies that are otherwise independent from the promotional influence of the supporting company and those that are not. The FDA emphasized that it does not intend to regulate industry-supported programs that are independent and nonpromotional. The distinction becomes important because programs that are not deemed independent and nonpromotional are subject to labeling and advertising restrictions, meaning in part that off-label uses may not be discussed and the "true statement" requirements apply, including "fair balance."

The guidance lists several factors the FDA will consider in evaluating whether an activity is independent. One factor is the degree of control the company has over the content of the program. Funding by a manufacturer for an educational program should be provided to a third party who conducts the program independently from the manufacturer. The manufacturer should not have a voice in determining program content in a truly independent program. Manufacturers commonly suggest the presenters, often academicians or clinical practitioners, to the third party, and this practice is completely permissible provided the content is objective and not influenced by the manufacturer. Other important factors include whether there was adequate disclosure during the program of the company's funding support; the company's relationship to the presenters; whether any unapproved uses will be discussed; whether the focus of the program is on educational content and free from commercial influence or bias; whether the audience was selected by the company, for example, as a reward to high prescribers, dispensers, or decision makers; and whether there are promotional activities, such as presentations or exhibits in the meeting room. In addition, although not required, a written agreement between the provider and the supporting company is encouraged to demonstrate that the sponsoring company has no involvement in the control or content of the symposia.

The guidance was challenged in *Washington Legal Foundation v. Friedman*, 13 F. Supp. 2d 51 (D.C. 1998), by a public interest group alleging that it violated the First Amendment (see the discussion in the case studies section). The court agreed that the guidance was overly restrictive and enjoined the FDA from prohibiting companies from being involved in the symposia content and discussing off-label uses as long as there is disclosure that the use is unapproved. The FDA appealed this decision in *Washington Legal Foundation v. Henney*, 202 F.3d 331 (C.A.D.C. 2000), arguing that a violation of the guidance is not illegal per se. Rather, continued the FDA, the guidance only serves as a "safe harbor," informing manufacturers of conduct that would not be challenged by the agency. On this basis, the court found that no constitutional issue existed, vacating the district court's decision that the guidance was unconstitutional. (Also see *Washington Legal Foundation v. Henney*, 36 F. Supp. 2d 418 (D.C. 1999).)

The Department of Health and Human Service's Office of Inspector General voiced its opinion about manufacturer-funded educational activities in a document titled "OIG Compliance Program Guidance for Pharmaceutical Manufacturers" (68 Fed. Reg. 23731, May 5, 2003). In this voluntary compliance guidance, the OIG noted that manufacturers should ensure that they are not using educational activities to channel improper remuneration to health care providers in a position to generate business for the manufacturer. The OIG also stated that the manufacturer should have no control over the speaker or the content of the program. To do otherwise creates a risk that the manufacturer might violate the federal antikickback statute.

Very aware that the government and the American public perceives the drug industry as ethically challenged in its relations with health care professionals, the Pharmaceutical Research and Manufacturers of America (PhRMA) drafted and published a voluntary guide called Code on Interactions with Healthcare Professionals, first in 2002 and updated in 2009 (http://www.phrma.org/about/principles-guidelines/code-interactions-healthcare-professionals). The Code prohibits companies from what used to be a common practice of providing entertainment and recreational activities to health care professionals, either separate from or in conjunction with an informational or educational program. Companies may provide financial support for CE programs but only through a CE provider, and the company may not provide advice or guidance to the CE provider. Although the company should not provide meals directly, the CE provider may choose to do so from the financial support provided to it from the company. Speaker expenses and honorariums are to be paid by the CE provider. The Code also prohibits providing health care professionals either directly or at programs with items, even of minimal value, that do not advance education, such as pens, note pads, mugs, or even stethoscopes.

FDA's Bad Ad Program

In 2010, the FDA implemented the "Bad Ad Program," with the intent of enlisting healt care professionals to help ensure that company promotion of prescription drugs is truthful (http://www.fda.gov/Drugs/GuidanceComplianceRegulatoryInformation/Surveillance/DrugMarketingAdvertisingandCommunications/ucm209384.htm). The FDA noted that its ability to monitor promotional activities in settings such as prescriber's offices, at local dinner programs, and at promotional speaker programs is limited. Thus, the agency asks health care professionals to assist it by recognizing misleading promotional activities and reporting them. One year after the program's implementation, the FDA announced that complaints against drug companies tripled. Based upon the success of the program, the FDA plans to develop education courses for prescribers, nurses, and pharmacists.

PRESCRIPTION DRUG ADVERTISING: MANUFACTURER TO CONSUMER

Manufacturer to consumer, known as direct-to-consumer (DTC), prescription drug advertising began in the early 1980s, breaking a tradition of advertising prescription drugs only to health care professionals. DTC advertising has become increasingly popular with drug manufacturers, touching off considerable controversy. Proponents contend that DTC advertising will benefit consumers by providing education, promoting awareness of potential health problems, improving compliance with drug therapies, and lowering drug prices. Pharmacists may benefit, according to the proponents, through increased prescription business and greater public recognition that they are the most knowledgeable and accessible source of additional prescription drug information. Opponents of DTC advertising contend that the practice will raise the cost of health care, create an inappropriate demand for medications and a demand for inappropriate medications, confuse patients, and jeopardize the physician–patient relationship.

There are no federal regulations that specifically address DTC advertising, meaning that essentially the advertising laws and regulations apply the same for DTC advertising, even though they were intended to regulate advertising to health care professionals, not consumers. Requiring the same criteria of a "true statement," a "brief summary," and "fair balance" creates problems as to whether these advertisements can be written in a manner that ordinary consumers can understand, especially because many manufacturers often use the same information regardless of the intended audience. In an effort to provide some direction and guidance to drug sponsors and ensure that consumers receive adequate communication of risk information, the FDA published a draft guidance in 1997 (notice at 62 Fed. Reg. 43171) and the final guidance in August 1999 (notice at 64 Fed. Reg. 43197). Of particular importance, the agency clarified what would satisfy the "adequate provision" requirement for DTC advertising through broadcast media. Advertisers may provide a summary of risks in audio and/or video form as long as there is "adequate provision" for the consumer to obtain full labeling information through a multifaceted approach from four sources: (1) a toll-free number, (2) an Internet webpage address, (3) referral to a print advertisement in a concurrently running print publication or by providing brochures in convenient outlets, and (4) referral to a health care provider. The FDA suggests that manufacturers should use all four sources of information. Although the regulations require that the approved product labeling (package insert) must be disseminated in connection with broadcast advertisements, the agency has instead asked manufacturers to consider translating the required information into language comprehensible to the general public.

Regarding DTC print advertising, the FDA announced in a 2004 draft guidance that it does not intend to hold manufacturers to the "brief summary" requirement, and in fact feels this level of information is not appropriate or useful for patients (http://www.fda.gov/Drugs/GuidanceComplianceRegulatoryInformation/Guidances/ucm064956.htm). The draft guidance is intended to encourage manufacturers to present key risk information in consumer-friendly ways. The guidance emphasizes that DTC ads should list only the most serious and most common risks associated with the product. The FDA indicates two ways of doing this are by using a modification of FDA-approved patient labeling, such as patient package inserts, or MedGuides. Or, at least until the FDA promulgates a regulation on this issue, manufacturers can include the information contained in the Highlights section of the package insert.

DTC advertising falls into one of three categories: product claim ads, reminder ads, or help-seeking ads. Product claim ads name the drug and the condition it treats and are subject to the regulations. Reminder ads give the drug's name, but not its uses, and are not subject to the regulation. Help-seeking ads are educational in nature and do not mention the name of the product, only the name of the company. These advertisements generally inform the consumer about diseases, mentioning that a physician can treat a particular condition with medications, and urge the consumer to see a physician. These ads need not conform to FDA labeling and advertising requirements. In an effort to encourage manufacturers to disseminate information about untreated and inadequately treated health conditions, the FDA published a draft guidance to help manufacturers distinguish between these "educational" type messages and "promotional" type messages (http://www.fda.gov/Drugs/GuidanceComplianceRegulatoryInformation/Guidances/ucm064956.htm).

Just as the FDA scrutinizes advertising directed to health care professionals, it also evaluates advertising directed to consumers, and has taken enforcement actions. In 1991, for example, Ciba-Geigy was forced to discontinue its DTC advertising of Actigall, a drug used in an effort to dissolve certain kinds of gallstones, in response to FDA concerns. The FDA believed that the advertisements misled consumers by intimating that surgery was the only other choice of treatment when there are newer, less obtrusive forms of treatment available. At the same time, Ciba-Geigy agreed to cease using celebrities to promote its products.

In November 2006, the U.S. Government Accountability Office (GAO) issued a report titled *Prescription Drugs: Improvements Needed in FDA's Oversight of Direct-to-Consumer Advertising* (http://www.gao.gov/cgi-bin/getrpt?GAO-07-54). As the title indicates, the GAO's report criticized the FDA for several weaknesses. The GAO noted that DTC advertising had increased twice as fast from 1997 through 2005 as spending on promotion to physicians or on research and development, and the number of DTC materials the FTC received had doubled. The GAO reported that although the agency said it prioritizes all this material, the GAO could find no documented criteria for prioritization. The report noted that informal criteria being used by FDA reviewers is not systematically applied to all DTC materials. The GAO report further found that the FDA's process for drafting and issuing violation letters takes longer, that the agency issues fewer letters, and that the effectiveness of the letters is limited.

The FDAAA has provided the FDA additional authority by allowing it to require a preview of DTC ads. Because the First Amendment precludes censorship, the FDA's authority after preview is limited to providing recommendations to the company. The FDA may, however, require a change in an ad if the change addresses serious risks associated with the drug's use.

Recently the FDA has been concerned about distracting ads, both print and broadcast, which divert the consumer's attention from the drug's risks. The agency issued a draft guidance in May 2009 to advise the drug industry of the agency's expectations as to how risk information should be presented (*Presenting Risk Information in Prescription Drug and Medical Device Promotion*, http://www.fda.gov/downloads/Drugs/GuidanceComplianceRegulatoryInformation/Guidances/UCM155480.pdf). The FDA warned advertisers about busy scenes, frequent scene changes, and speeding up of an announcer's description of risks as detracting from the consumer's comprehension. The FDA gave as one example a TV ad for a cholesterol-lowering drug that contains factually accurate risk information but is accompanied by loud upbeat music and quick scene changes showing comforting visual images of patients benefiting from the drug. The guidance indicates that the FDA will look at the "net impression" that the ad conveys from the perspective of a reasonable consumer.

Ultimately, the courts may have a significant influence as to the type of information a company must provide to consumers. The Supreme Court of New Jersey has held that when a manufacturer advertises its prescription product to consumers, it owes a legal duty to the consumer to properly warn of its product's risks (*Perez v. Wyeth Laboratories, Inc.*, 734 A.2d 1245 (N.J. 1999)). Historically, a company's duty to warn of a prescription product's risks is owed only to the health care professional, not the consumer.

PROMOTING PRESCRIPTION DRUGS FOR OFF-LABEL USES

The promotion of off-label uses (also termed unapproved or unlabeled uses) most likely represents the FDA's greatest concern within the area of advertising. The term *off-label* use refers to indications other than those approved by the FDA and thus that could not be included in the labeling. The FDA historically has been concerned that adverse health consequences could result if health care professionals and consumers are led to believe that a product is safe and effective for a use not approved by the agency. Thus, the agency had actively policed and basically prohibited any efforts by companies to disseminate off-label use information, even in the form of peer-reviewed journal articles, unless specifically requested by the health care practitioner (guidance published at 61 Fed. Reg. 52800 (1996)).

The FDAMA (§ 551 and § 552), however, relaxed FDA policy allowing companies to provide written information about off-label uses under certain conditions to health care professionals and certain entities such as pharmacy benefit managers, health insurance plans, and group health plans. The written information had to be in the form of unabridged peer-reviewed articles in scientific or medical journals or reference publications that had not been influenced by the company. The conditions for disseminating this information included that the company must (1) have filed an application for approval for the use; (2) submit to the agency 60 days before dissemination a copy of the information to be disseminated and any clinical trial information the company has; and (3) include with the disseminated information a disclosure that the use has not been approved, a copy of the official labeling for the product, any other products or treatments that have been approved for the use, the funding source for any studies relating to the use, and a bibliography of scientific publications regarding the use.

Some of these restrictions provided in the FDAMA had been ruled unconstitutional on First Amendment grounds by the *Washington Legal Foundation v. Friedman* and *Washington Legal Foundation v. Henney* cases mentioned previously and discussed in the case studies section. However, the court of appeals allowed the provisions to remain after the FDA changed its position to assert that the FDAMA provisions were not requirements, but merely established a "safe harbor."

The FDAMA provisions related to off-label use dissemination, however, expired on September 30, 2006, prompting the FDA to issue a proposed guidance document in February 2008 and the final guidance in January 2009, reflecting the agency's position on this issue (http://www.fda.gov/OHRMS/DOCKETS/98fr/FDA-2008-D-0053-gdl.pdf). The FDA noted that although the FDCA generally prohibits manufacturers from distributing products for unapproved uses, drugs are legally and commonly prescribed and dispensed by health care professionals for off-label use. Therefore, it is important in the interests of public health that health care professionals be able to receive truthful and nonmisleading publications about off-label uses.

Similar to the FDAMA provisions, the guidance document allows companies to distribute unabridged peer-reviewed articles published in scientific or medical journals or reference publications that have not been influenced by the company. The articles should address well-controlled clinical investigations considered by experts as scientifically sound. Similar to FDAMA provisions, the articles should be accompanied by the approved labeling, accompanied by a comprehensive bibliography of publications regarding the use (if available), disseminated with a representative publication (if in existence) that reaches contrary or different conclusions, distributed separately from promotional information, accompanied by a disclosure that the use has not been approved by the FDA, accompanied by a disclosure of any relationship between the company and the author of the article, and accompanied by a disclosure of any known significant risks or safety concerns not discussed in the article.

Conspicuously different from the FDAMA dissemination requirements, the guidance document does not require that the company must have filed an NDA for the use, or have submitted a copy of the article and related clinical information to the FDA 60 days prior to dissemination. Some consumer watchdog organizations and members of Congress soundly criticized the FDA for continuing to allow manufacturers to disseminate off-label use information and especially for dropping the additional FDAMA restrictions. It is unlikely that the agency appeased those critics when it replied that it never enforced those requirements anyway (most likely because of concerns that the requirements might violate the First Amendment).

NONPRESCRIPTION DRUG ADVERTISING BY MANUFACTURERS

As noted earlier, the FTC regulates nonprescription drug advertising under the Federal Trade Commission Act. The act allows the FTC to prohibit unfair methods of competition and unfair or deceptive acts or practices and to regulate advertising for foods, OTC drugs, and medical devices. The FTC cannot require companies to submit advertising to it for premarket approval but rather must act after the fact. The agency devotes top priority to advertisements in which the accuracy of the claims is difficult for consumers to verify; OTC drug advertisements often fall under this category. Moreover, the deceptive advertising claims of OTC products warrant priority on the basis that they can result in adverse health consequences and economic loss.

The FTC considers an advertisement deceptive when it contains a statement (or omission) of information that is likely to mislead reasonable consumers to their detriment. With this approach, the FTC need not prove that consumers were actually misled, only that they are likely to be misled. Advertising claims must have a reasonable basis. For example, if the advertisement states that the drug has been medically proven effective for a particular condition, the FTC expects the company to produce evidence to support the statement. The amount of verification that the FTC expects from the company depends on the type of advertising claim made, the type of product, the consequences of the false claim, the degree of reliance by consumers, and similar factors.

In *Porter & Dietsch, Inc. v. Federal Trade Commission*, 605 F.2d 294 (7th Cir.1979), the FTC challenged the advertising claims that the manufacturer made for X-11 diet tablets. The FTC contended that the advertisements were false and misleading because they proclaimed that users of the tablets can lose weight without changing their eating habits, that users will lose a significant amount of weight, and that X-11 contains a unique ingredient. The FTC also argued that the advertisements contained material omissions, including the information that persons with certain diseases should use X-11 tablets only as directed by a physician. The court decided in favor of the FTC because the company could produce no scientific basis for its claim of weight loss. As to the unique ingredient claim, the court agreed with the FTC that phenylpropanolamine had been in use for years and was hardly unique. Furthermore, the FTC admitted evidence showing that phenylpropanolamine could produce adverse effects in individuals with certain medical conditions, and the court agreed that this omission in the advertisements made them false and misleading.

In *Warner-Lambert Co. v. Federal Trade Commission*, 562 F.2d 749 (D.C. Cir. 1977), the FTC ordered Warner-Lambert to cease and desist misrepresenting the efficacy of Listerine mouthwash against the common cold. The company appealed the FTC's findings in court, arguing that the FTC did not have the evidence to sustain a finding of false and misleading advertising. The court found for the FTC, however, after the agency introduced several facts into evidence including:

- The ingredients of Listerine are not present in sufficient quantities to have any therapeutic effect.
- It is impossible for Listerine to reach critical areas of the body in significant concentration through the process of gargling.
- Even if the active ingredients in Listerine could reach critical sites in significant quantities, they could not penetrate tissue cells and, thus, could not affect the viruses.
- Warner-Lambert's clinical studies were unreliable.
- Even if Listerine kills millions of germs, as the advertisements claimed, it would be of no medical significance because these germs play no role in colds.

The FTC not only has the authority to issue cease-and-desist orders but also can order companies to issue corrective advertising. In *Warner-Lambert*, the court upheld the agency's order requiring the company to include this statement in every advertisement: "Listerine will not help prevent colds or sore throats or lessen their severity." The court also supported the FTC's order that this disclosure continue until the company had expended in Listerine advertising a sum equal to the average annual advertising budget for Listerine over a 10-year period, which amounted to approximately $10 million. The court viewed the corrective advertising as a necessary remedy for the erroneous consumer beliefs that the earlier advertising had fostered but cautioned that, because of the First Amendment, FTC restrictions may not be greater than necessary.

The FTC also has the authority to require advertisers to make affirmative disclosures when necessary to qualify certain statements (half truths) or to disclose certain adverse consequences of a drug. Often, the FTC collaborates with the FDA to determine whether there is a reasonable basis for a manufacturer's claims regarding an OTC drug or whether it is permissible for a manufacturer to make a therapeutic claim about a food product. The FTC and FDA have an agreement through which the FTC regulates food advertising and the FDA regulates food labeling. The FTC allows manufacturers to make therapeutic claims about food products as long as the claims are properly qualified and there is a reasonable basis for the claim. Occasionally, this policy places the FTC at odds with the FDA, which may oppose the therapeutic claim on the label, contending that the claim makes the food a drug.

The Lanham Trademark Act

Frequently, one company objects to the advertising claims made by another company for a competing product. The objecting party may attempt to persuade the FTC to bring an action against its competitor, or it may bring an action itself under the Lanham Trademark Act, which prohibits the use of "any false description or representation, including words or symbols" in connection with the sale of any goods or services (15 U.S.C. § 1125).

The Lanham Act allows for a private cause of action and the recovery of monetary damages, as well as injunctive relief. It is not uncommon to find OTC drug manufacturers battling each other in court under the Lanham Act. For example, in *American Home Products Corporation v. Johnson & Johnson*, 654 F. Supp. 568 (S.D.N.Y. 1987), American Home Products, which markets Advil (ibuprofen), and Johnson & Johnson, which markets Tylenol (acetaminophen), sued each other for false advertising claims. Clearly annoyed at the two feuding companies, the judge commented that the lawsuit represents an endless war between two titans of the drug industry and involves more resources than small nations have used to fight for their very survival.

In the lawsuit, American Home Products claimed that Johnson & Johnson published false printed materials and broadcast false television commercials that unfavorably compared ibuprofen with acetaminophen. Johnson & Johnson, in turn, countersued American Home Products for false comparative advertising of Advil and two of its other OTC analgesic products, Anacin and Anacin-3. After hearing several expert witnesses and reviewing thousands of pages of exhibits and briefs, the court concluded that each party was guilty of misleading advertising, and it was too complex to determine the damages to each party caused by lost sales, profits, and goodwill.

Although plaintiffs usually bring an action under the Lanham Act for their own self-interest, the consumer benefits from these actions when they result in the removal of false and misleading advertising. The Lanham Act does not protect the consumer, however, if manufacturers conspire to advertise in their best interests rather than in the best interests of the consumer. Thus, the Federal Trade Commission Act has a more important role in protecting the consumer against false and misleading advertising.

© Stockbyte/Thinkstock

STUDY SCENARIOS AND QUESTIONS

1. You are the only pharmacist at a meeting with other health care professionals. A physician brings up the topic of direct-to-consumer drug ads on television and in magazines, lamenting that the ads are so seductive and misleading that some of his patients practically demand he prescribe the drugs for them. The physician and the other attendees wonder if the FDA regulates these ads. Explain to the group in attendance the requirements for drug advertising for broadcast and print media.
2. Xecor makes several drugs including Anxless, approved by the FDA for the treatment of anxiety. Recent studies sponsored by Xecor indicate that Anxless may be a promising treatment for hypertension. Dr. Mabel is a pharmacy professor whom Xecor approached to see if she would be willing to present hypertension C.E. programs. The company told Dr. Mabel it would pay her $2,000 per one-hour program, and the company would give her the slides to use. Dr. Mabel agreed, and Xecor sponsored a C.E. program at a local restaurant personally inviting the pharmacists. Most of the program was about the recent studies demonstrating how effective Anxless is for hypertension. The company also distributed articles to attendees discussing these studies. The FDA monitored the program and issued warning letters to Xecor and Mabel. Explain the legal and social policy arguments as to why this program might violate FDA guidelines and why it might not. What legal violation might Xecor and Mabel have committed?

BIBLIOGRAPHY

Adams, D. G., et al. *Fundamentals of Law and Regulations. An In-Depth Look at Therapeutic Products.* Washington, DC: Food and Drug Law Institute, 1997.

American Pharmacists Association. Legislative and Regulatory Updates. Available at: http://www.pharmacist.com

American Society for Pharmacy Law. Available at: http://www.aspl.org

HPUS. Definition of Homeopathy. Available at: http://www.homeopathicdoctor.com/page8.html

Hutt, P. B. Investigations and reports respecting FDA regulation of new drugs: Parts 1 and 2. *Clinical Pharmacology and Therapeutics* 33 (1983): 537–548, 674–687.

Hutt, P. B., and R. A. Merrill. *Food and Drug Law.* 2nd ed. Westbury, NY: Foundation Press, 1991.

Hyman, P. U.S. food and drug law and FDA—A historical background. In: *A Practical Guide to Food and Drug Law and Regulation.* Washington, DC: Food and Drug Law Institute, 2002.

Hyman, P., and P. C. McNamara. Food and Drug Administration Amendments Act of 2007. Available at: http://www.hymanphelps.com

Janssen, W. F. Pharmacy and the food and drug law. *American Pharmacy* NS21 (1981): 212–221.

National Community Pharmacists Association. Governmental Affairs/Legal Proceedings. Available at: http://www.ncpanet.org

Pina, K. R., and W. L. Pines. *A Practical Guide to Food and Drug Law and Regulation*. 3rd ed. Washington, DC: Food and Drug Law Institute, 2008.

U.S. Food and Drug Administration. *Guidance for Industry. Brief Summary: Disclosing Risk Information in Consumer-Directed Print Advertisements*, January 2004a. Available at: http://www.fda.gov/downloads/Drugs/GuidanceComplianceRegulatoryInformation/Guidances/ucm069984.pdf

U.S. Food and Drug Administration. *Guidance for Industry. "Help-Seeking" and Other Disease Awareness Communications by or on Behalf of Drug and Device Firms*, January 2004b. Available at: http://www.fda.gov/downloads/Drugs/GuidanceComplianceRegulatoryInformation/Guidances/ucm070068.pdf

U.S. Food and Drug Administration. *An Introduction to FDA Drug Regulation: A Manual for Pharmacists.* Rockville, MD: Department of Health and Human Services, 1990.

U.S. Food and Drug Administration. *Managing the Risks from Medical Product Use: Creating a Risk Management Framework.* Rockville, MD: Department of Health and Human Services, 1999.

U.S. Food and Drug Administration. *Manufacture, Distribution, and Promotion of Adulterated, Misbranded, or Unapproved New Drugs for Human Use by State Licensed Pharmacies.* Compliance Policy 7132.16. Rockville, MD: Office of Enforcement, Division of Compliance Policy, March 16, 1992.

U.S. Food and Drug Administration. New Drug Development in the United States, January 30, 2007. Available at: http://www.fda.gov/cder/learn/CDERLearn/default.htm

U.S. Food and Drug Administration. FDA website. Available at: http://www.fda.gov

U.S. Government Accountability Office. *Prescription Drugs: Improvements Needed in FDA's Oversight of Direct-to-Consumer Advertising*, available at http://www.gao.gov/assets/260/253778.pdf

Valentino, J. Practical uses for the USP: A legal perspective. *American Journal of Pharmaceutical Education* 51 (1987): 80–81.

Von Eschenbach, A. C. The FDA Amendments Act: Reauthorization of the FDA 2008. *Food and Drug Law Journal* 63 (2008): 579.

Welage, L. S., et. al. Understanding the scientific issues embedded in the generic drug approval process. *Journal of the American Pharmaceutical Association* 41 no. 6 (2001): 856–867.

CASE STUDIES

CASE 2-1 **_Nutrilab, Inc., et al. v. Schweiker_, 713 F.2d 335 (7th Cir. 1983)**

Issue

Is a product derived from a food source and promoted for the purpose of weight reduction by blocking the body's digestion of starch a food or a drug?

Overview

In this case, the court confronted the issue of whether a product is really a food or a drug under the FDCA. Often courts are faced with ambiguous statutes and have to draw on their perception of legislative intent. Distinguishing a food from a drug has very significant regulatory implications. Food products are not subject to the premarket approval process as are drugs. Thus, in most cases if the FDA has objections over the promotion of a food product, the agency has the burden of proving its claim, during which time the product continues to be marketed. On the other hand, the FDA can withdraw a product from the market deemed to be a drug simply because it is an unapproved new drug. The agency also would have no difficulty establishing that the product is misbranded because the product's label would not be in compliance with drug labeling requirements.

As the definition of drug indicates, the critical issue in distinguishing whether a product is a drug is the intended use of the product. In determining the intended use of a product, courts will consider evidence beyond the label and labeling. Thus, a court considers advertising from television, radio, magazines, the Internet, and so forth. Because the health, safety, and welfare of the public are often at stake in these cases, courts will often apply the definition of drug liberally in favor of the FDA.

As you read this case, consider the difference in the intent and meaning of Section 321(g)(1)(B) and Section 321(g)(1)(C) of the drug definition. Why are foods specifically excluded from being drugs under part C and not part B? How did the court ultimately define food for the purpose of part C? If this case were brought today, would the product be considered a dietary supplement under DSHEA?

The court first described the facts of the case:

> Plaintiffs manufacture and market a product known as "starch blockers" which "block" the human body's digestion of starch as an aid in controlling weight. On July 1, 1982, the Food and Drug Administration ("FDA") classified starch blockers as "drugs" and requested that all such products be removed from the market until FDA approval was received. The next day plaintiffs filed two separate complaints in the district court seeking declaratory judgments that these products are foods under 21 U.S.C. 321(f) and not drugs under 21 U.S.C. 321(g). On October 5, 1982, the district court held that starch blockers were drugs under 21 U.S.C. 321(g), plaintiffs were permanently enjoined from manufacturing and distributing the products, and they were ordered to destroy existing inventories. The portion of the order requiring destruction of the products was stayed pending appeal.
>
> The only issue on appeal is whether starch blockers are foods or drugs under the Federal Food, Drug, and Cosmetic Act. Starch blocker tablets and capsules consist of a protein which is extracted from a certain type of raw kidney bean. That particular protein functions as an alpha-amylase inhibitor; alpha-amylase is an enzyme produced by the body which is utilized in digesting starch. When starch blockers are ingested during a meal, the protein acts to prevent the alpha-amylase enzyme from acting, thus allowing the undigested starch to pass through the body and avoiding the calories that would be realized from its digestion.
>
> Kidney beans, from which alpha-amylase inhibitor is derived, are dangerous if eaten raw. By August 1982, FDA had received 75 reports of adverse effects on people who had taken starch blockers, including complaints of gastrointestinal distress such as bloating, nausea, abdominal pain, constipation, and vomiting. Because plaintiffs consider starch blockers to be food, no testing as required to obtain FDA approval as a new drug has taken place. If starch blockers were drugs, the manufacturers would be required to file a new drug application pursuant to 21 U.S.C. 355 and remove the product from the marketplace until approved as a drug by the FDA.

After noting the facts and articulating the issue, the court proceeded to identify the relevant statutes, ascertain their meaning, and apply them to the facts of this case.

> The statutory scheme under the Food, Drug, and Cosmetic Act is a complicated one. Section 321(g)(1) provides that the term "drug" means ***(B) articles intended for use in the diagnosis, cure, mitigation, treatment, or prevention of disease in man or other animals; and (C) articles (other than food) intended to affect the structure or any function of the body of man or other animals; and (D) articles intended for use as a component of any article specified in clauses (A), (B), or (C) of this paragraph; but does not include devices or their components, parts, or accessories.
>
> The term "food" as defined in Section 321(f) means (1) articles used for food or drink for man or other animals, (2) chewing gum, and (3) articles used for components of any such article.
>
> Section 321(g)(1)(C) was added to the statute in 1938 to expand the definition of "drug." The amendment was necessary because certain articles intended by manufacturers to

be used as drugs did not fit within the "disease" requirement of Section 321(g)(1)(B). Obesity in particular was not considered a disease. Thus "anti-fat remedies" marketed with claims of "slenderizing effects" had escaped regulation under the prior definition. The purpose of part C in Section 321(g)(1) was "to make possible the regulation of a great many products that have been found on the market that cannot be alleged to be treatments for diseased conditions."

It is well established that the definitions of food and drug are normally not mutually exclusive; an article that happens to be a food but is intended for use in the treatment of disease fits squarely within the drug definition in part B of Section 321(g)(1) and may be regulated as such. Under part C of the statutory drug definition, however, "articles (other than food)" are expressly excluded from the drug definition (as are devices) in Section 321(g)(1). In order to decide if starch blockers are drugs under Section 321(g)(1)(C), therefore, we must decide if they are foods within the meaning of the part C "other than food" parenthetical exception to Section 321(g)(1)(C). And in order to decide the meaning of "food" in that parenthetical exception, we must first decide the meaning of "food" in Section 321(f).

Congress defined "food" in Section 321(f) as "articles used as food." This definition is not too helpful, but it does emphasize that "food" is to be defined in terms of its function as food, rather than in terms of its source, biochemical composition, or ingestibility. Plaintiffs' argument that starch blockers are food because they are derived from food—kidney beans—is not convincing; if Congress intended food to mean articles derived from food it would have so specified. Indeed some articles that are derived from food are indisputably not food, such as caffeine and penicillin. In addition, all articles that are classed biochemically as proteins cannot be food either, because, for example, insulin, botulism toxin, human hair, and influenza virus are proteins that are clearly not food.

If defining food in terms of its source or defining it in terms of its biochemical composition is clearly wrong, defining food as articles intended by the manufacturer to be used as food is problematic. When Congress meant to define a drug in terms of its intended use, it explicitly incorporated that element into its statutory definition. For example, Section 321(g)(1)(B) defines drugs as articles "intended for use" in, among other things, the treatment of disease; Section 321(g)(1)(C) defines drugs as "articles (other than food) intended to affect the structure or any function of the body of man or other animals." The definition of food in Section 321(f) omits any reference to intent. Further, a manufacturer cannot avoid the reach of the FDA by claiming that a product which looks like food and smells like food is not food because it was not intended for consumption.

Although it is easy to reject the proffered food definitions, it is difficult to arrive at a satisfactory one. In the absence of clear cut Congressional guidance, it is best to rely on statutory language and common sense. The statute evidently uses the word "food" in two different ways. The statutory definition of "food" in Section 321(f) is a term of art and is clearly intended to be broader than the common sense definition of food, because the statutory definition of "food" also includes chewing gum and food additives. Yet the statutory definition of "food" also includes in Section 321(f)(1) the common sense definition of food. When the statute defines "food" as "articles used for food," it means that the statutory definition of "food" includes articles used by people in the ordinary way most people use food—primarily for taste, aroma, or nutritive value. To hold as did the district court that articles used as food are articles used solely for taste, aroma, or nutritive value is unduly restrictive since some products such as coffee or prune juice are undoubtedly food but may be consumed on occasion for reasons other than taste, aroma, or nutritive value.

This double use of the word "food" in Section 321(f) makes it difficult to interpret the parenthetical "other than food" exclusion in the Section 321(g)(1)(C) drug definition.

As shown by that exclusion, Congress obviously meant a drug to be something "other than food," but was it referring to "food" as a term of art in the statutory sense or to foods in their ordinary meaning? Because all such foods are "intended to affect the structure or any function of the body of man or other animals" and would thus come within the part C drug definition, presumably Congress meant to exclude common sense foods. Fortunately, it is not necessary to decide this question here because starch blockers are not food in either sense. The tablets and pills at issue are not consumed primarily for taste, aroma, or nutritive value under Section 321(f)(1); in fact, as noted earlier, they are taken for their ability to block the digestion of food and aid in weight loss. In addition, starch blockers are not chewing gum under Section 321(f)(2) and are not components of food under Section 321(f)(3). To qualify as a drug under Section 321(g)(1)(C), the articles must not only be articles "other than food" but must also be "intended to affect the structure or any function of the body of man or other animals." Starch blockers indisputably satisfy this requirement for they are intended to affect digestion in the people who take them. Therefore, starch blockers are drugs under Section 321(g)(1)(C) of the Food, Drug, and Cosmetic Act.

The court affirmed the decision of the district court, finding against the plaintiffs.

Notes on *Nutrilab v. Schweiker*

1. *Nutrilab* points out the difference between part B of the drug definition and part C is that part C broadens the term drug to include articles intended to affect the structure or function of the body. If part C did not exist, the starch blockers would not likely be drugs because they were not promoted for the prevention or treatment of a disease. Foods were excluded under part C because all foods affect the function of the body. The question then becomes whether a product is a food for the purposes of part C. This raises a corollary issue of whether a product could be a food under the definition of food but not be a food for the purposes of part C. The court resolved the issue by concluding that the product was not a food at all, and thus subject to part C. The court refused to expand its analysis to whether part C excludes any product defined as a food or just common sense foods.

2. Under DSHEA, structure/function claims about a dietary supplement made pursuant to the law are excluded from the drug definition. Would the starch blockers be a dietary supplement under DSHEA? They might, under the definition of dietary supplement, providing two conditions could be established: that they are a botanical and that they are meant to supplement the diet.

CASE 2-2   *United States v. Hiland*, 909 F.2d 1114 (8th Cir. 1990)

Issue

Whether the defendants violated the FDCA by introducing a misbranded, unapproved, "new drug" into interstate commerce and whether they intended to mislead or defraud.

Overview

Like the *Nutrilab* case, this is a case in which a product becomes a drug on the basis of the intended use of the product by the sellers. Unlike *Nutrilab*, the defendants in this case committed a felony by allowing greed to blind their regard for public safety. Fortunately, a case like *Hiland* does not occur often. Note that this case highlights the fact that individual officers can be held individually accountable for their actions under the FDCA. As you read this case, consider when a violation of the FDCA evolves from a misdemeanor to a felony.

Because of the many infants killed or seriously injured by the defendants' vitamin E product, E-Ferol, this case often is mentioned as a reason why the FDA should have more, not less, authority over dietary supplements. As you read this case, ask yourself when does one intentionally violate the law as opposed to unintentionally violate the law, and what is the difference in consequences? About the time E-Ferol was being distributed, had the FDA allowed other unapproved drugs to be marketed? If so, on what basis, and why was this not a valid defense in this case? Also consider whether E-Ferol would be considered a dietary supplement today under DSHEA. Is there any way to prevent situations like this from occurring in the future? Are the penalties imposed on the defendants under the FDCA severe enough in light of the consequences of their crime?

The court related the facts of the case:

> Carter-Glogau, located in Glendale, Arizona, was a manufacturer of generic injectable drugs. Carter was the corporation's president and chief operating officer. OJF, located in Maryland Heights, Missouri, was a distributor of prescription pharmaceutical products, primarily generic drugs. Hiland was OJF's president and Madison was its executive vice-president of operations. Almost all of the injectable drugs distributed by OJF were manufactured by Carter-Glogau. In most cases, the drugs manufactured by Carter-Glogau for OJF were generic copies of innovator drugs that were formulated by other companies and approved by the FDA.

> In April 1982, one of Carter-Glogau's customers wrote Carter to ask whether an intravenous form of vitamin E could be developed, noting that "[t]here must be a Hell of a market out there." Carter expressed a reluctance to develop such a product. In his responses to the customer's inquiry, he stated that the amount of polysorbates needed "may be detrimental," and pointed out that "fat emulsions for IV use . . . are very tricky products and fraught with particular size problems."

At the time, there was a significant need for an intravenous form of vitamin E to combat retrolental fibroplasia (RLF), a disease that causes impaired vision or permanent blindness in premature infants. Even though not approved by the FDA for this use, many neonatologists considered vitamin E to be useful in reducing the incidence and severity of RLF. However, both the intramuscular and oral dosage forms currently available as nutritional supplements had drawbacks for administration to premature infants.

> In August 1982, Madison wrote Carter to see if he could develop for OJF a high potency intravenous form of vitamin E for use in premature infants. He informed Carter that Hoffmann-LaRoche, a large pharmaceutical company, was testing an injectable vitamin E product for the treatment of RLF in an effort to obtain FDA approval of the product. Madison wrote that he was "afraid that when Roche gets their vitamin E approved, we will lose the business, unless you can come up with something." Madison's letter clearly indicated that the primary purpose of the product he was proposing would be to treat RLF, and stated, "We could always label it for vitamin E supplementation." Hiland received a copy of this letter.

> In his responses to Madison's inquiries, Carter expressed serious safety concerns regarding the development of an intravenous vitamin E product, stating in part: "If we make some attempt to solubilize the vitamin E and use the wrong proportions and kill a few infants, we'd have some serious problems."

> Carter was specifically concerned about developing such a product without proper clinical testing. He wrote Madison that: "The administration of this product intravenously in neonatals without appropriate clinical work concerning toxicity will undoubtedly lead to an exposure in terms of product liability which neither you nor we may wish to assume."

Notwithstanding these safety concerns, after further dialogue with Madison, Carter proceeded to develop a high-potency intravenous vitamin E product called E-Ferol for OJF in the summer of 1983. Carter made the decisions as to the types and proportions of polysorbate the product would contain, admitting he did not know what levels were safe for premature infants. Moreover, neither he nor OJF did any testing to determine whether his formulation was safe and effective for premature infants. Later that summer Madison recommended to Hiland that E-Ferol be added to its product line for the treatment of RLF, and Hiland approved.

Carter and Madison then prepared the labeling for E-Ferol using the IM (nutrient supplement) label as the model, but adding a reference in the package insert about the product's use in treating RLF. The labeling indicated the dosage at the level used to treat RLF.

In September 1983, OJF conducted a massive mailing campaign for E-Ferol, mailing out "Dear Doctor" letters accompanied by a brochure and package insert. The group targeted was involved in the treatment of RLF, but the promotional information did not indicate that E-Ferol had never been tested for safety and efficacy. At trial, the physicians and pharmacists testified that E-Ferol's labeling led them to believe that the product was promoted to treat RLF in premature infants and that the product had been proven safe and effective. During the months that E-Ferol was on the market, OJF received various reports from hospitals and physicians of adverse reactions associated with the product, including infant deaths. After a report from a neonatologist in Spokane, Washington, in January 1984 regarding the death of three premature infants with excessively high levels of vitamin E, Hiland halted the distribution of E-Ferol and began an investigation. No effort was made to advise other users of the product of the reported deaths. Twelve days after the distribution of E-Ferol had been suspended, Hiland made the decision to resume all shipments of the product. The shipments continued until April 1984, despite further reports of infant deaths, at which time OJF recalled E-Ferol from the market.

A grand jury indicted Carter-Glogau, Carter, Hiland, Madison, and others. A trial was then begun resulting in the defendants being convicted of violating the FDCA on the basis of introducing into interstate commerce an unapproved "new drug" with the intent to defraud and mislead. The defendants also were convicted of misbranding E-Ferol on several counts including that the labeling omitted material facts, failed to bear adequate directions for use, failed to bear adequate warnings, and suggested uses dangerous to the health of premature infants. The basis of the fraud charge was that the defendants intentionally represented the E-Ferol as safe and effective despite no testing and continued to do so even after the adverse incident reports.

Madison and two other defendants plead guilty during the trial and were fined and given jail sentences. Carter and Hiland were each sentenced to 9 years imprisonment, all but 6 months of which was suspended, and fined $130,000. Carter-Glogau was also fined $130,000. Carter-Glogau, Carter, and Hiland appealed.

> Carter argues that his conviction on the new drug counts violated due process because (1) FDA policy actively led him to believe that E-Ferol could be marketed lawfully without a new drug approval, and (2) this same policy was so vague and indefinite as to deprive him of fair warning that his conduct was illegal.

The court then proceeded to analyze the merits of the defendants' arguments, first noting that the FDCA prohibits the introduction of any new drug into interstate commerce without FDA approval of safety and efficacy. Carter acknowledged this fact but argued that an FDA compliance policy guide (CPG 7132c.02) specified that the FDA would defer enforcement action against unapproved drugs marketed after 1962 that were identical or similar to existing pre-1962 drugs (DESI drugs) of unresolved regulatory status, unless there was some reason to question the safety and efficacy of the drug.

The FDA applied this same policy (termed "ISR policy") to drugs not included in the DESI review, such as vitamin E products. Because of this ISR policy, Carter stated he was led to believe that E-Ferol could be marketed without approval because it was similar to existing pre-1962 drugs.

The court, however, found no merit in the argument because Carter was allowed to introduce extensive evidence on this issue at trial and the jury did not believe he relied on or was misled by the policy. The court also found other reasons to reject Carter's argument.

> There are additional reasons why Carter's argument must fail, aside from the jury's rejection of his defense. The FDA's ISR policy did not purport to modify existing statutory requirements. The policy in no way suggested that it was lawful under the FDCA to market a new drug without an approved NDA. It simply established a set of enforcement priorities in an effort to best allocate limited FDA resources. Indeed, CPG 7132c.02 was adopted by the FDA after a federal court decision overturned its prior policy of permitting certain classes of new drugs to be marketed without an approved NDA. CPG 7132c.02 expressly recognized that "all drugs in the DESI review are 'new drugs' under the law," and stated further:

> It has been decided to reaffirm that all products marketed as drugs under the DESI program are new drugs and therefore require an approved NDA or ANDA [abbreviated new drug application] for marketing. In view of this reaffirmation of this policy, it is necessary that the Agency proceed to remove from the market any current DESI-effective prescription products not subject of an approved NDA or ANDA, and to prevent in the future the marketing of any such unapproved products.

> Finally, we note that even if the ISR policy could somehow have been construed as making it legal to market certain new drugs without an approved NDA, it certainly could not have been read as making such action lawful when done with the intent to defraud or mislead.

Losing on this argument, Carter and Hiland claimed another defense.

> Carter and Hiland contend that their convictions on the FDCA counts must be reversed because the district court denied their request to instruct the jury that (1) knowledge that E-Ferol was an unapproved "new drug" was an essential element of the new drug offense, and (2) knowledge that E-Ferol was "misbranded" was an essential element of the misbranding offense. The court instructed the jury that the essential elements of the new drug offense were (1) the defendants introduced E-Ferol into interstate commerce; (2) E-Ferol was an unapproved new drug; and (3) the defendants acted with the intent to defraud or mislead. The elements instruction for the misbranding offense was the same except that the court substituted the term "misbranded" for "unapproved new drug."

Under Section 333(a)(1), neither knowledge nor intent is required for a misdemeanor violation. However, under Section 333(a)(2), there must be an intent to defraud or mislead for a felony violation. The defendants contended then that they could not violate Section 333(a)(2) unless it could be established that they had knowledge that E-Ferol was an unapproved drug and knowledge that E-Ferol was misbranded. The government, however, argued that the knowledge requirement of (a)(2) applies to the intent to defraud or mislead, not to the Section 331 violations. The court replied:

> Given the fraud that the government alleged and sought to prove in the instant case, we think it is quite clear that Carter and Hiland could not have acted with the intent to defraud or mislead absent (1) knowledge that E-Ferol was a "drug" which was not approved by the FDA and had not been established as safe and effective for use in premature infants to treat RLF (i.e., was an unapproved "new drug"); and

(2) knowledge that E-Ferol's labeling contained misrepresentations and misleading omissions (i.e., was "misbranded"). Thus, we need not decide whether knowledge of the facts constituting the misdemeanor violation of 331 would be a separate and essential element of a 333(a)(2) violation in a case where the defendants could have acted with the intent to defraud or mislead without such knowledge. Our inquiry here is whether the court's instructions were adequate to prevent the jury from convicting Carter and Hiland on the FDCA counts without finding that they had the knowledge necessary for the intent required by 333(a)(2).

Although not a model of clarity, we conclude that when viewed as a whole and in the context of the entire trial, the district court's instructions fairly advised the jury that Carter and Hiland could not have acted with the intent to defraud or mislead without knowledge that E-Ferol was an unapproved new drug and misbranded.

Carter and Hiland also argued that the district court committed reversible error by giving a willful blindness instruction to the jury.

In essence, a willful blindness instruction "allows the jury to impute knowledge to [the defendant] of what should be obvious to him, if it found, beyond a reasonable doubt, a conscious purpose to avoid enlightenment." As the First Circuit has noted, "[t]he purpose of the willful blindness theory is to impose criminal liability on people who, recognizing the likelihood of wrongdoing, nonetheless consciously refuse to take basic investigatory steps."

We find no reversible error in the language used to instruct the jury on willful blindness. Viewed in the context of the entire jury charge, which included instructions on acts done knowingly, specific intent, and intent to defraud, the district court's willful blindness instruction did not permit the jury to convict the defendants on the basis of negligent conduct. We reject Carter's assertion that such an instruction must specifically state that a defendant has knowledge of a certain fact only if he is aware of a high probability of its existence, unless he actually believes that it does not exist.

Although the evidence in this regard was not overwhelming, taken as a whole it provided the jury with a reasonable basis for inferring that if Carter and Hiland did not actually know E-Ferol was dangerous and falsely labeled, it was only because they consciously chose to be ignorant of those facts. This inference could reasonably be drawn from the evidence concerning their responses to serious indications that E-Ferol was associated with the illness and deaths of premature infants.

Decision of the court: The court affirmed the lower court's ruling against the defendants.

Notes on *United States v. Hiland*

1. The FDCA imposes a strict liability (misdemeanor) requirement on product sellers, meaning that the mere introduction into interstate commerce of an unapproved or misbranded drug violates the law, regardless of whether the seller had any knowledge to this effect. The defendants tried to argue that intent to mislead or defraud (a criminal charge) cannot be established unless the government can prove they had knowledge that the product was an unapproved new drug and was misbranded. Usually in a fraud case, the prosecution must show knowledge. The government, however, argued that because knowledge to this effect is not required for the misdemeanor violation, it cannot be required for the fraud violation. The only elements required, argued the government, are that the defendants unknowingly committed the acts and had an intent to defraud. The court dodged the issue of whether knowledge must be proven or not by holding that

the facts clearly showed that the defendants knew their product was promoted as a drug and was mislabeled.

2. The defendants contended that they thought they could market their product without approval on the basis of FDA policy. During the DESI review, the FDA had allowed generic drug manufacturers to continue marketing their products pending a determination of efficacy. This policy was voided, however, by a federal court. Even had the policy been valid, it would not have applied to E-Ferol because it only applied to generics whose parent drug had been proven safe and effective. E-Ferol had no parent drug.

3. It is conceivable that if this case was brought today, the defendants would argue that the product is a dietary supplement, not a drug. This argument would not likely prevail, however. First, E-Ferol is intended for injection, and DSHEA defines a dietary supplement as one intended for ingestion. Second, the defendants clearly intended that the IV E-Ferol be used to treat RLF, a disease.

CASE 2-3 **United States v. Rutherford, 442 U.S. 544 (1979)**

Issue

Whether the federal FDCA precludes terminally ill cancer patients from obtaining Laetrile, a drug not recognized as "safe and effective" within the meaning of 201(p)(1) of the act.

Overview

The FDA has historically been criticized for taking too long to approve new drugs for market; especially drugs intended for use in the terminally ill, where any delay is critical. In the 1970s and early 1980s, Laetrile gained considerable notoriety as a possible cure for cancer, despite little good scientific evidence as to its safety and efficacy. In fact, 17 states had legalized the use of Laetrile within their borders. The FDA, however, considered the product an unapproved drug and thus would not allow the interstate shipment of the drug. The plaintiffs in this case, terminally ill patients, argued that the FDCA does not prevent the availability of Laetrile for use for the terminally ill. A federal district court and court of appeals both agreed, although for different reasons, and the FDA appealed to the U.S. Supreme Court. This case raises some important policy issues. Should terminally ill patients have access to any medical treatment they want? In other words, what are we protecting terminally ill patients from by denying them access to the medical treatment of their choice? Would the public health still be protected if unapproved drugs for the terminally ill were legally available on the market but labeled with mandatory disclaimers that they were unapproved for safety and efficacy? Alternatively, should the drug approval process at least be expedited for drugs intended to treat life-threatening diseases? If the Supreme Court had agreed with the lower courts' decisions, what effect might this have had on the commercial market for cancer treatments?

The Supreme Court first addressed the facts and applicable law:

> Section 505 of the Federal Food, Drug, and Cosmetic Act prohibits interstate distribution of any "new drug" unless the Secretary of Health, Education, and Welfare approves an application supported by substantial evidence of the drug's safety and effectiveness. As defined in 201(p)(1) of the Act, 21 U.S.C. 321(p)(1), the term "new drug" includes "[a]ny drug ... not generally recognized, among experts qualified by scientific training and experience to evaluate the safety and effectiveness of drugs, as safe and effective for use under the conditions prescribed, recommended, or suggested in the labeling...."

In 1975, terminally ill cancer patients and their spouses brought this action to enjoin the Government from interfering with the interstate shipment and sale of Laetrile, a drug not approved for distribution under the Act. Finding that Laetrile, in proper dosages, was nontoxic and effective, the District Court ordered the Government to permit limited purchases of the drug by one of the named plaintiffs. On appeal by the Government, the Court of Appeals for the Tenth Circuit did not disturb the injunction. However, it instructed the District Court to remand the case to the Food and Drug Administration for determination whether Laetrile was a "new drug" under 201(p)(1), and, if so, whether it was exempt from remarketing approval under either of the Act's grandfather clauses.

After the administrative hearings order by the court, the FDA found that Laetrile was a new drug because it was not generally recognized among experts as safe and effective for its prescribed use. The agency further found that Laetrile was not exempt from premarketing approval under either the 1938 or 1962 grandfather provisions.

Reviewing the commissioner's decision, the district court agreed that Laetrile was a new drug, but it ruled that Laetrile was exempt from the premarketing approval requirements, and also concluded that denying patients the right to use Laetrile infringed on their constitutionally protected privacy interests. The district court then granted an injunction, thus permitting the plaintiffs the use of Laetrile. The court of appeals approved the district court's injunction against the FDA, but on different grounds. The appellate court found that the terms safety and effectiveness have no relevance to the terminally ill. These patients will die regardless of the treatment and thus there are no standards on which to judge the safety and efficacy for these patients. The court of appeals did, however, limit the availability of Laetrile to intravenous use only under physician supervision.

The Supreme Court then provided its analysis of the issue.

The Federal Food, Drug, and Cosmetic Act makes no special provision for drugs used to treat terminally ill patients. By its terms, 505 of the Act requires premarketing approval for "any new drug" unless it is intended solely for investigative use or is exempt under one of the Act's grandfather provisions. And 201(p)(1) defines "new drug" to encompass "[a]ny drug . . . not generally recognized . . . as safe and effective for use under the conditions prescribed, recommended, or suggested in the labeling."

Nothing in the history of the 1938 Food, Drug, and Cosmetic Act, which first established procedures for review of drug safety, or of the 1962 Amendments, which added the current safety and effectiveness standards in 201(p)(1), suggests that Congress intended protection only for persons suffering from curable diseases. To the contrary, in deliberations preceding the 1938 Act, Congress expressed concern that individuals with fatal illnesses, such as cancer, should be shielded from fraudulent cures. Similarly, proponents of the 1962 Amendments to the Act, including Senator Kefauver, one of the bill's sponsors, indicated an understanding that experimental drugs used to treat cancer "in its last stages" were within the ambit of the statute.

In implementing the statutory scheme, the FDA has never made exception for drugs used by the terminally ill. As this Court has often recognized, the construction of a statute by those charged with its administration is entitled to substantial deference.

In the Court of Appeals' view, an implied exemption from the Act was justified because the safety and effectiveness standards set forth in 201(p)(1) could have "no reasonable application" to terminally ill patients. We disagree. Under our constitutional framework, federal courts do not sit as councils of revision, empowered to rewrite legislation in accord with their own conceptions of prudent public policy. Only when a literal construction of a statute yields results so manifestly unreasonable that they could not fairly be attributed to congressional design will an exception to statutory language be judicially implied. Here, however, we have no license to depart from the plain language of the Act, for Congress could reasonably have intended to shield terminal patients from ineffectual or unsafe drugs.

A drug is effective within the meaning of 201(p)(1) if there is general recognition among experts, founded on substantial evidence, that the drug in fact produces the results claimed for it under prescribed conditions. Contrary to the Court of Appeals' apparent assumption, effectiveness does not necessarily denote capacity to cure. In the treatment of any illness, terminal or otherwise, a drug is effective if it fulfills, by objective indices, its sponsor's claims of prolonged life, improved physical condition, or reduced pain.

So too, the concept of safety under 201(p)(1) is not without meaning for terminal patients. Few if any drugs are completely safe in the sense that they may be taken by all persons in all circumstances without risk. Thus, the Commissioner generally considers a drug safe when the expected therapeutic gain justifies the risk entailed by its use. For the terminally ill, as for anyone else, a drug is unsafe if its potential for inflicting death or physical injury is not offset by the possibility of therapeutic benefit. Indeed, the Court of Appeals implicitly acknowledged that safety considerations have relevance for terminal cancer patients by restricting authorized use of Laetrile to intravenous injections for persons under a doctor's supervision.

Moreover, there is a special sense in which the relationship between drug effectiveness and safety has meaning in the context of incurable illnesses. An otherwise harmless drug can be dangerous to any patient if it does not produce its purported therapeutic effect. But if an individual suffering from a potentially fatal disease rejects conventional therapy in favor of a drug with no demonstrable curative properties, the consequences can be irreversible. For this reason, even before the 1962 Amendments incorporated an efficacy standard into new drug application procedures, the FDA considered effectiveness when reviewing the safety of drugs used to treat terminal illness. The FDA's practice also reflects the recognition, amply supported by expert medical testimony in this case, that with diseases such as cancer it is often impossible to identify a patient as terminally ill except in retrospect. Cancers vary considerably in behavior and in responsiveness to different forms of therapy. Even critically ill individuals may have unexpected remissions and may respond to conventional treatment. Thus, as the Commissioner concluded, to exempt from the Act drugs with no proved effectiveness in the treatment of cancer "would lead to needless deaths and suffering among . . . patients characterized as 'terminal' who could actually be helped by legitimate therapy."

The Court then noted that accepting the court of appeal's logic would have broad consequences.

It bears emphasis that although the Court of Appeals' ruling was limited to Laetrile, its reasoning cannot be so readily confined. To accept the proposition that the safety and efficacy standards of the Act have no relevance for terminal patients is to deny the Commissioner's authority over all drugs, however toxic or ineffectual, for such individuals. If history is any guide, this new market would not be long overlooked. Since the turn of the century, resourceful entrepreneurs have advertised a wide variety of purportedly simple and painless cures for cancer, including liniments of turpentine, mustard, oil, eggs, and ammonia; peat moss; arrangements of colored flood lamps; pastes made from glycerin and limburger cheese; mineral tablets; and "Fountain of Youth" mixtures of spices, oil, and suet. In citing these examples, we do not, of course, intend to deprecate the sincerity of Laetrile's current proponents, or to imply any opinion on whether that drug may ultimately prove safe and effective for cancer treatment. But this historical experience does suggest why Congress could reasonably have determined to protect the terminally ill, no less than other patients, from the vast range of self styled panaceas that inventive minds can devise.

The Supreme Court reversed the decision of the court of appeals, finding in favor of the FDA.

Notes on *United States v. Rutherford*

1. The Supreme Court held that the requirements of the FDCA must be applied equally to all drugs, regardless of their intended use. At first impression it does seem bizarre that the government seeks to protect terminally ill patients from drugs not safe and effective when they are going to die anyway. The government's restriction appears more reasonable considering that patients might forgo legitimate treatments, which might be effective, for worthless cures and that unscrupulous individuals would benefit at the expense of the helpless and desperate. Some First Amendment advocates would respond, however, that patients should have the right to choose any treatment they wish, provided that unapproved drugs are labeled with adequate warnings and disclaimers. A significant concern to the Court was the broad effect its decision would have on the commercial market, beyond Laetrile. If it agreed with the lower courts' decisions, the Court was fearful it would give a green light to unscrupulous entrepreneurs to prey on desperate people.

2. The fact that the FDA opposed the plaintiffs in *Rutherford* does not imply that the FDA was unsympathetic to the plights of the terminally ill. The FDA has continuously studied the issue of how the approval system could better accommodate the needs of those with life-threatening illness and yet still protect them from products that might worsen their situation and from quackery. As discussed earlier, the agency did enact regulations to allow the use of investigational drugs and expedite the approval of drugs for serious and life-threatening diseases, and these regulations were ultimately codified in the FDAMA.

3. Although the plaintiffs raised the constitutional issue that their right of privacy was violated, both the court of appeals and the Supreme Court did not address it. This is common because courts will not address complex constitutional issues if the controversy can be decided on other grounds.

CASE 2-4   *Washington Legal Foundation v. Friedman*, 13 F. Supp. 2d 51 (D.C. 1998)

Issue

Whether the FDA's guidance publications restricting the use of textbook and journal reprints and educational seminars promoting off-label uses violate the First Amendment.

Overview

As noted in the advertising and promotions section of this chapter, the First Amendment is a significant factor in any governmental attempt to regulate in this area. At issue in this case is the constitutionality of two FDA policy guidances, one of which establishes restrictions for drug manufacturers disseminating textbooks and journal articles related to off-label uses and the other of which restricts a company from discussing the off-label uses of its drug at educational symposia that it sponsors. (Refer to the advertising section in this chapter for a discussion of the guidance policies.) Because the FDAMA was enacted after the guidance regulating the dissemination of written materials was published, supplanting the guidance, the constitutionality of the FDAMA provisions became an issue in a subsequent decision discussed in the notes after the case. The plaintiffs in this case contend that the guidance policies are too restrictive and thus violate the First Amendment.

As you read this case, ask: What is the primary reason why manufacturers want to notify health care providers of off-label uses? Has the FDA gone too far in its restrictions of discussing and disseminating off-label uses, or are the restrictions really necessary to protect the public? What alternatives did the court suggest that would be less restrictive than the FDA's off-label use policy, yet still protect the public? Does this case mean that the FDA cannot in any way restrict manufacturer promotion of off-label uses? Although this decision was appealed and the constitutional issues dismissed, this decision raises valid concerns and highlights the delicate relationship between government regulation and First Amendment rights.

The court started its analysis with a discussion of the facts.

> Plaintiff Washington Legal Foundation ("WLF") is a nonprofit public interest law and policy center that defends "the rights of individuals and businesses to go about their affairs without undue influence from government regulators." In this action, WLF seeks to enjoin the Food and Drug Administration ("FDA") and the Department of Health and Human Services ("HHS") from enforcing policies restricting certain forms of manufacturer promotion of off-label uses for FDA-approved drugs and devices. The policies at issue—expressed through Guidance Documents—concern manufacturer distribution of reprints of medical textbooks and peer-reviewed journal articles ("enduring materials"), and manufacturer involvement in continuing medical education seminars and symposia ("CME").

> Plaintiff seeks a declaratory judgment that the FDA policies expressed in the Guidance Documents violate the rights of its members under the First Amendment of the Constitution. It further requests that the court enter preliminary and permanent injunctions against defendants, preventing them from enforcing, relying upon, or otherwise giving effect to the Guidance Documents.

The court then reviewed the regulatory framework for drug approval, finding that the FDCA clearly proscribes the labeling of off-label uses by manufacturers. The court noted that 21 U.S.C. § 321(p) makes it clear that drugs must be proven safe and effective for "use under the conditions prescribed," meaning that a drug must have FDA approval for each use. Otherwise the use is unapproved and considered to be off-label. Manufacturer promotion of off-label uses constitutes misbranding under 21 U.S.C. § 352. The court, however, also noted a significant discrepancy between the regulatory framework and medical practice.

> Central to this litigation is that what a manufacturer may lawfully claim that a drug does under the statutory and regulatory scheme, and what a physician may prescribe a drug for, do not match. Once a drug has been approved by the FDA for marketing for any use, the actual prescription choices regarding those drugs are left to the discretion of the physician. A physician may prescribe an approved drug for any medical condition, irrespective of whether FDA has determined that the drug is safe and effective with respect to that illness. The FDA contends that it accepts the practice of off-label use by physicians as part of its enforcement discretion, though it appears to be an open question as to whether the FDA could currently regulate this aspect of the practice of medicine if it wished to do so.

In light of this discrepancy, the court considered the merits of off-label use, noting that it is an accepted aspect of a physician's prescribing regimen and that even the FDA has acknowledged that off-label use constitutes good medical practice in appropriate situations. The court also noted that the FDA has stated that physicians need current and reliable information about off-label uses, but that off-label prescribing can pose problems to the public.

The plaintiffs did not disagree with the FDA completely but argued that the guidance documents are too restrictive under the First Amendment, because one guidance prohibits entirely the discussion of off-label uses at company-sponsored promotional symposia and the other prohibits the unsolicited distribution of articles and texts addressing off-label uses. (The court noted that the FDAMA subsequently replaced this guidance, permitting distribution provided that the manufacturer submits an application to have the new use approved by the FDA. Nonetheless, the court included this guidance in its ruling.) The court then launched its First Amendment analysis of the guidance restrictions starting with the issue of how to classify the speech being regulated.

> Plaintiff argues that it is scientific and academic speech, which is entitled to the highest level of First Amendment protection. Defendants challenge this assertion by first making a somewhat difficult to discern argument that the Guidance Documents regulate conduct. A closer examination demonstrates that what the FDA is actually contending is that because the federal government has the broad power to regulate the pharmaceutical industry, the Guidance Documents are incidental encroachments upon speech and entirely compatible with the First Amendment. In the alternative, FDA claims that the Guidance Documents at most regulate commercial speech, which is subject to a more relaxed inquiry than core First Amendment speech.

The court had no difficulty concluding that the guidance documents regulate speech, not conduct. The conduct, stated the court, is the off-label prescribing by physicians, but the guidance documents regulate the off-label dissemination activities by the manufacturers, which encourage the conduct, and are speech. The issue of whether the speech is pure speech or commercial speech gave the court more difficulty.

> The resolution of this question is not an easy one, as the communications present one of those "complex mixtures of commercial and non-commercial elements." Typical "commercial speech" is authored and/or uttered directly by the commercial entity that wishes to financially benefit from the message. A purveyor of goods or services makes claim about his products in order to induce a purchase. In this instance, by contrast, the speech that the manufacturers wish to "communicate" is the speech of others—the work product of scientists, physicians and other academics.

Nonetheless, the court found that the purpose of the manufacturer's dissemination of pure speech by others is to influence prescribers and in turn increase sales. Therefore, the court concluded the speech is commercial. The court then proceeded to analyze whether the government regulation of this commercial speech is constitutional under *Central Hudson*'s four-prong test (see summary of *Hudson* earlier in this chapter).

Hudson's first prong is that the speech must be neither unlawful nor inherently misleading. Regarding the unlawful issue, the court found it could not be unlawful because the speech promotes the conduct of prescribing drugs for off-label uses, a lawful activity. As for the inherently misleading component, the court noted that the speech must be "more likely to deceive the public than to inform it," stating:

> In asserting that any and all scientific claims about the safety, effectiveness, contra-indications, side effects, and the like regarding prescription drugs are presumptively untruthful or misleading until the FDA has had the opportunity to evaluate them, FDA exaggerates its overall place in the universe.

> To categorize the speech at issue here as "inherently misleading" is particularly unsupportable when one considers all the controls available to FDA to ensure that the information manufacturers wish to distribute is scientifically reliable, and therefore less likely to even be "potentially misleading."

The court listed the controls that the FDA retains over off-label use promotion after its decision, which would allow the FDA to:

- Require a disclaimer that the uses have not been approved by the FDA
- Require that reprinted articles come from a bona fide peer-review journal
- Require that textbook reprints be published by a "bona fide independent publisher"
- Require that for CME seminars and symposia, the sponsor must be an "independent program provider"
- Require manufacturers that sponsor or provide financial support for the dissemination of articles or reference textbooks or for seminars and symposia to disclose (a) their interest in the product promoted and (b) the fact that the use discussed has not been approved by the FDA
- Enforce any rules, regulations, guidance, statutes, or other provisions of law that sanction the dissemination or redistribution of material that is false or misleading

Finding that the manufacturers' speech is neither unlawful nor inherently misleading, the court addressed the second prong, whether the government's interest is substantial. The court noted that the government has two interests: one, that physicians receive accurate and unbiased information; and two, that manufacturers receive ample incentive to get the unapproved uses approved. The first reason, stated the court, is not legitimate. The government cannot assume paternalistically that the public will use truthful, nonmisleading information unwisely, especially in this situation, where the public is physicians who possess the knowledge and sophistication to make informed choices and are capable of evaluating the materials distributed to them. As for the second reason, the court did find that the government has a substantial interest in compelling manufacturers to seek approval for off-label uses because the FDCA requires it.

The court then addressed the third prong of the *Hudson* test, whether the guidance documents advance a substantial government interest "in a direct and material way" by requiring manufacturers to submit supplemental applications to obtain approval for new uses. The court held that they did, noting that manufacturers would otherwise avoid submitting approved drugs for subsequent approval because of the time and cost involved and the fact that the drugs were already on the market.

The court last analyzed the fourth prong, whether the guidance documents restrict more extensively than is necessary, concluding that the restrictions were more extensive than necessary to achieve the government's substantial interest of encouraging manufacturers to get new uses approved.

> This determination is based in large part upon the fact that there exist less burdensome alternatives to this restriction on commercial speech. The most obvious alternative is full, complete, and unambiguous disclosure by the manufacturer. Full disclosure not only addresses all of the concerns advanced by the FDA but addresses them more effectively. It is less restrictive on speech, while at the same time deals more precisely with the concerns of the FDA and Congress.

Full disclosure, concluded the court, will assuage concerns that the manufacturer's promotions are inherently misleading because physicians would know that the product has not been approved for the use promoted. In addition, stated the court, manufacturers would still have adequate incentives to obtain approval for new uses for several reasons:

- They are proscribed from producing and distributing marketing materials for off-label use.
- They cannot be involved in seminars unless conducted by an independent program provider.

- They cannot initiate person-to-person contact with a physician about the off-label use.
- They cannot advertise off-label uses to consumers.

Also, noted the court, because of malpractice concerns, FDA approval is important to physicians.

The court granted the plaintiff's motion, enjoining the FDA from restricting any company from disseminating to health care professionals peer-reviewed published articles or reference textbooks that discuss off-label uses. The agency also may not prevent companies from suggesting content or speakers to independent educational symposia regarding off-label uses. The FDA is permitted to impose the six controls previously stated.

Notes on *Washington Legal Foundation v. Friedman*

1. In applying the *Hudson* test to this case, the judge found that the company's dissemination of off-label use information was not unlawful because the speech is intended to promote the activity of prescribing drugs for off-label use, which is lawful. Could it not be equally valid that the speech is intended by the manufacturers to further the activity of marketing drugs for unapproved uses, an illegal use? Should the decision turn on the conduct of the physicians or the conduct of the manufacturers?

2. After the decision, the FDA filed a motion with the court to confine the injunction to the policy guidance only and not to the FDAMA, which became effective after the decision. The WLF challenged this motion and the court found for the WLF, stating that the injunction applied to the pertinent policies contained in the FDAMA, not just the guidance documents (*Washington Legal Foundation v. Friedman*, 36 F. Supp. 2d 16 (D.C. 1999)). Otherwise, stated the court, the FDAMA would render its decision meaningless. The court stopped short of declaring any specific portion of the FDAMA unconstitutional, however, until after the parties submitted briefs and adjudicated the matter.

3. The matter was then adjudicated in *Washington Legal Foundation v. Henney*, 36 F. Supp. 2d 418 (D.C. 1999), where the judge, after reviewing the FDAMA's restrictions on manufacturer dissemination of peer-reviewed articles and texts, declared that insofar as the restrictions perpetuated policies previously determined unconstitutional, those portions of the FDAMA must also be unconstitutional. In particular, the court found disfavor with the FDAMA requirement that off-label use information could be disseminated only if a supplemental application has been submitted for approval. Stated the court, "The supplemental application requirement amounts to a kind of constitutional blackmail—comply with the statute or sacrifice your First Amendment rights. It should go without saying that this tactic cannot survive judicial scrutiny." The court continued by noting that the supplemental application requirement is unnecessary in light of the numerous other incentives that exist for manufacturers to seek approval for off-label uses as determined in the *Friedman* decision.

4. The FDA appealed the *Friedman* and *Henney* decisions in *WLF v. Henney*, No. 99 5304 (D.C. 2000), insofar as the decisions declared unconstitutional the CME guidance and the FDAMA provisions regulating the dissemination of articles and textbooks. (The FDA conceded that the FDAMA superseded the guidances related to regulating the dissemination of articles.) The appellate court was prepared to consider the constitutional issue, when in a surprise move, the FDA asserted that it had no authority to regulate manufacturer speech. Instead, argued

the agency, the requirements contained in the FDAMA and CME guidance only establish a "safe harbor," ensuring that certain forms of conduct would not be used against manufacturers. Thus, continued the FDA, neither the FDAMA nor CME guidance authorize the FDA to prohibit or to sanction speech. If a company wants to disseminate off-label use information in violation of the FDAMA or CME guidance, that would not be a per se violation of the law and would not trigger agency sanction. The FDA, however, would retain the right to use the conduct as evidence in a misbranding or intended use enforcement action. In light of this "new" position by the FDA, both parties then agreed that the FDAMA and CME guidance do not facially violate the First Amendment. In light of this agreement, the court found a constitutional controversy no longer existed. It therefore refused to consider the merits of the district court's decision as requested by WLF, dismissing the FDA's appeal and vacating the district court's decisions holding the FDAMA and CME guidance unconstitutional.

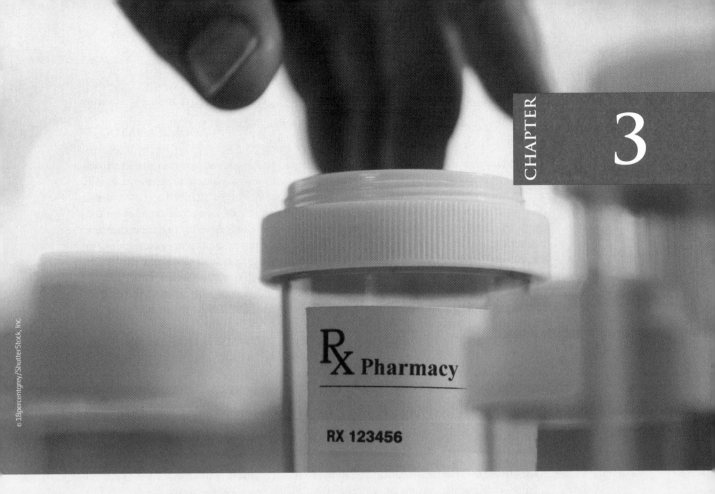

FEDERAL REGULATION OF MEDICATIONS: DISPENSING

CHAPTER OBJECTIVES

Upon completing this chapter, the reader will be able to:

- ▸ Discuss the criteria by which a drug is determined to be prescription or over-the-counter (OTC).
- ▸ Understand how the provisions of the Durham-Humphrey Amendment affect drug classification and pharmacy practice.
- ▸ Describe the FDA's role in regulating written patient information.
- ▸ Identify the issues associated with unlabeled drug uses.
- ▸ Distinguish pharmacy compounding from manufacturing.
- ▸ Determine the role and use of the Orange Book in pharmacy practice.
- ▸ Identify the scope and implications of the Prescription Drug Marketing Act.

- ▸ Recognize the requirements established in the Poison Prevention Packaging Act.
- ▸ Understand the legal issues related to pharmacies advertising prescription and nonprescription drugs.

The federal Food, Drug, and Cosmetic Act (FDCA) adopts a regulatory approach that emphasizes the elimination, or at least limitation, of risks throughout the drug distribution chain—from the time a scientist first imagines that a molecule might be effective as a drug through the ingestion by a patient of a product containing that drug. Pharmacists are involved with every aspect of drug development, production, marketing, and distribution. However, the primary focus of pharmacy practice is drug dispensing. In contemporary pharmacy practice, dispensing includes more than order processing. Dispensing is a comprehensive activity that incorporates drug therapy monitoring and patient education as well as drug distribution. Because most pharmacists perform dispensing functions, the aspects of the FDCA that relate specifically to dispensing are particularly relevant to pharmacy practice.

This chapter discusses regulatory activities of the Food and Drug Administration (FDA) that have particular significance to those who are directly involved in the dispensing function and in other patient care activities.

THE DURHAM-HUMPHREY AMENDMENT OF 1951

As discussed in Chapter 2, section 502 of the FDCA establishes different labeling requirements for drugs, depending on whether they are prescription or nonprescription. The questions then become, "How did it happen that we have two classes of drugs instead of one or three?" "What determines if a drug is a prescription drug?" These answers can be found in the Durham-Humphrey Amendment, also known as the Prescription Drug Amendment (§ 503; 21 U.S.C. § 353).

Cosponsored by two pharmacist-legislators, Senator Hubert Humphrey and Congressman Carl Durham, this important amendment to the FDCA created the first statutory distinction between prescription and nonprescription drugs. Legislative history of the amendment discloses that the prescription distinction from OTC was not the primary focus of the bill leading to this important law. Legalization of the verbal transmission of prescriptions (as opposed to the traditional method of writing them) and the legal right for pharmacists to honor refill authorizations indicated by physicians in the initial prescription were the key provisions of the bill. The full impact of a clear dichotomy between prescription and OTC drugs may not have been fully appreciated at the time. Although the Durham-Humphrey Amendment recognized pharmacists as being instrumental in the distribution of drugs, it failed to acknowledge that pharmacists may play a significant role in drug therapy.

THE LAW

The amendment, as subsequently amended by the Food and Drug Administration Modernization Act of 1997 (FDAMA), provides in part

(b)(1) A drug intended for use by man which—

(A) because of its toxicity or other potentiality for harmful effect, or the method of its use, or the collateral measures necessary to its use, is not safe for use except under the supervision of a practitioner licensed by law to administer such drug; or

(B) is limited by an approved application under section 505 to use under the professional supervision of a practitioner licensed by law to administer such drug;

shall be dispensed only (i) upon a written prescription of a practitioner licensed by law to administer such drug, or (ii) upon an oral prescription of such practitioner which is reduced promptly to writing and filed by the pharmacist, or (iii) by refilling any such written or oral prescription if such refilling is authorized by the prescriber either in the original prescription or by oral order which is reduced promptly to writing and filed by the pharmacist. The act of dispensing a drug contrary to the provisions of this paragraph shall be deemed to be an act which results in the drug being misbranded while held for sale.

(2) Any drug dispensed by filling or refilling a written or oral prescription of a practitioner licensed by law to administer such drug shall be exempt from the requirements of section 502, except paragraphs (a), (i)(2) and (3), (k), and (l), and the packaging requirements of paragraphs (g), (h), and (p), if the drug bears a label containing the name and address of the dispenser, the serial number and date of the prescription or of its filling, the name of the prescriber, and, if stated in the prescription, the name of the patient, and the directions for use and cautionary statements, if any, contained in such prescription. This exemption shall not apply to any drug dispensed in the course of the conduct of a business of dispensing drugs pursuant to diagnosis by mail, or to a drug dispensed in violation of paragraph (1) of this subsection.

(3) The Secretary may by regulation remove drugs subject to section 505 from the requirements of paragraph (1) of this subsection when such requirements are not necessary for the protection of the public health.

(4)(A) A drug which is subject to paragraph (1) of this subsection shall be deemed to be misbranded if at any time prior to dispensing the label of the drug fails to bear, at a minimum, the symbol "Rx only."

(B) A drug to which paragraph (1) of this subsection does not apply shall be deemed to be misbranded if at any time prior to dispensing the label of the drug bears the symbol described in subparagraph (A).

EXPLANATION OF THE DURHAM-HUMPHREY AMENDMENT

Before the passage of the Durham-Humphrey Amendment, drug manufacturers generally determined whether their products were prescription or OTC drugs. If the FDA disagreed with the manufacturer's choice, it had to sue the manufacturer for misbranding. There was a great deal of confusion for health care practitioners and patients, however, because one manufacturer could label an active ingredient a prescription drug, whereas another manufacturer labeled the same ingredient an OTC drug. The amendment resolved this situation by establishing criteria for the classification of prescription drugs. All other drugs were, of course, considered nonprescription drugs. Thus, the amendment officially established two classes of drugs: prescription and OTC.

Prescription Versus Over-the-Counter Drugs

Subsection (b)(1) of the amendment provides that the FDA has the authority to categorize as prescription drugs those that are

- Unsafe for use except under the supervision of a practitioner because of the toxicity, the method of use, or the collateral measures necessary to use the drug
- Subject to the new drug application (NDA) approval process

(*Note:* Before the FDAMA this subsection also listed habit-forming drugs as those that the FDA could categorize as prescription.)

The issue of if a drug requires the supervision of a practitioner for its use under subsection (b)(1)(A) and, thus, should be a prescription drug, was addressed in *United States v. Article of Drug—Decholin*, 264 F. Supp. 473 (E.D. Mich. 1967). In *Decholin*, the court established that the FDA must prove two issues to change the status of a drug from OTC to prescription: (1) that the toxicity and method of use require practitioner supervision, and (2) that the collateral measures necessary to use the drug require supervision.

Addressing the toxicity and method of use issue, the court stated that the FDA must show that the pharmacological and toxic effect of the drug is such that, unless it is taken pursuant to a physician's directions, it may harm the patient. This requires evidence of the seriousness of harm resulting from the unsupervised use, including the dosage level that is likely to cause this harm, the immediacy of the harm, the effect of prolonging treatment by a physician, and the patient's ability to recognize that the drug is not helping before real harm occurs.

Examining the collateral measures issue, the court concluded that the government also must establish that a patient who takes the drug for a condition that the drug cannot cure will suffer harm because of the postponement of a visit to the physician in reliance on the drug. This requires the government to show the seriousness of the harm resulting from the delay, the length of delay that is detrimental, the quality of advice contained on the label (e.g., whether it alerts a patient to the possibility that professional attention may be required), and the possibility that the drug may alleviate the symptoms, making a patient think that the condition has been cured when it has not.

Dispensing Written, Oral, and Electronic Prescriptions

Subsection (b)(1) also stipulates that prescription drugs may be dispensed pursuant to written or oral prescriptions promptly reduced to writing and filed. Before the Durham-Humphrey Amendment, oral prescriptions were not valid nor were refills recognized. This subsection allows for refills, as long as they are authorized either in the original prescription or by oral order.

Note that the Durham-Humphrey Amendment does not specifically authorize the electronic transmission of prescriptions. Obviously, when Congress enacted the Durham-Humphrey Amendment it could not have contemplated electronic prescriptions (e-prescribing). Nonetheless, most states have enacted laws and regulations authorizing the transmission of prescriptions by both image transmission (fax) and data transmission, and historically the FDA has regarded electronic prescriptions very favorably. The Medicare prescription drug law (part D) specifically permits e-prescribing and preempts any contrary state restriction. The issue is more complicated with controlled substance prescriptions. Drug Enforcement Administration (DEA) regulations allow the faxing of controlled substance prescriptions, but not data transmission. The DEA, however, has proposed a regulation to allow for data transmission prescriptions.

The legitimacy of electronic records and electronic signatures received a boost in 2000. In that year, Congress enacted the Electronic Signatures in Global and National Commerce Act, known as E-Sign (P.L. 106-229). E-Sign provides that electronic records, signatures, or contracts in interstate commerce are legally valid. If a law requires a signature to be in writing, an electronic signature satisfies the law. E-Sign preempts inconsistent state laws. It is not completely clear as to the extent in which E-Sign preempts laws related to prescriptions and prescription records. If completely applicable, state and federal laws requiring pharmacies to keep paper records would be invalid if the pharmacies can maintain those records electronically. Moreover, if applicable, E-Sign would invalidate laws that require prescriptions to be handwritten or signed in writing by the prescriber.

Labeling Requirements

Without the Durham-Humphrey Amendment, pharmacists would be required to label every dispensed prescription drug pursuant to the same requirements that manufacturers must meet. Subsection (b)(2), however, recognizes that some of the information mandated by section 502 would be impractical for drugs dispensed pursuant to prescription and should fall under the discretion of the health care provider. Thus, subsection (b)(2) exempts the dispensing pharmacist from the labeling requirements of section 502 except for the following:

- The label must not be false or misleading.
- The drug dispensed must not be an imitation drug.
- The drug must not be sold under the name of another drug.
- The packaging and labeling must conform to official compendia standards.
- If it is a drug liable to deterioration, it must be packaged and labeled appropriately.
- It must be packaged in conformance with the Poison Prevention Packaging Act (15 U.S.C. § 1571 et seq.).

In the case of the *Pharmaceutical Manufacturers Association v. Food and Drug Administration* (reported in the case studies section), the physician and pharmacist plaintiffs unsuccessfully argued that the exemption accorded in subsection (b)(2) precludes the government from mandating that health care providers distribute written information to patients for certain prescription drugs. The plaintiffs argued that because subsection (b)(2) gives them discretion as to what information to provide to a patient, the government could not mandate that they provide written information to patients. The court disagreed, finding that it was not the intent of the provision to give complete discretion to health care providers to the exclusion of the government.

Subsection (b)(2) also specifies the minimum information that the pharmacist must include on the label of a dispensed drug. Most state laws require additional information on the label such as

- The name, initials, or license number of the dispensing pharmacist
- The expiration date of the drug, if any
- The drug's name and strength
- The address of the patient
- The name of the manufacturer or distributor
- The lot or control number

State Standardized Prescription Labels

Recently, there has been increased awareness that many patients cannot read or understand the label effectively, thus leading to adverse drug events. A 2006 study published in the *Annals of Internal Medicine* revealed that 46 percent of patients misunderstood one or more instructions printed on the container labels of five commonly prescribed medications. In an effort to improve this situation, the USP (http://www.usp.org) and the National Association of Boards of Pharmacy (NABP) (http://www.nabp.net) have proposed that states develop standards to establish patient-centered standardized labels. California and New York have done so. Generally, this means that the label should be organized in a patient-centered manner such that critical information (i.e., name of patient, name and strength of drug, directions for use, purpose or condition) is grouped together, prominently displayed, and clear; that the critical information should be in an appropriate font size; that directions for use should be standardized and explicitly describe dosage and intervals; and when possible the labeling should be in the patient's preferred language. California and New York require that the label be interpreted in certain languages other than English.

Other Subsection (b)(2) Considerations

Subsection (b)(2) also used to provide that if the dispensed drug was an antibiotic or insulin product subject to batch certification, then the product must have come from a batch-certified source. However, the FDAMA eliminated batch certification requirements.

Subsection (b)(2) does not exempt drugs from section 502 if they are dispensed pursuant to diagnosis by mail. The purpose of this provision is to help protect the consumer against fraud and quackery. It does not apply to the typical mail-order drug outlets. This provision may, however, apply to situations in which patients, who have never established a legitimate, personal physician–patient relationship, are being diagnosed and prescribed for by means of the Internet. Neither the FDA nor the courts have ever considered the application of this clause to Internet prescriptions, however.

Expiration or Beyond-Use Dating

The manufacturer is required to include the expiration date on the label of its product. This date identifies the time during which the drug may be expected to meet the requirements of the United States Pharmacopeia (USP) monograph for the drug. Correspondingly, almost every state requires that the pharmacist include an expiration date on the label of the dispensed drug product; however, this date may or may not be the same date as the manufacturer's expiration date, depending on state law and other factors. The USP states that "The dispenser shall place on the label of the prescription container a suitable beyond-use date (emphasis added) . . ." (USP 29/NF 24, p. 11). The "beyond-use date" is defined as the date after which the drug should not be used, and it must not exceed the manufacturer's expiration date. The USP provides that in determining the beyond-use date, the pharmacist shall take into account the nature of the drug, the container in which it was packaged by the manufacturer, the characteristics of the dispensed container, expected storage conditions, and other factors.

The USP further states that for multiple-unit containers (the typical prescription vial), absent data to the contrary, the beyond-use date "shall not be later than (a) the expiration date on the manufacturer's container, or (b) 1 year from the date the drug is dispensed, whichever is earlier." When nonsterile solid and liquid drug products are repackaged into unit-dose or single-unit containers, USP guidelines provide that the pharmacist should affix a beyond-use date that is the earlier of 1 year from the date of repackaging or the expiration date on the original bulk container. Pharmacists should use an even earlier date, of course, if stability data or the manufacturer's labeling indicates otherwise.

Many pharmacies have adopted the USP beyond-use date guidelines, leading to some consumer confusion. A good example of this occurred in about 2003 in California. State law in California requires the label to contain "The expiration date of the effectiveness of the drug dispensed" (CA B&P Code 4076(a)(9)). Rite Aid pharmacies typically affixed on the label the expiration date as being one year from the date of dispensing or the manufacturer's expiration date if it was sooner, pursuant to the USP. At the behest of a group of consumers, the State of California brought a lawsuit against Rite Aid contending the chain engaged in consumer fraud for placing a misleading expiration date on the label. The suit alleged that the misleading date induced consumers to discard their medications prior to the manufacturer's expiration date and replace them, thus unfairly generating more business for Rite Aid. (A similar suit was filed directly by consumers against Walgreens in Illinois in 2003.) Once Rite Aid pointed out it was merely conforming to the USP standards, the suit was dropped.

It is likely that state boards of pharmacy will accept either the USP's beyond-use date or the manufacturer's expiration date. However, state law is determinate, and pharmacists must conform to the law in their particular state on this issue.

SWITCH OF PRESCRIPTION DRUGS TO OVER-THE-COUNTER DRUGS

As discussed earlier, subsection 503(b)(3) of the Durham-Humphrey Amendment authorizes the FDA to switch prescription drugs to OTC status by regulation when the conditions warrant. A switch may occur in three ways:

1. The manufacturer may request the switch by submitting a supplemental application to its approved NDA.
2. The manufacturer may petition the FDA.
3. The FDA may add or amend an OTC monograph.

The OTC drug review process was initially the primary mechanism by which drugs were switched from prescription to OTC status. Under the review process, the advisory review panels may recommend such a switch to the FDA. If the agency agrees, it publishes a final OTC drug monograph to this effect, which becomes binding on manufacturers of that active ingredient. Today most switches occur through the SNDA. Using this manner generally allows the manufacturer to obtain market exclusivity for the product.

Some switches have justifiably confused pharmacists because on occasion a product from one manufacturer is a prescription drug and an identical product from another manufacturer is an OTC drug. (*Note:* Differentiate this issue from how adequate directions for use labeling can cause a drug to be both OTC and prescription.) This situation can result when a switch to OTC status occurs through FDA approval of a manufacturer's supplemental application to its NDA. Approval for one NDA holder to switch does not automatically apply to other manufacturers of products containing the same ingredients. Each manufacturer must submit a supplement for approval. Therefore, switches for identical products can occur at different times. Pharmacists must abide by the label and not sell a legend drug without a prescription, even though the competitor's product may be sold OTC. A switch in status pursuant to a monograph, on the other hand, generally applies to all other manufacturers' products at the same time.

The petition route to a switch had essentially been a nonissue until Blue Cross (now WellPoint Health Networks) submitted a citizen petition to switch the nonsedating antihistamines (Allegra, Claritin, and Zyrtec) from prescription to OTC in 2001. Although the regulations do not specify who may petition, no party other than a product's manufacturer had ever submitted a petition. WellPoint's petition raised the issue of whether the FDA could legally approve a petition by a party other than the manufacturer over the manufacturer's objections. Ultimately an FDA panel voted to support the petition, but the FDA took no action, leaving it up to the manufacturers. Schering-Plough switched Claritin in 2002 and Zyrtec was switched in 2007.

Third Class of Drugs/Behind-the-Counter/Nonprescription Under Conditions of Safe Use

Since at least the 1970s, pharmacy organizations and others have contemplated a "third class of drugs." Although the exact definition for a third class of drugs has varied, it was generally agreed that it would include certain nonprescription drugs that could be sold only by a pharmacist. The rationale for a third class of drugs included that some of the drugs being switched could jeopardize a patient's health unless a pharmacist provided appropriate consultation and that such a class of drugs would allow the FDA to switch drugs that could not otherwise be switched because of safety concerns. Some examples of a third class of drugs do exist presently, including the sale of some Schedule V drugs in states that permit their sale as exempt narcotics and Plan B for emergency contraception, discussed later.

Some question has always existed as to if an amendment to the Durham-Humphrey Amendment would be necessary to establish a third class of drugs on a national basis or if the FDA has the statutory authority to do so by regulation. The FDAMA included provisions for the national uniformity of nonprescription drugs, thus making it unlikely that a state would have the authority to establish a third class of drugs. Regardless, the FDA traditionally had opposed pharmacists on this issue. In 1974, FDA Commissioner A. M. Schmidt issued a policy statement that was later summarized in a 1984 petition response:

> It would be inappropriate to restrict the sale of OTC drugs to pharmacies based on anything less than proof that a significant safety issue was involved. Restricting certain OTC drugs to pharmacies only could decrease the number of outlets where the consumer could purchase OTC drug products, limit competition, and raise some OTC drug prices, with no attendant public health benefit. Recognizing at all times the important contribution of pharmacists to the health care system, the FDA has continued to conclude that limiting certain drugs to sale-by-pharmacists only is unnecessary because a public need for such a limitation has not been demonstrated. (Poole, 1991)

The FDA, however, first signaled a likely change in its position in 2007 by announcing a public meeting to obtain comments regarding the creation of a "behind-the-counter (BTC)" class of drugs (renamed from third class of drugs) (72 Fed. Reg. 56769, Oct. 4, 2007). The hearing was held in November 2007 where organized pharmacy spoke in favor of a BTC category of drugs, while some other organizations, most notably the American Medical Association, opposed the category. Subsequently, the General Accounting Office (GAO) issued a report on the BTC issue in 2009, comparing the U.S. regulation of nonprescription drugs to four European Union countries (available at http://www.gao.gov/search?q=nonprescription+drugs&search_type=Solr&now_sort= score%20desc). The report describes arguments pro and con and identifies important policy considerations but concludes: "The classification of drugs in other countries and the existence of other classes provide little insight into the likely effect of a BTC drug class on nonprescription drug availability in the United States."

In February 2012, without mentioning the BTC discussions, the FDA announced that it is considering the creation of a class of nonprescription drugs that could be made available to patients "under conditions for safe use" (77 Fed. Reg. 12059, Feb. 28, 2012). The FDA noted that conditions for safe use would be specific to the drug product and could include various means, such as requiring pharmacist intervention, or using innovative technologies, like diagnostics, in the pharmacy or other settings. The agency held hearings in March 2012, where predictably pharmacy and insurance organizations supported the concept and medical organizations opposed it.

PROFESSIONAL PRACTICE CONSIDERATIONS

The Durham-Humphrey Amendment directly or indirectly raises several issues of importance to professional pharmacy practice, as discussed here. State laws address many of these issues with much more specificity.

Prescription Refill Authorization

As stated in the law, a prescription may not be refilled unless there is specific authorization, either orally or in writing, from the prescriber. A physician's employee or agent, including office nurse, cannot legally authorize a refill of a prescription unless state law has specifically granted the person this authority, nor can a prescriber legally delegate authority to an employee or agent not authorized by state law. The physician's employee or agent may, however (state law permitting), simply transmit or communicate the refill authorization (or new prescription) from the prescriber. In practice, this means that if a pharmacist calls a prescriber's office for refill authorization and speaks to an employee of the prescriber who immediately grants authorization, the pharmacist should question who is really authorizing the refill.

Prescriptive Authority

The Durham-Humphrey Amendment provides that legend drugs may be prescribed by a practitioner "licensed by law to administer such drug." Health care practitioners are not licensed by federal law, however, but by state law. Thus, each state determines if a practitioner in that state has the authority to prescribe. Some states have granted various degrees of prescriptive authority not only to allopathic physicians (MDs), osteopathic physicians (DOs), dentists, podiatrists, and veterinarians but also to nurse practitioners, physician's assistants, optometrists, naturopathic doctors, and pharmacists. Pharmacists must know which categories of practitioners can prescribe in their state and be able to distinguish who falls into those categories. For example, pharmacists must understand the legal difference in their state between registered nurses and nurse practitioners or advance practice nurses. Depending upon state laws, nurse practitioners or advance practice nurses may have either independent or collaborative prescriptive authority.

In addition to ascertaining if a health care practitioner has prescriptive authority, a pharmacist must consider the practitioner's scope of prescriptive authority. State law (called state practice acts) defines a practitioner's scope of practice to diagnose and treat, which, in turn, determines the practitioner's scope of prescriptive authority. State laws grant physicians broad treatment authority and thus the authority to prescribe almost any drug. This applies even to specialists such as psychiatrists and radiologists who, because they are physicians, can legally treat conditions outside their specialty. Other prescribers such as dentists, veterinarians, and podiatrists have much narrower treatment and prescriptive authority. For example, a dentist who treats a patient for acne has very likely exceeded the scope of practice for dentistry. If the dentist then prescribed tetracycline for the treatment of the acne, the prescription would be invalid, and the pharmacist who knowingly dispensed the drug might then be in violation of the state practice act.

In reality, because a pharmacist is not usually privy to the diagnosis, determining if a practitioner is prescribing within the scope of his or her authority might be difficult to impossible in some cases. Thus, a pharmacist would not likely be held legally accountable for dispensing a prescription from a prescriber who has exceeded his or her prescriptive authority, if the pharmacist dispensed the prescription in good faith after making an attempt to ascertain the condition for which the drug was prescribed. It is important that pharmacists contact the prescriber when aware that a prescription might be outside the prescriber's scope of practice, if merely to determine if the correct drug has been prescribed.

In states that authorize nurse practitioners, physician's assistants, or optometrists to prescribe medication, there are generally certain limits on the prescriptive authority of these professionals. The pharmacist must be aware of these limits.

Emergency Contraception (Plan B)

An example of a situation that involves pharmacist independent prescriptive authority in some states, and a third class of drugs in all states, is emergency contraception (EC). The first approved EC product was Plan B, marketed by Barr Laboratories (now Teva), containing a high dosage (0.75 mg) of levonorgestrel, which is a synthetic hormone used in lower dosages as an oral contraceptive. EC is a method of preventing pregnancy after contraception fails or after unprotected sex and is not intended for routine use. The products work like birth control drugs and should not be confused with abortion drugs. The FDA approved Plan B as a prescription-only medication in 1999 and since that time the product has enjoyed a colorful history.

In 2001 several medical, public health and reproductive organizations filed a citizen petition with the FDA asking the agency to switch Plan B to OTC status without age restrictions. Later, in 2003, Barr submitted a supplemental new drug application (SNDA) to the FDA requesting a switch of the drug to OTC status without age restrictions. Despite approval for the switch by two FDA advisory committees for all age groups, the FDA rejected the SNDA application. The FDA's decision raised public outcry by many over whether politics outweighed science. The FDA, however, suggested that Barr could reapply by presenting evidence that girls under the age of 16 could use the drug over the counter safely. Barr then submitted another SNDA in 2004. The FDA then replied that it could not reach a decision because of three issues: (1) Whether the same active ingredient could be marketed both Rx and OTC based solely on the age of the user (rather than different indications); (2) whether and how age-based distinctions could be enforced; and (3) whether the Rx and OTC versions may be marketed in a single package.

After considerable public controversy and FDA deliberations with Barr, the agency announced, in 2006, that it had approved the amended version of Barr's SNDA application. The FDA acknowledged that Barr had submitted adequate information to demonstrate that Plan B is safe and effective for use under the labeling conditions established. Those conditions included that Plan B will be sold only from behind the counter in pharmacies staffed by a licensed pharmacist, and that the purchaser must present personal identification showing proof of age (18 or older). Although no counseling, special forms, or fact sheets need be provided, pharmacists should provide counseling and information to the patient.

The FDA set the OTC age at 18 or older despite the fact that FDA staff agreed that Barr's SNDA established that the drug was safe and effective for 17-year-olds. Meanwhile, after a 5-year delay, the FDA denied the citizen's petition that had been filed in 2001 seeking that the drug be available OTC for all ages. This denial prompted a lawsuit by the petitioners (*Tummino v. Torti*, 603 F.Supp2d 519 (E.D.N.Y 2009)). Finding for the plaintiffs, the court found that the FDA's decision had been influenced by political and ideological considerations and it had acted in bad faith and abused its discretion in denying the petition. The court ordered the FDA to make the drug available to 17-year-olds and also ordered the agency to reconsider if it should be available for all ages without prescription.

Subsequently, in February 2011, Teva Women's Health Inc. submitted an SNDA seeking to make the product available OTC for all girls of reproductive age. In December 2011, the commissioner of the FDA approved the SNDA; however, the secretary of Health and Human Services overruled the commissioner's decision (http://www.hhs.gov/news/press/2011pres/12/20111207a.html). The commissioner agreed with FDA experts that well-supported, science-based evidence existed that established Plan B is safe and effective for use in all females of child-bearing potential. Nonetheless, the secretary felt there was not enough data presented considering the significant cognitive and behavioral differences among girls of different ages.

Some states have enacted legislation allowing pharmacists to independently prescribe EC directly to girls younger than age 17, provided that the pharmacist meets state-specified education and training requirements and follows certain protocols.

Conscientious Objection

Prescriptions for emergency contraceptive drugs, abortifacient drugs, and oral contraceptives have raised a very contentious issue: if the pharmacist has a right to refuse to dispense prescriptions to which the pharmacist has moral or religious opposition. This issue has been labeled as one of conscientious objection, and has been the subject of discussion among the media, Congress, state legislators, and professional organizations. It has resulted in legislation and/or board of pharmacy regulations in many states as well as professional organization guidelines; however, no consensus has really emerged. Some states have passed laws or regulations requiring pharmacists to dispense prescriptions regardless of their moral beliefs. Some states have enacted laws establishing "conscience clauses," such that pharmacists may refuse to dispense prescriptions that violate their conscience.

Professional organizations and state boards of pharmacy generally have taken a compromise position, attempting to respect the pharmacist's beliefs, while ensuring that patients receive the medications to which they have a legal right. Under this philosophy, a pharmacist should notify the employer in advance in writing of his or her objections to dispense particular drugs. The employer, provided it can do so without undue hardship, should develop procedures such that the pharmacist is not placed in a situation where he or she would be required to dispense the objectionable prescriptions, and yet that still allow the patient to receive the drug with minimal inconvenience. For example, another pharmacist on duty could dispense the medication, or the patient could be referred to a nearby pharmacy.

In no situation should a pharmacist obstruct a patient's legal right to receive a lawful medication. In the case of *Noesen v. State, Dept. of Regulation and Licensing*, 754 N.W.2d 849 (WI 2008), a Wisconsin pharmacist informed the employer of his conscientious objection to dispense birth control prescriptions, but did not tell the employer that he would not transfer refills upon the request of another pharmacy. When a patient attempted to refill her birth control prescription, the pharmacist told her he could not dispense it and that there was no other pharmacist on duty. The patient then went to another pharmacy but the pharmacist refused to transfer the prescription to the pharmacy, resulting in the patient missing a dose. The State Board of Pharmacy found the pharmacist guilty of unprofessional conduct because his failure to transfer the prescription constituted a danger to the health and safety of the patient and substantially departed from the standard of care of a pharmacist. The Board ordered that the pharmacist inform all future employers in writing that he would not dispense birth control prescriptions and outline the steps he would take to ensure that a patient has access to the medication. The pharmacist sued the Board, but the Wisconsin court of appeals upheld the Board's decision.

However, in a situation in Idaho, a prescriber phoned in a prescription to a pharmacist for Methergine, a drug generally used for the prevention and control of postpartum hemorrhage. The pharmacist asked if the drug was for postabortion care, and the prescriber replied that she could not disclose that information because of confidentiality. The pharmacist said she would not dispense the prescription and hung up when the prescriber requested a referral to another pharmacy. A complaint was filed with the

Board of Pharmacy that found no violation of Idaho pharmacy laws or regulations under Idaho's conscience clause law (*NABP Newsletter*, 2011).

In a state of Washington case, the issue centered upon whether Board of Pharmacy regulations requiring pharmacies to dispense lawfully prescribed drugs except under certain circumstances violated the plaintiff pharmacists' constitutional rights (*Stormans, Inc. v. Selecky*, 844 F.Supp.2d 1172 (W.D.Wash. Feb. 22, 2012)). After 4 years of litigation, a federal district court determined that the Washington regulation violated the plaintiff pharmacy's and pharmacists' First Amendment rights to the free exercise of religion as well as their rights to equal protection under the Fourteenth Amendment.

Collaborative Practice Agreements

Pharmacists do not have general independent prescriptive authority in any state. However, most states have enacted legislation allowing pharmacists to initiate or adjust drug therapies in collaboration with a physician. This collaborative arrangement requires a written contractual agreement in the form of protocols and procedures. The extent to which a pharmacist may engage in drug therapy management often depends upon state law, the collaborative agreement, and the practice setting. Authority granted to the pharmacist can range from following a restrictive drug formulary to having complete discretion to select any drug the pharmacist deems best.

Authority to Dispense Prescription Drugs

The FDCA does not specify who may or may not dispense prescription drugs; this again is the jurisdiction of the states. Pharmacists licensed to practice under state law may dispense prescription drugs, of course, as may any other practitioner who is authorized to do so under a state's laws, including physicians.

Physician dispensing increased significantly in the 1980s as physicians sought ways to supplement their incomes, lowered as the result of both managed care and governmental cost containment efforts. Pharmacists strongly oppose physician dispensing on economic and ethical grounds and were particularly irked that physicians in many states did not conform to the same dispensing standards required of pharmacists. Some physicians, for example, poured tablets and capsules in sacks and either wrote the directions on the sack or merely told the patient the directions. Looking for ways to curb the practice of physician dispensing, or at least to hold physicians to dispensing standards, pharmacists asked the FDA to step in and apply the Durham-Humphrey Amendment's standards to physicians. On the basis of its interpretation of congressional intent, however, the FDA took the position that the labeling requirements of the law apply only to pharmacists, not physicians.

The wisdom of the FDA's interpretation aside, many states enacted legislation in the 1980s mandating that dispensing physicians must meet the same or similar dispensing requirements as pharmacists. One state pharmacy board went a step further, and proposed regulations placing greater dispensing restrictions on physicians than pharmacists. This prompted the Federal Trade Commission (FTC) to threaten legal action against the pharmacy board. The FTC viewed the proposed regulations as anticompetitive in violation of the antitrust laws because one group of competing professionals was unduly restricting another group of competitors for economic advantage. The board subsequently amended its regulations to impose the same restrictions on physicians as pharmacists.

Federal law does place some restrictions on physician dispensing through the Medicare/Medicaid fraud and abuse statutes. Federal law also prohibits physicians from referring Medicare and Medicaid patients to pharmacies that they own.

© Stockbyte/Thinkstock

STUDY SCENARIOS AND QUESTIONS

1. A prescription drug container from the manufacturer contains an expiration date of 12/09. The pharmacist dispenses the prescription on 3/21/07 in the same container; however, the pharmacy labels the expiration date as 3/21/08. The patient asks the pharmacist why the dates differ. What explanation should the pharmacist provide?
2. A pharmacist received a prescription from a psychiatrist for a cardiac antiarrhythmia drug. Explain if it would violate the law to dispense this prescription and the procedure that the pharmacist should follow in this situation.
3. A pharmacist received a prescription from a dentist for an antibiotic written to take tid for a urinary infection. Explain if it would violate the law to dispense this prescription and the procedure that the pharmacist should follow in this situation. How would this situation differ from the previous one?
4. You are a pharmacist. A 17-year-old female approaches you and asks that you sell her Plan B over the counter. Explain if you can sell her the drug, and the requirements to do so. Law aside, should the patient be counseled?

PRESCRIPTION DRUG LABELING INFORMATION FOR THE PATIENT

As you learned in Chapter 2 and the discussion of the Durham–Humphrey Amendment, prescription drug labeling by manufacturers is directed at the health care professional, not the patient. There are, however, two types of labeling mandated by federal law that manufacturers must supply for the patient—patient package inserts and medication guides.

PATIENT PACKAGE INSERTS

Until the late 1960s the FDA had not devoted much attention to the issue of manufacturers providing prescription drug labeling directed to the patient. The FDA's inattention to this issue changed dramatically in 1970 when it issued a regulation requiring that information for the patient, called patient package inserts or PPIs, accompany oral contraceptive drugs, explaining the drugs' uses, the risks, and the precautions (21 C.F.R. § 310.501). The agency initiated this action because of the widespread popularity of oral contraceptives and the relative unawareness by women of the drugs' potential serious adverse effects, especially thrombophlebitis and pulmonary embolism. If this information is not contained on or in the product package, it must be provided as leaflets with the product. Furthermore, the manufacturer must instruct the pharmacist to distribute a leaflet with each prescription.

On the heels of this regulation, the FDA enacted regulations in 1977 requiring PPIs for estrogen-containing drugs (21 C.F.R. § 310.515) such as conjugated estrogens and diethylstilbestrol (DES) not intended for oral contraceptive use, and progestational drugs (21 C.F.R. § 310.516). The PPI requirement for progestational drugs was repealed in 1999; however, if a progestational drug is intended for use as an oral contraceptive, then the oral contraceptive PPI is required. (*Note:* The FDA issued a draft guidance for noncontraceptive estrogen drug products in November 2005 [http://www.fda.gov/downloads/Drugs/GuidanceComplianceRegulatoryInformation/Guidances/

UCM075090.pdf], recommending that manufacturers comply with specified prescriber and patient labeling information contained in the guidance.) The authority of the FDA to promulgate these regulations was upheld in the case of *Pharmaceutical Manufacturers Association v. Food and Drug Administration* (discussed in detail in the case studies section of this chapter).

Manufacturers must include a PPI for each package that it intends will be distributed to the patient, and in turn, pharmacists must include a PPI with each container dispensed, regardless of whether it is initially dispensed or a refill. Failure to do so is misbranding. Patient package insert regulations apply not only to community pharmacies but also, in a modified form, to institutions. An institution may provide the insert to the inpatient the same as an ambulatory patient, or it may provide the insert before the administration of the first dose and then once every 30 days thereafter. In *Schlieter v. Carlos*, Nos. 87-0955 SC, 11592 SC (D.N.M. Aug. 1989), an inpatient contended that the hospital was negligent in not providing her with a PPI when she was given estrogen (Premarin). The defendant hospital argued that it had a right to rely on the treating physician to provide the PPI if the physician so wished. The court disagreed, establishing that an institution cannot delegate its responsibility for providing a PPI to the prescribing physician. The court concluded that the intent of the regulation is that patients, not physicians, must be given the information.

Firmly believing in the importance of written drug information for patients, the FDA in 1980 enacted regulations requiring PPIs for all prescription drugs (45 Fed. Reg. 60754, Sept. 12, 1980). The proposal received strong opposition, however, from physician and pharmacy organizations on the grounds that the program would be unduly expensive and burdensome for providers and would not achieve the patient outcomes desired. Many of these organizations then proposed alternative means of providing information to the patient, causing the FDA to agree that private sector initiatives were preferable to a government-mandated program and to revoke the regulations (47 Fed. Reg. 39147, Sept. 7, 1982).

USEFUL WRITTEN PATIENT INFORMATION AND MEDICATION GUIDES

Not satisfied, however, with private sector efforts to provide prescription drug information to patients, the FDA in 1995 published a proposed rule that would implement a new patient information program (60 Fed. Reg. 44182, Aug. 24, 1995). The program consisted of two parts. One part would require that manufacturers provide Medication Guides, called "MedGuides," for a few specifically designated drugs that pose a "serious and significant" concern to public health. The second part mandated that "useful" written patient information (now called consumer medication information (CMI) be given to the patient for every drug each time a new prescription is dispensed.

The goal of the program was to ensure that all patients receive comprehensive written information about their prescribed drugs to supplement oral counseling from health care professionals. The FDA believes that this patient information is necessary for patients to use drug products safely and effectively. In turn, commented the agency, substantial health care cost savings would result by "reducing the harm caused by inappropriate drug use and enhancing the benefits of drugs by facilitating their proper use."

Consumer Medication Information (CMI)

Regarding the second part of the program that useful written patient information (CMI) accompany every new prescription, the agency proposed distribution goals and performance standards for patient information and left it up to the private sector to accomplish them. If the private sector failed to reach these goals and meet the standards, the agency indicated that it would then become necessary to federally establish a comprehensive patient information program.

The program proposal generated considerable controversy, especially among pharmacy organizations and pharmaceutical manufacturers who resented the FDA's intrusion. Shortly thereafter, Congress enacted legislation that established a voluntary private-sector process under which national organizations of health care providers, consumers, pharmaceutical companies, and others could collaborate to achieve the program's goals but without the threat of a federally mandated program (P.L. 104-180, Sept. 30, 1996). The law requires that 95 percent of patients receiving new prescriptions must receive useful written information about their medications by 2006. Failure of the private sector to implement a program within 4 years of the law's passage would result in reinstatement of the original FDA-mandated proposal. Pursuant to this requirement, private sector stakeholders met to assess the effectiveness of current oral and written patient information, developed guidelines based upon this assessment, and developed a process to continually evaluate the quality and frequency of the information provided to patients. This collaboration program was completed and its plan accepted by the FDA prior to the deadline.

Assessing the progress of the private sector plan, an FDA commissioned study in 2001 found that although 89 percent of patients with new prescriptions received written information, the information was useful to patients only about 50 percent of the time. (This report is available at http://www.fda.gov/AboutFDA/CentersOffices/Office ofMedicalProductsandTobacco/CDER/ucm169753.htm.) In order to assist the private sector in meeting the 95 percent goal, the FDA published a guidance titled "Guidance: Useful Written Consumer Medication Information (CMI)" in July 2006 (available at http://www.fda.gov/downloads/Drugs/GuidanceComplianceRegulatoryInformation/ Guidances/UCM080602.pdf). The guidance provides recommendations on what information should be provided and how it should be provided. The FDA noted that failure of pharmacies and others to meet these CMI standards voluntarily could result in the FDA resorting again to mandatory measures. In December of 2008 the FDA released the results of a follow-up study (http://www.fda.gov/AboutFDA/Centers Offices/OfficeofMedicalProductsandTobacco/CDER/ReportsBudgets/ucm163777. htm) showing that although more consumers are receiving CMI (94 percent), only about 71 percent of this information meets the minimum standard criteria for usefulness. (Recall the law requires 95 percent.) An FDA official remarked: "The current voluntary system has failed to provide consumers with the quality information they need in order to use medicines effectively and safely" (Janet Woodcock, MD, director of CDER, *FDA News*, December 16, 2008). Flaws in current CMI include formatting that is too small and crowded; inconsistent word counts with some CMI being extremely lengthy and repetitive; lack of clear action steps patients should take in the result of an adverse event; lack of clear organization and prioritization of information; and cluttering of important information with unnecessary verbiage. Since the law's target compliance levels have not been attained, FDA must now evaluate alternative actions.

Medication Guides

After passage of the 1996 law, the FDA acknowledged that the law had stripped it of its authority to establish a comprehensive private sector patient information program for all drugs. It felt, however, that it retained the authority to mandate the Medication Guide program for drugs posing a "serious and significant concern," and therefore enacted a final regulation to this effect in 1998 (63 Fed. Reg. 66378; 21 C.F.R. parts 201, 208, 314, 601, and 610). Under the final regulation, patient labeling for a product is required if the FDA determines that one or more of the following circumstances exists regarding a drug product: (1) that patient labeling could help prevent serious adverse effects; (2) that the product has serious risks relative to its benefits of which the patient should be aware to decide whether to use or continue to use the product; and (3) that patient adherence to directions is crucial to the drug's effectiveness. The FDA acknowledged that the MedGuides would be required for very few products, "no more than 5 to 10 products per year." In November 2011, the FDA published a guidance document explaining when the agency will require that a MedGuide be provided to a health care professional for administration to the patient and when a MedGuide will be required as part of REMS (available at http://www.fda.gov/downloads/Drugs/GuidanceComplianceRegulatoryInformation/Guidances/UCM244570.pdf).

Pursuant to the regulation, MedGuides must be written in nontechnical language and in a uniform format, containing the approved uses for the product, circumstances when the product should not be used, serious adverse reactions, proper use, cautions, and other general information. The manufacturer of the drug product for which a MedGuide is required must obtain FDA approval before the guide is distributed with the product. Manufacturers must provide directly, or supply the means to provide, sufficient numbers of the MedGuides to the distributor or dispenser of the product. The dispenser, in turn, must provide the guide to the patient each time the medication is dispensed, unless an exemption applies. It is important to note that other written drug information the pharmacy may distribute does not replace the MedGuide. A study conducted in 2005 revealed that only 1 of 21 Pennsylvania pharmacies surveyed distributed the required MedGuide for celecoxib (Sasich, JD, and Sukkari, SR, 2006).

The FDA has significantly increased the number of drugs subject to MedGuides over the past few years, now requiring more than 180 drugs to have MedGuides. A list of those drugs can be accessed at http://www.fda.gov/Drugs/DrugSafety/ucm085729.htm. The number of MedGuides has raised concerns from pharmacy organizations over the administrative burdens and distribution difficulties MedGuides cause pharmacies and their impact on pharmacy workflow. Because of the concern over MedGuides and the fact that Congressional goals had not been met for CMI, the FDA convened the Risk Communication Advisory Committee in February 2009 and encouraged public participation. The Agency also held a public workshop in September 2009 seeking answers as to the best ways to provide useful prescription information to consumers. The goal is ultimately to develop a single, easy-to-read document that incorporates PPIs, CMI, and MedGuides. In 2011, the FDA announced that it plans to test single-page consumer information guides as soon as it obtains funding from the Office of Management and Budget (http://on.wsj.com/kip0jb).

Risk Management Programs for Very High Risk Drugs

For a few drugs the FDA has determined that black box warnings, PPIs, and MedGuides are simply inadequate to protect the patient. In these situations the FDA has required manufacturers to develop approved risk management programs called Risk Evaluation and Mitigation Strategies (REMS). (The FDAAA significantly expanded the FDA's authority to require REMS postmarket.) The iPLEDGE program for isotretinoin (Accutane) was a notable example of a REMS program. But as restrictive as that REMS program was, it could not effectively enough prevent the occurrence of adverse events and ultimately the drug had to be withdrawn from the market. Some other drugs for which the FDA has required risk management programs well prior to the FDAAA include Plan B, Thalidomide, clozapine (Clozaril), olosetron (Lotronex), and alendrolate (Fosamax).

DRUG INFORMATION WEBSITE FOR PHARMACISTS: DRUG INFO ROUNDS

At the FDA website, pharmacists can access "Drug Info Rounds," which is a series of training videos providing important and timely drug information to pharmacists so as to assist them in helping patients make better medication decisions.

DRUG INFORMATION WEBSITE FOR CONSUMERS: DRUGS@FDA

In addition to the patient-directed labeling required of manufacturers, the FDA provides its own source of drug information for consumers. Accessible through the FDA's home page or directly at http://www.accessdata.fda.gov/scripts/cder/drugsatfda, the website, called Drugs@FDA, provides consumers with a searchable database that includes information on approved prescription drugs, some OTC drugs, and even discontinued drugs. Consumers can search by drug name or active ingredient and obtain essentially all relevant labeling information about the drug, including therapeutically equivalent drugs and the approval history.

© Stockbyte/Thinkstock

STUDY SCENARIO

A pharmacist dispenses prescriptions to a patient for Premarin, Coumadin, and amoxicillin. Discuss whether written patient information is required for each of these drugs, and if so, whether the pharmacy-generated patient information will suffice for each.

APPROVED DRUGS FOR UNLABELED INDICATIONS

When manufacturers can promote drug products for off-label uses is subject to significant restrictions. Nonetheless, health care professionals commonly prescribe and dispense many drugs for indications other than those listed in the approved labeling. This is especially true in the treatment of cancer and human immunodeficiency virus (HIV) infection. There are many reasons why some indications for a drug's use are not included in the approved labeling. One reason is that practitioners find promising uses for drugs much faster than the drug regulatory system can approve those uses. Another reason is that manufacturers commonly seek NDA approvals for a minimal number of indications so that they can expedite the approval process and market their drugs as soon as possible, generally with the intent to submit an abbreviated or supplemental new drug application to have the additional indications added to the labeling at a later date.

Any time a drug is prescribed for a condition not listed in its official labeling, that use is considered off-label, unlabeled, or unapproved. The FDA has taken the position that a drug may be legally prescribed and dispensed for an unlabeled indication or dosage. In a 1972 proposal statement, the FDA announced:

> If an approved new drug is shipped in interstate commerce with the approved package insert and neither the shipper nor the recipient intends that it be used for an unapproved purpose, the requirements of section 505 of the Act are satisfied. Once the new drug is in a local pharmacy after interstate shipment, the physician may, as part of the practice of medicine, lawfully prescribe a different dosage for his patient, or may otherwise vary the conditions of use from those approved in the package insert, without informing or obtaining the approval of the Food and Drug Administration. (37 Fed. Reg. 16503, Aug. 15, 1972)

This proposal was never finalized, but in response to physician requests for more formal guidance, the FDA published additional statements recognizing that accepted medical practice includes the use of drugs for off-label indications. The Omnibus Budget Reconciliation Act of 1990 (OBRA '90) also seems to recognize the medical importance of off-label indications by accepting information in professional compendia (which often list a drug's off-label indications in addition to its labeled indications) as a standard in determining appropriate drug use for Medicaid patients. Some contend, however, that OBRA '90 actually restricts off-label indications because many off-label indications are not stated in compendia sources.

Clearly, the act of prescribing and dispensing approved drugs for off-label indications is less an issue of labeling than it is an issue of eliminating unreasonable risks. From a practical perspective, pharmacists must exercise professional judgment. If a drug is prescribed for either a labeled or an off-label indication and there is no unreasonable risk to the patient, the pharmacist may dispense the drug. If the risk to the patient is unreasonable, the pharmacist has a duty to take additional action. The pharmacist should contact the prescriber to confirm that the proper drug or dosage has been prescribed. In situations in which the patient is at significant risk of harm, the prescriber may have to justify the decision to the pharmacist. These actions are important both to protect the patient and to reduce the risk of civil liability because the use of a drug for unlabeled indications may create a greater risk of civil liability in the event of patient injury. In *Mulder v. Parke-Davis & Co.,* 181 N.W.2d 882 (Minn. 1970), the court considered the package insert as prima facie evidence of negligence, shifting to the physician the burden of establishing why he or she deviated from the labeling. Recent decisions, however, such as *Ramon v. Farr*, 770 P.2d 131 (Utah 1989), reported in the case studies section of the chapter, hold that the package insert is only evidence of the standard of care.

As another practical matter, pharmacists must be aware that certain third-party insurance and managed health care plans will not compensate providers for drugs prescribed and dispensed for off-label indications.

Pharmacists who provide drug information to other health care providers regarding off-label indications generally need not fear violating the FDCA as long as the intent of the information is advisory or educational, not promotional. In *United States v. Evers*, 643 F.2d 1043 (5th Cir. 1981), the court held that a physician who publicly advocated calcium disodium edetate (calcium EDTA) for unapproved use as a chelating agent did not violate the FDCA. The physician was not selling the drug to other physicians or pharmacies but merely distributing the drug to his own patients within his own practice of medicine.

STUDY SCENARIO AND QUESTIONS

Dr. Bill is a hospital pharmacist making rounds with a physician, Dr. Jake. One of Dr. Jake's patients had just been admitted to the hospital in premature labor. Unable to reduce the contractions, Dr. Jake consulted with Dr. Bill about administering terbutaline sulfate. The drug has FDA approval only for use in bronchial asthma but was also being widely used as a tocolytic agent because it relaxes smooth muscles. Dr. Bill had reservations because the labeling for terbutaline states

> . . . is indicated for the prevention and reversal of bronchospasm in patients with bronchial asthma and reversible bronchospasm associated with bronchitis and emphysema. *** Terbutaline sulfate should not be used for tocolysis. Serious adverse reactions may occur after administration of terbutaline sulfate to women in labor. In the mother, these include increased heart rate, transient hyperglycemia, hypokalemia, cardiac arrhythmias, pulmonary edema, and myocardial ischemia.

Nonetheless, Dr. Bill agreed with Dr. Jake that this was the best course of therapy. After 48 hours of dosing, the contractions stopped. Shortly thereafter, the patient suffered a heart attack, delivered a healthy baby, and underwent open-heart surgery. The patient subsequently sued both Dr. Bill and Dr. Jake.

1. Did Dr. Bill or Dr. Jake violate the FDCA?
2. If you were Dr. Bill, what would you have done?
3. Should the patient have been told of the risks?
4. Should the patient have been told the drug was being used off-label?
5. When would you not dispense or prescribe a drug for an off-label use?
6. How much evidentiary weight should the labeling be given in the malpractice lawsuit?

PHARMACY COMPOUNDING VERSUS MANUFACTURING

Long before the existence of pharmaceutical manufacturers, pharmacists compounded medications for their patients. Eventually, however, manufacturers began producing an ever-increasing number of products in finished form, obviating the need for pharmacy compounding in most situations. Nonetheless, compounding has enjoyed a resurgence of popularity as pharmacists prepare significant numbers of intravenous products, radiopharmaceuticals, chemotherapeutic agents, topical preparations, suppositories, veterinary medications, and even tablets and capsules.

Section 510(g) of the FDCA provides in part that pharmacies are exempt from registering as manufacturers if they

> do not manufacture, prepare, propagate, compound or process drugs or devices for sale other than in the regular course of their business of dispensing or selling drugs or devices at retail. (§ 510(g); 21 U.S.C. § 360(g))

Section 510(g) recognizes that the traditional compounding by pharmacists, which is regulated by state law, is not manufacturing. The pharmacy exception provided by this section is important because a pharmacy that is deemed a manufacturer must obtain a license from the FDA, most likely obtain an approved IND application, and conform to the regulations regarding current good manufacturing practice. Pharmacies that repackage OTC products or in any way change the container, wrapper, or labeling of these products for resale must also register as manufacturers (§ 510(a)(1)). Thus, pharmacies in the business of repackaging prescription drug products for sale to other health care providers must register as manufacturers. Pharmacists who dispense to long-term care facilities (LTCFs) have expressed concern as to whether they violate federal and state laws when they repackage and relabel drugs dispensed by another pharmacy. This situation may occur when a patient is admitted to the LTCF and brings along medications the patient has been taking at home. The LTCF might then send the patient's medications to the contracting pharmacy for repackaging into packaging compliant with the LTCF's policies. Although the FDA has never issued an opinion on this practice under federal law, some states have enacted laws or regulations to authorize the practice.

Historically there has been considerable friction between the FDA and the pharmacy profession over the interpretation of the compounding exemption. The FDA became quite concerned about pharmacy compounding in light of problems that resulted in patient injuries. In 1989, for example, a Pittsburgh pharmacist prepared indomethacin eye drops that resulted in eye infections in 12 patients. Two of these patients had to have an eye surgically removed. The same year, patients died because a hospital pharmacy in Lincoln, Nebraska, prepared surgical solutions that became microbially infected. As a result, the FDA published an Alert Letter on compounding in November 1990, expressing concern that some pharmacies were using incorrect procedures and controls when compounding sterile products (Bloom, 1991). The FDA emphasized that pharmacists who prepare batches of sterile drug products are responsible for conforming to current good manufacturing practice and for using safe packaging to ensure continued sterility during use. The letter also warned pharmacists to balance their need to prepare batches of sterile products with their capacity for doing so. The FDA concluded that it did not wish to discourage pharmacists from compounding, but offered the letter as a "strong reminder" to pharmacists of the seriousness of batch-producing sterile drugs.

FDA 1992 COMPLIANCE POLICY GUIDE

After the Alert Letter, state and national pharmacy organizations became concerned that the FDA was intent on eliminating the right of pharmacists to compound medications as part of their ordinary practice. This concern led to several meetings between pharmacy organizations and the FDA, resulting in the publication of Compliance Policy Guide 7132.16 on March 16, 1992. The Compliance Policy Guide emphasized that the FDA had no intention of regulating pharmacy's historic exemption to compound drugs extemporaneously in reasonable quantities pursuant to prescription. The guide also stated that pharmacists may also prepare "very limited quantities" of drugs before receiving valid prescriptions, provided that these anticipated quantities can be documented historically with prescriptions on file. However, the FDA stated:

> FDA believes that an increasing number of establishments with retail pharmacy licenses are engaged in manufacturing, distributing, and promoting unapproved new drugs for human use in a manner that is clearly outside the bounds of traditional pharmacy practice and that constitute violations of the Act. (Compliance Policy Guide 7132.16 at 2)

Many compounding pharmacists believed that this last statement really set the tone for how the agency felt about pharmacist compounding and that the FDA's enforcement activities were too intrusive. In part Congress agreed, and somewhat reduced the FDA's authority over drugs compounded in pharmacies in FDAMA.

FDAMA'S COMPOUNDING PROVISIONS

FDAMA amended the FDCA (§ 503A; 21 U.S.C. 353a), effectively rescinding the 1992 Compliance Policy Guide. The compounding law helped clarify for pharmacists those activities that would be considered as compounding and those activities that would constitute manufacturing. The law essentially reflected the FDA's prior policies, except for one very important departure. Prior to the law, the FDA had always contended that drugs compounded in the pharmacy are exempt from the misbranding and adulteration provisions of the FDCA, but not the new drug provision (§ 505). In other words, the FDA held the position that compounded drugs are "new drugs," thus giving the agency the authority to regulate the products if it chose to do so, regardless that the pharmacy was not manufacturing. The FDAMA compounding law took this authority away from the agency.

The compounding law was short lived, however, because it contained two requirements that the U.S. Supreme Court held were unconstitutional. The first requirement stated that the prescription could not be solicited. The second offending requirement provided that pharmacies and physicians could promote and advertise that they compound, but that they could not advertise or promote the compounding of any particular drug, class of drug, or type of drug. A group of compounding pharmacists challenged the constitutionality of these restrictions, prevailing in both federal district court and in the court of appeals. The Supreme Court affirmed the court of appeal's decision, ruling the two requirements unconstitutional because they amounted to an impermissible regulation of commercial speech under the First Amendment (*Thompson v. Western States Medical Center*, 122 S.Ct. 1497 (2002)). The Court found that the FDA had available less intrusive means of achieving its goals than restricting speech in this manner. After the Court's decision, it was generally regarded that the entire compounding law was invalidated because the court of appeals decided that the offending clauses were not severable and the Supreme Court neither agreed nor disagreed with that particular conclusion.

FDA 2002 COMPLIANCE POLICY GUIDE (CPG)

In reaction to the Supreme Court's decision, the FDA drafted a new compliance policy guide on May 29, 2002 (http://www.fda.gov/downloads/Drugs/GuidanceCompliance RegulatoryInformation/Guidances/UCM124736.pdf), essentially reinstating by policy many of the provisions in the invalidated compounding law. In the guidance, the FDA stated that pharmacists have traditionally compounded drugs extemporaneously in reasonable quantities pursuant to a prescription for an individual patient, and that this activity is not the subject of the CPG. However, the FDA continued by noting that it believes an increasing number of pharmacies are engaging in manufacturing and distributing unapproved new drugs clearly outside of traditional pharmacy compounding, and these pharmacies are the subject of the guide. The agency noted that it would continue to defer to state authorities for less significant violations of the act, but would consider direct enforcement action against significant violations.

In determining if to initiate an enforcement action against a pharmacy, the FDA will consider if the pharmacy engages in any of the following nine acts:

1. Compounding in anticipation of receiving prescriptions, except in very limited quantities. (Although the FDA has traditionally allowed pharmacists to compound "in anticipation" of prescriptions, the amount compounded must be legitimately based on the established practice history among the prescriber, pharmacist, and patients. For example, if every day the pharmacist dispenses between four and eight prescriptions for a particular compounded drug, the pharmacist

could prepare at least this amount ahead of time. What constitutes a limited quantity depends on the circumstances, such as how many prescriptions a day can be expected and the stability of the compound.)

2. Compounding drugs withdrawn or removed from the market for safety reasons.
3. Compounding from bulk ingredients not approved by the FDA.
4. Receiving, storing, or using drugs without first obtaining written assurance from the supplier that each lot of the drug was made in an FDA-registered facility.
5. Receiving, storing, or using drug components not guaranteed or determined to meet compendia requirements.
6. Using commercial-scale manufacturing or testing equipment.
7. Compounding for third parties for resale.
8. Compounding drugs that are commercially available or that are essentially copies of commercially available products. A pharmacist may compound a small quantity of a drug that is only slightly different than the commercially available product provided that there is a medical need for the variation for the particular patient.
9. Failing to operate in conformance with applicable state law.

The FDA emphasized that this list is not intended to be exhaustive and that other factors may be considered, depending upon the particular case.

Subsequent to issuing the CPG, the jurisdiction of the FDA to inspect a pharmacy for compounding violations was challenged in the case of *Wedgewood Village Pharmacy, Inc. v. U.S.*, 421 F.3d 263 (2005). Based upon a number of concerns, including that the pharmacy was compounding drugs that were essentially copies of commercially available products and using commercial-scale manufacturing equipment, the FDA obtained a warrant and commenced inspection. After 3 days of inspection, however, the pharmacy filed a motion to quash the warrant on the basis that the FDA had no jurisdiction over state-licensed pharmacies. The pharmacy pointed to language in the FDCA that specifically excludes pharmacies from FDA inspection if they do not manufacture or compound drugs or devices other than in the regular course of business. Thus, argued the pharmacy, pharmacies are exempt from FDA inspection. Ruling for the FDA, however, the court stated that Congress intended that the FDA must be granted the authority to generally inspect pharmacies in order to determine if the exemption applies. Otherwise, the FDA would have to rely on the representations of the pharmacies and essentially be powerless to enforce the law. The court found that the law prohibits the FDA from inspecting the records of the pharmacy unless the general inspection reveals that the pharmacy is manufacturing and thus does not qualify for the exemption. Regarding whether the FDA had probable cause to conclude that Wedgewood was not exempt from further inspection on the basis of the provisions of the 2002 compliance guide, the court agreed that the FDA could reasonably rely on the guide for its conclusions.

Demonstrating that it will apply the provisions of the CPG, the FDA sent warning letters in January 2008 to certain pharmacies that compound hormonal replacement products stating that any claims they make about the safety and efficacy of these products are unsupported and would be considered as false and misleading (http://www.fda.gov/NewsEvents/Newsroom/PressAnnouncements/2008/ucm116832.htm). The FDA warned that the use of the term "Bio-identical Hormone Replacement Therapy (BHRT)," implying the drugs are identical to hormones made in the body, is misleading. The FDA further warned against compounding products containing estriol since estriol is not approved by the FDA.

Surprisingly there is no federal definition of compounding. Rather, FDAMA and the 2002 compliance guide essentially provide examples of activities that are not compounding. Is a pharmacy that measures out a prescribed amount of a bulk active ingredient into a single-dose container with a separately packaged appropriate amount of saline for the consumer to mix with the powder compounding? This was the issue involving a Colorado pharmacy that imported HGH and dispensed prescriptions for it in this manner (*U.S. v. Bader*, 2009 WL 2219258 (D.Colo. 2009)). The pharmacist imported the HGH from another country by representing that it was for compounding. On this basis FDA inspectors allowed the drug into the country as an "Active Pharmaceutical Ingredient (API)." If the drug was to be sold as a finished drug, it could not be imported. The FDA contended that the pharmacist made false representations since it did not compound the HGH but sold it as a finished drug, and charged him with conspiracy to facilitate the sale of smuggled goods. The federal district court, noting the lack of a federal definition and the FDA's traditional practice of deferring to state regulation of compounded drugs, determined that Colorado's definition of compounding should apply; and Colorado's definition includes repackaging as compounding. The court's decision is only an initial victory for the pharmacy because at trial the government could likely establish that the pharmacy violated FDAMA or the compliance guide (for example compounding a copy of a commercially available product or using an unapproved active ingredient) that would make the compounded products new drugs.

NEW DRUG ISSUE

As noted, prior to FDAMA the FDA maintained that a pharmacy-compounded drug is a new drug; however, FDAMA reversed the FDA's position. Once the FDAMA compounding law was invalidated, however, the FDA resumed its position that a pharmacy-compounded drug is a new drug. A group of 10 compounding pharmacies brought legal action against the FDA seeking declarative and injunctive relief from (among other things) the FDA's policy of considering lawfully compounded drugs as new drugs. In a 2006 federal district court decision (*Medical Center Pharmacy v. Gonzales*, 451 F.Supp.2d 854 (W.D. Tex. 2006)), the court agreed with the plaintiffs, finding that the nonadvertising provisions are severable, thus leaving FDAMA in effect. The court also held that compounded drugs created for an individual patient pursuant to a prescription are "implicitly exempt from the new drug definitions. . . ." The basis for the court's conclusion was that FDAMA's provision stating that compounded drugs are not new drugs remains effective and demonstrates the intent of Congress. The court further supported its decision by noting that if compounded drugs were required to undergo the NDA process, patients requiring individually tailored prescription drugs would not be able to receive them due to the cost and time necessary to obtain FDA approval. The court made it clear that if a pharmacy crossed the line from compounding to manufacturing, the new drug definition would be applicable.

On appeal, the fifth circuit court of appeals voided the district court's decision, but in essence reached a very similar result (*Medical Center Pharmacy v. Mukasey*, 536 F.3d 383 (5th Cir. 2008)). The court agreed that the nonadvertising provisions were severable but held that pharmacy compounded drugs are new drugs but "are neither uniformly exempt from the new drug approval requirements nor uniformly subject to them." In other words, the court held that compounded drugs are exempt provided the pharmacy meets all the conditions established in FDAMA. The fifth circuit's decision means that the FDA is prohibited from treating compounded drugs as new drugs in Louisiana, Mississippi, and Texas (the jurisdiction of the court) but can treat compounded drugs as new drugs in the rest of the country.

More recently, the FDA attempted to enjoin a pharmacy from compounding medications for animals from bulk ingredients. In *U.S. v. Franck's Lab, Inc.*, 816 F.Supp.2d 1209 (M.D.Fla. Sept. 12, 2011), the FDA contended that any medications compounded for animals from bulk substances, even pursuant to a prescription from a veterinarian, are new drugs and violate the FDCA. In denying the injunction the court noted that the FDA seeks to eradicate the line between manufacturing and traditional pharmacy compounding contrary to congressional intent. Thus, the court concluded that the agency lacks the statutory authority to regulate the traditional pharmacy compounding of animal drugs. The FDA has appealed.

Some pharmacies compound herbal products pursuant to prescription. This practice raises some interesting issues. If the product is intended to treat a disease, it could transform the product from a dietary supplement to a drug. If this is the case, the bulk ingredients used must conform to USP or NF standards. Very few herbals could meet this requirement, and if they do not, the compounded product could well be considered a new drug.

Occasionally, consumers ask a pharmacist to prepare a nonprescription drug compound for their own use. Technically, such a product may be considered a new drug under the act, and would constitute dispensing a prescription drug without a prescription in some states. In an Iowa case, a patient complained to the pharmacist about nasal irritation (*Houck v. Iowa Bd. of Pharmacy Examiners*, 752 N.W.2d 114 (Iowa 2008)). The pharmacist compounded a nasal spray using several nonprescription drug ingredients. The product worsened the patient's condition and he filed a compliant with the Iowa Board of Pharmacy. The Board found the pharmacist had unlawfully manufactured and dispensed a compounded drug without a prescription and the court upheld the Board's interpretation that OTC compounded drugs require a prescription. Pharmacists, of course, cannot dispense a compounded product with any prescription ingredients without a prescription and should be aware of their increased risk of civil liability when dispensing any compounded product.

Patent Issues

Occasionally, compounding by pharmacists can create patent problems with a manufacturer, as did the compounding of minoxidil topical solutions in the 1980s. A legal patent right will supersede pharmacy compounding rights. The Upjohn Company first marketed minoxidil in tablet form for oral use as an antihypertensive. A side effect of minoxidil is hair growth, and Upjohn holds use patents that enable the company to label minoxidil exclusively for this purpose. Before Upjohn could market the product for hair growth, however, it had to obtain FDA approval. While Upjohn was waiting for FDA approval to market minoxidil in a topical form, many physicians were already prescribing the drug in topical form for this use, and pharmacists were compounding the prescriptions. Upjohn took no action against the pharmacies at that time, even though it held the use patents, because it could not market the drug topically for this purpose anyway and had nothing to gain. Ultimately, the FDA granted Upjohn approval to market the topical form for hair growth, and Upjohn began marketing it under the name Rogaine. Upjohn then issued letters to the pharmacies that were compounding minoxidil, warning them that the company would bring legal action unless they stopped the compounding; most pharmacies complied.

The case of minoxidil is somewhat unique in that the use patents for this drug are more enforceable than are those for many other drugs. For example, if a company manufactures a particular drug product in a 25-mg oral tablet and holds a use patent for that product for one indication, it would be difficult or impossible for the company to enforce its use patents if pharmacies compounded the drug in 25-mg oral tablets pursuant to prescription. The prescribers and pharmacies could simply contend that the drug was being prescribed for indications other than the one patented. Although the company might be able to prove otherwise, it would not likely be worth the company's efforts to attempt to enforce its patents in this situation, especially if the drug is, in fact, used for other indications. In contrast, there is only one clear use for topical minoxidil—hair growth.

© Stockbyte/Thinkstock

STUDY SCENARIO

Compoundit Pharmacy is near a clinic with three dermatologists, and as a result receives several prescriptions a week for various topical prescription ointments, creams, and gels. Most of the ointments, creams, and gels are available commercially, but Compoundit prefers to compound them because of the greater profits. Compoundit makes about a week's supply of the various topical drugs at a time. Other pharmacies in the area also get prescriptions for these topicals, but dispense the commercially made products. Compoundit approached these pharmacies, offering to make and sell them the topicals at a less expensive price than they pay from the manufacturers. The pharmacies agreed to purchase the products from Compoundit.

The FDA and board of pharmacy launch an investigation of Compoundit. Analyze and discuss each of the activities presented in this scenario and whether each activity constitutes compounding or manufacturing.

THE ORANGE BOOK AND GENERIC SUBSTITUTION

STATE GENERIC SUBSTITUTION LAWS

Today, every state has enacted generic drug substitution laws, expanding the scope of pharmacy practice to allow pharmacists to substitute a generically equivalent drug for the prescribed drug, subject to certain requirements and restrictions. Prior to the early 1970s, few states permitted generic substitution; pharmacists were compelled by law to dispense the brand prescribed by the physician, even if a less expensive and therapeutically equivalent generic product was available. These antisubstitution laws were imposed in the 1940s and 1950s to address abuses by some pharmacists who substituted low-quality and counterfeit drugs for the prescribed drugs. As more and more generic drugs became approved in the late 1960s and early 1970s, however, the public's awareness of and demand for lower cost generic drugs correspondingly increased. In addition, the Department of Health, Education and Welfare implemented the Medicaid Maximum Allowable Cost Program in 1974, which encouraged pharmacists to substitute generics by setting upper reimbursement limits on certain multisource drugs. State antisubstitution laws, however, obstructed both patient access to generic drugs and state participation in the Medicaid drug program, prompting state legislative action to allow pharmacists the authority to engage in generic substitutions.

Drug product selection laws vary significantly among states. In "mandatory" substitution states, pharmacists must substitute a less expensive generic drug for the brand-name drug unless the prescriber writes "dispense as written," "brand necessary," or a similar notation on the prescription. In "permissive" substitution states, a pharmacist may choose to substitute if the prescriber issues the prescription in a way that permits substitution. Without the prescriber's permission, either express or tacit, substitution is not allowed in most states, even if the consumer wishes a substitute.

Drug product selection rules apply only when a specific product has been prescribed, usually through the use of a brand-name. If a prescription is written generically, the selection is not subject to the drug product selection law. In this situation the pharmacist may dispense any product in the generic drug class, subject to the ever-present requirement for good professional judgment.

It would constitute misbranding under both state and federal law in most situations if a pharmacist labeled a substituted generic drug with the brand-name drug. Other legal violations may also result, such as in *Agbogun v. State*, 756 S.W.2d 1 (Tex. Crim. App. 1988), where a pharmacist was found guilty of the misdemeanor offense of deceptive business practices. The record showed that the patient had presented a prescription for Flagyl and that the pharmacist had substituted a generic drug but had labeled the vial with the trade name. The jury apparently disbelieved the pharmacist's explanation that he thought the physician had given him permission to label the bottle of generic tablets inaccurately with the trade name.

IMPORTANCE OF THE ORANGE BOOK IN GENERIC SUBSTITUTION

Pharmacists are responsible for ensuring that the substituted generic drug product is bioequivalent to the prescribed product. Bioequivalence basically means that the products display comparable bioavailability (rate and extent of absorption) at the site of action under similar conditions. Despite the enactment of state generic substitution laws, the proliferation of generic drugs in the late 1970s, and pressure from government and consumers to substitute generics, physicians and pharmacists were reluctant to substitute because of bioequivalence concerns. To assist pharmacists, other health care professionals, health care agencies and organizations, and others with this problem, the FDA published a book entitled Approved Drug Products with Therapeutic Equivalence Evaluations. First published in 1979 and republished annually with periodic updates, it quickly became known as the Orange Book because of its orange cover. The Orange Book, which can be accessed at the FDA's website at http://www.fda.gov/cder/ob, lists thousands of currently marketed multisource drug products that the FDA has approved as safe and effective. Note that the Orange Book only includes approved drug products; marketed unapproved drug products are not included.

Approved drug products that are "pharmaceutical equivalents" (defined by the FDA as products that contain the same active ingredients and are identical in strength and are of the same dosage form) are rated in the publication for "therapeutic equivalence." Therapeutic equivalence is defined as pharmaceutical equivalents that can be expected to have the same clinical effect and safety. Pharmaceutical equivalents that are bioequivalent are presumed by the FDA to be therapeutically equivalent. (*Note:* Do not confuse therapeutic equivalence as used in the Orange Book with the separate issue of therapeutic substitution, which refers to substituting different therapeutic agents that may be used for the same condition, such as amoxicillin for penicillin.) The issue of whether a generic drug with a different sustained-release system than the reference drug should be considered a pharmaceutical equivalent arose in the case of *Pfizer, Inc. v. Shalala*, 1 F. Supp. 2d 38 (D.C. 1998). In this case (which is reported in the case studies section of this chapter), Pfizer challenged the FDA's acceptance of an abbreviated new drug application (ANDA) from Mylan for a drug with the same active ingredient but a different sustained-release system as Pfizer's drug. Pfizer argued that the drugs are not the same dosage form and thus could not be considered as generic equivalents.

The court, however, finding for the FDA, concluded that the FDA's interpretation of what constitutes the same dosage form is reasonable.

The FDA uses a two-letter coding system for the therapeutic equivalence evaluations of multisource drug products. The first letter of the code is either an A or a B. Products rated with the first letter A are considered therapeutically equivalent to a reference drug product. Products rated with the first letter B are not considered to be therapeutically equivalent for various reasons, including that they may have documented bioequivalence problems to a reference drug product or there may be a significant potential for such problems and no adequate studies demonstrating bioequivalence. Ratings of B may also indicate that the quality standards are inadequate, or the FDA has insufficient data to determine therapeutic equivalence, or the drug product is still under review. The second letter of the code more specifically describes the dosage form or nature of the product. The list includes:

- AA: Drugs that are available in conventional dosage forms and have no bioequivalence problems.
- AB: Drugs identified by the FDA as having actual or potential bioequivalence problems, but which have been resolved by adequate scientific evidence. (In contrast, drugs placed in AA, AN, AO, AP, and AT have no known or suspected bioequivalence problems.)
- AN: Bioequivalent solutions and powders for aerosolization.
- AO: Bioequivalent injectable oil solutions.
- AP: Bioequivalent injectable aqueous solutions and some intravenous nonaqueous solutions.
- AT: Bioequivalent topical drug with no known bioequivalence problems.
- BC: Drugs in extended-release dosage forms with bioequivalence issues.
- BD: Active ingredients and dosage forms with documented bioequivalence problems.
- BE: Delayed-release oral dosage forms with potential bioequivalence problems.
- BN: Products in aerosol-nebulizer drug delivery systems unless proven bioequivalent.
- BP: Active ingredients and dosage forms with potential bioequivalence problems.
- BR: Suppositories or enemas that deliver drugs for systemic absorption unless proven bioequivalent.
- BS: Products having drug standard deficiencies.
- BT: Topical drug products with bioequivalence issues.
- BX: Products for which the data are insufficient to determine therapeutic equivalence.
- B★: Drugs for which no determination of therapeutic equivalence will be made until certain questions have been resolved.

Generic drugs marketed after 1984 and approved under an ANDA should all have an A rating because the PTRA requires that the generic drug must demonstrate proof of bioequivalence before approval.

The Orange Book has important implications for pharmacists involved in generic substitution and drug formulary decision making. For example, if the Orange Book lists four pharmaceutically equivalent drugs, two with a B rating and two with an A rating, the pharmacist may interchange the two drugs with A ratings. An interchange of the drugs with B ratings, either with the A-rated drugs or with one another, carries a risk the products will not produce the same clinical effects, however.

In some situations there may be more than one pharmaceutically equivalent reference drug that have not been determined to be bioequivalent to each other. This situation occurs because the pharmaceutically equivalent products have received approved NDAs and thus must demonstrate bioavailability, not bioequivalence. For these products the FDA implemented a three-character code such as AB1, AB2, and AB3. If a generic drug product establishes bioequivalence to one of the reference drugs, it will receive the same three-character code as that reference drug. For example, Adalat CC and Procardia XL are both extended-release nifedipine tablets with approved NDAs but are not rated as bioequivalent. A generic product to be approved must establish bioequivalence to either Adalat CC or Procardia XL (or both). So health care professionals know which generic products are bioequivalent to which reference drug, Adalat CC is assigned a rating of AB1 and Procardia XL a rating of AB2. Generic products that are bioequivalent to Adalat CC receive a rating of AB1, and those bioequivalent to Procardia XL receive a rating of AB2. Looking at the Orange Book under nifedipine products will reveal four generic products rated either AB1 or AB2. AB1-rated drugs are not considered bioequivalent to AB2-rated drugs.

Pharmacists should not switch pharmaceutically equivalent products without consulting the Orange Book. Switching refers to the practice of substituting a pharmaceutically equivalent product for the drug the patient has been taking and thus has become stabilized on. Switching B-rated products and drugs not included in the Orange Book requires a pharmacist's professional care and judgment because the switch could result in significant blood level differences in the patient. If a switch must be made, pharmacists should consult with the physician and counsel the patient as to the potential risks. (Many state laws require this.) Similarly, formularies should be constructed with an awareness of which drug products carry a B rating or which might not be bioequivalent. Too often, the inflexibility of a formulary or the reimbursement mandates of a third-party payer frustrate the exercise of professional judgment.

A pharmacist who substitutes a B-rated drug product for the drug prescribed does not violate the FDCA because the Orange Book is not a mandate; it is merely a guide. The pharmacist might violate state law, however. In most states, substitution or switching is allowed only if the drug is therapeutically equivalent or bioequivalent to the prescribed drug. In addition, switching a B-rated product without evaluating and balancing the clinical risks increases the pharmacist's risk of civil liability should a patient suffer injury.

NARROW THERAPEUTIC INDEX (NTI) DRUGS

In addition to B-rated drugs and pre-1938 drugs, pharmacists should also recognize the somewhat controversial category of drugs commonly called narrow therapeutic index (NTI) drugs, or as referred to in FDA regulations, narrow therapeutic ratio (NTR) drugs (21 C.F.R. 320.33(c)). An NTI or NTR drug is defined as one where there is less than a two-fold difference between the median lethal dose and the median effective dose, or where there is less than a two-fold difference between the minimum toxic concentrations and the minimum effective concentrations in the blood. Safe and effective use of these drugs requires careful titration and patient monitoring. Some examples of NTI drugs listed by the FDA in guidance documents include carbamazepine, clonidine, levothyroxine, lithium, minoxidil, phenytoin, theophylline, and warfarin.

Some drug manufacturers and health care providers have expressed concern that the FDA's bioequivalence standards allowing a range of 80 to 125 percent are not precise enough for NTI drugs. These critics have argued for more stringent criteria. Historically, the FDA has rejected such arguments, stating that it has reviewed no clinical data that would warrant narrowing this interval. However, in 2010 the agency reconsidered and presented the issue to an advisory committee that voted nearly unanimously that bioequivalence requirements are not adequate for NTI drugs. Subsequently, the advisory committee met in 2011 and voted that the FDA should adopt new guidelines for NTI drugs including narrowing the potency range to 95 to 105 percent, which the agency is in the process of drafting.

This means that pharmacists should exercise professional judgment when switching even A-rated NTI drugs, inform patients of the switch, and alert patients to contact them if they notice any physiological changes. B–rated NTI drugs should not be switched without notifying the prescriber and informing the patient. Pharmacists also must be aware of state laws that may restrict the substitution of some of these products.

© Stockbyte/Thinkstock

STUDY SCENARIO AND QUESTIONS

Sally, a pharmacist at SuperClinic Pharmacy, received a prescription from a patient, Mr. Lee, for Menton. Mr. Lee asked if there was a less expensive generic drug available because he had to pay for his medications personally. Sally knew that there was a generic product available but that it had a B rating to Menton in the FDA's Orange Book. Sally was uncertain whether to dispense the generic or not.

1. How is it possible that the generic is not bioequivalent to Menton?
2. Should the fact that the generic is B rated affect Sally's substitution decision? Explain how Sally should proceed.
3. Would switching to the generic present more or less risk to Mr. Lee if he had previously been taking Menton?
4. Explain whether substituting the generic for Menton would violate federal law or the law in your state. If so, how could Sally legally substitute the drugs?
5. If a substitution is made, what should Sally tell the patient?

PRESCRIPTION DRUG MARKETING ACT OF 1987

Enacted in 1987 (P.L. 100-293), the Prescription Drug Marketing Act (PDMA) amends the FDCA to

- Require states to license wholesale distributors of prescription drugs
- Ban the reimportation of prescription drugs, except by the manufacturer or for emergency use
- Ban the sale, trade, or purchase of drug samples
- Mandate storage, handling, and recordkeeping requirements for drug samples
- Ban the trafficking in or counterfeiting of drug coupons
- Prohibit the resale of prescription drugs purchased by hospitals or health care facilities, with certain exceptions

The PDMA was passed after 2 years of congressional hearings, during which it was established that many prescription drug products were being misbranded and adulterated because they were being diverted from the normal stream of distribution. Congress concluded that the U.S. public could no longer purchase prescription drugs with the certainty that the products were safe and effective unless legislation was enacted. The FDA issued final regulations implementing the PDMA in 1999 (64 Fed. Reg. 67720).

REGULATION OF PRESCRIPTION DRUG SAMPLES

Congressional investigators discovered that drug manufacturers' representatives commonly left large quantities of samples at hospitals, physicians' offices, clinics, and other locations. They kept few records of distribution, and there was no quality control for the storage of these samples. This situation was exacerbated by individuals who gathered up the samples, combined them into stock bottles, relabeled the bottles, and sold them to community and hospital pharmacies. The pharmacies then dispensed and sold the samples to patients. Often, the drugs had been improperly stored under hot and unsanitary conditions, improperly labeled, and mixed with other drug lots. The consumer had no assurance that the drugs were unadulterated or labeled properly. To prevent these abuses, the PDMA prohibits the sale, purchase, or trade of samples. The same restrictions apply to coupons used to redeem the drug at no cost or at a reduced cost.

A sample is defined as a unit of drug intended not to be sold but rather to promote the sale of the drug. Starter packs distributed by manufacturers free to pharmacies are not considered samples because they are not labeled as such and could be sold. Samples from manufacturers and distributors may be distributed only to practitioners licensed to prescribe or to pharmacies of hospitals or health care entities (i.e., organizations that provide diagnostic, medical, surgical, or dental treatment but do not include a retail pharmacy) at the written request of the prescriber on a form that includes the information specified by law. The practitioner must make the request each time; a standing request is not acceptable. If the distribution is by mail or common carrier, the recipient must execute a written receipt for the sample on delivery, and the receipt must be returned to the manufacturer or authorized distributor. The manufacturer and distributor must store the samples under proper conditions. They also must keep annual inventories of samples in the possession of company representatives.

Proposed regulations by the FDA (59 Fed. Reg. 11842, March 14, 1994) emphasized that retail pharmacies are barred from receiving any sample prescription drug, and provided that the mere presence of any sample prescription drug in a retail pharmacy shall be considered evidence that the sample was obtained illegally. Although this strong language was not included in the final regulations, the final regulations clearly do not allow retail pharmacies to receive samples (59 Fed. Reg. 67720, 1999). The pharmacy of a hospital or health care entity may receive samples at the request of a licensed practitioner, provided there is a receipt containing:

- The name and address of the requesting prescriber
- The name and address of the hospital or health care entity designated to receive the drug sample
- The name, address, title, and signature of the person acknowledging delivery of the drug sample
- The proprietary or established name and strength of the drug sample
- The quantity and lot or control number
- The date of delivery

PURCHASES AND RESALES BY HOSPITALS AND HEALTH CARE ENTITIES

Diversionary markets did not involve only drug samples. Congressional investigators discovered that prescription drugs were diverted when hospitals and health care entities resold their excess purchases. Because of their nonprofit status, cooperative bidding practices, and restrictive formularies, hospitals, health maintenance organizations (HMOs), and other health are entities often are able to purchase drugs at prices much lower than community pharmacies must pay for the same drugs. Some health care entities were reselling their purchases at a markup to brokers, retail pharmacies, and even wholesalers. This practice created misbranding and adulteration problems because the drugs were often improperly stored under unsanitary conditions in garages and automobile trunks for large periods of time. In addition, some drugs were repackaged from large containers into smaller, improperly labeled containers under unsanitary conditions. Such schemes also led to unfair competition because those pharmacies that purchased the drugs in the diversionary market obtained a price advantage over those that did not participate.

In an attempt to stop this diversionary market, the PDMA prohibits the sale, purchase, or trade (or offer to do so) of prescription drugs that have been purchased by a hospital, health care entity, or charitable organization. Very important exceptions to this general rule include:

- A hospital's purchases from a group purchasing organization or from other member hospitals for its own use
- Sales or purchases to nonprofit affiliates
- Sales or purchases among hospitals or health care entities under common control
- Sales or purchases for emergency medical reasons (e.g., transfers allowed between health care entities or from a health care entity to a community pharmacy to alleviate a temporary shortage of a prescription drug)
- Selling or dispensing prescription drugs pursuant to prescriptions

PRODUCT RETURNS

Shortly after passage of the law, there was some confusion as to whether hospitals and health care entities could legally return mistakenly ordered and outdated prescription drug products to wholesalers and manufacturers or whether these transactions would constitute a sale or trade. After considerable debate, the FDA agreed to permit legitimate returns, provided that the drugs are properly stored and handled and proper records are kept (21 C.F.R. part 205).

WHOLESALE DISTRIBUTORS

Under the Prescription Drug Marketing Act, all persons engaged in the wholesale distribution of prescription drugs must be licensed by the state in accordance with prescribed guidelines. Wholesale distribution is defined as distribution to anyone other than the consumer. The intent of this provision is to prevent individuals who can obtain drugs at lower prices from reselling those drugs unless they are licensed as a wholesaler. Through licensure, the states can ensure that those functioning as wholesalers meet the required standards. In 1990, the FDA established uniform standards that wholesale distributors of prescription drugs must meet to be licensed (21 C.F.R. part 205). (Some of these standards were subsequently amended by the 1999 regulations.) Because of the counterfeit drug problem (discussed next) and the threat of terrorism, some associations have argued that state regulation does not work for interstate wholesalers and that the FDA should assume the licensure of wholesalers.

PEDIGREES AND COUNTERFEITING

The PDMA granted the FDA the authority to require wholesalers that are not manufacturers and that are not authorized by a manufacturer of the drug to maintain a record that identifies each prior sale, purchase, or trade of the drugs they receive and distribute. Today this type of record is generally called a pedigree since it contains information on each transaction changing the ownership of the drug. Wholesalers not authorized by a manufacturer are generally called secondary wholesalers. Secondary wholesalers are a legal and important component of the drug distribution system and far outnumber authorized wholesalers. The PDMA limited the pedigree requirement to secondary wholesalers because at the time Congress found that most of the problems of counterfeiting and diversion occurred in the secondary market.

Interpreting what the PDMA meant by "each prior sale," the FDA issued a final regulation to implement the pedigree requirement in 1999 (64 Fed. Reg. 67720), requiring each secondary wholesaler to receive and distribute a pedigree that includes a record of ownership back to the "original" manufacturer. The FDA, however, then delayed implementation because of concerns from the wholesale industry regarding the cost and burden of maintaining a paper pedigree on each drug. Now, however, electronic technologies exist via radio frequency identification (RFID) to make pedigrees workable. RFID technology allows drug product packages to be tagged with tiny chips containing an electronic product code or unique electronic serial number. Using RFIDs the history of a drug can be traced from the manufacturer to the final dispenser.

The FDA announced in June 2006 that the regulation would no longer be delayed and would become effective December 1, 2006 (71 Fed. Reg. 34249). Subsequently the FDA published a compliance policy guide, "Prescription Drug Marketing Act Pedigree Requirements Under 21 CFR Part 203," intended to clarify how the FDA plans to prioritize enforcement of the pedigree requirements. However, on November 30, 2006, one day before the regulation's effective date, a federal district court issued a preliminary injunction against DHHS preventing the regulation's implementation, and the court of appeals affirmed the decision in 2008 (*RxUSA Wholesale, Inc., et al. v. DHHS*, 467 F.Supp.2d 285 (E.D.N.Y. 2006); aff'd. 285 Fed.Appx.809 (C.A.2 (N.Y.) 2008)). The court agreed with the secondary wholesaler plaintiffs that if the regulation became effective, they would suffer irreparable harm and that the PDMA pedigree requirement likely violates the U.S. Constitution's equal protection clause. The reason for the court's ruling was that the regulation (in conformance with the PDMA) requires only secondary wholesalers to have records tracing the drug back to the original manufacturer. Secondary wholesalers generally purchase from authorized wholesalers who do not have to keep these records and thus would not have them to pass on to the secondary wholesalers. This would mean that the secondary wholesalers could not obtain a record of ownership from the original manufacturer, would be powerless to comply with the regulation, and would go out of business as a result. Both the district court and appellate court found that the PDMA does not specifically require that the pedigree must extend back to the original manufacturer or if it need go back only to the last authorized distributor. Based upon the court decisions, the FDA issued a proposed regulation in July 2011 that would instead require secondary wholesalers to identify the last authorized distributor (76 Fed. Reg. 41434).

The reason that the FDA and most state pharmacy boards are now anxious to implement the pedigree requirement is not just because of advances in technology, but because counterfeit drugs have allegedly become a growing and significant problem. This is also the reason that some states enacted legislation in the past few years to require pedigree tracking at some future date by everyone in the chain of distribution, including pharmacies. The FDA has noted that the number of counterfeit cases increased from 6 in 2000 to 72 in 2010 and then dropped down somewhat to 59 in 2011. Counterfeit drugs have found their way into the legitimate U.S. drug distribution system and onto the shelves of pharmacies. Although the three largest wholesalers in this country sell 90 percent of all drugs in the United States and buy primarily from manufacturers, there are over 7,000 smaller secondary wholesalers in this country that buy drugs from several sources and sell to several difference sources, including the three largest wholesalers. There are multiple opportunities for counterfeiters to introduce their products into this system, and thus government regulators are putting great faith in RFID technology to reduce the counterfeiting problem.

For these reasons, Congress included in the 2007 FDAAA a mandate that the FDA, by March 2010, prioritize and develop standards to identify, authenticate, and track and trace prescription drugs; develop a standard numerical identifier to be applied to the drug by the manufacturer; and utilize promising technologies such as RFID, nanotechnology, and encryption. The FDA has solicited public comments since 2008 for the purpose of developing these standards. In 2010, the FDA issued a guidance document regarding the development of standardized numerical identifiers (SNIs) for prescription drug packages as its initial step in complying with the FDAAA mandate (http://www.fda. gov/RegulatoryInformation/Guidances/ucm125505.htm). The guidance states that the SNI would be required at the package level (defined as the smallest unit sold by the manufacturer to a dispenser) and should be a serialized National Drug Code (sNDC). The FDA Safety and Innovation Act enacted in 2012 was to have included the standards for a national track and trace system; however, disagreement among legislators, manufacturers, wholesalers, and pharmacies caused it to be deleted.

REIMPORTATION OF PRESCRIPTION DRUGS

Generally speaking, the importation of prescription drugs from another country is illegal because the FDA has likely not approved the drug or else not approved the manufacturer to manufacture the drug. The PDMA does allow the reimportation of prescription drugs, but only by the original manufacturer or for emergency use. The Medicare Prescription Drug, Improvement and Modernization Act (MMA) allows the Secretary of Health and Human Services (HHS) to promulgate regulations that facilitate the wholesale importation of prescription medications from Canada. The secretary may only do so, however, if the secretary can certify the program would pose no additional risk to public health or safety and would significantly reduce cost. To date the secretary has refused to recognize any certification.

Under a compassionate use policy in place for several years, the FDA has permitted the personal importation of small amounts of drugs, but only if they are not approved in the United States and are used for the treatment of a serious condition for which no satisfactory treatment is available in this country. The drug must not represent an unreasonable risk and the patient seeking to import the drug must provide the name of the licensed U.S. physician responsible for treating the patient with the unapproved drug. Under a provision in the Department of Homeland Security Appropriations Act of 2007, however, an individual patient may import an FDA-approved prescription drug from Canada (P.L. No. 109-295). The exemption applies only to individuals transporting the drug on their person in a quantity not to exceed a 90-day supply. Moreover, the drug may not be a controlled substance or biological product. The Controlled Substances Act and regulations do allow for a personal use exemption for controlled substances, regardless of the country. The exemption only allows for a total combined quantity of 50 dosage units that must be transported personally—not shipped—across the border (21 U.S.C. § 956, 21 C.F.R. § (1301.26)). The drug must be in the original, dispensed container and must be declared at customs. The 50-dosage–unit limitation does not apply to controlled substances lawfully dispensed in the United States by a DEA registrant.

Nonetheless, many U.S. patients have for years crossed the borders of Canada and Mexico to have their prescriptions dispensed in those countries at lower prices, and the FDA has generally not taken any action. In recent years, Internet as well as brick-and-mortar businesses have offered patients nationwide the option of purchasing their medications through Canadian pharmacies. (Canada has become the country of choice because of easier availability of drugs and fewer fears of counterfeiting, adulteration, and misbranding.) Even some states and cities have authorized or proposed prescription benefit plans that allow patients to purchase the drugs from Canada. Rhode Island has gone so far as to legalize the state board of pharmacy to license Canadian pharmacies. Vermont filed a petition with the FDA to allow its state employee benefit plan to import prescription medications, but the FDA rejected the petition. Vermont then sued HHS and the FDA contending that the MMA was unconstitutional because it delegated Congressional authority to approve importation to the secretary. Vermont also asked for the prompt issuance of regulations allowing for importation. The court found that the Vermont plan violates the FDCA and that the MMA establishes an "intelligible principle" directing the secretary to certify safety and costs, and as such the delegation is not illegal (*State of Vermont v. Leavitt*, 405 F.Supp.2d 466 (D.Vt., Sept. 19, 2005)).

The FDA has staunchly maintained that although it sympathizes with consumer and local government efforts to obtain drugs at lower prices, the practice of importing prescription drugs from other countries for U.S. patients violates the PDMA (21 U.S.C. § 381(d)(1)). In *U.S. v. Rx Depot, Inc.*, 2003 WL 22519473 (N.D. Okla., Nov. 6, 2003), the FDA brought an injunction action against a company engaged in this practice. The defendant, Rx Depot, operated stores throughout the United States, and solicited patients to mail, fax, or deliver their prescriptions to one of its stores. Rx Depot would then transmit the prescription and a medical history form it required the patient to provide to a participating pharmacy in Canada. A Canadian doctor would rewrite the prescription, and the Canadian pharmacy would fill and ship it directly to the patient in the United States. Rx Depot would receive a 10 to 12 percent commission for each sale. The court concluded that it was sympathetic to patients who cannot afford prescription drugs at U.S. prices, but that Rx Depot was violating the law and thus granted the FDA's motion for an injunction, requiring that the defendant cease its operations.

The FDA has promised enforcement action against businesses engaged in these activities because of public health concerns. The agency maintains that most drugs sold outside the United States, including in Canada, have not received FDA approval. Many drugs produced for foreign markets are made by firms that have not applied for FDA approval. Even if a manufacturer has FDA approval for a particular drug in this country, the FDA contends that the version produced for other markets usually does not meet all the requirements for U.S. approval. As a result, the agency is greatly concerned that foreign products risk being adulterated or misbranded as well as counterfeited. After a 1-year investigation, a DHHS Task Force issued a report in December 2004 finding that drug reimportation presents significant risks (http://www.hhs.gov/importtaskforce). Nonetheless, at present, Congress is considering measures to legalize the importation of prescription drugs from Canada.

PENALTIES

The penalty provision in the PDMA is extensive and specific. There are several different penalties, including up to 10 years in prison, a $250,000 fine, or both for first offenses.

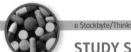

© Stockbyte/Thinkstock

STUDY SCENARIOS AND QUESTIONS

1. Through the power of its purchasing cooperative and its nonprofit status, Mercy Hospital's pharmacy is able to purchase prescription drugs at much lower prices than community pharmacies. The director of the pharmacy decided to purchase more inventory than the pharmacy needed and to sell the excess inventory to community pharmacies. The hospital benefited by making extra profit and the pharmacies benefited by purchasing the drugs at less than their direct cost from the manufacturer. Explain if this activity is legal, and why. What if, instead of Mercy Hospital purchasing and reselling the drugs, it was a chain pharmacy? Would your answer change, and why?

2. Tom and Mary are a middle-aged couple who pay out of pocket nearly $2,000 per month for prescription drugs in your pharmacy. One of their friends told them that they could buy the drugs in Canada for about half that price. Tom and Mary ask you if they could legally buy the drugs in Canada. If so, they wonder how they could do this and ask if maybe you could get the drugs for them and their friends. Provide Tom and Mary with accurate information on this subject.

INSPECTIONS UNDER THE FEDERAL FOOD, DRUG, AND COSMETIC ACT

The FDA does not routinely inspect pharmacies. Section 704 of the FDCA states that FDA inspectors may inspect facilities where drugs are held at reasonable times, within reasonable limits, and in a reasonable manner. However, section 704 exempts from FDA inspection authority pharmacies that regularly dispense prescriptions and that do not manufacture, prepare, or compound drugs or devices for sale other than in the regular course of their retail business. Nonetheless, the agency has always assumed it has the authority to inspect pharmacies, especially when it has reason to believe that the pharmacy may be engaging in manufacturing or repackaging activities, and has done so. As discussed in the compounding section of this chapter, the federal courts have supported the FDA's position. Courts have held that the FDA can generally inspect a pharmacy to determine whether it meets the pharmacy exemption or is engaging in manufacturing. If the FDA has probable cause to believe the pharmacy is manufacturing, the FDA can extend the search to the pharmacy's records. FDA agents do not need a warrant under the statute but merely must show their credentials and a notice of inspection. They do not even need to state the reason for the inspection. The U.S. Supreme Court has never considered the constitutionality of the warrantless search statute; however, a pharmacist would be wise not to refuse an agent without a warrant. Refusing entry to FDA inspectors could result in a penalty of up to 1 year in prison, a $1,000 fine, or both (FDCA §§ 301(f) and 303(a)).

RELATED LAWS TO THE FDCA

USE OF ALCOHOL IN PHARMACY PRACTICE

Pharmacists handle several kinds of alcohol, depending on their practice setting. These include denatured alcohols (rubbing alcohol and alcohols used in compounding external medications), ethyl alcohols (used in compounding internal and external medications, flavoring agents, etc.), and isopropyl alcohol. Tax-paid ethyl alcohol is the beverage liquor sold in such retail outlets as liquor stores, grocery stores, and pharmacies. Anyone selling federally taxed alcohol at retail must conform to the licensing and tax requirements established by the Bureau of Alcohol, Tobacco and Firearms and the Internal Revenue Service. Community pharmacies that use alcohol to compound prescriptions commonly use tax-paid ethyl alcohol, usually 190-proof grain alcohol, purchased from an authorized retail or wholesale outlet.

In contrast, some entities are entitled to use 190-proof ethyl alcohol that is not taxed by the federal government (called tax-free alcohol). Tax-free alcohol may be used by the following entities for the following purposes (27 C.F.R. Part 22):

- State or political subdivisions for scientific and mechanical purposes
- Educational institutions for scientific and mechanical purposes
- Laboratories for scientific research
- Hospitals, blood banks, and sanitariums for scientific, mechanical, and medicinal purposes, and in the treatment of patients
- Pathology laboratories in connection with hospitals and sanitariums for scientific, mechanical, and medicinal purposes and in the treatment of patients
- Nonprofit clinics for scientific, mechanical, and medicinal purposes and in the treatment of patients

Community pharmacies cannot legally obtain or use tax-free alcohol. Hospitals that purchase tax-free alcohol may use it only for medicinal, mechanical, and scientific purposes and in the treatment of patients. Tax-free alcohol may never be used in beverages or food products, and medicines made with tax-free alcohol may not be sold to outpatients. Medicines compounded on hospital premises for inpatients may be sold if a separate charge is made. Outpatient charity clinics may furnish medicines made with tax-free alcohol to outpatients if they do not charge. The sale of tax-free alcohol by hospitals to retail pharmacies and physicians' offices is prohibited.

Tax-free alcohol must be stored in a securely locked storeroom with the labels and markings on the containers intact. After the containers are empty, the labels and markings must be obliterated before discarding.

POISON PREVENTION PACKAGING ACT

Congress enacted the Poison Prevention Packaging Act (PPPA) in 1970 (15 U.S.C. §§ 1471–1474) with the intent of protecting children from accidental poisonings with "household substances." The law defines a "household substance" as any substance that is customarily produced for or used in the household and is designated:

- A hazardous substance in the federal Hazardous Substances Act
- An economic poison under the federal Insecticide, Fungicide and Rodenticide Act
- A food, drug, or cosmetic under the FDCA
- A household fuel when stored in a portable container

The FDA enforced the PPPA until 1973, when this responsibility was placed with the Consumer Product Safety Commission (CPSC). The CPSC has noted that the PPPA has resulted in remarkable declines in the reported deaths of children as the result of accidental ingestion of household substances. The CPSC also cautions, however, that among children younger than 5 years of age there are still an average of 50 deaths a year and 85,000 who are seen in emergency rooms following poisonings. (See *Poison Prevention Packaging: A Guide for Healthcare Professionals* at http://www.cpsc.gov/cpscpub/pubs/384.pdf.)

The act requires the use of child-resistant containers for packaging most OTC drugs and nearly all prescription drugs that the pharmacist will dispense directly to the consumer. These containers must be manufactured such that 80 percent of the children less than 5 years of age cannot open them, whereas at least 90 percent of adults can.

A drug may be dispensed only one time in a child-resistant container or vial because continued use compromises the effectiveness of the container. If the container is glass or threaded plastic, however, the Consumer Product Safety Commission permits reuse of the container as long as it is dispensed with a new safety closure. The commission has indicated that the pharmacist may dispense drugs in reversible containers (those with closures that are child-resistant when used on one side and not child-resistant on the other), as long as they are dispensed in the child-resistant mode. However, the commission continues, this practice is strongly discouraged because it could result in the use of the noncomplying packaging by those able to use the child-resistant packaging without difficulty.

Although pharmacists must normally dispense oral prescription drugs in child-resistant packaging, the law exempts drugs dispensed pursuant to prescription from the packaging requirement if either the physician prescribing the drug or the patient receiving the drug requests noncompliant containers. These requests may be oral, although the pharmacist may be wise to document each request. Preferably, the pharmacist should have the patient sign a statement that the patient requested a noncompliant container. Patients may make a blanket request that all their medications be dispensed in noncompliant packaging; prescribers, however, may not, except for refills of the prescription. Blanket requests by patients should be in writing and the pharmacist should periodically check with the patient to ensure that the patient continues to prefer noncompliant packaging. The commission has indicated that it would be legal, but not preferable, for prescribers simply to check a box on a prescription blank to indicate that the drug be dispensed in a noncompliant package. This practice could encourage excessive use of noncompliant packages.

As another exemption, the Poison Prevention Packaging Act allows manufacturers to market one size of an OTC product for elderly or handicapped individuals in noncompliant packaging. The package must contain the statement, "This Package for Households Without Young Children." If the label is too small for this statement, it may contain the warning, "Package Not Child-Resistant." If the size marketed in noncompliant packaging happens to be a popular size, the manufacturer must also market it in child-resistant packaging.

Drugs dispensed to institutionalized patients are exempt from the act if they are to be administered by the institution's employees.

All legend drugs and controlled substances must be packaged in child-resistant containers except

- Sublingual dosage forms of nitroglycerin
- Sublingual and chewable forms of isosorbide dinitrate in strengths of 10 mg or less
- Sodium fluoride products containing not more than 264 mg of sodium fluoride per package
- Anhydrous cholestyramine in powder form
- Methylprednisolone tablets containing not more than 84 mg of the drug per package

- Mebendazole tablets containing not more than 600 mg of the drug per package
- Betamethasone tablets containing not more than 12.6 mg of the drug per package
- Potassium supplements in unit dose forms, including effervescent tablets, unit dose vials of liquid potassium, and powdered potassium in unit dose packets containing not more than 50 mEq per unit dose
- Erythromycin ethylsuccinate granules for oral suspension and oral suspensions in packages containing not more than 8 g of the equivalent of erythromycin
- Colestipol in powder form up to 5 g in a packet
- Erythromycin ethylsuccinate tablets in packages containing no more than 16 g of the drug
- Preparations in aerosol containers intended for inhalation therapy
- Pancrelipase preparations
- Prednisone tablets containing not more than 105 mg per package
- Cyclically administered oral contraceptives, conjugated estrogens, and norethindrone acetate tablets in manufacturer's memory-aid (mnemonic) dispenser packages
- Medroxyprogesterone acetate tablets
- Sucrase preparations in a solution of glycerol and water
- Oral dosage form products containing aspirin and acetaminophen must comply with the act's packaging requirements, except
  - Effervescent tablets containing aspirin or acetaminophen, other than those intended for pediatric use. The dry tablet must contain less than 15 percent of aspirin or acetaminophen, the tablet must have an oral LD50 in rates of greater than 5 g/kg body weight, and the tablet placed in water must release at least 85 ml of carbon dioxide per grain in the dry tablet when measured stoichiometrically at standard conditions.
  - Unflavored aspirin- or acetaminophen-containing preparations in powder form, not intended for pediatric use, that are packaged in unit doses providing not more than 15.4 grains of aspirin or 13 grains of acetaminophen per unit dose and that contain no other substances subject to the provisions of the act.

The PPPA also allows for a procedure to obtain exemptions from child-resistant packaging in the form of a formal petition. Most such petitions come from the manufacturer of the product and generally for a specific package size of an oral prescription drug.

A few other products covered by the Poison Prevention Packaging Act, subject to specified requirements, include

- Furniture polish
- Methyl salicylate
- Sodium and potassium hydroxide
- Turpentine
- Kindling and illuminating preparations
- Methyl alcohol
- Sulfuric acid
- Ethylene glycol
- Iron-containing drugs
- Dietary supplements containing iron
- Solvents for paint or other similar surface-coating material

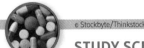
© Stockbyte/Thinkstock

STUDY SCENARIO AND QUESTIONS

Mr. Thomas is an elderly patient who requests non–child-resistant containers when he can remember. When he cannot remember, the pharmacy dispenses his medications in child-resistant containers. One day he complained to his physician. When the physician called in a new prescription for Mr. Thomas he told the pharmacy to dispense all of Mr. Thomas's prescriptions in non–child-resistant containers.

Is it permissible for the physician to do this? If not, what should the pharmacy do to prevent Mr. Thomas from receiving child-resistant containers in the future?

DRUG ADVERTISING BY PHARMACIES

This section examines drug advertising by pharmacies. In contrast to manufacturers, pharmacists are not usually interested in advertising the merits of drug products, but rather the prices of these products. Price advertising by pharmacists is regulated primarily by state laws and regulatory agencies, but the First Amendment applies no less to pharmacy advertising than it does to manufacturer advertising.

Price Advertising

The FDA considers the advertising of prescription prices by pharmacists to be reminder advertising. Under 21 C.F.R. § 200.200, prescription drug reminder advertisements intended to provide price information to consumers are exempt from the requirements of the advertising regulations (21 C.F.R. § 202.1), provided certain conditions are met:

- The only purpose of the advertising is to provide information on price, not information on the drug's safety, efficacy, or indications for use.
- The advertising contains the proprietary name of the drug, if any; the established name (generic), if any; the drug's strength; the dosage form; and the price charged for a specific quantity of the drug.
- The advertising may include other information, such as the availability of professional or other types of services, as long as it is not misleading.
- The price stated in the advertising shall include all charges to the consumer; mailing fees and delivery fees, if any, may be stated separately. Any reminder advertising that is not in compliance with the regulations may be the subject of regulatory action.

Product Advertising: Strict Liability

Occasionally, pharmacists become involved in the advertising of OTC products that is not reminder advertising. In these situations, the Federal Trade Commission Act is most applicable and, in fact, establishes a strict liability standard for those who participate in false advertising. (Recall that the FTC Act prohibits deceptive or false advertising.) In *Porter & Dietsch, Inc. v. Federal Trade Commission*, 605 F.2d 294 (7th Cir. 1979), the FTC brought action not only against the manufacturer of the X-11 tablets but also against the Pay'n Save drugstore chain. Pay'n Save's only connection with the X-11 advertising was its participation in Porter & Dietsch's cooperative advertising program, through which it received advertising materials for publication under Pay'n Save's name. Pay'n Save had no knowledge that the advertisements were false or unsubstantiated.

Pay'n Save argued that it should not be held liable for its use of advertisements prepared by others. The court, however, found the drugstore chain liable and cited section 12(a) of the act, which provides, "It shall be unlawful for any person, partnership, or corporation to disseminate, or cause to be disseminated, any false advertisement." Stated the court, "The statute does not make mental state an element of violation and creates no exemption from liability for parties not involved in the creation of the false advertising or for unwitting disseminators of false advertising" (605 F.2d at 309).

The FTC has recently signaled an aggressive position against the deceptive and false marketing of dietary supplements, testifying before a Senate committee in 2009 that marketers of dietary supplements and other products have become very bold in their medical benefit claims causing health and safety concerns. In 2009, the FTC announced that Rite Aid agreed to pay $500,000 to settle charges for the deceptive advertising of its product "Germ Defense" for touting the product as able to prevent, treat, or reduce the severity of colds and flu. This settlement came after an FTC action and a consumer class action lawsuit against Airborne Health for the false advertising of its cold prevention products that Airborne agreed to settle for $30 million in 2008. A consumer class action suit against Walgreens for its generic equivalent of Airborne resulted in a settlement in 2009 where the chain agreed to pay each claimant consumer up to $14.97 or a free flu shot. These actions indicate that pharmacies must not only be concerned with a more aggressive FTC but class action lawsuits by consumers as well.

State Advertising Laws: The *Virginia* Case and the First Amendment

Before 1976, many state laws prohibited pharmacists from advertising prescription drug prices. Attempts by chain pharmacies to invalidate these laws as not reasonably related to the public health, safety, and welfare generally failed. (See *Supermarkets General Corporation v. Sills*, 225 A.2d 728 (N.S. Super 1966); *Patterson Drug Co. v. Kingery*, 305 F. Supp. 821 (W.D. Va. 1969); and *Mississippi State Board of Pharmacy v. Steele*, 317 So.2d 33 (Miss. 1975).) In 1976, however, in the landmark case *Virginia State Board of Pharmacy v. Virginia Citizens Consumer Council, Inc.*, 425 U.S. 748 (1976), the U.S. Supreme Court held that such state statutes violate the First Amendment protection of free speech. In a reversal of previous decisions, the Court found that commercial speech does enjoy limited First Amendment protection.

At issue in *Virginia* was the constitutionality of a Virginia statute that declared the publishing, advertising, or promoting of any amount, fee, premium, discount, or rebate for any prescription drug to be unprofessional conduct. The plaintiffs-appellees in the case were consumers who contended that the law violated the First Amendment of the U.S. Constitution. *Virginia* raised two unique issues to the Court: (1) Does the First Amendment right of free speech apply to the listeners or recipients of the speech? (2) Does the First Amendment apply to commercial speech?

In answer to the first issue, the Court stated, "If there is a right to advertise, there is a reciprocal right to receive the advertising and it may be asserted by these appellees" (425 U.S. at 757). Regarding the second issue, the Court found that, even if an advertiser's interest is purely economic, the advertiser does not lose First Amendment protection. In fact, continued the Court, the consumer may have as keen an interest in the free flow of commercial information as in the most urgent political debate. The Court was impressed by the consumers' arguments that prescription prices vary greatly from pharmacy to pharmacy and that those most affected by the suppression of prescription drug price information are the poor, the sick, and, particularly, the aged. These groups tend to spend a disproportionate amount of their income on prescription drugs, yet they are the least able to ascertain by shopping at the various pharmacies where they should spend their scarce dollars. Stated the Court, "It is a matter of public interest that those [consumer] decisions, in the aggregate, be intelligent and well informed. To this end, the free flow of commercial information is indispensable" (425 U.S. at 765).

The Virginia pharmacy board contended that allowing price advertising would drive the service-oriented pharmacies out of business; encourage consumers to shop around, thus making medication monitoring impossible; and damage the professional image of the pharmacist. The Court rejected all the state pharmacy board's reasons for the advertising ban and replied that the state appeared to be protecting its citizens by keeping them ignorant. The Court felt that the advertising ban would not achieve the state's objectives:

> There is, of course, an alternative to this highly paternalistic approach. That alternative is to assume that this information is not in itself harmful, that people will perceive their own best interests if only they are well enough informed, and that the best means to that end is to open the channels of communication rather than to close them. If they are truly open, nothing prevents the "professional" pharmacist from marketing his own assertedly superior product, and contrasting it with that of the low-cost, high-volume prescription drug retailer. But the choice among these alternative approaches is not ours to make or the Virginia General Assembly's. It is precisely this kind of choice, between the dangers of suppressing information, and the dangers of its misuse if it is freely available, that the First Amendment makes for us. Virginia is free to require whatever professional standards it wishes of its pharmacists; it may subsidize them or protect them from competition in other ways. But it may not do so by keeping the public in ignorance of the entirely lawful terms that competing pharmacists are offering. (425 U.S. at 770)

The *Virginia* decision not only opened the doors for pharmacists to advertise prescription drug prices but also ultimately affected the other professions as well. For example, in a subsequent Supreme Court decision, *Bates v. State Bar of Arizona*, 443 U.S. 350 (1977), the Court declared state laws that prohibited the advertising of legal services unconstitutional.

Although the Court did not hold in *Virginia* that pharmacists must advertise prescription price information, some states have chosen to mandate that pharmacists must provide such information on the request of the consumer. The *Virginia* decision does not prohibit states from regulating the false and misleading advertising of pharmacy goods and services, and nearly all state laws prohibit such advertising. In addition, some states prohibit pharmacists from advertising professional superiority.

The *Virginia* decision does not bar a state from making it illegal for pharmacists to offer discounts or rebates in connection with the sale of drugs. In the matter of *CVS Pharmacy Wayne*, 561 A.2d 1160 (N.J. 1989), the CVS pharmacy chain distributed mail circulars advertising a special 1-week price of $3.00 for prescription drugs. The state board of pharmacy ruled that the chain was guilty of unprofessional conduct for violating a New Jersey law that prohibited the distribution of discounts, premiums, or rebates, except for trading stamps and except to those more than 62 years of age. The pharmacy first brought legal action, arguing that the New Jersey law unconstitutionally restricted its right of free speech but was unsuccessful (*in re Board of Pharmacy*, 465 A.2d 522 (N.J. Super. Ct. App. Div. 1983); cert. denied 470 A.2d 413 (N.J. 1983)). In state court, CVS argued that the law was unconstitutional on other grounds, especially because it discriminated between those less than and those older than 62 years of age. The state court, while acknowledging that the law has several flaws and may not be the best method of achieving the legislative purpose, sustained the validity of the law. The court established an insurmountable burden of proof for CVS by stating that it would presume that every state statute attempts to protect the public health, safety, and welfare as long as it attempts to do so in a reasonable manner.

As *Virginia* demonstrates, any government attempt, federal or state, to regulate advertising to protect consumers or protect competition must be weighed against the advertisers' and consumers' First Amendment rights.

© Stockbyte/Thinkstock

STUDY SCENARIO

Blevco Pharmacy and Dietco, the manufacturer of an OTC diet product, entered into a contract whereby in local promotional television ads, Dietco would tout Blevco as the place to purchase the product. In those ads, unknown to Blevco, Dietco engaged in false and misleading advertising. The FTC brought action against both Blevco and Dietco. Explain the liability or lack thereof of each party.

REFERENCES

U.S. Consumer Product Safety Commission website. Available at: http://www.cpsc.gov
U.S. Food and Drug Administration website. Available at: http://www.fda.gov

BIBLIOGRAPHY

Abood, R. Prescription Drug Marketing Act and the hospital pharmacy. *Pharmacy Management Adviser* 1, no. 6 (1994): 1–3, 10–11.
American Pharmacists Association. Legislative and Regulatory Updates. Available at: http://www.pharmacist.com
American Society for Pharmacy Law. Available at: http://www.aspl.org
Bloom, M. Z. Compounding in today's practice. *American Pharmacy* NS 31, no. 10 (October 1991): 31–37.
Crane, V. S. New perspectives on preventing medication errors and adverse drug events. *American Journal of Health-System Pharmacy* 57 (2000): 690–697.
Fink, J. L. Dispensing FDA-approved drugs for non-approved uses. *U.S. Pharmacist* 2 (1977): 24, 26. Reported in Drug Topics, April 3, 2006.
Food and Drug Administration. *An Introduction to FDA Drug Regulation: A Manual for Pharmacists.* Rockville, MD: U.S. Department of Health and Human Services, 1990.
Food and Drug Administration. *Approved Drug Products with Therapeutic Equivalence Evaluations.* Washington, DC: U.S. Government Printing Office, 1979 (annual updates).
Generic Drug Entry Prior to Patent Expiration, an FTC Study (July 2002). Available at: http://www.ftc.gov/os/2002/07/genericdrugstudy.pdf
Hutt, P. B. Investigations and reports respecting FDA regulation of new drugs: Parts 1 and 2. *Clinical Pharmacology and Therapeutics* 33 (1983): 537–548, 674–687.
Janssen, W. F. Pharmacy and the food and drug law. *American Pharmacy* NS 21 (1981): 212–221.
Knoben, J. E., et al. An overview of the FDA publication approved drug products with therapeutic equivalence evaluations. *American Journal of Hospital Pharmacy* 47 (1990): 2696–2700.
National Association of Boards of Pharmacy. *NABP Newsletter* 40 (2011): 76–77, 82. Available at: http://www.nabp.net/publications/assets/April11.pdf
National Community Pharmacists Association. *Governmental Affairs/Legal Proceedings.* Available at: http://www.ncpanet.org

Poole, B. W. Letter from Barry W. Poole, FDA Consumer Safety Officer. *Pharmacist Planning Service Newsletter* (Autumn 1991).

Valentino, J. Practical uses for the USP: A legal perspective. *American Journal of Pharmaceutical Education* 51 (1987): 80–81.

 CASE STUDIES

CASE 3-1   *Pharmaceutical Manufacturers Association v. Food and Drug Administration,* **484 F. Supp. 1179 (D. Del. 1980)**

Issue

Whether the FDA has the authority to promulgate a regulation requiring that patient information (patient package inserts [PPIs]) be provided to patients for whom estrogen-containing drugs are prescribed.

Overview

Package inserts are labeling directed at health care professionals. Historically, the FDCA had left it up to prescribers and dispensers to determine what written drug information should be provided to patients for prescription drugs. This policy changed somewhat in the mid-1970s, however, because the FDA believed that patient package inserts (termed "PPIs") should be mandated for certain prescription drugs, and enacted regulations to this effect. The regulations angered pharmacy organizations, which were primarily concerned about the logistics, the cost, and the effort of storing and distributing these PPIs. As you read this case, consider if PPIs are necessary to protect the health and safety of patients prescribed estrogen drugs. Is it an unjust governmental intrusion for the government to dictate to health care providers what information they should tell patients? On what basis does the FDA have the regulatory authority to require patient information? Should PPIs be required for all prescription drugs? Is there a need for uniformity in the written information provided to patients by pharmacists? How does the Medication Guide program differ from the PPI program? Should pharmacy be supportive of or opposed to the Medication Guide program, and why?

The court related the facts of the case as follows:

> In this case, plaintiffs, the Pharmaceutical Manufacturers Association, the American College of Obstetricians and Gynecologists, the National Association of Chain Drug Stores, Inc., Private Medical Care Foundation, and others challenge the validity of a regulation promulgated by the Food and Drug Administration which requires certain information to be provided to patients for whom drugs containing estrogens are prescribed.

> The agency's action came as a result of several studies published in 1975 that indicated an association between the use of conjugated estrogens and an increased risk of endometrial cancer in women.

The FDA published the rule in July 1977. Before the rule would take effect on September 20, 1977, however, the plaintiffs brought suit seeking a motion for a preliminary injunction. That motion rejected, they then filed this motion for a summary judgment.

> Plaintiffs and plaintiff-intervenors raise a number of challenges to the regulation. First, they contend that the FDA lacks statutory authority to require patient

packaging inserts for prescription drugs. They next assert that such a requirement is an unconstitutional interference with the practice of medicine. Finally, they challenge the adequacy of the FDA's findings and conclusions embodied in the preamble to the regulation and argue that, based on the administrative record, the regulation is "arbitrary, capricious, an abuse of discretion. . . ."

The court began its analysis by first noting that the FDA has broad rule-making authority under section 701(a) of the FDCA, and then took account of the relevant statutes.

Section 502 reads in pertinent part:

A drug or device shall be deemed to be misbranded

(a) If its labeling is false or misleading in any particular.

(f) Unless its labeling bears (1) adequate directions for use; and (2) such adequate warnings against use. . . .

Section 201, 21 U.S.C. § 321, the "Definition" section of the Act, describes the concept of "misleading" in the following terms:

(n) If an article is alleged to be misbranded because the labeling is misleading, then in determining whether the labeling is misleading there shall be taken into account (among other things) not only representations made or suggested by statement, word, design, device, or any combination thereof but also the extent to which the labeling fails to reveal facts material in the light of such representations or material with respect to consequences which may result from the use of the article. . . .

Reading the statutes together with the FDA's authority under section 701(a), the court felt there was sufficient support for the regulation on the basis of congressional intent that users of both prescription and nonprescription drugs should receive information material to the consequences of using the drug. The plaintiffs disagreed.

The plaintiffs acknowledge that Sections 201 and 502 may be read in this manner, but maintain that this reading is contrary to the legislative history of the 1938 Act and is specifically precluded by the enactment of the Durham-Humphrey Amendments to the Act in 1951.

Relying on the legislative history of the 1938 Act, the plaintiffs assert that Section 502(a) was never intended to apply to drugs dispensed on prescription. I find nothing in that legislative history to support this position. Indeed, all the evidence persuades me that the opposite is true. Despite a number of requests from representatives of the medical profession that prescription drugs be exempted from all labeling requirements, the final version of the Act provided an exemption only with respect to certain identified requirements. Section 503(b) exempted any drug dispensed on a written prescription from the labeling requirements of Section 502(b) (relating to quantity of contents) and 502(e) (relating to common names), and exempted prescription narcotics from the requirement that the label carry a warning that the drug may be habit forming, so long as the prescription was not refillable. It did not, however, exempt prescription drugs from the requirements of either 502(a) or 502(f), and both were understood to apply fully to all drug preparations.

The plaintiffs continued by arguing that section 503(b) of the Durham–Humphrey Amendment exempts prescription drugs from the "warnings against misuse" and "adequate directions for use" requirements of section 502 when the drugs are prescribed by physicians and dispensed and labeled pursuant to law. The court found this to be true and that it is the intent of 503(b) that physicians be the primary source of adequate directions for use and adequate warnings against misuse. However, continued the court, this does not mean that Congress meant to strip the commissioner of regulatory authority.

> Plaintiffs' argument glosses over the fact that while prescription drugs were exempted from the requirements of Section 502(f) in 1951, they were not exempted from the requirement of Section 502(a), that their labels not be misleading.

> Thus, while plaintiffs are correct in pointing out that the effect of the Section 503(b)(2) exemption as enacted in 1951 was to make the prescribing physician the primary source of information available to a consumer of a prescription drug, this does not mean that Congress intended to leave this matter to the unregulated discretion of the prescribing physician. The retention of Section 502(a) as a regulatory provision applicable to prescription drugs precludes one from attributing that intention to Congress. The long and short of the matter is that Congress intended patients using prescription drugs, as well as those using over-the-counter drugs, to receive "facts material with respect to consequences which may result from the use of the (drug) . . . under the conditions of use prescribed in the labeling or under such conditions of use as are customary and usual."

The court then addressed the plaintiffs' constitutional challenges. The plaintiffs first advanced that the practice of medicine is within the police powers of the state and not the federal government. The court quickly rejected this argument, however, finding that the federal government also has jurisdiction in this area as a reasonable exercise of the power vested in Congress by the Constitution.

The plaintiffs next argued that mandating PPIs unconstitutionally interferes with the practice of medicine and strips the physician of the right to exercise professional judgment.

> Turning to plaintiff's view of a physician's right to exercise professional judgment, it is important to focus on what the challenged regulation does not do. The regulation at issue here does not forbid a physician from prescribing conjugated estrogen drugs, or limit the physician's exercise of professional judgment in that regard. Nor does it limit the information the physician may impart to his or her patients concerning estrogens. If the physician disagrees with a perceived "slant" of the labeling provided by the manufacturer, or with the facts stated therein, he or she is free to discuss the matter fully with the patient, noting his own disagreement and views. The sample labeling encourages the patient to have this kind of open discussion with her doctor.

> When these limitations on the effect of the challenged regulation are considered, it becomes apparent that the plaintiffs urge recognition not of a right to exercise judgment in prescribing treatment, but rather of a right to control patient access to information. As I pointed out in my earlier Opinion, labeling is only one of many sources from which patients receive information about drugs, and the control which the plaintiffs claim to have possessed prior to the challenged regulation is largely illusory. But there is a more fundamental problem with their position. There simply is no constitutional basis for recognition of a right on the part of physicians to control patient access to information concerning the possible side effects of prescription drugs.

> By holding that physicians do not possess the constitutional right which plaintiffs claim, I do not overlook the affidavits of numerous experienced physicians who foresee patient anxiety and ruptured physician-patient relationships as a result of the implementation of the regulation. These matters are clearly relevant to an evaluation of the wisdom of the regulation. They do not, however, render it constitutionally infirm.

Dispensing with the constitutional issue, the court lastly turned its attention to the issue of whether the FDA provided a basis and purpose for the regulation as required by administrative law. The plaintiffs felt the regulation was promulgated arbitrarily and capriciously (an abuse of administrative discretion) because the regulation did not provide an exception for those situations in which the physician might want to withhold the information from the patient. The court replied that whether the regulation is arbitrary and capricious depends on whether the regulation was "based on a consideration of the relevant factors and whether there has been a clear error of judgment." The court then found that the agency had given considerable attention to whether to include the option.

> Given the purposes of the Act and its mislabeling provisions, the touchstone of any decision of the Commissioner is the safety and health of the patient. With this touchstone in mind, the primary factors to be weighed in deciding to grant or deny the option for which plaintiffs press are (1) the extent and character of the risk involved in using estrogen drugs, (2) the efficacy of, or the benefit to be derived from, providing patients with information concerning that risk, and (3) the extent and character of any risk involved in exposing all patients to that information. The Commissioner explains his views in each of these areas. First, it is apparent that he considers the risk associated with the use of estrogen drugs to be great, in terms of both the number of users and the gravity of the consequences to those who are adversely affected. Second, he explains that he finds this to be an area where patients are capable of understanding the advantages and risk of use and where most patients because of the nature of the condition for which the drug is prescribed, have a real option to use or not to use it. And, finally, on the other side of the balance, the Commissioner states that, unlike the situation with respect to some other drugs, he finds no likelihood of a substantial adverse effect on patients from exposure to the information provided by the labeling.

> If a patient decides to follow the instruction of her physician, the Commissioner does not believe that patient labeling will significantly increase the incidence of sugges-tion-induced side effects. Suggestion effects, moreover, seem to play a minimal role in determining serious adverse reactions. It is, in any event, possible to hypothesize beneficial as well as negative effects of suggestion. Clear expectations about the effects of drug therapy, reinforced by patient labeling, may make patients more sen-sitive and aware of certain physical or psychological reactions. Effects which might otherwise go unnoticed may be identified as drug related. Although this may have the effect of nominally increasing the reported incidence of less serious adverse reaction, it also may have beneficial results. Patients may be more sensitive to "warning sig-nals" of serious adverse effect. . . . It is the Commissioner's opinion that the possible positive effects of supplying accurate side-effect information outweigh the possible negative effects.

> While reasonable minds might reach different conclusions, this explanation of the Commissioner's reasoning is sufficient to demonstrate that the challenged regulation is the product of a rational process.

The court granted the FDA's motion for summary judgment finding that the FDA does have statutory authority to require patient labeling, that the regulation does not interfere with any constitutionally protected rights of physicians, and that the agency's reasoning is sufficiently articulated and supported.

Notes on *Pharmaceutical Manufacturers Association v. Food and Drug Administration*

1. The plaintiffs attempted to distort the intent of the Durham–Humphrey Amendment, which in part exempts prescription drugs from section 502. If not for the amendment, pharmacists would have to label every drug dispensed in conformance with all the requirements of section 502—not a practical proposition. The amendment recognizes that prescription drugs cannot be

labeled with adequate directions for use, thus requiring the guidance of health care professionals. Its intent is not to provide health care professionals with total discretion to control patient information. The plaintiffs also adopted an extremely paternalistic position by arguing that only they are qualified to determine what information should be provided to patients. In fact, taking this position and denying the government's right to require patient information is contrary to the ethical and legal principle that patients have a right to be informed. Moreover, the fact that the physicians asserted they have a constitutional right to practice medicine without government interference of their professional judgment completely overstates their role. If anything, it is the patient who may really have a constitutional right to receive drug information.

2. The FDA had proposed in the 1970s to make PPIs mandatory for several drugs, but because of tremendous opposition, dropped this plan. The agency made no further directives regarding patient information until the Medication Guide program was proposed. Somewhat surprisingly, the MedGuide program also faced vigorous opposition by health care professionals, even in a present climate in which patients are demanding drug information. The agency's interest in the MedGuide program also was somewhat surprising considering the passage of OBRA '90 and the offer to counsel requirement. However, OBRA '90 does not mandate that patients receive written information about their drugs, and the agency was obviously dissatisfied with the information health care providers were providing patients. One problem with the written information distributed by pharmacies is a lack of standardization, a problem the FDA would like to rectify.

3. Many pharmacies now routinely provide patients with some type of written information. In fact, one can make a strong case that providing written information constitutes the legal standard of care. In a lawsuit by a patient alleging that the pharmacist had a legal duty to warn of the adverse effect suffered by the patient, providing written information that contains the warning would mitigate the probability of the pharmacist being found negligent.

CASE 3-2   *Ramon v. Farr*, 770 P.2d 131 (Utah 1989)

Issue

Whether the package insert constitutes prima facie evidence of the standard of care.

Overview

It is not uncommon for health care practitioners to prescribe and dispense medications for off-label uses or dosages. As discussed earlier, it is not a violation of federal or state law to do so. However, deviating from a drug's labeling can present civil liability concerns in the event of a bad outcome. As you read this case, consider why it is that many drugs have off-label uses. What role does the product's labeling play in determining liability? Should patients be informed that the drug is being prescribed for an off-label use? Does the health care provider face a greater risk of liability when deviating from the labeling? If so, how can that risk of liability be minimized?

The court first described the facts of the case, which can be summarized as follows. Dr. Boyd Farr, who was the attending physician for Alicia Ramon during the delivery of her baby, performed a cervical block by injecting Ramon in the cervical region with Marcaine approximately 1 hour before the birth.

At birth, Jaime appeared to be a normal, healthy child, but he began to show symptoms of serious problems several hours later. He was transferred to an intensive care unit and later suffered grand mal seizures. The parties agree that Jaime has serious permanent physical and mental defects and can never be expected to reach normal ranges of mental or physical development.

Ramon and her husband sued the hospital and Dr. Farr on behalf of their son, and the hospital settled out of court. The trial court, finding for Dr. Farr, refused to give the jury the instructions requested by the Ramons that would have made the manufacturer's package insert prima facie evidence of the applicable standard of care. The Ramons appealed, claiming that the trial court erred in refusing to give the jury the instructions.

The Ramons' first claim arises from the trial court's refusal to submit their second theory to the jury. That theory apparently was that the mere injection of the mother and not the child with Marcaine was negligent and caused Jaime's condition. The trial court refused to give a proposed jury instruction pertinent to that theory. The instruction stated that the use of Marcaine for a paracervical block when that use was not recommended by the manufacturer is prima facie evidence of negligence. Both the package insert that was shipped with the Marcaine and the 1980 (34th ed.) *Physician's Desk Reference* ("PDR") at page 695 read: "Until further clinical experience is gained, paracervical block with Marcaine is not recommended." The Ramons claim that the trial court erred in rejecting the proposed instruction.

The appellate court found that the trial court was justified in its determination because the Ramons failed to present sufficient evidence that the Marcaine caused the injury. The court went on to note:

But even if there were sufficient evidence of causation to submit the Ramons' second theory to the jury, we have another reason for upholding the trial court's refusal to give the proposed instruction: we decline to adopt the legal rule that it states. The Ramons observe that the Utah courts have not settled the question of the legal effect to be given recommendations that are issued by drug manufacturers in the form of package inserts and PDR entries. They argue that we should follow the rule that the insert constitutes prima facie evidence of the applicable standard of care. In other words, they ask us to hold that the mere introduction in evidence of an insert or PDR entry shifts the burden of proof on the standard of care to the defendant physician.

In response, Dr. Farr first observes that the insert language at issue did not contraindicate the use of Marcaine for paracervical blocks, but simply stated that the manufacturer was not recommending the use of the drug without further testing. He urges us to hold that the package insert is only some evidence that the jury can take into account in determining the standard of care and that the plaintiff in a medical malpractice action usually bears the burden of introducing evidence on the standard of care in the form of expert testimony. In support of this position, Dr. Farr argues that the decision to use a particular drug is always a matter of judgment for the physician based on all information available, including medical journals, advice from colleagues, professional experience, and the information provided by manufacturers. He contends that it would be unrealistic to straitjacket a physician's treatment choices with package inserts.

The court continued by recognizing that decisions differ on whether the package insert should be prima facie evidence of the standard of care.

One line of authority relied on by the Ramons is represented by *Mulder v. Parke Davis & Co.*, 288 Minn. 332, 181 N.W.2d 882 (1970). In *Mulder*, the Minnesota Supreme Court held that when a drug manufacturer provides recommendations concerning the administration and proper dosage of a prescription drug and also warns of the dangers inherent in its use, a physician's "deviation from such recommendations is prima facie evidence of negligence if there is competent medical testimony that his patient's injury or death resulted from the doctor's failure to adhere to the recommendations." *Mulder* has been followed by the courts of only a few other states. And the Minnesota courts have since retreated somewhat from the *Mulder* standard. Minnesota presently requires a *Mulder* prima facie negligence instruction only when the manufacturer's instructions contain a clear and explicit warning against the type of use that is alleged and a deviation from that recommendation caused the injury. In the present case, the manufacturer did not make such a clear and explicit recommendation against the use of Marcaine for a paracervical block. Rather, it simply did not recommend its use until further studies were performed. Thus, even under the current Minnesota rule, the Ramons would not be entitled to their proposed jury instruction.

In any event, we decline to follow the *Mulder* rule, either as originally articulated or in its current incarnation. Rather, we think the better rule is that manufacturers' inserts and parallel PDR entries do not by themselves set the standard of care, even as a prima facie matter. A manufacturer's recommendations are, however, some evidence that the finder of fact may consider along with expert testimony on the standard of care.

The court noted that this is the favored approach of most other jurisdictions as well.

Although package inserts may provide useful information, they are not designed to establish a standard of medical practice, and their conflicting purposes make it extremely unlikely that they could be so designed. We therefore conclude that the trial court acted properly in refusing to give the Ramons' requested jury instruction on the effect of the insert. The judgment was affirmed.

Notes on *Ramon v. Farr*

1. Manufacturers often market a drug product with a minimum number of indications in order to get the product marketed as quickly as possible. Subsequently they will obtain approval for additional indications. Moreover, for liability reasons, manufacturers actually may tend to over-warn in some instances. Therefore, prescribers often prescribe drugs for off-label uses or dosages, or contrary to warnings in the labeling, when their professional judgment warrants.

2. *Ramon* represents how most courts would determine the role of the package insert in determining a legal standard of care. In *Morlino v. Medical Center of Ocean County*, a physician prescribed ciprofloxacin for an infection in a pregnant woman even though the package insert warned against the use in pregnant women. The plaintiff alleged that the ciprofloxacin caused the death of her fetus. The physician knew the risk, but determined that the benefit of prescribing ciprofloxacin outweighed the risk in this case. Finding for the physician, the court ruled that the package insert can be admitted into evidence to show the standard of care as long as expert testimony is presented to explain the standard to the jury.

3. The real issue for a pharmacist confronted with a prescription for a drug prescribed for an unlabeled use or dosage is to exercise professional judgment. This means researching the issue to determine if there is a risk of harm to the patient and just how likely and how great that harm might be. The next step is to contact the prescriber to determine first whether the prescriber intended the drug to be used in the manner prescribed and second to apprise the prescriber of the risks as determined from the research. If the risk to the patient is likely and/or potentially of great magnitude, the pharmacist should ask the

prescriber to justify his or her decision to use the drug in the manner prescribed (e.g., by reference to referred articles in scientific journals). If the use cannot be justified, or if the risk to the patient just appears too great, the pharmacist may decide to not dispense the drug. If, on the other hand, after researching the issue and discussing the issue with the prescriber, the benefit appears to outweigh the risk, the pharmacist then should dispense the drug but only after counseling the patient about the benefits and risks. At this point, the patient might decide not to take the drug. Finally, the pharmacist must document his or her intervention.

CASE 3-3	*Pfizer, Inc. v. Shalala*, 1 F. Supp. 2d 38 (D.C. 1998)

Issue

Is a generic drug with a different sustained-release system from the parent drug a generic equivalent to the parent drug?

Overview

The Patent Term Restoration Act facilitated the marketing of generic drugs by allowing generic drug sponsors to file ANDAs rather than NDAs. This case provides additional insight into the procedures followed by the FDA to determine if a product is similar enough to the parent drug such that the sponsor may file an ANDA. The plaintiff, Pfizer, contends that the products are not similar enough and of course has the ulterior motive of restraining competition. At issue in this case is whether two drug products can be considered generically equivalent if the manner in which they release the active ingredient is substantially different. This is a controversial issue with drug manufacturers because dosage-form technology has advanced tremendously in the past few years. As you read this case ask yourself, is the FDA's position correct? The FDA is essentially saying, the means in which the generic product releases the active ingredient in the body is irrelevant, as long as the generic drug product establishes bioequivalence to the parent. In other words, the end is more important than the means. Is there a public health problem with this interpretation? Also, consider what the effect on generic competition would be if Pfizer's position is correct. Would companies just continually redesign the dosage forms of their products to subvert competition? Finally, if Pfizer's position is rejected, what effect will this have on the science of dosage-form design? Will companies have any market incentive to expend money on innovative dosage-form technology if competitor products without the technology are deemed generically equivalent?

The court first provided the facts of the case.

The FDA accepted an abbreviated new drug application (ANDA) from Mylan Pharmaceuticals for a generic version of a sustained-release nifedipine tablet. Pfizer is the company that first developed the nongeneric or pioneer version of this drug. Plaintiff Pfizer, Inc., brought this summary judgment action to convince the court to order the FDA to reject Mylan's ANDA on the basis that Mylan's drug does not have the same type of extended-release system as its drug and thus is not an identical dosage form.

> Pfizer's pioneer drug, Procardia XL, is a controlled release drug in which the full dose of the active ingredient in the drug, nifedipine, is released slowly, over time. There are several mechanisms used in controlled release oral drugs in order to regulate the release of a drug's active ingredients. Procardia XL uses a patented oral osmotic pump release mechanism to release the nifedipine it contains. Osmotic release systems

function by slowly releasing the drug's active ingredients from a shell; a pump or push component inside the shell swells when gastrointestinal fluid enters the shell to expel the active ingredient. Procardia XL's osmotic pump device is covered by four patents, and the size of the nifedipine crystals used in the drug is also patented. (Unlike Procardia XL, Mylan's nifedipine product is a "conventionally-pressed" tablet that uses an extended-release system other than an osmotic pump to release its active ingredients.)

The court then proceeded to examine the relevant statutes and regulations applicable to the NDA process, noting that Congress passed the Drug Price Competition and Patent Term Restoration Act of 1984 to provide for an expedited review process (the ANDA). The court noted that under the FDCA and FDA regulations, the ANDA procedure is only available after the FDA makes a "threshold determination that the ANDA is sufficiently complete to permit a substantive review." Substantive review will only occur if, on its face, the ANDA indicates that the generic drug's active ingredients, route of administration, dosage form, and strength are the same as the pioneer drug. If a generic drug is similar, but not identical to, the pioneer drug on those factors, the applicant must first file a "suitability petition" to allow the FDA to assess the differences. If approved, the applicant may then file an ANDA.

If the FDA accepts an ANDA as being properly filed, either because it is sufficiently complete on its face or because a suitability petition has been approved, the FDA then proceeds to the substantive review stage. During the substantive review stage, the FDA goes beyond its preliminary threshold determination and this time thoroughly reviews the sufficiency of the ANDA's information. The applicant must show, interalia, that the generic product (1) has the same active ingredients, route of administration, dosage form and strength as the pioneer drug, (2) is bioequivalent to the pioneer drug, and (3) is safe under the conditions prescribed, or, in the case of an ANDA that has been filed subsequent to the approval of a suitability petition, the ANDA must contain sufficient information about the particular aspect of the drug that is different from the pioneer drug.

If the FDA finds that the information in the ANDA is sufficient under the FDCA and FDA regulations, it will approve the ANDA and issue a notice that the generic imitation is therapeutically equivalent to the reference listed drug.

If the FDA decides at any point that a proposed generic product varies from the pioneer drug in any of the four statutory categories (active ingredients, rate of administration, dosage form, or strength), it must conclude that the generic drug is only a "pharmaceutical alternative," not a "pharmaceutical equivalent" (21 C.F.R. § 320.1(c) and (d)). This is a great disadvantage to a generic product manufacturer because many state laws require a generic product to be pharmaceutically equivalent to the pioneer drug before it may be substituted for the pioneer drug. It is important to note that any drug manufacturer that seeks approval of a suitability petition before filing an ANDA is relinquishing the "pharmaceutical equivalence" label for its proposed generic product. Generic drugs that are approved through the suitability petition process can only meet the definition of a "pharmaceutical alternative" because the very filing of a suitability petition is an admission that the drug's active ingredients, route of administration, dosage form, or strength is different from that of the pioneer drug.

After reviewing the regulatory framework, the court then focused on the issue of whether the FDA acted properly in accepting Mylan's ANDA on the basis that the generic drug had the same dosage form as Procardia XL. Pfizer contended that the dosage forms of the drugs cannot be the same because they have different release systems. The FDA, however, argued that for the purpose of accepting an ANDA application, the fact that each drug is an extended-release tablet makes them have the same dosage form. Stated the FDA:

> The 74 dosage form descriptions, including the descriptions "extended-release tablet" and "extended-release capsule," that are currently listed in the Orange Book have effectively served the public, the Agency, and the industry. The categories are useful in that they are sufficiently differentiated to make a reasonable distinction based on dosage form, which includes the appearance of the drug. However, the categories are also useful in that they are not so narrow as to be virtually product-specific. As a result, these categories have allowed the FDA to make threshold determinations that products have the same dosage form while encouraging manufacturers to develop innovative release technologies and allowing the public the benefit of safe and effective generic drug products.

The court agreed that the FDA's view is reasonable and not inconsistent with the FDCA. The court stated that when a statute fails to define a relevant term, such as dosage form, its role is to determine whether the FDA's definition is a permissible construction, rational, and consistent with the statute. Taking issue with Pfizer's contention that the FDA's decision that extended-release dosage forms can be properly categorized on the basis of appearance and route of administration rather than on the basis of the drug's release or delivery mechanism is irrational and outmoded, the court remarked:

> The FDA has offered a more than rational explanation for interpreting "dosage form" the way it has for so many years and for maintaining its current dosage form classification system. Although neither the Congress in the FDCA nor the FDA itself in its regulations has specifically defined the term "dosage form," the manner in which the FDA defines dosage form and applies its definition is rational. It is governed primarily by a list of 74 dosage forms set forth in Appendix C of the FDA's Approved Drug Product with Therapeutic Equivalence Evaluation, 17th ed., commonly known as the "Orange Book." The FDA admits that while this list is not binding on it or on the pharmaceutical industry, it does serve as informal guidance to a generic company on what is considered to be the "same" or "identical" dosage form.
>
> Under the current system, if two drugs fall into the same dosage form in the Orange Book, such as "extended-release tablet," the FDA makes a threshold determination that their dosage forms are the "same" and, all other information being sufficient, it will then accept a generic drug company's ANDA as being filed. In this case, the FDA has preliminarily decided that Mylan's ANDA contained enough information to enable the FDA to make a threshold determination that the dosage form of Mylan's drug (among other things) is the "same" dosage form as Procardia XL, an extended-release tablet.
>
> Under the current FDA regime, an ANDA sponsor therefore may submit an ANDA for a generic drug that has the same active ingredients, route of administration, strength, and dosage form as the pioneer drug but a different formulation and, thus, a different release mechanism as the pioneer drug. In fact, under FDA regulations, the definition of "pharmaceutical equivalents" is "drug products that contain identical amounts of the identical active drug ingredient . . . in identical dosage forms, but not necessarily containing the same inactive ingredients." This makes sense. If, for instance, a generic tablet that does not use the osmotic pump can perform the same extended release functions as Procardia XL, and can perform them safely, then it is logical that the generic drug would be approved as a generic equivalent of Procardia XL. What else would a generic drug be?
>
> Despite plaintiff's claims to the contrary, there is nothing in the Federal Food, Drug, and Cosmetic Act to indicate that Congress intended the FDA to develop a dosage form classification system based on a drug's release mechanism. When Congress

passed the Waxman-Hatch Amendments, the FDA already had an abbreviated drug application procedure in place that utilized a dosage form classification system that was not based on release mechanism differences. Congress' choice not to address or revisit the ongoing FDA system of classifying dosage forms strongly suggests both that it was aware of the system and that it did not intend to change it. Indeed, in light of the principal objectives of the Waxman-Hatch Amendments, this Court sees no reason why Congress would want to change the FDA's interpretation of dosage form or the application of that interpretation.

The court denied Pfizer's claim and awarded summary judgment for the FDA.

Notes on *Pfizer, Inc. v. Shalala*

1. To support his decision, the judge concluded that the purpose of the Waxman-Hatch Amendments, to make more low-cost generic drugs available, would be defeated if Pfizer prevailed. He called Pfizer's interpretation of the law "transparently self-serving," in that such an interpretation would suppress generic competition for years.

2. It is important to realize that this decision does not hold that Mylan's product has the same dosage form as Pfizer's. Rather, the court has ruled that the FDA's interpretation of the drug dosage form classification system is reasonable and permissible. In fact, at the time of this trial, the FDA had only accepted Mylan's ANDA for filing and had not even considered the merits of the ANDA yet. It is conceivable that the FDA, in the process of reviewing the ANDA, could yet find that the two products are indeed not identical dosage forms. The court recognized this and refused to allow Pfizer to challenge the FDA's acceptance of the ANDA on the basis of ripeness. In other words, courts will not permit judicial review before an agency makes a final determination and until the plaintiff has exhausted all remedies within the administrative agency. If Pfizer had prevailed in this case, Mylan would have been forced to submit a suitability petition, which would have precluded their product from ever being approved as a pharmaceutical equivalent.

3. It is important financially to innovator drug manufacturers that generic drug competitors not be "A" rated to their product. In this situation, the manufacturer can actively market to health care providers that their product should not be substituted. In addition, many state laws prohibit the interchange of drugs that are not bioequivalent without specific authorization from the prescriber.

CASE 3-4   *Winn Dixie of Montgomery, Inc. v. Colburn*, 709 So.2d 1222 (Ala. 1998)

Issue

Whether the damage award to a plaintiff injured as a result of a pharmacist substituting a drug that was not generically equivalent to the drug prescribed was appropriate.

Overview

Even though this case is not an FDCA case and is really about damages, it highlights important issues under the FDCA, including substitution without authorization and the issue of generic and therapeutic substitution. In this case, the pharmacist substituted what he thought was a generic equivalent to the drug prescribed, even though the prescriber refused to authorize substitution. The substituted drug was not a generic equivalent and the patient sustained harm. This case demonstrates the importance of making certain that the products are generic equivalents, but it also raises the broader issue of when might substitution present a greater risk of harm to the patient, and thus a greater risk of liability for the pharmacist. As you read this case, consider these issues: Does your state allow substitution without prescriber authorization? Can a pharmacist substitute if a patient requests but the physician refuses authorization? Should a pharmacist be able to rely on software? Are there any types of drugs in which generic substitution might cause harm to a patient and thus increase legal risk? What is the difference between generic substitution and therapeutic substitution? Does therapeutic substitution present a greater risk?

The court stated the facts of the case as follows:

> Mary Catherine Colburn sued Winn Dixie of Montgomery, Inc., and Robert Hagan, alleging that they were negligent or wanton in filling a prescription for her. Specifically, Colburn claimed that Robert Hagan, the pharmacist at a store operated by Winn Dixie of Montgomery, wantonly or negligently dispensed Fiorinal No. 3 as a substitute medication for a prescription of Sedapap. The jury returned a general verdict for Colburn and against Winn Dixie and Hagan, awarding damages of $130,000. The trial court entered a judgment on that verdict.

> Winn Dixie and Hagan claim that the judgment should be reversed because the evidence was insufficient to support the damages award. They also argue that the judgment is excessive.

> Viewed in the light most favorable to Colburn, the evidence suggests the following: Colburn consulted Dr. Mildred Howell, complaining of migraine headaches. Dr. Howell, knowing that Colburn was allergic to codeine, prescribed Sedapap, which does not contain codeine, to treat Colburn's migraine headaches. Dr. Howell signed the prescription form over a line that stated "product selection permitted"; that statement means that a generic equivalent could be substituted for the name-brand product. Colburn took her prescription to a pharmacy at a Winn Dixie supermarket to have it filled. The Winn Dixie pharmacy did not have Sedapap in stock. Hagan testified at trial that he looked up Sedapap on the Winn Dixie computer drug profile, and that it reported that Sedapap and Fiorinal No. 3 were identical. However, Fiorinal No. 3, which was substituted for Sedapap, is not a generic equivalent to Sedapap; in fact, it contains codeine, the very thing to which Colburn was allergic. In his prescription-error report, Hagan wrote that he had substituted the Fiorinal No. 3 because it was the "closest formula" to Sedapap and he felt certain that the physician would allow the substitution. In addition, at trial Colburn presented evidence indicating that Hagan telephoned Dr. Howell to ask if he could substitute Fiorinal No. 3 for Sedapap, and that Dr. Howell had her assistant tell him that it could not be substituted.

After taking the medication, Colburn went into anaphylactic shock and was rushed to the hospital emergency room, nearly dying on the way. After treatment, she returned home that night but continued to feel the side effects, including a severe headache that lasted several days. She presented evidence indicating that but for her husband's swift reaction, she likely would have died of anaphylactic shock. She testified that she is still afraid to take prescription drugs.

> Winn Dixie and Hagan contend that because Colburn suffered no permanent physical injury the $130,000 award is out of proportion to her injury. Winn Dixie and Hagan do not address the propriety of the jury's finding of liability. They simply argue that the amount of the award bears no reasonable relationship to the harm suffered by the plaintiff. However, Winn Dixie and Hagan consented to the jury's use of a general verdict form that did not delineate separate amounts of compensatory damages and

punitive damages. Therefore, this Court has no way to determine what portion of the award was intended as punitive damages. In fact, the jury may have intended the entire amount to be compensatory damages.

In fairness to Winn Dixie and Hagan, however, the court decided to consider that part of the $130,000 was punitive in nature and then proceeded to apply the three "guideposts" articulated by the U.S. Supreme Court in BMW of *North America, Inc. v. Gore*, to determine whether the punitive award was excessive.

The first "guidepost" is the reprehensibility of the defendant's conduct. In BMW, the Supreme Court indicated that "indifference to or reckless disregard for the health and safety of others" is an aggravating factor associated with particularly reprehensible conduct. Clearly, this aggravating factor was present in this case. There was evidence that Hagan telephoned Colburn's physician to ask if he could substitute Fiorinal No. 3 for Sedapap and that the physician had her assistant tell him that it could not be substituted. Thus, the jury could have found that the pharmacist received specific instructions from the physician not to substitute the medication but did so anyway; thus, the jury could have found that Hagan acted with a reckless disregard for Colburn's safety. Further, the Winn Dixie computer drug profile erroneously reported that Sedapap and Fiorinal No. 3 were identical; and the evidence indicates that, even once the error was discovered, Winn Dixie did not correct the information in the computer, thereby increasing the risk of further harm to its customers. This evidence supports a finding of reprehensibility on the part of Hagan and Winn Dixie that would warrant a large punitive damages award.

The second BMW guidepost for determining whether an award of punitive damages is excessive is the ratio of punitive damages to the actual harm inflicted upon the plaintiff. Because the jury awarded general damages, we cannot determine with certainty the ratio of punitive damages to compensatory damages. It is important to note that we do not consider that any compensatory award was based solely on economic loss; rather, we consider it to be based largely upon the obvious mental and emotional distress that Colburn endured because of her life-threatening experience. We conclude that it was well within the right of the jury to award Colburn $130,000 because she experienced the natural terror associated with what she believed to be imminent death.

Finally, the last guidepost BMW gives for determining whether a punitive damages award was excessive is a comparison of the punitive award to the civil or criminal penalties that could be imposed for similar misconduct. In this present case, the maximum penalty under Alabama law for dispensing a different drug or different brand drug in lieu of that ordered or prescribed, without the express permission of the person ordering or prescribing the drug, is a $1,000 fine (Ala. Code 1975, 34-23-8). We must point out that the dispensing of prescription drugs is a matter of public trust and that one who dispenses them carelessly endangers the health and safety of the consumer. A $1,000 fine is a meager sanction for such a serious offense and provides little basis for determining a meaningful punitive damages award.

We affirm that portion of the judgment imposing liability. However, we remand this case for the trial court to make written findings on the issue of excessiveness of the punitive damages award, if, indeed, it determines that any of the award was punitive in nature.

Notes on *Winn Dixie of Montgomery, Inc. v. Colburn*

1. Although the drug substitution laws do vary from state to state, certain aspects do not. Pharmacists may not legally substitute when prescribers specifically

prohibit substitution, and pharmacists may not legally substitute unless the drugs are generically equivalent. The pharmacist did not make a generic substitution but a therapeutic substitution. The products are in the same therapeutic class but are not generically equivalent. For the most part, therapeutic substitution by a pharmacist without specific authorization from the prescriber is illegal. The pharmacist in this case intentionally violated the law, permitting a jury to conclude that the pharmacist's behavior was more than just negligent, but reprehensible, leading to punitive or punishment damages. Pharmacists who violate laws, even unintentionally, run a significantly greater risk of being found liable in a negligence case. Pharmacists who violate laws intentionally risk punitive damages as well.

2. The pharmacist relied on software in this case, but it is unlikely that a court would ever find that a pharmacist can forgo professional judgment on the basis of relying on software. Software is only a tool to help pharmacists, not a replacement for judgment.

3. In most cases, generic substitution would not present any patient risk. Some generics, however, might present patient risk such as drugs with B ratings in the Orange Book and pre-1938 drugs where there is not sufficient evidence of bioequivalence. Some contend that even narrow therapeutic index drugs with A ratings are risky to substitute. Pharmacists should not switch patients stabilized on one generically equivalent drug with another unless the products are bioequivalent. If a substitution among nonbioequivalent drug products is necessary, the prescriber should be contacted to authorize the substitution (this would be the law in many states), and the patient must be counseled.

CASE 3-5   *Kennedy v. Kentucky Board of Pharmacy*, 799 S.W.2d 58 (Ky. App. 1990)

Issue

Whether a pharmacist who resells drugs from the hospital pharmacy inventory to a wholesaler is a wholesaler and whether by doing so has engaged in unprofessional conduct.

Overview

In this case, a hospital pharmacist regularly resold his excess inventory to a drug wholesaler. Although the Prescription Drug Marketing Act (PDMA) was not an issue in this case, perhaps it should have been. The PDMA was passed in 1987 in part to prevent hospitals from reselling prescription drugs that they purchased at preferred prices. Some organizations and individuals made considerable profits engaging in this secondary market and in the process jeopardized public health and safety by selling adulterated and misbranded drugs. As you read this case, consider whether this is the type of situation the PDMA meant to prohibit. Does it matter under the PDMA whether the pharmacist or the pharmacy profited or not from the resales? What might the outcome have been under the PDMA? Consider the two charges made by the board of pharmacy against the pharmacist. What evidence would the board have to bring to win on those two charges—or could the board win?

The court narrated the facts of this case as follows:

John Kennedy appealed from the judgment of the Clay Circuit Court which affirmed the decision of the appellee, Kentucky Board of Pharmacy, to suspend his license for

1 year and which imposed a $4,000 fine. The board found that Kennedy, a licensed pharmacist, violated KRS 315.036(1) and 315.036(2), and engaged in unethical conduct as contemplated by KRS 315.121(1)(f). We agree with Kennedy that the board erred as a matter of law, necessitating reversal of its findings and conclusions.

The facts are well known to the parties and need not be set out at length in this opinion. Briefly, Kennedy has been a licensed pharmacist for many years and had a permit from the board to operate the Red Bird Hospital Pharmacy. Four times a year Kennedy gathered up his excess drugs [and sold them to a drug wholesaler, Elite Supply Company]. Included in these sales were birth control pills, the invoices for which were stamped by the manufacturer, Wyeth Laboratories, "For clinic use only. This specifically priced merchandise is not intended for resale or distribution outside the clinic."

The court then noted the relevant statutes that included KRS 315.010(6), (7), (10), and (12):

(6) "Manufacturer" means any person, except a pharmacist, within the Commonwealth engaged in the commercial production, preparation, propagation, compounding, conversion, or processing of a drug, either directly or indirectly, by extraction from substances of natural origin or independently by means of chemical synthesis, or both, and includes any packaging or repackaging of a drug or the labeling or relabeling of its container.

(7) "Pharmacist" means a natural person licensed by this state to engage in the practice of the profession of pharmacy.

(10) "Practice of pharmacy" means a health service which includes the dispensing, storage, and instruction as to the proper use of drugs, including radioactive substances, and related devices, the maintenance and management of health and the encouragement of safety and efficacy in those activities.

(12) "Wholesaler" means any person, except a pharmacist, within the Commonwealth who legally buys drugs for resale and distribution to persons other than patients or consumers.

The two statutory provisions that Kennedy was found to have violated were 315.036(1) and (2), which require that manufacturers and wholesalers register with the board, obtain a permit and pay a fee, and maintain adequate records of all drugs manufactured, received, and sold.

The court then proceeded with its analysis of the case.

Kennedy's argument, with which we agree, is that the board erred in disciplining him under the statutes pertaining to manufacturers and wholesalers as, by definition, he is neither a manufacturer nor wholesaler. In clear, plain terms the definitions previously set forth specifically exclude a pharmacist from the category consisting of manufacturers and wholesalers. The board argues, and the circuit court agreed, that Kennedy is not entitled to be excluded from the category of a manufacturer or wholesaler when acting as a pharmacist as defined in KRS 315.010(10). We are not persuaded the argument supports the board's decision for two reasons. First, it seems quite reasonable to us that selling excess drugs before they become stale or expire is conduct that would fall within the definition of the "practice of pharmacy." At least there was no evidence to the contrary. Secondly, there are other statutory provisions in the chapter applicable to pharmacists, specifically KRS 315.035 and KRS 315.121, which permit the board to set standards of conduct and to regulate the practice of pharmacy. If Kennedy's conduct in selling excess prescription drugs offended any statute or regulation pertaining to pharmacists, the board has yet to so allege.

It is basic that in construing a statute the courts must examine and give effect to each word, clause or sentence that allows for reasonableness. We must assume the legislature had a purpose for differentiating between "pharmacists" and "wholesalers." To ignore the difference, as did the board, does violence to the well-established principle that words specifically defined by statute "must be given the meaning prescribed by the legislature in construing the statute." Thus we conclude the board erred as a matter of law in disciplining Kennedy for his failure to get a wholesaler's license.

We also agree with Kennedy that the board erred in concluding that his conduct was "unethical or unprofessional" and of a "character likely to deceive, defraud or harm the public." This charge was predicated on the resale of the birth control pills originally obtained from Wyeth Laboratories under invoices indicating the medication was not intended for resale.

Kennedy's claim in this regard is that the statute is unconstitutionally vague. However, we need not reach that issue as there is simply no evidence in support of the board's finding that the public was being, or was likely to be, deceived, defrauded or harmed. Kennedy's explanation for the resale of the birth control pills was that he was required to purchase larger quantities than the Red Bird Pharmacy could handle in order to get a price his customers could afford to pay. The board offered no evidence whatsoever contradicting Kennedy's motives. There is not the slightest evidence that Kennedy personally benefited, financially or otherwise, from these transactions.

Conceivably Kennedy was defrauding Wyeth Laboratories (although the record before the board does not establish the elements of fraud), or perhaps his conduct constituted a breach of his contract with that firm. But Wyeth did not participate in the hearing. As far as we know, Wyeth has never lodged any complaint against Kennedy before any tribunal, administrative or judicial. In any event Kennedy's actions vis a vis Wyeth did not amount to unprofessional conduct as contemplated by the legislature in KRS 315.121(1)(f). Never was the conduct of reselling the birth control pills to another drug company shown to deceive, defraud or harm the public. Such a showing is essential, we believe, to any charge of unprofessional conduct, again by reference to the plain words of the statute.

The court reversed the circuit court's decision and remanded the case back to the board of pharmacy for dismissal of the charges.

Notes on *Kennedy v. Kentucky Board of Pharmacy*

1. The PDMA prohibits the resale of prescription drugs by hospitals except under specified circumstances. It would appear that Kennedy violated the PDMA because reselling to a wholesaler is not one of the specified exceptions. Drug returns are not considered a sale or trade for the purpose of the PDMA, but Kennedy was not engaging in product returns. Although Kennedy appeared to be acting with no intent to profit from the resale, the PDMA does not include profit as a criterion. The PDMA was enacted to invalidate this type of situation and prevent a secondary distribution market. As this case demonstrates, state law was inadequate, and Kennedy may have been fortunate that the FDA did not bring the action.

2. Notice that the state law provides that a wholesaler is any person except a pharmacist. Could a pharmacist thus ever be considered a wholesaler under Kentucky law? Moreover, the statute says a wholesaler is a person who buys the drugs for resale. Was Kennedy buying the drugs originally for resale? He admitted that he

purchased more product than necessary in order to get the best price. What else could he do with the excess other than resell? State boards have historically used unprofessional conduct charges as a catchall for acts that the board deems offensive but that the law does not specifically prohibit.

3. In Kennedy's defense, the PDMA was intended to prevent drug diversion because of fear of adulterated and misbranded products and unfair competition. None of these problems would seem to be outcomes from Kennedy's resale. However, violation of the PDMA does not require proof of injury or bad consequences.

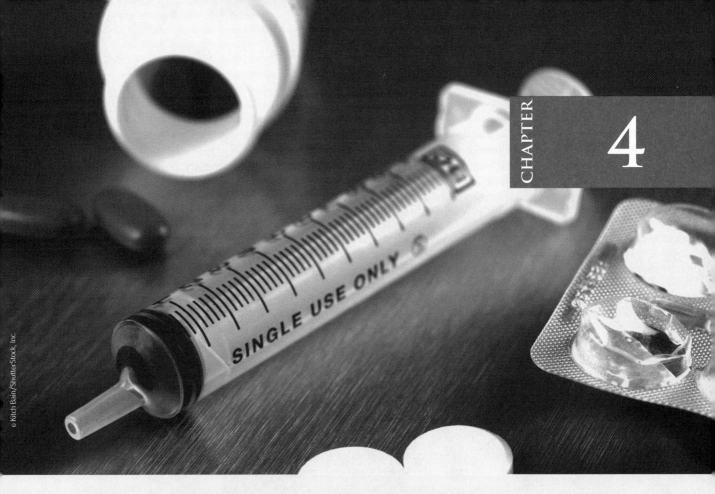

THE CLOSED SYSTEM OF CONTROLLED SUBSTANCE DISTRIBUTION

CHAPTER OBJECTIVES

Upon completing this chapter, the reader will be able to:

▸ Distinguish the five schedules of controlled substances.

▸ Understand which activities require registration with the Drug Enforcement Administration (DEA).

▸ Recognize the general requirements for opioid treatment programs and for treating addicts outside of treatment programs.

▸ Identify the penalties for violating the Controlled Substances Act.

▸ Discuss the authority and scope of a DEA inspection of a pharmacy.

▸ Describe laws related to the Controlled Substances Act.

Society has determined that certain drugs warrant stricter regulation and control than do other drugs. Called controlled substances or scheduled drugs, these drugs have the potential for addiction and abuse. This chapter outlines the general rules that govern the distribution of controlled substances.

The primary federal law that regulates this class of drugs is called the Federal Comprehensive Drug Abuse Prevention and Control Act of 1970, more commonly known as the Controlled Substances Act (CSA) (21 U.S.C. §§ 801–970).

The act consists of three titles:

- Title I establishes rehabilitation programs for drug abusers.
- Title II provides for the registration and distribution of controlled substances.
- Title III addresses the importation and exportation of controlled substances.

Title II and its regulations are applicable to pharmacy practice.

Replacing several federal laws that haphazardly regulated these drugs in one fashion or another, the law establishes a "closed" system for the manufacturing, distributing, and dispensing of controlled substances. Thus, only those persons or entities registered with the Drug Enforcement Administration (DEA), an agency of the U.S. Department of Justice, may legally engage in these activities. The intent of this closed system is to reduce the diversion of controlled substances to illicit markets.

As part of the intent to reduce diversion, the CSA's system of national registration, as opposed to state registration, is designed to achieve uniformity. For example, in *State v. Rasmussen*, 213 N.W.2d 661 (Iowa 1973), reported in the case studies section of the chapter, the Iowa Supreme Court ruled that, because of the CSA's objective to establish national uniformity, the Iowa Board of Pharmacy could not prohibit Iowa pharmacies from dispensing controlled substance prescriptions from out-of-state physicians.

The DEA is charged with administering all parts of the CSA. The DEA's website at http://www.usdoj.gov/dea provides access to considerable information related to controlled substances, including the CSA, *Federal Register*, *Code of Federal Regulations*, and the *Pharmacist's Manual* containing summaries of relevant laws and regulations. Because controlled substances are drugs, they are also subject to the Food, Drug and Cosmetic Act (FDCA), often necessitating that the DEA coordinate its activities with the Food and Drug Administration (FDA). Created in 1973 by means of a presidential reorganization, the DEA replaced the Bureau of Narcotics and Dangerous Drugs, the Office for Drug Abuse Law Enforcement, the Office of National Narcotic Intelligence, and various departments of other agencies.

STATE VERSUS FEDERAL AUTHORITY

A state may regulate controlled substances under its police powers as long as the state law does not conflict with the federal law. Therefore, the state law should not be less strict than its federal counterpart, or the state law might be invalidated under the preemption doctrine. Many times, however, pharmacists are faced with conflicting state and federal laws. Under California law, for example, the address and DEA number of a prescriber need not be written on the controlled substance prescription itself, provided that the information is readily retrievable. Federal law, however, mandates that this information be on the prescription itself. Pharmacists who do not comply with the stricter federal law risk prosecution by the DEA.

In *Lemmon Company v. State Board of Medical Examiners*, 417 A.2d 568 (D.J. Super. 1980), reported in the case studies section of the chapter, two drug manufacturers challenged the validity of a New Jersey regulation that prohibited the use of certain amphetamines and amphetamine-type controlled drugs in the treatment of obesity. One of the arguments advanced by the plaintiffs was that the regulation conflicted with federal law because federal law does not so restrict the use of these drugs. The court, however, disagreed with the plaintiffs, finding that the regulation was not inconsistent with federal law and was reasonably related to the legitimate objective of controlling the traffic in controlled substances.

The DEA works closely with many state boards of pharmacy and frequently leaves the routine investigation of pharmacies to the state boards. If controlled substance violations are found, the pharmacy board often informs the DEA of the situation. Although the DEA may then choose to investigate, it may allow the state board to proceed in the further investigation and enforcement of the incident. The federal government has the authority to regulate drugs through the Interstate Commerce Clause of the U.S. Constitution. The CSA, however, reaches into intrastate commerce as well. Under section 801 of the act, Congress made clear its position that intrastate transactions involving controlled substances have a "substantial and direct" effect on interstate commerce. Sections 801(5) and (6) of the act further provide that the interstate manufacture and distribution of controlled substances cannot be distinguished from intrastate manufacture and distribution. As a result, federal regulation of intrastate traffic of controlled substances is essential to the effective regulation of the interstate traffic.

The courts have upheld this presumption of an impact on interstate commerce. In *United States v. Lopez*, 459 F.2d 949 (5th Cir. 1972), the appellants contended that section 801 was unconstitutional because Congress exceeded the scope of the Interstate Commerce Clause. The court, however, held that Congress is justified in its actions, and no attempt at differentiation is necessary when separating interstate activities from intrastate activities would be futile and obstruct justice, such as with controlled substances.

CLASSIFICATION OF CONTROLLED SUBSTANCES

In several provisions, the CSA refers specifically to narcotic controlled substances. Thus, the distinction between narcotic and nonnarcotic controlled substances is important. A narcotic controlled substance is defined as a natural or synthetic opium or opiate and any derivative, such as poppy straw, coca leaves, cocaine, and ecgonine (21 C.F.R. § 1300.01(b)(30)). Section 812 of the CSA provides for five schedules of controlled substances. A drug is placed into one of the schedules according to the listed criteria.

SCHEDULE I (DRUGS AND OTHER SUBSTANCES)

Drugs and other substances are placed in schedule I based upon the following criteria:

- Have a high potential for abuse.
- Have no currently accepted medical use in treatment in the United States.
- Lack accepted information on the safety of their use, even under medical supervision.

Among those substances listed in schedule I are some opiates and opiate derivatives, such as dihydromorphine, heroin, and morphine methylbromide; and hallucinogenic substances, such as marijuana, certain synthetic cannabinoids (known as herbal incense), certain synthetic cathinones (known as bath salts), lysergic acid diethylamide (LSD), peyote, mescaline, psilocybin, and tetrahydrocannabinol (THC). Methaqualone, also in schedule I, in a relatively few years worked its way from unscheduled, then to schedule II, and ultimately to schedule I because of its extremely high potential for abuse. Gamma hydroxybutyric acid (GHB), known as the date rape drug, is placed in this schedule if it is a GHB product not approved by the FDA. (If it is a GHB product that has been approved by the FDA, it is listed in schedule III.) Schedule I drugs have no accepted medical use and, thus, cannot be manufactured, prescribed, or dispensed, except as approved by the DEA for investigation purposes.

Medical Marijuana

Marijuana has many supporters who firmly believe in its medicinal value, especially for relieving pain and nausea in terminal illness, and who argue that it should not be listed in schedule I. (*Note:* Dronabinol, which contains an active ingredient of marijuana, is available as an oral schedule III drug. However, most patients who use marijuana medically do not regard it as being as effective as marijuana.) In *Seeley v. State of Washington*, 940 P.2d 604 (Wash. 1997), reported in the case studies section of this chapter, a terminally ill patient sued the state of Washington, contending that the state violated his constitutional rights by not allowing him to be prescribed marijuana by his physician. The court, however, rejected the plaintiff's argument, finding that Washington's placement of marijuana into schedule I was reasonably related to its purpose of preventing drug abuse.

As of early 2012, 16 states plus the District of Columbia have enacted laws allowing patients with a legitimate medical need as certified by a physician the right to possess or grow marijuana, and 14 other states have pending bills. These state laws, however, do not change the fact that marijuana is a schedule I drug under federal law. The laws also do not allow marijuana to be dispensed by pharmacists, nor could they without putting pharmacists in a conflict of law dilemma. States that authorize medical marijuana place patients who wish to possess and use the drug in a similar conflict of law position. Patients face arrest by the federal government for illegal possession of a schedule I drug, even though their conduct would be legal under state law.

In the case of *Gonzales v. Raich*, 545 U.S. 1 (June 6, 2005), sheriff's deputies and DEA agents raided the home of a terminally ill patient in California and found six marijuana plants. The deputies concluded that the plants were legal under California law and took no action. The DEA agents, however, destroyed the plants. Fearing future federal action, the patient and her caregivers brought an injunction action against the U.S. attorney general, contending that the CSA is unconstitutional to the extent it prevents them from the intrastate cultivation and possession of marijuana for personal medical use. Plaintiffs emphasized that the marijuana is locally cultivated and used domestically, rather than being sold on the open market and that, therefore, federal regulation violates the Interstate Commerce Clause. The district court found for the government and denied the injunction. Overruling the district court, the 9th Circuit Court of Appeals allowed the injunction. The court found that the plaintiffs had a strong likelihood of success on the merits and that a denial of the injunction would cause them a significant hardship. On appeal to the U.S. Supreme Court, however, the Court overturned the court of appeals decision and found for the government. The Court held that, based upon precedent, the government can regulate intrastate marijuana because failure to do so could undercut interstate regulation of the substance and because it would be difficult for law enforcement to differentiate intrastate from interstate marijuana.

The *Raich* decision places patients in medical marijuana states in the situation of being able to legally possess the plants under state law but not under federal law.

State medical marijuana laws create additional dilemmas for patients as well. Although the laws allow qualified patients to possess or grow marijuana, some do not define how much medical marijuana a patient may legally possess, resulting in some patients being arrested by the state for growing too many plants. Obtaining the drug or the plants creates additional problems because many patients cannot grow their own. In response, cannabis buyer cooperatives materialized for the purpose of manufacturing and distributing the marijuana to the patients. State and local governments generally tolerate the cooperatives unless a cooperative crosses the line and sells marijuana for nonmedical uses as well. The U.S. Justice Department challenged the legality of one of these cooperatives under federal law, ultimately leading to a U.S. Supreme Court decision that the cooperative violated the CSA by manufacturing and distributing marijuana (*United States v. Oakland Cannabis Buyer's Co-op*, 532 U.S. 483 (2001)). Combining this decision with the *Raich* decision leaves no question that medical marijuana users may not lawfully possess, purchase, or sell the substance under federal law.

Under President George W. Bush, the federal government aggressively attempted to enforce federal law and limit the effect of state medical marijuana laws. The U.S. Justice Department issued a policy that any physician who recommended marijuana to a patient could face revocation of the physician's DEA registration. The 9th Circuit Court of Appeals, however, ruled in the case of *Conant v. Walters*, 309 F.3d 629 (9th Cir. 2002) that this policy violated the First Amendment rights of physicians. After that failed attempt, the DEA issued letters to the landlords of medical marijuana dispensaries warning that under federal law they could be imprisoned and forced to forfeit their buildings. The Obama administration signaled in 2009 that it would not interfere with state medical marijuana laws. However, since that announcement, the Department of Justice has proceeded to enforce federal law against medical marijuana dispensaries and has threatened landlords of dispensaries with legal action.

SCHEDULE II (DRUGS AND OTHER SUBSTANCES)

Drugs and other substances are placed in schedule II based upon the following criteria:

- Have a high potential for abuse.
- Have a currently accepted medical use in treatment in the United States or a currently accepted medical use with severe restrictions.
- Abuse of the drug or other substance may lead to severe physical or psychological dependence.

Schedule II drugs include opium and various other narcotics, such as morphine, codeine, fentanyl, hydromorphone, oxycodone, methadone, meperidine, dihydrocodeine, diphenoxylate, and cocaine; certain stimulants, such as amphetamine, methamphetamine, phenmetrazine, and methylphenidate; and certain depressants, such as amobarbital, glutethimide, pentobarbital, secobarbital, and phencyclidine.

SCHEDULE III (DRUGS AND OTHER SUBSTANCES)

Schedule III includes those drugs and other substances that

- Have a potential for abuse less than that of the drugs or other substances in schedules I and II.
- Have a currently accepted medical use in treatment in the United States.
- When abused may lead to moderate or low physical dependence or high psychological dependence.

Schedule III drugs include many whose active ingredient is listed in schedule II; however, because the active ingredient is compounded with another ingredient or is in a smaller dosage, the drug's abuse potential is not great enough to warrant a schedule II classification. Examples of schedule III drugs are depressants, such as amobarbital, secobarbital, and pentobarbital in any mixture or preparation, as well as lysergic acid and methyprylone in suppository form; narcotic drugs, such as aspirin with codeine and acetaminophen with codeine; nalorphine; certain stimulants, benzphetamine, chlorphentermine, clortermine, and phendimetrazine; anabolic steroids; dronabinol; ketamine; GHB approved by the FDA; and paregoric.

A narcotic schedule III drug may not contain more than

- 1.8 g of codeine or dihydrocodeine per 100 ml, or not more than 90 mg per dosage unit.
- 300 mg of dihydrocodeinone and ethylmorphine per 100 ml, or not more than 15 mg per dosage unit.
- 500 mg of opium per 100 ml or per 100 g, or not more than 25 mg per dosage unit.
- 50 mg of morphine per 100 ml or per 100 g.

SCHEDULE IV (DRUGS AND OTHER SUBSTANCES)

Schedule IV drugs and other substances include those that

- Have a low potential for abuse relative to the drugs or other substances in schedule III.
- Have a currently accepted medical use in treatment in the United States.
- When abused may lead to limited physical dependence or psychological dependence relative to the drugs or other substances in schedule III.

Schedule IV drugs include narcotics, such as dextropropoxyphene and products that contain not more than 1 mg of difenoxin and not less than 25 mcg of atropine sulfate per dosage unit; depressants, such as alprazolam, barbital, chloral hydrate, chlordiazepoxide, diazepam, flurazepam, lorazepam, meprobamate, oxazepam, phenobarbital, and triazolam; stimulants, such as diethylpropion and phentermine; pentazocine; and a muscle relaxant, carisoprodol (effective January 11, 2012).

SCHEDULE V (DRUGS AND OTHER SUBSTANCES)

Schedule V drugs and other substances include those that

- Have a low potential for abuse relative to the drugs or other substances in schedule IV.
- Have a currently accepted medical use in treatment in the United States.
- When abused may lead to limited physical dependence or psychological dependence relative to the drugs or other substances in schedule IV.

Schedule V includes primarily antitussive preparations that contain codeine and antidiarrheal products that contain an opiate. A schedule V drug cannot contain more than

- 200 mg of codeine per 100 ml or 100 g.
- 100 mg of dihydrocodeine, ethylmorphine, or opium per 100 ml or 100 g.

- 2.5 mg of diphenoxylate and not less than 25 mcg of atropine sulfate per dosage unit.
- 0.5 mg of difenoxin and not less than 25 mcg of atropine sulfate per dosage unit.

Section 812 and the regulations (21 C.F.R. §§ 1308.11–1308.15) provide a complete list of all drugs in each schedule.

AUTHORITY FOR SCHEDULING

Section 811 of the CSA grants the attorney general of the United States the authority to place an unscheduled drug into a schedule, place a scheduled drug into a different schedule, or remove a drug from scheduling. Such a determination, however, must be based on the record after opportunity for a hearing.

Before initiating any proceedings, the attorney general must request from the Secretary of the Department of Health and Human Services (DHHS) a scientific and medical evaluation of the drug and a recommendation as to if the drug should be controlled. The secretary and attorney general must base the ultimate decision on these factors:

- Actual or relative potential for abuse
- Scientific evidence of its pharmacological effect, if known
- The state of current scientific knowledge regarding the drug or other substance
- History and current pattern of abuse
- Scope, duration, and significance of abuse
- Risk to the public health
- Physiological or psychic dependence liability
- Whether the substance is an immediate precursor of a substance already controlled

The recommendations of the secretary in regard to scientific and medical matters are binding on the attorney general. If the secretary recommends that a drug not be controlled, the attorney general must comply. If the attorney general finds that a drug must be placed into schedule I to avoid an "imminent hazard to the public safety," however, the attorney general may so schedule the drug without consulting the secretary of DHHS (§ 811(h)).

Whenever a manufacturer submits a new drug application to the secretary for any drug having a stimulant, depressant, or hallucinogenic effect on the central nervous system, the secretary must forward this information to the attorney general if it appears that the drug has abuse potential (§ 811(f)).

MANUFACTURER LABELING AND PACKAGING

All commercial containers of a controlled substance must be labeled with identification symbols designating the schedule in which the drug has been placed (§ 825). The symbols are generally C-I, C-II, C-III, C-IV, and C-V. Alternately, the symbol may be a C with the schedule designation inside it.

This symbol must be prominently located on the label or labeling of the commercial container. The symbol or labels must be clear and large enough to provide easy identification of the drug product's schedule on inspection without removal from the shelf. The symbol on all other labeling shall be clear and large enough to afford prompt identification on inspection of the labeling (21 C.F.R. § 1302.04).

REGISTRATION

Many of the narcotic laws that preceded the CSA provided for the control and accountability of controlled substances by means of a tax, much as alcohol is taxed today. The CSA, however, achieves control and accountability by requiring those who manufacture, distribute, or dispense a controlled substance, or who propose to engage in any of these activities, to register with the attorney general. Manufacturers and distributors must register annually. As for dispensers, the law allows the attorney general to determine the period of time for which registrations remain in effect as long as this period of time is not less than 1 year or more than 3 years. Under the current regulation (21 C.F.R. § 1301.13(d)), the registration for dispensers is effective for 3 years.

EXEMPTIONS

The CSA specifically allows the following persons to possess controlled substances without registration:

- An agent or employee of any registered manufacturer, distributor, or dispenser of any controlled substance if such agent or employee is acting in the usual course of his business or employment
- A common or contract carrier or warehouseman, or an employee thereof, whose possession of the controlled substance is in the usual course of his business or employment
- An ultimate user who possesses such substance for a lawful purpose (§ 822(c))

Under the first exemption, pharmacists employed by a registered pharmacy or institution need not be individually registered. Therefore, the standard practice is for the pharmacy in which a pharmacist works to be registered with the DEA, but not for an individual pharmacist to be registered.

Individual Practitioners as Agents or Employees

An individual practitioner is defined as a physician, dentist, veterinarian, or other individual licensed or registered to dispense controlled substances in the jurisdiction in which he or she practices, but the term does not include a pharmacist, pharmacy, or institutional practitioner (21 C.F.R. § 1300.01(b)(17)). An individual practitioner must ordinarily be registered with the DEA to prescribe controlled substances. Under regulations amended in 1995, however, individual practitioners who are agents or employees of another individual practitioner, other than a mid-level practitioner (e.g., nurse practitioner, nurse midwife, physician assistant), who is registered to dispense controlled substances may, when acting within the normal course of their employment, administer or dispense—but not prescribe—controlled substances using the registration of the employer (in accordance with state law) (21 C.F.R. § 1301.22(b)).

If the individual practitioner is an agent or employee of a hospital or other institution, the individual practitioner may, when acting in the normal course of business or employment, administer, dispense, and prescribe controlled substances under the registration of the hospital or institution provided that

1. The dispensing, administering, or prescribing is done in the usual course of professional practice;
2. The individual practitioner is authorized or permitted to do so by the jurisdiction in which he is practicing;

3. The hospital or other institution by whom he is employed has verified that the individual practitioner is so permitted to dispense, administer, or prescribe drugs within the jurisdiction;
4. Such individual practitioner is acting only within the scope of his employment in the hospital or institution;
5. The hospital or other institution authorizes the intern, resident, or foreign-trained physician to dispense or prescribe under the hospital registration and designates a specific internal code number for each intern, resident, or foreign-trained physician so authorized. The code number shall consist of numbers, letters, or a combination thereof and shall be a suffix to the institution's DEA registration number, preceded by a hyphen (e.g., APO123456-10 or APO123456-A12); and
6. A current list of internal codes and the corresponding individual practitioners is kept by the hospital or other institution and is made available at all times to other registrants and law enforcement agencies upon request for the purpose of verifying the authority of the prescribing individual practitioner. (21 C.F.R. § 1301.22(c))

Before 1995, this regulation was much more restrictive, authorizing only individual practitioners who were interns, residents, foreign-trained physicians, or physicians on the staff of a Veterans Administration facility to use the hospital or institutional DEA registration number. Now, however, any individual practitioner may do so, provided of course they meet the regulation's requirements. Prescriptions issued by these individual practitioners are valid at community pharmacies and may be dispensed by community pharmacies. In practice, these prescriptions can present difficulties for community pharmacists who must attempt to ascertain the validity of questionable prescriptions and who, in some instances, cannot determine who wrote the prescription.

Other Exemptions from Registration

The regulations also exempt from registration officials of the armed services, public health service, or bureau of prisons, who are authorized to prescribe, dispense, or administer controlled substances in the usual course of their official duties. They may not purchase controlled substances, however. Furthermore, if they engage in private activities involving controlled substances, they must be individually registered (21 C.F.R. § 1301.23). Exemptions also are made for law enforcement officials engaged in the performance of their duties (21 C.F.R. § 1301.24).

ACTIVITIES THAT REQUIRE REGISTRATION

Each of the following independent activities requires a separate registration, except where regulations allow for "coincidental activities" (21 C.F.R. § 1301.13 (e)):

- Manufacturing schedules I–V controlled substances
- Distributing schedules I–V controlled substances
- Reverse distributing controlled substances
- Dispensing schedules II–V controlled substances or instructing
- Conducting research with schedule I controlled substances
- Conducting research with schedules II–V controlled substances
- Conducting a narcotic treatment program (including a compounder) using any narcotic drug listed in schedules II–V
- Conducting chemical analyses with controlled substances
- Importing controlled substances
- Exporting controlled substances

The CSA defines each of the activities for which registration is necessary. Because the act requires registration according to the nature of the activity rather than the individual's status, pharmacists must be cautious not to engage inadvertently in activities that constitute manufacturing or distributing because these activities have more costly and onerous storage, security, and recordkeeping requirements.

Dispensing

Under section 802(10) of the act, the term "dispense" means

> to deliver a controlled substance to an ultimate user or research subject by, or pursuant to the lawful order of, a practitioner, including the prescribing and administering of a controlled substance and the packaging, labeling, or compounding necessary to prepare the substance for such delivery. The term "dispenser" means a practitioner who so delivers a controlled substance to an ultimate user or research subject. (§ 802(10))

The term "practitioner" is then defined as

> a physician, dentist, veterinarian, scientific investigator, pharmacy, hospital, or other person licensed, registered, or otherwise permitted, by the United States or the jurisdiction in which he practices or does research, to distribute, dispense, conduct research with respect to, administer, or use in teaching or chemical analysis, a controlled substance in the course of professional practice or research. (§ 802(21))

Thus, from the definition of practitioner, a pharmacy is a practitioner. Because a pharmacy delivers controlled substances to ultimate users, a pharmacy (including a pharmacist) is a dispenser and would register as such. The regulation defining the term dispenser confirms this logic by stating that a dispenser is an individual practitioner, institutional practitioner, pharmacy, or pharmacist. The broad definition of dispensing includes the functions of prescribing and administering. Therefore, when an individual practitioner prescribes or administers a controlled substance, that person is regarded by the law as dispensing the substance and registers as a dispenser.

The fact that a pharmacy is defined as a practitioner, which includes the function of prescribing, does not necessarily mean that a pharmacist can prescribe. Pharmacists may perform only those functions that state law authorizes them to perform, regardless of the federal definitions.

Although a practitioner by definition, a pharmacy is not an individual practitioner, nor is it an institutional practitioner. Regulations define an institutional practitioner as

> a hospital or other person (other than an individual) licensed, registered, or otherwise permitted, by the United States or the jurisdiction in which it practices, to dispense a controlled substance in the course of professional practice, but does not include a pharmacy (21 C.F.R. § 1300.01(b)(18)).

Pursuant to an institutional registration, the hospital pharmacy may dispense controlled substances without a separate registration, and hospital staff authorized by law may dispense, administer, or prescribe controlled substances to patients.

Regulations enacted in June 1993 specifically recognize mid-level practitioners as individual practitioners who may register as dispensers, providing state law has granted them independent or collaborative prescriptive authority (21 C.F.R. § 1300.01(b)(28)). Included in this group are individual practitioners other than physicians, dentists, veterinarians, or podiatrists, such as nurse practitioners, nurse midwives, nurse anesthetists, clinical nurse specialists, and physician assistants. Most recently the DEA has recognized that in some states pharmacists who are engaged in collaborative practice agreements may register as mid-level practitioners. Pharmacists in these states generally have the authority to administer, initiate, and modify drug therapy in accordance with collaborative practice requirements.

Mid-level practitioners not engaged in prescribing activities need not be separately registered if they are agents or employees of a registrant (e.g., a physician), provided that the registrant is not another mid-level practitioner. Coincidental activities permitted under a dispensing registration include research and instructional activities, but mid-level practitioners may conduct research only to the extent expressly authorized by state law (21 C.F.R. § 1301.13(e)(l)(iii)).

Manufacturing

Under section 802(15) of the CSA, "manufacture" means the production, preparation, propagation, compounding, or processing of a drug, either directly or indirectly, either by extraction from natural origin or by chemical synthesis. Manufacture also includes any packaging, repackaging, labeling, or relabeling. The term does not include the activities of practitioners that are incidental to the administering or dispensing of controlled drugs within the course of their professional practice.

A manufacturer may lawfully distribute that substance or class of drugs it is registered to manufacture (21 C.F.R. § 1301.13(e)(l)(i)). Other coincidental activities to a manufacturer registration are chemical analysis and preclinical research.

On the basis of the definition of the term manufacture, pharmacists engaged in the ordinary practice of pharmacy need not worry about registering as manufacturers. Those engaged in compounding, repackaging, or relabeling controlled substances must be so concerned, however. The regulations allow a pharmacist to manufacture and distribute to other practitioners (without registering as a manufacturer) an aqueous or oleaginous solution or solid dosage form containing a narcotic substance in a preparation not exceeding 20 percent of the complete product (21 C.F.R. § 1301.13(e)(l)(iii)).

Manufacturing activities permitted by pharmacies under the CSA seem to differ from manufacturing under the FDCA, as interpreted by the FDA. FDA policy guidelines provide that a pharmacy that compounds and distributes a product to other practitioners is manufacturing and must register as such. The CSA would seem to permit pharmacies to do so without registering as a manufacturer, provided that the product does not exceed 20 percent of a narcotic substance.

Distributing

To distribute means to deliver (other than by administering or dispensing) a controlled substance (§ 802(11)). Wholesalers of course must register as distributors, as must reverse distributors (those distributors that handle unwanted, unusable, or outdated controlled substances acquired from another DEA registrant; 21 C.F.R. §1301.13). Practitioners registered to dispense may distribute, without being registered as distributors, controlled substances to other practitioners for the purpose of general dispensing by these practitioners to their patients, provided that

- The practitioner to whom the drug is distributed is registered to dispense.
- The distribution is recorded with the proper information by the distributing and receiving practitioners.
- If the drug is a schedule I or II drug, the triplicate federal order form (DEA Form 222) is executed.
- The total number of dosage units distributed does not exceed 5 percent of the total units of controlled substances distributed and dispensed in 1 year (21 C.F.R. §§ 1307.11(a)(1)(i), (ii), (iii), (iv)).

Practitioners who return controlled substances to the supplier or manufacturer are also exempt from registering as distributors under the regulations (21 C.F.R. § 1307.12), provided that a written record is maintained indicating

- The date of the transaction
- The name, form, and quantity of the substance
- The name, address, and registration number, if any, of the person making the distribution
- The name, address, and registration number, if known, of the supplier or manufacturer

A DEA Form 222 must be used for the return of any schedule I or II controlled substances.

Registered distributors (and manufacturers) are required to design and operate a system that is able to detect suspicious orders of controlled substances and inform the DEA upon discovery of suspicious orders. In 2005, the DEA established the Distributor Initiative Program to facilitate the enforcement of this requirement. For example, in 2007 the DEA charged Cardinal Health with distributing millions of dosage units of opioid drugs to rogue Internet pharmacies and community pharmacies that dispensed these drugs pursuant to nonlegitimate prescriptions. The DEA then suspended the operations of 7 of Cardinal's 27 distribution facilities. Ultimately, Cardinal agreed to pay $34 million to settle the claims. The DEA also temporarily suspended the license of an Amerisource-Bergen Distribution Center in 2007 and in the same year alleged that McKesson filled suspicious orders that it did not report. In 2012, the DEA suspended Cardinal's authority to distribute controlled substances from a Florida distribution center based upon the distribution center supplying very large quantities of opioids to four area pharmacies.

Distributing Versus Dispensing (Constructive Delivery)

The DEA has taken the controversial position that a compounding pharmacy that delivers a compounded controlled substance medication to the prescribing practitioner, rather than the patient, for administration to the patient by the prescriber is distributing, not dispensing. In *Wedgewood Village Pharmacy v. Drug Enforcement Administration*, 509 F.3d 541 (U.S.D.C. (2007)), a pharmacy challenged the DEA's revocation of its registration, which the agency had revoked for two reasons. First, the DEA determined that the pharmacy was manufacturing, not compounding, and also distributing in excess of the 5% rule, by dispensing medications for veterinarians pursuant to prescriptions that were not written for an ultimate user. The veterinarians issued the prescriptions in their own names for general office use and would later administer the medications to horses at where they were stabled. Second, the DEA determined that because the pharmacy delivered the medications to the veterinarians, not the patients (ultimate users), this constituted distributing rather than dispensing.

The court found for the pharmacy, vacating the revocation, and remanded the case back to the DEA for reconsideration. The court found the DEA's analysis for its conclusion to revoke inadequate. Regarding that the prescriptions were written for office use, determined the court, requires that the DEA examine if this is necessary for veterinary practice. The court also found troubling the DEA's conclusion that delivery to the veterinarians constitutes distributing, not dispensing. The court noted that the law § 802(10) defines dispensing as the delivery of a controlled substance to an ultimate user, including any compounding necessary for the deliver. Moreover, the law § 802(8) defines delivery as including actual, *constructive* or attempted transfer. The court took issue with the DEA's determination that constructive delivery could not include the act of delivering the compounded product to the practitioner.

On remand and after a hearing, the DEA again concluded in 2009 to deny the pharmacy's registration. To avoid protracted litigation, the parties agreed to a settlement in May 2010 (http://www.wedgewoodpharmacy.com/news/press-room/wedgewood-pharmacy-s-dea-registration-to-dispense-controlled-substances-is-restored-0.html).

The pharmacy agreed to abide by the DEA's interpretation of the law, but specifically provided it does not agree with the DEA's position.

Subsequently, the DEA warned pharmacies that compounding morphine, even pursuant to a prescription for a particular patient, and then delivering it to the prescribing physician for intrathecal administration to the patient is distributing, not dispensing, and that the pharmacy must register as a manufacturer. One pharmacy involved sued the DEA, challenging the agency's position. The court, however, ruled that the DEA has not yet taken any enforcement action directly against the pharmacy and thus it does not have subject matter jurisdiction until there is final agency action (*Anazaohealth Corporation v. Holder*, 2011 WL 41914 (M.D.Fla.)).

In a 2010 joint letter to the DEA, several pharmacy organizations requested that the DEA reconsider its interpretation of constructive delivery (http://www.nhia.org/working_for_you/2012/w4u_032212.cfm).

Conducting Research

As mentioned earlier, dispensers are allowed to conduct research with substances listed in schedules II through V without registering separately as researchers. Research using schedule I drugs, however, requires that the applicant submit a protocol with the application, including such information as

- The name and qualifications of the investigator
- The institutional affiliation
- A description of the project
- If the research is to be clinical, copies of the investigational new drug notice and a description of the security precautions to be implemented (21 C.F.R. § 1301.18)

Separate Registrations

Each principal place of business or professional practice where controlled substances are manufactured, distributed, or dispensed requires a separate registration (§ 822(e); 21 C.F.R. § 1301.12(a)). Thus, a chain pharmacy must have a registration for each store. It is not necessary, however, to have separate registrations for warehouses where controlled substances are stored by or for a registrant (unless the substances are distributed to locations other than the registrant's). It also is not necessary for practitioners to maintain more than one registration when prescribing from more than one office, provided that the practitioner only prescribes controlled substances and does not administer, dispense, or store them in more than one office.

APPLICATIONS FOR REGISTRATION AND REREGISTRATION

No person may engage in an activity for which registration is required until the application for registration is granted and a Certificate of Registration is issued (21 C.F.R. § 1301.13(a)). This is an important consideration for those planning to start new pharmacies or to purchase existing pharmacies.

Each current registrant will receive in the mail a registration form from the DEA approximately 50 days before the expiration date on the existing registration certificate. The DEA advises that if the registrant has not received the form by 30 days before the expiration date, the registrant should promptly give notice and request the forms in writing from the branch DEA office. A corporation that owns or operates a chain of pharmacies may submit a single affidavit form (DEA Form 224b) rather than a separate form for each pharmacy registration.

Any person wishing to register with the DEA as a dispenser must complete DEA Form 224 (see **Figure 4-1**), which is available online at the DEA's website (http://www.deadiversion.usdoj.gov/drugreg/reg_apps/index.html).

Form 224	APPLICATION FOR REGISTRATION Under the Controlled Substances Act	APPROVED OMB NO 1117-0014 FORM DEA-224 (10-06) Previous editions are obsolete

INSTRUCTIONS

Save time - apply on-line at *www.deadiversion.usdoj.gov*

1. To apply by mail complete this application. Keep a copy for your records.
2. Print clearly, using black or blue ink, or use a typewriter.
3. Mail this form to the address provided in Section 7 or use enclosed envelope.
4. Include the correct payment amount. FEE IS NON-REFUNDABLE.
5. If you have any questions call 800-882-9539 prior to submitting your application.

IMPORTANT: DO NOT SEND THIS APPLICATION **AND** APPLY ON-LINE.

DEA OFFICIAL USE :

Do you have other DEA egistration numbers?

☐ NO   ☐ YES

MAIL-TO ADDRESS   Please print mailing address changes to the right of the address in this box.

FEE FOR THREE (3) YEARS IS $551
FEE IS NON-REFUNDABLE

SECTION 1   APPLICANT IDENTIFICATION   ☐ Individual Registration   ☐ Business Registration

Name 1   (Last Name of individual -OR- Business or Facility Name)

Name 2   (First Name and Middle Name of individual -OR- Continuation of business name)

Street Address Line 1 (if applying for fee exemption, this must be address of the fee exempt institution)

Address Line 2

City   State   Zip Code

Business Phone Number   Point of Contact

Business Fax Number   E-mail Address

DEBT COLLECTION INFORMATION

Mandatory pursuant to Debt Collection Improvements Act

Social Security Number (*if registration is for individual*)

Provide SSN or TIN.
See additional information
note #3 on page 4.

Tax Identification Number (*if registration is for business*)

FOR Practitioner or MLP ONLY:

Professional Degree : *select from list only*

Professional School :

Year of Graduation :

National Provider Identification:

Date of Birth (*MM-DD-YYYY*):

M M - D D - Y Y Y Y

SECTION 2 BUSINESS ACTIVITY

Check one business activity box only

☐ Central Fill Pharmacy

☐ Retail Pharmacy

☐ Nursing Home

☐ Automated Dispensing System

☐ Practitioner (DDS, DMD, DO, DPM, DVM, MD or PHD)

☐ Practitioner Military (DDS, DMD, DO, DPM, DVM, MD or PHD)

☐ Mid-level Prectitioner (MLP) (DOM, HMD, MP, ND, NP, OD, PA or RPH)

☐ Euthanasia Technician

☐ Ambulance Service

☐ Animal Shelter

☐ Hospital/Clinic

☐ Teaching Institution

FOR Automated Dispensing System (ADS) ONLY:

DEA Registration # of Retail Pharmacy for this ADS

An ADS is automatically fee-exempt. Skip Section 6 and Section 7 on page 2. You must attach a notarized affidavit.

SECTION 3 DRUG SCHEDULES
Check all that apply

☐ Schedule II Narcotic

☐ Schedule II Non-Narcotic

☐ Schedule III Narcotic

☐ Schedule III Non-Narcotic

☐ Schedule IV

☐ Schedule V

☐ Check this box if you require official order forms - for purchase or transfer of schedule 2 narcotic and/or schedule 2 non-narcotic controlled substances.

NEW - Page 1

SECTION 4 You MUST be currently authorized to prescribe, distribute, dispense, conduct research, or otherwise handle the controlled substances in the schedules for which you are applying under the laws of the **state** or jurisdiction in which you are operating or propose to operate.

STATE LICENSE(S)
Be sure to include both state license numbers if applicable

State License Number (required) | Expiration Date (required) / / MM - DD - YYYY

What state was this license issued in? _____

State Controlled Substance License Number (if required) | Expiration Date / / MM - DD - YYYY

What state was this license issued in? _____

SECTION 5

LIABILITY

IMPORTANT
All questions in this section must be answered.

1. Has the applicant ever been **convicted of a crime** in connection with controlled substance(s) under state or federal law, or is any such action pending? YES NO
Date(s) of incident MM-DD-YYYY:

2. Has the applicant ever surrendered (for cause) or had a **federal** controlled substance registration revoked, suspended, restricted, or denied, or is any such action pending? YES NO
Date(s) of incident MM-DD-YYYY:

3. Has the applicant ever surrendered (for cause) or had a **state** professional license or controlled substance registration revoked, suspended, denied, restricted, or placed on probation, or is any such action pending? YES NO
Date(s) of incident MM-DD-YYYY:

4. If the applicant is a **corporation** (other than a corporation whose stock is owned and traded by the public), association, partnership, or pharmacy, has any officer, partner, stockholder, or proprietor been **convicted of a crime** in connection with controlled substance(s) under state or federal law, or ever surrendered, for cause, or had a **federal** controlled substance registration revoked, suspended, restricted, denied, or ever had a **state** professional license or controlled substance registration revoked, suspended, denied, restricted or placed on probation, or is any such action pending? YES NO
Date(s) of incident MM-DD-YYYY:
Note: If question 4 does not apply to you, be sure to mark 'NO'. It will slow down processing of your application if you leave it blank.

EXPLANATION OF "YES" ANSWERS

Applicants who have answered "YES" to any of the four questions above **must provide a statement to explain each "YES" answer.** Use this space or attach a separate sheet and return with application

Liability question # _____ Location(s) of incident: _____

Nature of incident:

Disposition of incident:

SECTION 6 **EXEMPTION FROM APPLICATION FEE**

☐ Check this box if the applicant is a federal, state, or local government official or institution. Does not apply to contractor-operated institutions.

Business or Facility Name of Fee Exempt Institution. **Be sure to enter the address of this exempt institution in Section 1.**

The undersigned hereby certifies that the applicant named hereon is a federal, state or local government official or institution, and is exempt from payment of the application fee.

FEE EXEMPT CERTIFIER
Provide the name and phone number of the certifying official

Signature of certifying official (**other than applicant**) | Date

Print or type name and title of certifying official | Telephone No. (required for verification)

SECTION 7

METHOD OF PAYMENT
Check one form of payment only

☐ Check Make check payable to: **Drug Enforcement Administration** See page 4 of instructions for important information.

☐ American Express ☐ Discover ☐ Master Card ☐ Visa

Credit Card Number | Expiration Date

Mail this form with payment to:

U.S. Department of Justice
Drug Enforcement Administration
P.O. Box 28083
Washington, DC 20038-8083

Sign if paying by credit card

Signature of Card Holder

Printed Name of Card Holder

FEE IS NON-REFUNDABLE

SECTION 8

APPLICANT'S SIGNATURE
Sign in ink

I certify that the foregoing information furnished on this application is true and correct.

Signature of applicant (sign in ink) | Date

Print or type name and title of applicant

WARNING: Section 843(a)(4)(A) of Title 21, United States Code states that any person who knowingly or intentionally furnishes false or fraudulent information in the application is subject to imprisonment for not more than four years, a fine of not more than $30,000, or both.

NEW - Page 2

(continues)

Form 224	APPLICATION FOR REGISTRATION	Supplementary Instructions and Information

SECTION 1. APPLICANT IDENTIFICATION Information must be typed or printed in the blocks provided to help reduce data entry errors. A physical address is required in address line 1; a post office box or continuation of address may be entered in address line 2. Fee exempt applicant must list the address of the fee exempt institution.

Applicant must enter a valid social security number (SSN), or a tax identification number (TIN) if applying as a business entity. *Debt collection information is mandatory pursuant to the Debt Collection Improvement Act of 1996.*

The email address, point of contact, national provider ID, date of birth, year graduated, and professional school are new data items that are in the process of OMB approval and will soon be mandatory. They are requested in order to facilitate communication or as required by inter-agency data sharing requirements.

Practitioner must enter one degree from this list: DDS, DMD, DO, DPM, DVM, MD, or PHD.

Mid-level practitioner must enter one degree from this list: DOM, HMD, MP, ND, NP, OD, PA, or RPH.

SECTION 2. BUSINESS ACTIVITY Indicate only one. Practitioner or mid-level practitioner must enter the degree conferred and are requested to enter the last professional school of matriculation and the year graduated.

> ADS must provide current DEA registration number of parent retail pharmacy or hospital and attach a notarized affidavit in accordance with 21 CFR part 1301.17. Affidavit must include:
>
> 1) Name of parent retail pharmacy or hospital and complete address
>
> 2) Name of Long-term Care (LTC) facility and complete address
>
> 3) Permit or license number(s) and date issued of State certification to operate ADS at named LTC facility
>
> 4) Required statement:
>
> > *This affidavit is submitted to obtain a DEA registration number. If any material information is false, the Administrator may commence proceedings to deny the application under section 304 of the Act (21 USC 822a). Any false or fraudulent material information contained in this affidavit may subject the person signing this affidavit, and the named corporation/partnership/business, to prosecution under section 403 of the Act (21 USC 843).*
>
> 5) Name of corporation operating the retail pharmacy or hospital
>
> 6) Name and title of corporate officer signing affidavit
>
> 7) Signature of authorized officer

SECTION 3. DRUG SCHEDULES Applicant should check all drug schedules to be handled. However, applicant must still comply with state requirements; federal registration does not overrule state restrictions. Check the order form box only if you intend to purchase or to transfer schedule 2 controlled substances. Order forms will be mailed to the registered address following issuance of a Certificate of Registration. The following list of drug codes are examples of controlled substances for schedules 2, 3, 4, and 5. Refer to the CFR for a complete list of basic classes

SCHEDULE 2 NARCOTIC	BASIC CLASS
Alphaprodine (Nisente)	9010
Anileridine (Leritine)	9020
Cocaine (Methyl Benzoylecgonine)	9041
Codeine (Morphine methyl ester)	9050
Dextropropoxyphene, bulk	9273
Diphenoxylate	9170
Diprenorphine (M50-50)	9058
Ethylmorpine (Dionin)	9190
Etorphine HCL (M-99)	9059
Glutethimide (Doriden, Dorimide)	2550
Hydrocodone (Dihydrocodeinone)	9193
Hydromorphone (Dilaudid)	9150
Levo-alphacetylmethadol (LAAM)	9648
Levorphanol (Levo-Dromoran)	9220
Meperidine (Demerol, Mepergan)	9230
Methadone (Dolophine, Methadose)	9250
Morphine (MS Contin, Roxanol)	9300
Opium, powdered	9639
Opium, raw	9600
Oxycodone (Oxycontin, Percocet)	9143
Oxymorphone (Numorphan)	9652
Opium Poppy/Poppy Straw	9650
Poppy Straw Concentrate	9670
Thebaine	9333

SCHEDULE 2 NON-NARCOTIC	BASIC CLASS
Amobarbital (Amytal, Tuinal)	2125
Amphetamine (Dexedrine, Adderall)	1100
Methamphetamine (Desoxyn)	1105
Methylphenidate (Concerta, Ritalin)	1724
Pentobarbital (Nembutal)	2270
Phencyclidine	7471
Phenmetrazine (Preludin)	1631
Phenylacetone	8501
Secobarbital (Seconal)	2315

SCHEDULE 3 NARCOTIC	BASIC CLASS
Buprenorphine (Buprenex, Temgesic, Subutex)	9064
Codeine combo product 90 mg/du (Empirin)	9804
Dihydrocodeine combo prod 90 mg/du (Compal)	9807
Ethylmorphine combo product 15 mg/du	9808
Hydrocodone combo product (Lorcet, Vicodin)	9806
Morphine combo product 50 mg/100 ml or gm	9810
Opium combo product 25 mg/du (Paregoric)	9809

SCHEDULE 3 NON-NARCOTIC	BASIC CLASS
Anabolic Steroids	4000
Benzphetamine (Didrex, Inapetyl)	1228
Butalbital (Fiorinal, Butalbital w/aspirin)	2100/2165
Dronabinol in sesame oil with soft gelatin capsule	7369
Gamma Hydroxybutyric Acid preps (Zyrem)	2012
Ketamine (Ketaset)	7285
Methyprylon (Noludar)	2575
Pentobarbital suppository du and noncontrolled active ingred (FP-3, WANS)	2271
Phendimetrazine (Plegine, Bontril, Statobex)	1615
Secobarbital suppository du and noncontrolled active ingredients	2316
Thiopental (Pentothal)	2100/2329
Vinbarbital (Delvinal)	2100/2329

SCHEDULE 5	BASIC CLASS
Codeine Cough Preparation (Cosanyl, Pediacof)	9050
Difenoxin Preparation (Motofen)	9167
Dihydrocodeine Preparation (Cophene-S)	9120

SCHEDULE 4	BASIC CLASS
Alprazolam (Xanax)	2882
Barbital (Veronal, Plexonal, Barbitone)	2145
Chloral Hydrate (Noctec)	2465
Chlordiazepoxide (Librium, Libritabs)	2744
Clorazepate (Tranxene)	2768
Dextropropoxyphene du (Darvon)	9278
Diazepam (Valium, Diastat)	2765
Diethylpropion (Tenuate, Tepanil)	1610
Difenoxin 1 mg/25ug ATSO4/du (Motofen)	9167
Fenfluramine (Pondimin, Dexfenfluramine)	1670
Flurazepam (Dalmane)	2767
Halazepam (Paxipam)	2762
Lorzaepam (Ativan)	2885
Mazindol (Sanorex, Mazanor)	1605
Mebutamate (Capla)	2800
Meprobamate (Miltown, Equanil)	2820
Methohexital (Brevital)	2264
Methylphenobarbital (Mebaral)	2250
Midazolam (Versed)	2884
Oxazepam (Serax, Serenid-D)	2835
Paraldehyde (Paral)	2585
Pemoline (Cylert)	1530
Pentazocine (Talwin, Talacen)	9709
Phenobarbital (Luminal, Donnatal)	2285
Phentermine (Ionamin, Fastin, Zantryl)	1640
Prazepam (Centrax)	2764
Quazepam (Doral)	2881
Temazepam (Restoril)	2925
Triazolam (Halcion)	2887
Zolpidem (Ambiem, Ivadal, Stilnox)	2783

SCHEDULE 5	BASIC CLASS
Diphenoxylate Preparation (Lomotil, Logen)	9170
Ethylmorphine Preparation	9190

Form 224	**APPLICATION FOR REGISTRATION**	**Supplementary Instructions and Information**
	- CONTINUED -	

SECTION 4. STATE LICENSE(S) Federal registration by DEA is based upon the applicant's compliance with applicable state and local laws. Applicant should contact the local state licensing authority prior to completing this application. If your state requires a separate controlled substance number, provide that number on this application.

SECTION 5. LIABILITY Applicant must answer all four questions for the application to be accepted for processing. If you answer "Yes" to a question, provide an explanation in the space provided. If you answer "Yes" to several of the questions, then you must provide a separate explanation describing the location, nature, and result of incident for each "Yes" answer. If additional space is required, you may attach a separate page.

SECTION 6. EXEMPTION FROM APPLICATION FEE Exemption from payment of application fee is limited to federal, state or local government official or institution. The applicant's superior or agency officer must certify exempt status. The signature, authority title, and telephone number of the certifying official (other than the applicant) must be provided. The address of the fee exempt institution must appear in Section 1.

SECTION 7. METHOD OF PAYMENT Indicate the desired method of payment. Make checks payable to "Drug Enforcement Administration". Third-party checks or checks drawn on foreign banks will not be accepted. ***FEES ARE NON-REFUNDABLE.***

SECTION 8. APPLICANT'S SIGNATURE Applicant must sign in this section or application will be returned. Card holder signature in Section 7 does not fulfill this requirement.

Notice to Registrants Making Payment by Check

Authorization to Convert Your Check: If you send us a check to make your payment, your check will be converted into an electronic fund transfer. "Electronic fund transfer" is the term used to refer to the process in which we electronically instruct your financial institution to transfer funds from your account to our account, rather than processing your check. By sending your completed, signed check to us, you authorize us to copy your check and to use the account information from your check to make an electronic fund transfer from your account for the same amount as the check. If the electronic fund transfer cannot be processed for technical reasons, you authorize us to process the copy of your check.

Insufficient Funds: The electronic funds transfer from your account will usually occur within 24 hours, which is faster than a check is normally processed. Therefore, make sure there are sufficient funds available in your checking account when you send us your check. If the electronic funds transfer cannot be completed because of insufficient funds, we may try to make the transfer up to two more times.

Transaction Information: The electronic fund transfer from your account will be on the account statement you receive from your financial institution. However, the transfer may be in a different place on your statement than the place where your checks normally appear. For example, it may appear under "other withdrawals" or "other transactions." You will not receive your original check back from your financial institution. For security reasons, we will destroy your original check, but we will keep a copy of the check for record-keeping purposes.

Your Rights: You should contact your financial institution immediately if you believe that the electronic fund transfer reported on your account statement was not properly authorized or is otherwise incorrect. Consumers have protections under Federal law called the Electronic Fund Transfer Act for an unauthorized or incorrect electronic fund transfer.

ADDITIONAL INFORMATION
1. No registration will be issued unless a completed application form has been received (21 CFR 1301. 13).
2. In accordance with the Paperwork Reduction Act of 1995, no person is required to respond to a collection of information unless it displays a valid OMB control number. The OMB number for this collection is 1117-0014. Public reporting burden for this collection of information is estimated to average 15 minutes per response, including the time for reviewing instructions, searching existing data sources, gathering and maintaining the data needed, and completing and reviewing the information.
3. The Debt Collection Improvements Act of 1996 (PL 104-134) requires that you furnish your Taxpayer Identification Number and/or Social Security Number on this application. This number is required for debt collection procedures if your fee is not collectible.
4. PRIVACY ACT INFORMATION
   AUTHORITY: Section 302 and 303 of the Controlled Substances Act of 1970 (PL 91-513) and Debt Collection Improvements Act of 1966 (PL 104-134) for SSN and/or TIN
   PURPOSE: To obtain information required to register applicants pursuant to the Controlled Substances Act of 1970
   ROUTINE USES: The Controlled Substances Act registration system produces special reports as required for statistical analytical purposes. Disclosures of information from this system are made to the following:
          A. Other federal law enforcement and regulatory agencies for law enforcement and regulatory purposes
          B. State and local law enforcement and regulatory agencies for law enforcement and regulatory purposes
          C. Persons registered under the Controlled Substances Act (PL 91-513) for the purpose of verifying registration
   EFFECT: Failure to complete form will preclude processing of the application.

INTERNET:
www.deadiversion.usdoj.gov

TELEPHONE:
HQ Call Center (800)882-9539

WRITTEN INQUIRIES:
DEA
P.O. Box 28083
Washington, D.C. 29938-8083

FIGURE 4-1 DEA Form 224.

Source: U.S. Department of Justice, Drug Enforcement Administration

The form may be completed interactively online and printed by the applicant, or the blank form may be printed and completed manually. Manufacturers, distributors, and narcotic treatment programs must complete DEA Form 225, also available online.

MODIFICATION, TRANSFER, AND TERMINATION OF REGISTRATION

A registrant who wishes to modify the registration (e.g., change a name or address) may apply to the DEA online or in writing. If the modification is approved, a new certificate will be issued, and the registrant must maintain it with the old certificate until expiration (21 C.F.R. § 1301.51).

If a person (including natural person and corporation) dies, ceases legal existence, or discontinues the business or professional practice, the DEA must be notified and the registration terminated (21 C.F.R. § 1301.52(a)). No registration can be assigned or transferred except with the approval of the DEA after submitting a written request and providing full details of the proposed transfer (21 C.F.R. § 1301.52(b)). If the registrant discontinues business (and does not transfer the business to another), the certificate of registration must be returned to the DEA, together with any unexecuted order forms (21 C.F.R. § 1301.52(c)). Any controlled substances in the registrant's possession must be disposed of in accordance with DEA requirements.

When a pharmacy is sold to another person as an ongoing business and wishes to transfer the registration to another person, the registrant must submit the proposal for transfer in person or by registered or certified mail, return receipt requested, to the special agent of the DEA in charge in the registrant's area. The proposal must be submitted at least 14 days in advance of the planned transfer, unless this requirement is waived by the special agent in charge. The following information must be included:

- The name, address, registration number, and authorized business activity of the registrant discontinuing business and that of the person acquiring the business
- Whether the business activities currently registered will be continued at the present address or at another specified address
- Whether the transferor has a quota to manufacture or procure any controlled substance in schedules I or II
- The date on which the transfer of controlled substances will occur

Unless the regional administrator of the DEA notifies the transferor that the transfer may not occur, the transferor may distribute the controlled substances to the transferee. A complete inventory of all controlled substances must be taken on the date of transfer, and transfers of any schedule I or II substances must be pursuant to DEA Form 222 (or electronic equivalent). Furthermore, all required records must be transferred on the date of transfer. Although responsibility for the accuracy of the records remains with the transferor, responsibility for their custody and maintenance rests with the transferee (21 C.F.R. § 1301.52(d)).

DENIAL, REVOCATION, OR SUSPENSION OF REGISTRATION

The attorney general may deny a practitioner-applicant a registration to dispense or conduct research with controlled substances if it is determined that the registration would not be in the public interest (§ 823(f)). In this determination, the attorney general must consider

- The recommendation of the appropriate state licensing board
- The applicant's experience

- The applicant's conviction record with respect to controlled substances
- The applicant's compliance with applicable state, federal, or local laws
- Any other conduct by the applicant that may threaten the public health and safety

A registration to manufacture, distribute, or dispense controlled substances may be suspended or revoked by the attorney general on a finding that the applicant (§ 824(a))

- Has materially falsified any application
- Has been convicted of a felony relative to controlled substances
- Has had a state license or registration suspended, revoked, or denied
- Has committed acts inconsistent with public interest (as described earlier)
- Has been excluded from participation in a Medicaid or Medicare program

SECURITY REQUIREMENTS

The extent of the security that a registrant must provide depends on whether the registrant is a practitioner or a nonpractitioner. Practitioners who stock controlled substances must provide for the security of these drugs. The regulations specify that "[a]ll applicants and registrants shall provide effective controls and procedures to guard against theft and diversion of controlled substances" (21 C.F.R. § 1301.71(a)).

When evaluating if the overall security system of a registrant or applicant is adequate, the DEA may consider any of the following:

- The type of activity conducted
- The type and form of controlled substances handled
- The quantity of controlled substances handled
- The location of the premises
- The type of building construction and its general characteristics
- The type of vault, safe, and secure enclosures or other storage system
- The type of closures on vaults, safes, and secure enclosures
- The adequacy of key control systems or combination lock control systems
- The adequacy of electronic detection and alarm systems
- The extent of unsupervised public access to the facility, including the presence and characteristics of perimeter fencing, if any
- The adequacy of supervision over employees having access to manufacturing and storage areas
- The procedures for handling business guests, visitors, maintenance personnel, and nonemployee service personnel
- The availability of local police protection or security personnel
- The adequacy of the system used for monitoring the receipt, manufacture, distribution, and disposition of controlled substances

Practitioners must store schedule I drugs in a securely locked, substantially constructed cabinet (21 C.F.R. § 1301.75). Although individual practitioners must store schedules II, III, IV, and V drugs in the same manner, pharmacies and institutional practitioners may disperse these substances throughout their stock of noncontrolled substances in a manner that will obstruct theft or diversion. Etorphine hydrochloride and diprenorphine must be stored in a safe or steel cabinet equivalent to a U.S. Government Class V security container.

A practitioner may not employ any person who has been convicted of a felony related to controlled substances or who has had an application for registration denied, revoked, or surrendered for cause in a position that involves access to controlled substances (21 C.F.R. § 1301.76). The practitioner may seek a waiver to this requirement if the practitioner provides details as listed in the *Pharmacist's Manual*. Any theft or significant loss of any controlled substance must be reported to the DEA.

In addition to the requirements of section 1301.71(a), nonpractitioners must also meet the extensive security requirements contained in sections 1301.72 through 1301.74 and sections 1301.90 through 1301.93. In general, the requirements specify that all except a small amount of schedule I or II substances must be stored in a safe weighing more than 750 pounds and bolted or cemented to the floor. Schedule III through V substances must be stored in a secured area subject to stringent security regulations. Few pharmacies could meet the security requirements imposed on manufacturers and distributors.

PENALTIES

Violations of the CSA can result in severe penalties. The severity of the penalty often depends on the nature of the activity, the drug or drugs involved, and the defendant's prior record.

DRUG TRAFFICKING OFFENSES

Practitioners are not immune from being prosecuted as drug traffickers. Section 841 provides:

> (a) except as authorized by this subchapter, it shall be unlawful for any person knowingly or intentionally—
>   (1) to manufacture, distribute or dispense, or possess with intent to manufacture, distribute or dispense a controlled substance; or
>   (2) to create, distribute, or dispense, or possess with intent to distribute or dispense, a counterfeit substance.

The penalty for violating section 841 ranges from imprisonment of 10 years to life, a fine of up to $4 million if specified quantities of certain schedule I drugs and cocaine are involved, or both. With respect to other schedule I and schedule II drugs, the penalty is imprisonment of not more than 20 years, a fine of up to $1 million, or both. Penalties are less severe for schedules III, IV, and V drugs, and marijuana. Health care professionals who prescribe or dispense controlled substances outside the usual course of professional practice could face section 841 sanctions.

DISTRIBUTING OR DISPENSING IN VIOLATION OF THE CONTROLLED SUBSTANCES ACT

Section 842 provides that it is unlawful for registrants or their employees to distribute or dispense a controlled substance other than as prescribed by the CSA. This includes failing to make, keep, or furnish any required records or reports and not including on these records all required information. Thus, for example, a pharmacy could be in violation of section 842 for not including the prescriber's DEA number or address on the prescription. Congress amended section 842 in 1998 after the DEA began a zealous enforcement campaign resulting in individual pharmacies being fined hundreds of thousands of dollars for innocent, minor recordkeeping errors. Before the amendment, an unknowing or unintentional recordkeeping violation could result in a civil penalty of up to $25,000 for each violation. (For example, a pharmacy that did not include the address of the prescriber on 10 prescriptions could be fined $250,000.) Outraged pharmacy organizations convinced Congress to amend section 842 from its strict liability standard to a negligence standard. As the law now reads, if the violation is with knowledge or intent (i.e., voluntary or deliberate), the penalty is criminal—up to 1 year in prison, a fine of up to $25,000, or both for first offenses. If the recordkeeping violation is due to negligence, the violator is subject to a civil penalty of not more than $10,000. In *United States v. Little*, 59 F. Supp. 2d 177 (D. Mass. 1999), reported in the case studies section of this chapter, a pharmacy owner and his pharmacy were charged with recordkeeping violations under the strict liability standard of section 842. After the case was filed, Congress changed the law to the negligence standard and the defendants argued that the change should be made retroactive. The court, however, refused.

ORDER FORM 222 VIOLATION

Section 843 of the CSA, among other things, makes it unlawful for any registrant to distribute schedules I and II drugs knowingly and intentionally, except pursuant to a Form 222. The penalty is up to 4 years in prison and a fine of up to $30,000.

ILLEGAL POSSESSION

Section 844 prohibits any person from knowingly or intentionally possessing a controlled substance, except pursuant to a valid prescription or order issued by a practitioner in the usual course of professional practice or as otherwise authorized by the CSA. The penalty for first time violators is up to 1 year in prison and/or a fine of up to $1,000. Possession of cocaine carries much more serious penalties.

STATE BOARD DISCIPLINE

Pharmacists who are prosecuted under the CSA are also subject to disciplinary proceedings by the state board of pharmacy. As a result, the pharmacists and pharmacies involved not only could have their licenses revoked or suspended but also could be subject to a fine, depending on state law.

 © Stockbyte/Thinkstock

STUDY SCENARIOS AND QUESTIONS

1. Butrazid (fct) is a controlled substance placed in schedule II by the federal government. One state has been having abuse and diversion problems with Butrazid, especially among teenagers. The drug has proven to be addictive and has even caused deaths, including the death of the daughter of a state legislator. The legislator vowed to take Butrazid off the streets by introducing a bill classifying Butrazid as a schedule I drug. Butrazid also happens to be the most effective drug available for a particular neurological disorder. Without the drug, patients suffering this disorder would face a greatly diminished quality of life. Despite the vocal opposition of these patients, the law passed. The patients sued to invalidate the law. Discuss if this state law conflicts with the CSA and if the state law is unconstitutional. (*Note:* Be sure to consider the *Seeley* case [Case 4-3] in your answer.)

2. A pharmacist received a prescription from a physician employed at the county hospital. The prescription was written on a prescription form that contained the DEA registration number of the hospital, but not the physician. The pharmacist called the physician, who told the pharmacist that he had no DEA number and that he just uses the hospital number. Discuss if this practice is legal and what, if any, requirements must be met.

3. Mary decided to open a new pharmacy in a growing town. She applied for a pharmacy license from the state board, but is not sure how to get a DEA registration. She would like to open the pharmacy as soon as possible and wonders if she could purchase and dispense controlled substances while her

registration is pending. Advise Mary how to obtain registration with the DEA and if she could purchase and dispense controlled substances while her registration is pending.

4. John is a new pharmacist at XYZ Pharmacy. John noticed that the pharmacy kept the C-II drugs on the shelf interspersed with other drugs. All the other pharmacies where John had worked kept the C-IIs in a safe. John told the pharmacy manager that it was his understanding that the C-II drugs must be kept in a safe and that the pharmacy was violating the law. Discuss whether John is right or wrong.

5. Lim is a new pharmacist heavily in debt. A couple of Lim's patients at the pharmacy who regularly received prescriptions for controlled substances told Lim they could make it worth his while if he would simply dispense to them more tablets than what was prescribed. Lim did so and was caught. Explain the type of offense the DEA might charge Lim with under the penalty statutes.

PHARMACY INSPECTIONS

To determine whether pharmacies are complying with state and federal laws and regulations, administrative agencies have the authority to inspect pharmacies. Inspections may be routine and simply to confirm compliance with the law, or triggered by (1) a fear of an imminent danger to the public health, safety, and welfare; (2) a formal complaint; or (3) the belief that a specific violation has occurred or will occur.

Constitutional Requirements

The Fourth Amendment to the Constitution protects individuals from unreasonable searches and seizures. Search warrants are issued only to authorized law enforcement officers by judges. The amendment provides that no search warrant can be issued unless there is probable cause for the search; moreover, the warrant must particularly describe the place to be searched and the persons or things to be seized.

Law enforcement officers must be concerned that any search or seizure will withstand constitutional scrutiny. Under the "exclusionary rule," no evidence obtained pursuant to an illegal search can be used in court against a defendant. Because this evidence often is crucial to convicting a guilty defendant, the exclusion of evidence obtained in a search can be the difference between winning or losing the case.

The Fourth Amendment has been the subject of many U.S. Supreme Court cases. The Court often is called upon to determine whether officers were entitled to seize evidence without a warrant, whether officers exceeded the scope of a warrant, and whether the probable cause used to justify a warrant was sufficient. The case law on these issues is extensive and somewhat complicated, even confusing. Some authorities find it unfair that law enforcement officers must make instantaneous decisions in the heat of a criminal investigation, and yet the courts have years to analyze whether the officers' decisions were constitutional.

DEA Inspections Under the CSA

The CSA provides that the DEA may enter and inspect any place where controlled substance records are kept or persons are registered under the CSA (21 U.S.C. § 880; 21 C.F.R. §§ 1316.01–1316.13). Under the CSA, a DEA inspector is allowed to examine and copy all records and reports, to inspect the premises within reasonable limits, and to take an inventory of the controlled substances. Unless the owner or pharmacist in charge consents in writing, the inspector is not allowed to inspect financial data, sales data other than shipment data, or pricing data. In a normal audit, the inspector examines the records of the amount of drug(s) received and the records of the amount of drug(s) dispersed. The inventory should account for the difference in these amounts. Inspectors also examine records to determine their legitimacy, accuracy, and compliance with the law.

Before an inspection, the inspector is required to state the purpose of the inspection and present to the owner or pharmacist in charge the agent's credentials and a written notice of inspection. The notice contains the name of the owner or pharmacist in charge, the name and address of the business, the date and time of the inspection, and a statement that the notice has been given (see **Figure 4-2**).

U.S. DEPARTMENT OF JUSTICE
DRUG ENFORCEMENT ADMINISTRATION

NOTICE OF INSPECTION OF CONTROLLED PREMISES

DEA USE ONLY
FILE NUMBER

NAME OF INDIVIDUAL	TITLE	
NAME OF CONTROLLED PREMISES		DEA REGISTRATION NO.
NUMBER AND STREET		DATE
CITY AND STATE	ZIP CODE	TIME *(initial inspection)*

STATEMENT OF RIGHTS

1. You have a constitutional right not to have an administrative inspection made without an administrative inspection warrant.
2. You have the right to refuse to consent to this inspection.
3. Anything of an incriminating nature which may be found may be seized and used against you in a criminal prosecution.
4. You shall be presented with a copy of this Notice of Inspection.
5. You may withdraw your consent at any time during the course of the inspection.

ACKNOWLEDGEMENT AND CONSENT

1, ______________________________, have been advised of the above Statement of Rights
(Name)

by DEA ______________________________, who
(Title and Name)

has identified himself/herself to me with his/her credentials and presented me with this Notice of Inspection containing a copy of sections 302 (f) and 510(a), (b) and (c) of the Controlled Substances Act (21 U.S.C. 822(f) and 21 U.S.C. 880(a), (b) and (c), printed hereon, * authorizing an inspection of the above-described controlled premises. I hereby acknowledge receipt of this Notice of Inspection. In addition, I hereby certify that I am the ______________________________
(President) *(Manager)* *(Owner)*

for the premises described in this Notice of Inspection; that I have read the foregoing and understand its contents; that I have authority to act in this matter and have signed this Notice of Inspection pursuant to my authority.

I understand what my rights are concerning inspection. No threats or promises have been made to me and no pressure of any kind has been used against me. I voluntarily give consent for inspection of these controlled premises.

____
(Signature)

____
(Date)

WITNESSES:

______________________ ______________
(Signed) *(Date)*

______________________ ______________
(Signed) *(Date)*

FIGURE 4-2 Notice of inspection of controlled premises.
Source: U.S. Department of Justice, Drug Enforcement Administration

Consent Requirement

In addition, the inspector must obtain a written statement of informed consent to the search, signed by the owner or pharmacist in charge. The statement must note that the owner or pharmacist in charge has been informed of and understands the following:

- There is a constitutional right to refuse the inspection until an administrative inspection warrant has been obtained.
- Any incriminating evidence found may be seized and used against the owner or pharmacist in charge in a criminal prosecution.
- A notice of inspection has been presented.
- The consent is voluntary and not coerced.
- The consent may be withdrawn at any time during the course of inspection.

The written consent must be produced in duplicate; the inspector keeps the original and gives the copy to the person who consented to the inspection.

Courts have addressed the issue of whether a pharmacist's consent is voluntary or coerced. In *United States v. Enserro*, 401 F. Supp. 460 (W.D.N.Y. 1975), DEA officers responded to a complaint about the illegal distribution of drugs at the defendant's pharmacy. With a notice of inspection in hand, the agents approached the employee-pharmacist on duty and showed him a copy. They told the pharmacist that he "would face criminal penalties under Title 21 of the United States Code unless he signed a consent permitting the inspection" (401 F. Supp. at 462). Faced with that threat, the pharmacist signed the consent and permitted the inspection. The owner-defendant was subsequently charged with the illegal distribution of schedule II controlled substances, but the court found that the evidence had been obtained illegally because the consent was forced.

Rather than giving unconditional consent, the owner or pharmacist in charge may wish to give a limited consent, specifically excluding a particular part of the premises or particular records. The owner or pharmacist in charge should then document the limited nature of the consent in writing, and the documentation should be signed by both parties.

Use of an Administrative Inspection Warrant

As an alternative to presenting a notice of inspection an inspector may instead present the pharmacy with an administrative inspection warrant (AIW) or even a search warrant. Under either warrant consent is not required. An administrative inspection warrant as provided for in the CSA differs from a search warrant in one very important respect—the probable cause requirement. Although law enforcement officers must show probable cause for a judge to issue either type of warrant, the probable cause requirement is much easier to satisfy for an AIW. Probable cause for a search warrant requires law enforcement officers to convince a judge that a reasonable person would believe that a crime has been or will be committed on the premises to be searched or that evidence relevant to a crime exists at the premises. Under the CSA, probable cause for an AIW is defined as a "valid public interest." Several court cases have defined what constitutes a "valid public interest."

In *United States v. Shiffman*, 572 F.2d 1137 (5th Cir. 1978), officers arrested two men who possessed manufacturer stock bottles of 1,000 Seconal, Dexedrine, and Tuinal. An investigation by the DEA and the state board of pharmacy led them to the defendant's pharmacy as the source of the drugs. An inspection of the pharmacy by the state pharmacy board showed the pharmacy could not account for certain amounts of several controlled substances. Using this information as probable cause for an AIW, a DEA agent then inspected the defendant's pharmacy and arrested him. The pharmacist was subsequently convicted of conspiring to possess and distribute controlled substances, distributing controlled substances, and furnishing false information in his records. He appealed the conviction, however, contending that the information obtained from the state board of pharmacy and used to establish the probable cause for the AIW was illegally obtained. Thus, he continued, the warrant itself was illegally obtained and all the evidence should be inadmissible. The court disagreed with the pharmacist, stating that the legality of the evidence that established the probable cause for the warrant was irrelevant. The court stated that evidence of large purchases of controlled substances by itself constitutes probable cause for the purpose of the CSA. The court further noted that registrants should be aware that, as a condition of engaging in the manufacture or distribution of drugs, they are subject to the regulatory system imposed by the act, including administrative inspections by the DEA.

In addition to large purchases of controlled substances, other courts have held that merely a need to ensure compliance with the recordkeeping requirements of the act and the passage of a substantial period of time since the last inspection may constitute a "valid public interest."

The U.S. Supreme Court essentially created the AIW as an alternative to the search warrant when two Supreme Court cases—*See v. City of Seattle*, 387 U.S. 541 (1967), and *Camara v. Municipal Court*, 387 U.S. 523 (1967)—established that the Fourth Amendment applied to administrative inspections of commercial premises and, therefore, agents must have warrants to conduct such inspections. Before this time, courts had generally held that search warrants were not required for the administrative inspections of commercial premises because the need of the public to have businesses inspected outweighed the minimal intrusion into individual privacy that resulted. Requiring agents to have a search warrant to inspect commercial premises, however, would cause considerable difficulties. The probable cause required of a search warrant would in most cases preclude inspectors from conducting a routine investigation because they would have no evidence of a violation of the law. Recognizing this dilemma, the Court in *See* stated that a "valid public interest" can serve as a probable cause for an administrative search and justify the intrusion.

An administrative inspection warrant must contain

- The name and address of the premises to be inspected
- A statement of the statutory authority for the warrant
- A statement as to the nature and extent of the inspection including, when necessary, a request to seize specified items
- A statement that the premises either have not been previously inspected or were last inspected on a particular date

An AIW may only be served during regular business hours and must be completed in a reasonable manner. (A search warrant may be served day or night.) A registrant presented with an AIW may not refuse consent. A refusal of consent at this point is unlawful and carries a maximum penalty of a $25,000 fine, up to 1 year imprisonment, or both.

Exceptions to an Administrative Inspection Warrant

An inspector or officer does not normally need an AIW if

1. The inspection is an initial inspection of a new pharmacy for licensure purposes.
2. The records are ordered pursuant to an administrative subpoena.
3. The owner has given informed consent.

4. The situation presents an imminent danger to the public health and safety.
5. It is an exceptional or emergency situation where obtaining a warrant would be impractical because of lack of time or opportunity to obtain one.
6. It is a situation where a warrant is not constitutionally required. Some examples include:
   a. When a search is made incident to a lawful arrest.
   b. When the inspection is limited to areas of the commercial premises open to the public.
   c. When the evidence is in "plain view," providing the officer is legally in a place the officer should be and inadvertently sees the evidence. (21 C.F.R. § 1316.07)

State Pharmacy Board Inspections

State boards of pharmacy and the DEA often work collaboratively when controlled substances are the subject of a pharmacy investigation. The requirements of the CSA applicable to DEA inspectors do not apply to state board inspectors. Rather, state law dictates the procedures they must follow.

Unlike the federal CSA, some state laws allow the inspection of pharmacies without warrants. Although, as previously stated, the U.S. Supreme Court has held that a warrant is required for an administrative search, it has fashioned exceptions to this general rule. In *Colonnade Catering v. United States*, 397 U.S. 72 (1970), the Court upheld the legality of a federal law allowing warrantless inspections in the liquor industry. Noting that the law did not authorize forcible entry without a warrant and that the liquor industry has had a long history of close supervision and inspection by the government, the court felt that the law was constitutional. Similarly, in *United States v. Biswell*, 406 U.S. 311 (1972), the Court upheld the constitutionality of a warrantless inspection of a firearms dealer. The Court stated that inspections were a crucial part of the regulatory scheme and that a firearms dealer should have known in advance that such a business would be subject to inspection.

Essentially, the *Colonnade* and *Biswell* decisions constitute a "licensing exemption." Under this exemption, statutes that allow warrantless searches of licensed premises may be constitutional if

- The industry is one that is "pervasively regulated."
- The licensee's expectation of privacy is outweighed by the government interests of protecting the public health, safety, and welfare.
- The statute carefully limits the time, place, and scope of the inspection.

In a later decision (*Marshall v. Barlow's, Inc.*, 436 U.S. 307 (1978)), the Court reiterated its support for the "licensing exemption" doctrine, yet found that a warrantless search provision in the Occupational Safety and Health Act was unconstitutional because it did not limit the searches to closely regulated businesses.

The Supreme Court has never decided whether pharmacy is a pervasively regulated industry within the intent of these three decisions, but some state courts have. In *Stone et al. v. City of Stow et al.*, 593 N.E.2d 294 (1992), the Ohio Supreme Court upheld the right of police officers to conduct administrative searches of a pharmacy without a warrant, finding that pharmacy is a pervasively regulated industry and pharmacists should expect to be inspected. The Ohio decision was followed by a decision of the Vermont Supreme Court in *State of Vermont v. Welch*, 624 A.2d 1105 (1992) in which the court also held that warrantless searches of pharmacies were permissible because pharmacy is a pervasively regulated industry.

The "pervasively regulated industry" exception will not permit a warrantless search if an applicable statute specifies the necessity of a warrant. In the *Enserro* case discussed previously, DEA agents coerced a pharmacist into consenting to an inspection. The DEA argued that the fact that the pharmacist's consent was coerced was irrelevant because pharmacy is a pervasively regulated industry and no warrant was required. The court disagreed, noting that Congress has specifically provided in the CSA that an administrative inspection warrant is necessary if it is not possible to obtain informed consent: "A warrant remains the necessary standard procedure, since there is no statute defining specific standards for warrantless inspections in terms of time, place and scope unless and until Congress sees fit to change the statute" (p. 463).

PRACTICAL CONSIDERATIONS

When an agent or inspector visits the pharmacy for an inspection, the pharmacist should ascertain the purpose of the inspection and note the agent's credentials. Under normal circumstances pharmacists should not fear an inspection, especially if it is a routine state board inspection, and should be cordial and cooperative. If the inspection is not routine and is for the purpose of conducting a controlled substance accountability audit, the pharmacist should contact the employer or supervisor, who may wish to contact an attorney. If the inspector has an AIW or SW, the pharmacist should never refuse to allow the agent to inspect. If the inspector does not have an AIW or SW, the pharmacist must decide whether to consent to the inspection or not, depending upon the circumstances. (Remember, in some states, board inspectors do not need a warrant and consent would not be needed.) If the pharmacist denies consent but the agent insists on inspecting anyway, the pharmacist should document the conversation, obtain the agent's signature, and allow the agent to inspect. Resistance or interference could lead to arrest. The validity of the search would be determined at a later time.

Pharmacists should never lie to an agent, and generally the best course of action is to say as little as possible if the inspection is other than routine. Also, for other than routine board inspections, the pharmacist should document what is said and done during the inspection. In addition, a pharmacist should not sign anything presented by an agent unless the pharmacist completely understands what is being signed.

© Stockbyte/Thinkstock

STUDY SCENARIO

Two DEA agents walked into DrugCo Pharmacy and presented the pharmacist on duty with an administrative inspection warrant (AIW). The pharmacist informed the agents that she did not have the authority to allow them to search because the manager was not present. The agents informed her that they would proceed anyway. The audit conducted by the agents found inaccurate records of controlled substances and possible diversion. Later it was learned that the DEA inspected the pharmacy on the basis of an informant who had suspicions of diversion. The DEA charged the pharmacy with multiple violations of the CSA. The pharmacy sought to exclude all evidence obtained by the agents on the basis that the inspection was unconstitutional. The pharmacy argued no consent was given for the search, that the employee pharmacist did not have authority to allow the search, and that the agents should have produced a search warrant. Discuss these issues.

Assume now the same facts except that the inspectors were State Board of Pharmacy inspectors from your state board and they had no warrants. Based upon your state law, discuss if the search would have been legal.

OPIOID TREATMENT PROGRAMS

The incidence of illegal heroin addiction skyrocketed in the 1960s, bringing with it a host of social problems, including crime, disease, infections, and deaths. The medical community played a small role, except for a few individuals who experimented with the concept of administering methadone to addicts as a therapeutic alternative to heroin. The concept spread; however, no legal or medical standards existed to regulate methadone use and considerable diversion occurred. After intense policy debate, Congress enacted the Narcotic Addict Treatment Act of 1974, which legalized the practice and resulted in the medical community's involvement. The law required practitioners who wished to conduct maintenance or detoxification treatment for addicts using controlled substances to do so only by being separately registered by the DEA as narcotic treatment programs (NTPs). Only methadone, levo-alpha-acetyl-methadol (LAAM), buprenorphine sublingual, and buprenorphine-naloxone are approved for the treatment of narcotic addiction in these treatment programs. Physicians may not in the usual course of professional practice prescribe controlled substances to an addict in order to maintain or detoxify the addict (21 C.F.R. § 1306.07).

The law authorized the Department of Health and Human Services (actually the FDA) to establish treatment standards, and thus the FDA regulated NTPs with some overlap jurisdiction with the DEA. This system of regulation, however, was criticized as process, rather than outcome, oriented; outdated; rigid; diversion, rather than clinically oriented; and imposing unnecessary constraints on the exercise of clinical judgment. In response, the Clinton administration issued a notice of a proposed rule to address these concerns in July 1999. The regulation was published as final in March 2001 (66 Fed. Reg. 4076; 42 C.F.R. Part 8) and, after a delay while the George W. Bush administration assumed office, took effect in May 2001 (66 Fed. Reg. 15347).

The new regulation repealed FDA regulations, transferred enforcement to the Substance Abuse and Mental Health Services Administration (SAMHSA), and changed the name of the treatment programs from narcotic to opioid treatment programs (OTPs). The regulation created an entirely new system whereby practitioners intending to treat opioid addiction must apply for a certification. Certification is determined by an accreditation body that evaluates if the OTP meets the required standards. An OTP must be reaccredited and recertified every 3 years.

The regulations define detoxification treatment and maintenance treatment as follows:

> The term "detoxification treatment" means: the dispensing of an opioid agonist treatment medication in decreasing doses to an individual to alleviate adverse physiological or psychological effects incident to withdrawal from the continuous or sustained use of an opioid drug and as a method of bringing the individual to a narcotic drug-free state within such period. (Also see 21 C.F.R. § 1300.01(b)(10).)

> The term "maintenance treatment" means: the dispensing of an opioid agonist treatment medication at stable dosage levels for a period in excess of 21 days, in the treatment of an individual for opioid addiction. (Also see 21 C.F.R. § 1300.01(b)(26).)

The regulation defines opioid addiction as a cluster of cognitive, behavioral, and physiological symptoms in which the individual continues use of opiates despite significant opiate-induced problems. Opiate dependence is characterized by repeated self-administration that usually results in opiate tolerance, withdrawal symptoms, and compulsive drug taking. Dependence may occur with or without the physiological symptoms of tolerance and withdrawal.

Each person authorized or registered to engage in detoxification or maintenance activities must keep records of each narcotic controlled substance administered containing the information required by regulation (21 C.F.R. § 1304.24). More extensive recordkeeping requirements apply to compounded narcotic drugs (21 C.F.R. § 1304.25). A "compounder" is defined by regulation as any person who engages "in maintenance or detoxification treatment who also mixes, prepares, packages or changes the dosage form of a narcotic drug listed in schedules II, III, IV or V for use in maintenance or detoxification treatment by another narcotic treatment program" (21 C.F.R. § 1300.01(b)(7)).

The issue of treating addicts for their addiction within the context of differentiating addiction treatment from pain treatment is an issue of great significance in community pharmacy practice.

METHADONE

A synthetic narcotic analgesic listed in schedule II, methadone is used both for the treatment of severe pain and in the detoxification and maintenance of narcotic addicts in OTPs. In the 1970s, the FDA attempted to restrict the distribution of methadone to only a few pharmacies. The American Pharmaceutical Association successfully challenged the FDA's action in *American Pharmaceutical Association v. Weinberger*, 377 F. Supp. 824 (D.D.C. 1974), proving that the FDA did not have the authority to restrict the distribution of a prescription drug. As a result, any licensed, registered pharmacy may dispense methadone, but only for its analgesic indication. In January 2008, the DEA issued an advisory that manufacturers had voluntarily agreed to restrict the distribution of 40 mg methadone tablets to OTPs (http://www.deadiversion.usdoj.gov/pubs/advisories/methadone_advisory.htm). The restriction was imposed in an effort to curb an increase in adverse events. Some prescribers, not aware of the differences between methadone and other opioids, especially short-acting opioids, failed to dose patients properly, leading to toxic overdoses. Even though methadone is also an antitussive, it may not legally be prescribed or dispensed for this purpose. It cannot be overemphasized that the drug may not be prescribed or dispensed for the maintenance or detoxification of addicts in the regular course of medical practice.

TREATMENT OF ADDICTS OUTSIDE OF OTPS (DATA)

In 2000, Congress created a landmark exception to the rule that controlled substances may not be prescribed or dispensed for opioid addiction other than in OTPs by enacting a law called the Drug Addiction Treatment Act (DATA) (P.L. 106-310). The law resulted from concern that OTPs were not accessible to many addicts, especially those in more rural areas, and concern because many addicts shunned treatment for fear of stigmatization if seen at the clinic by people they know.

DATA provides for office-based treatment of opioid-dependent patients by amending the CSA to allow "qualifying physicians" to prescribe and dispense schedules III, IV, and V opioids that have been approved by the FDA for maintenance or detoxification treatment. The FDA did not approve any drug for this purpose until 2002, when it approved buprenorphine sublingual tablets (Subutex) and buprenorphine-naloxone tablets (Suboxone). A "qualifying physician" is defined in part as a physician board certified in addiction psychiatry or addiction medicine or, alternately, who has at least 8 hours of authorized training in the treatment and management of opioid-dependent patients. Each qualifying physician may not treat more than 30 opioid-dependent patients at a time for the first year. After 1 year, the physician can submit a notification of the need and intent to treat up to 100 opioid-dependent patients. To prescribe under DATA, the physicians must obtain a special DEA number. Because then-current DEA regulations did not allow practitioners to engage in the prescribing of controlled substances for the treatment of addicts, the DEA promulgated new regulations in order to comply with DATA. (See 70 Fed. Reg. 36338, June 23, 2005.)

Subutex is intended for beginning treatment and will likely be administered by physicians from their offices directly to the patient. Pharmacists should contact the physician for verification if they receive a prescription for Subutex. Community pharmacists more likely receive prescriptions for Suboxone, preferred for long-term therapy. (The naloxone is added to deter people from crushing and injecting the tablets.) If a patient presents prescriptions from more than one physician during the same time period, pharmacists should refuse to fill the prescriptions and notify the prescribers. Pharmacists and physicians can learn much more information about the use of Subutex and Suboxone for the treatment of addicts under DATA at http://buprenorphine.samhsa.gov/faq.html#A10.

© Stockbyte/Thinkstock

STUDY SCENARIO

A pharmacist received a prescription for methadone. Upon calling the prescriber, the pharmacist learned that the purpose of the prescription was to maintain an addiction. The physician informed the pharmacist he was treating the patient under DATA, but was not knowledgeable about the requirements to do so. Inform the physician of the requirements to be a qualifying physician and if methadone could be prescribed under this program.

LAWS RELATED TO THE CONTROLLED SUBSTANCES ACT

THE CONTROLLED SUBSTANCE REGISTRANT PROTECTION ACT OF 1984

Robberies, burglaries, and violent crimes are a constant threat to many pharmacists. In an effort to address these crimes, Congress passed the Controlled Substance Registrant Protection Act of 1984. Before the passage of this act, it was not a violation of federal law when a criminal robbed a pharmacy of controlled substances. Pharmacists were concerned that the convictions and punishments under state laws regarding controlled substance crimes were inadequate and had lobbied vigorously for the act's passage. The Controlled Substance Registrant Protection Act mandates that a federal investigation occur if any of the following conditions are met:

- The replacement cost of the controlled substances taken is $500 or greater.
- A registrant or other person is killed or suffers "significant" injury.
- Interstate or foreign commerce is involved in the planning or execution of the crime.

Originally, the act required that the replacement cost of the controlled substances taken be $5,000 or greater before a federal investigation would occur. Pharmacists complained that this threshold amount excluded most pharmacy crimes from the act and succeeded in having the amount reduced to $500.

Penalties under the act for robbery or burglary can result in a maximum of 20 years' imprisonment, a maximum $25,000 fine, or both. If a dangerous weapon is used in the commission of the crime, the penalty could be a maximum of 25 years' imprisonment, a fine up to $35,000, or both. If a death results from the crime, the penalty could be life imprisonment, a maximum fine of $50,000, or both.

THE CHEMICAL DIVERSION AND TRAFFICKING ACT OF 1988

In an effort to curb the illicit manufacture of controlled substances, Congress in 1988 passed the Chemical Diversion and Trafficking Act. This law places under federal control 20 chemicals and the tableting and encapsulating machines that are known to be commonly used in the illegal manufacture of controlled substances. Some of these chemicals, including their salts and isomers, are anthranilic acid, benzyl cyanide, ephedrine, ergotamine, ergonovine, norpseudoephedrine, phenylacetic acid, phenylpropanolamine, acetone, benzyl chloride, ethyl ether, and toluene. The act allows the federal government to add or delete chemicals by rulemaking if warranted.

Manufacturers and suppliers of these chemicals and machines must verify the legitimacy of customers before concluding transactions. They must also maintain records of transactions and report certain transactions to the DEA.

THE ANABOLIC STEROIDS ACT OF 2004

Chemically and pharmacologically related to testosterone, anabolic steroids promote muscle growth. Despite the fact that anabolic steroids are legend drugs, athletes have obtained them easily, with or without prescriptions. Moreover, many athletes extensively misused steroids in an attempt to increase their muscle mass and improve their athletic performance. The result for many athletes has been serious permanent physical injury and cancer.

The serious consequences of the abuse of anabolic steroids prompted Congress to amend the FDCA in 1988 to impose criminal penalties on anyone who distributed or possessed anabolic steroids for purposes other than the treatment of disease pursuant to prescription (21 U.S.C. § 333(e)). The amendment, however, failed to slow the abuse of anabolic steroids, forcing Congress to enact the Anabolic Steroids Control Act of 1990 (P.L. 101-647), making anabolic steroids for human use schedule III substances under the CSA. The 1990 law was in turn amended by the Anabolic Steroids Act of 2004 (P.L. 108-358), making several changes to the 1990 law including:

- Amending the definition of anabolic steroids, eliminating the requirement to prove muscle growth
- Replacing the list of 23 steroids with a list of 59 steroids, including precursors such as androstenedione (andro)
- Providing for automatic scheduling of salts, esters, and ethers of schedule III anabolic steroids without the need to prove they promote muscle growth
- Excluding certain OTC products from regulation

The 2004 law thus provides the DEA considerably more flexibility to immediately schedule steroid precursors, without having to play catch-up with every variation that enters the market.

The inclusion of anabolic steroids in schedule III has provided the government with more weapons to stem the abuse of these steroids. Nonetheless, anabolic steroids are an anomaly in schedule III. They have not been found to have moderate or low physical dependence, or high psychological dependence, as is the requirement for the other drugs in this schedule.

THE COMBAT METHAMPHETAMINE EPIDEMIC ACT (CMEA) OF 2005 AND THE METHAMPHETAMINE PREVENTION ACT OF 2008

Concern over the rampant illegal manufacture and use of methamphetamine resulted in Congress passing the Combat Methamphetamine Epidemic Act (CMEA) of 2005 (Title VII of the USA Patriot Improvement and Reauthorization Act, P.L. 109-177); amended in 2008 by the Methamphetamine Prevention Act (MPA) (P.L. 110-415). The CMEA regulates the OTC sale of any product containing ephedrine, pseudoephedrine (PSE), or phenylpropanolamine (PPA) by placing them into a new category of the CSA known as "scheduled listed chemical products (SLCP)." These products have been commonly purchased in large quantities as precursor chemicals to manufacture methamphetamine. For example, a pharmacy in California reportedly sold 550,000 PSE tablets to a single individual in five orders over a 3-month period. Pharmacists must reconcile the Combat Methamphetamine Epidemic Act with state laws. If state law is stricter, the state law must be followed.

Sale Quantity and Storage Restrictions

Under the CMEA, a regulated seller (i.e., a grocery store, general merchandise store, drug store) may not sell OTC more than 3.6 g of ephedrine base, PSE base, or PPA base to a single purchaser per day, regardless of the number of transactions. Additionally, no consumer may purchase more than 9 g of the listed products within a 30-day period, or 7.5 g within a 30-day period if purchased by mail order. (Conversion tables as to how many tablets or milliliters of base can legally be sold can be found at http://www .deadiversion.usdoj.gov/meth/cma2005.htm.) Generally, all nonliquid forms of the products must be sold in two-unit blister packs or unit dose packaging.

The products must be stored behind the counter or in a locked cabinet in an area where customers do not have direct access. (Some states have stricter laws, requiring that the products may only be sold from the pharmacy department.)

Recordkeeping Requirements

All sales, except those of 60 mg or less of PSE, must be recorded in a written or electronic logbook that identifies the product by name, the quantity sold, the name and address of the purchaser, and the date and time of the sale. The purchaser must sign the logbook. Although the CMEA does not mandate electronic logbooks, Congress hopes that all pharmacies will ultimately employ electronic logbooks and share the information with other pharmacies and law enforcement through a common electronic network. The MPA allows for federal grants to states to develop electronic logbook systems and to collaborate their logbook systems to prevent "smurfing" across state lines. Several states now require the electronic tracking of PSE sales.

Sellers may capture much of the required logbook information electronically by means of a bar code reader or similar technology. The seller or purchaser may enter the purchaser's name, address, and date and time of sale. If the purchaser enters the information, the seller must verify it. If the seller enters the information, the purchaser must verify that the information is correct. The seller may collect the purchaser's signature by any of three means:

- Signing an electronic signature device
- Signing a bound paper book where the signature is adjacent to a unique identifier number or printed sticker linking the signature to the logbook information
- Signing a document that the seller prints at the time of sale, displaying the required logbook information

The log must warn the purchaser of misrepresentation and include the maximum fine and term of imprisonment for misrepresentation. The log record must be maintained for 2 years after the last entry. Except for purchases of 60 mg or less of PSE, all purchasers must show a federal- or state-issued photographic identification or identification acceptable by the Immigration and Naturalization Service or Department of Homeland Security and the seller must verify that the name in the logbook corresponds to the name on the identification.

Self-Certification

The CMEA requires all sellers of SLCPs to annually self-certify. By self-certifying, the seller is attesting to the following:

- Employees engaged in the sale of SLCPs have undergone appropriate training (as designated by the DEA).
- Records of training are maintained.
- Sale quantity restrictions are followed.
- Nonliquid forms are packaged as required.
- SLCPs are stored behind the counter or locked in a cabinet.
- Recordkeeping requirements are followed and maintained.
- Logbook information is disclosed only as required by law.

Self-certification can occur only through the DEA's Diversion website (http://www.deadiversion.usdoj.gov). A certificate is generated upon receipt of the application that the seller may print, or the DEA will print and mail it to the seller. It is the seller's responsibility to renew the certificate annually before it expires.

U.S. POSTAL LAWS: MAILING CONTROLLED SUBSTANCES

In 1994 the U.S. Postal Service enacted final regulations removing restrictions on the mailing of controlled substances (59 Fed. Reg. 50690; 39 C.F.R. 111). Under current regulations controlled substances may be mailed with the U.S. Postal service provided the following preparation and packaging standards are met:

- The inner container of any parcel containing controlled substances must be marked and sealed pursuant to any relevant provisions in the CSA and its regulations, and placed in a plain outer container or securely wrapped in plain paper.
- If the controlled substances consist of prescription medicines, the inner container must also be labeled to show the name and address of the pharmacy, practitioner, or other person dispensing the prescription.
- The outside wrapper or container must be free of markings that would indicate the nature of the contents.

© Stockbyte/Thinkstock

STUDY SCENARIO

A consumer angrily approached the pharmacist on duty and asked where the pharmacy was hiding the PSE products. The pharmacist politely informed the patient that the pharmacy kept the drug behind the prescription counter in order to comply with the law. The patient then asked for four boxes of 30 tablets each of PSE HCl 30-mg tablets. Explain if the pharmacy can sell the patient this much drug and what legal requirements must be met to do so.

REFERENCES

U.S. Drug Enforcement Administration Diversion Control Program website: http://www.deadiversion.usdoj.gov

U.S. Department of Health and Human Services, Substance Abuse and Mental Health Services Administration (SAMHSA) website: http://www.samhsa.gov

BIBLIOGRAPHY

Alpers, A. Criminal act or palliative care? Prosecutions involving the care of the dying. *Journal of Law, Medicine and Ethics* 26 (1998): 308–331.

American Pharmacists Association. Legislative and Regulatory Updates. Available at: http://www.pharmacist.com

American Society for Pharmacy Law. Available at: http://www.aspl.org

Boatwright, D. E. Buprenorphine and addiction: Challenges for the pharmacist. *Journal of the American Pharmaceutical Association* 42, no. 3 (2002): 432–438.

Brody, R. Is the DEA on your case? *American Druggist* 203, no. 6 (1991): 27.

Molinari, S. P., J. R. Cooper, and D. J. Czechowicz. Federal regulation of clinical practice in narcotic addiction treatment: Purpose, status, and alternatives. *Journal of Law, Medicine and Ethics* 22 (1994): 231–239.

National Community Pharmacists Association. *Governmental Affairs/Legal Proceedings*. Available at: http://www.ncpanet.org

Uelmen, F. G., and V. G. Haddox. *Drug Abuse and the Law*. St. Paul, MN: West Publishing Co., 1974.

U.S. Department of Justice, Office of Diversion Control. *Pharmacist's Manual: An Informational Outline of the Controlled Substances Act of 1970*. Revised 2010. Available at: http://www.deadiversion.usdoj.gov/pubs/manuals/index.html.

© Junial Enterprises/ShutterStock, Inc.

CASE STUDIES

CASE 4-1   *State v. Rasmussen, 213 N.W.2d 661 (Iowa 1973)*

Issue

Whether the Iowa Uniform Controlled Substances Act prohibits Iowa pharmacies from dispensing controlled substances prescribed by nonresident physicians, not registered to prescribe controlled substances in Iowa.

Overview

Congress passed the federal Controlled Substances Act in 1970 with the purpose of establishing a uniform system of regulation of controlled substances in partnership with the states. In this case, an Iowa law has been interpreted by the board of pharmacy as prohibiting the filling of controlled substance prescriptions from out-of-state prescribers unless the prescribers were licensed in Iowa. As you read this case, consider: Why is it important that Iowa not be allowed to apply its interpretation of the law? Why is national uniformity important in the regulation of controlled substances? What might be the real motivation behind the board of pharmacy bringing this lawsuit?

The facts of this case are as follows:

> Defendant, Federal Prescription Service, Inc., is a pharmacy located at Madrid (Iowa), and is registered under both federal and Iowa law to dispense controlled substances. Defendant Rasmussen is the manager of the pharmacy. Defendant pharmacy receives prescriptions by mail, fills them and returns them by mail to the person to whom the prescription was issued. Some of such prescriptions received by mail are written by nonresident physicians who are not registered to prescribe controlled substances by the Iowa issuing authority, the Iowa Board of Pharmacy Examiners.

The Iowa attorney general on behalf of the Iowa Board of Pharmacy Examiners sought a permanent injunction to prevent the defendants from filling controlled substance prescriptions written by the nonresident physicians. The trial court found for the defendant pharmacy, deciding that the Iowa Uniform Controlled Substances Act was intended to regulate only intrastate transactions of controlled substances and that registration under the federal Controlled Substances Act constituted compliance with the Iowa Act. The state then appealed to the Iowa Supreme Court.

> The parties are in agreement that the Iowa Act prohibits the filling by Iowa pharmacists of prescriptions written by physicians resident in Iowa who are not registered by the Iowa authorities to prescribe controlled substances. We are asked to determine whether registration of a nonresident physician under the federal Act pertaining to drugs is sufficient to permit a resident pharmacist to fill a prescription of such nonresident physician, and whether the Iowa Uniform Controlled Substances Act is intended to regulate only intrastate transactions.

The court then proceeded with its analysis of the issue, starting with the relevant Iowa law and then examining the objectives of the federal CSA.

> Dispense "means to deliver a controlled substance to an ultimate user or research subject by or pursuant to the lawful order of a practitioner, including the prescribing, administering, packaging, labeling, or compounding necessary to prepare the substance for that delivery."

> "Practitioner" means either:

> "a. A physician, dentist, veterinarian, scientific investigator, or other person licensed, registered or otherwise permitted to distribute, dispense, conduct research with respect to or to administer a controlled substance in the course of professional practice or research in this state.

> b. A pharmacy, hospital or other institution licensed, registered, or otherwise permitted to distribute, dispense, conduct research with respect to or to administer a controlled substance in the course of professional practice or research in this state."

> The Uniform Controlled Substances Act was promulgated by the National Conference of Commissioners on Uniform State Laws at its annual conference at St. Louis in

August of 1970. The following is excerpted from the prefatory note to the Uniform Act then drafted by the Conference:

This Uniform Act was drafted to achieve uniformity between the laws of the several States and those of the Federal government. It has been designed to complement the new Federal narcotic and dangerous drug legislation and provide an interlocking trellis of Federal and State law to enable government at all levels to control more effectively the drug abuse problem.

Much of this major increase in drug use and abuse is attributable to the increased mobility of our citizens and their affluence. As modern American society becomes increasingly mobile, drugs clandestinely manufactured or illegally diverted from legitimate channels in one part of a State are easily transported for sale to another part of that State or even to another State. Nowhere is this mobility manifested with greater impact than in the legitimate pharmaceutical industry. The lines of distribution of the products of this major national industry cross in and out of a State innumerable times during the manufacturing or distribution processes. To assure the continued free movement of controlled substances between States, while at the same time securing such States against drug diversion from legitimate sources, it becomes critical to approach not only the control of illicit and legitimate traffic in these substances at the national and international levels but also to approach this problem at the State and local level on a uniform basis.

Another objective of this Act is to establish a closed regulatory system for the legitimate handlers of controlled drugs in order better to prevent illicit drug diversion. This system will require that these individuals register with a designated State agency, maintain records, and make biennial inventories of all controlled drug stocks.

We must presume the Iowa legislature, in adopting the Uniform Controlled Substances Act, intended to come within the scheme of complementary federal-state control of the distribution of drugs and to create an "interlocking trellis" to assure effectiveness of the Act.

Plaintiff argues the prescribing of drugs is an integral part of the practice of medicine, and that when a prescription is filled in Iowa by a pharmacist that such filling of prescription constitutes the practice of medicine in Iowa and that the practice should not be permitted to circumvent the licensing requirements of Iowa while carrying on a professional practice elsewhere. Plaintiff further argues that the State "cannot be certain that physicians who are registered by other states are competent to prescribe drugs which are dispensed by pharmacies in Iowa," and therefore the State of Iowa should be able to prohibit all practitioners not registered with the Iowa authorities from filling prescriptions in Iowa.

We conclude the construction placed upon the Iowa statute by plaintiff would bring about a positive conflict in policy so that the two statutes (the Iowa Act and the federal CSA) could not consistently stand together.

A holding by this court that the Iowa Act applies to all practitioners attempting to have their prescriptions filled in Iowa would present constitutional problems under the commerce clause of the United States Constitution, as such construction would impose unreasonable burdens on interstate commerce.

If a state statute, on its face, is for the protection of local economic benefit, such a statute is per se unconstitutional as it would place an undue burden on interstate commerce.

The Iowa statute does not discriminate in its language between foreign practitioners and those registered in Iowa—all are required to register under the provisions of the Iowa Act in order to dispense drugs in Iowa. We do not regard such a provision as being per se unconstitutional. However, if the effect of the law is to insulate in-state business against interstate competition (assuming for sake of argument no preemption problem), it is our responsibility to balance the purpose of the Act with its effect, and to assess the State's interest in adopting that particular statute in light of any reasonable alternatives available. In the absence of conflicting legislation by Congress, this court is the final arbiter of the competing demands of state and national interests.

The court noted that it does not question the right of a state to regulate the licensing standards of practitioners for the health and safety of its citizens. However, continued the court, this right of the state must be balanced against the need for national uniformity in controlling drug trafficking.

The need for national registration was anticipated by Congress, although it permitted the mechanics of registration to be adopted or at least supplemented by the several states. The federal authority issues licenses to dispense to accomplish the purposes of federal legislation for the control of drug abuse, and has therefore acted definitively with respect to the interstate prescriber of controlled substances. Such an interest clearly outweighs any local interest that Iowa might have in allowing only practitioners registered in this state to prescribe here, and for pharmacists in this state to fill prescriptions emanating from out-of-state.

We therefore affirm the trial court.

Notes on *State v. Rasmussen*

1. The Iowa court held that Congress did not intend to preempt state law by enacting the CSA and thus the states can pass their own controlled substance laws. A state has broad authority and considerable latitude to enact laws to protect the public health, safety, and welfare. There are limits, however, one being that the state law cannot conflict with the objective of a federal law. One objective of the CSA is to achieve national uniformity to prevent drug diversion. In this case the court felt that if the Iowa law was interpreted as the board intended, this would conflict with the objective of the CSA. The court, however, never completely articulated why. Ask yourself: How would prohibiting pharmacies from dispensing out-of-state controlled substance prescriptions frustrate this objective of the CSA? Would not the board's interpretation actually help prevent diversion because many pharmacists are leery to fill out-of-state controlled substance prescriptions because of fear that they might not be legitimate?

2. As part of the CSA's objective of achieving national uniformity, Congress has declared the jurisdiction of the act to include the intrastate manufacture and distribution of controlled substances. Normally, federal law can only regulate interstate commerce and only incidentally regulate intrastate commerce. However, Congress has determined, and the courts have agreed, that drug diversion is an issue of critical national importance and that intrastate activities are so integrated with interstate activities that differentiation is impossible.

3. One has to surmise that the real reason the board interpreted the Iowa law as it did was to obstruct the business of mail-order pharmacy. Notice that the court commented that a law that protects local economic benefit from interstate competition might impose an unreasonable burden on interstate commerce and thus be unconstitutional. However, after bringing up the interstate commerce issue, the court avoided it by deciding that the board's interpretation would conflict with the CSA. Thus, it never had to reach the interstate commerce determination, but most likely the court would have found against the state on this issue

as well. In fact, in the past few years, states have been warned that any law that imposes undue restrictions on mail-order pharmacies, such as requiring them to have state licensure, might violate the interstate commerce clause.

CASE 4-2	*Lemmon Company v. State Board of Medical Examiners*, 417 A.2d 568 (N.J. Super. 1980)

Issue

Whether a regulation enacted by the New Jersey Board of Medical Examiners proscribing the medical use of schedule II amphetamines or amphetamine-type drugs in the treatment of exogenous obesity is valid.

Overview

Medical boards have the authority to regulate the practice of medicine, in part through rulemaking. Technically speaking, administrative agencies cannot make new law through rulemaking. Rather, regulations must be based on a statute that grants the agency the authority to regulate that particular subject. Regulations then often are enacted to explain or add details to a law. Sometimes, however, it is difficult to tell whether the agency is acting pursuant to statute or indeed making law. Often courts give administrative agencies a fair amount of discretion when the means are necessary to achieve a governmental objective. In this case, the medical board has issued a regulation that would prevent prescribers from exercising individual professional judgment with respect to treating patients for weight loss with amphetamines. This use is permitted under both the FDCA and the CSA. As you read this case, consider the following: Has the board exceeded the scope of its authority with this regulation? In other words, does the statute cited by the court as authority for the regulation really grant the board this authority? Does the regulation conflict with federal law? Has the board gone too far in its proscription? On the basis of this decision, could a state board enact a regulation making amphetamines schedule I? On the basis of this decision, could a state board determine that schedule II opioids cannot be used to treat nonchronic pain?

The facts of this case can be summarized as follows:

The New Jersey Board of Medical Examiners enacted a regulation that provides that no physician shall use schedule II amphetamines or amphetamine-type drugs for weight management, dieting, or any other anorectic purpose. The appellants challenging the regulation include the Lemmon Company and Boehringer Inglehelm.

The court first noted the positions of the opposing parties as follows:

Without becoming overly involved in the factual-medical intricacies of the matter, the essential controversy reflected in the arguments made to us and the material on file with the Board concerns the relationship between the benefits to be derived from use of such drugs in the treatment of obesity and the hazards to the patient and to the public from the medically prescribed use of such drugs for such a condition. Those who oppose the regulation deplore what they view as the Draconian means to curb the abuse and unlawful trafficking in amphetamines by proscribing entirely its use in weight management. They point to approval of amphetamines by the Federal Food and Drug Administration as being effective and safe in weight control in short-term use and under careful medical supervision. Those in support of the regulation point to authoritative opinion, which we view as reflecting the clearly preponderant medical view on this record, that the benefits to be derived from the use of amphetamines and their schedule II counterparts are marginal, and are in any event clearly outweighed by the substantial risk of physical and psychic dependence by the patient and the abuse by others who unlawfully obtain the prescribed drug. Moreover, they refer to other drugs of equal effectiveness which are available as adjuncts to calorie control in weight management programs without subjecting the patient and public to risks associated with amphetamine use. The challenged regulation reflects the Board's adoption of this latter view and carefully limits the use of schedule II amphetamines and amphetamine-like drugs to a few syndromes unassociated with obesity for which they are recognized as being effective and proscribing entirely their use in the treatment of exogenous obesity.

The court then proceeded with its analysis of the issues.

The most fundamental challenge is to the Board's power to adopt the regulation. Appellants contend that the board's proscription against physician use of schedule II drugs in the treatment of obesity is unnecessary, is inconsistent with state and federal law, and is, accordingly, in conflict with the statute empowering the Board to adopt rules and regulations.

We disagree with all these contentions. The Board's rule-making power derives, in the final analysis, from its need to "perform the duties" and "transact the business" which the Legislature imposed upon it by specific statutory provision. A rule becomes necessary when it implements a Board obligation. As long as a rule is reasonably related to a legislatively imposed duty of the Board, it will be regarded by this court as complying with the "necessary" standard.

The court found that the board's power to adopt the regulation comes from section 45:1–13 of New Jersey law, which provides:

It shall be a valid ground for the refusal to grant, revocation or suspension of a license to practice a health care profession, subject to regulation in this State, including the practice of pharmacy, or for the refusal to admit to an examination a candidate for licensure, that the licensee has prescribed or dispensed a controlled dangerous substance or substances, as defined by the "New Jersey Controlled Dangerous Substances Act" (P.L. 1970, c. 226) (C. 24:21-1 et seq.), in an indiscriminate manner, or not in good faith, or without good cause, or where the licensee reasonably knows or should have known that the substance or substances prescribed are to be used for unauthorized or illicit consumption or distribution or that a substance or substances previously prescribed or dispensed were used by the patient for unauthorized or illicit consumption or distribution.

By the rule under discussion, the Board has endeavored to give advance notice to doctors and surgeons subject to its jurisdiction that it will not regard the treatment of exogenous obesity as "good cause" for the prescription of schedule II amphetamines or amphetamine-like drugs. In our view, the Board has power to discipline a physician for such conduct in the absence of a rule. Accordingly, it must have the power to advise physicians in advance, by rule, of what it proposes to do. The material on file with the Board overwhelmingly supports the Board's position reflected in this regulation.

We do not regard the regulation as being in conflict with federal law as appellants contend. That the Federal Food and Drug Administration has recognized the utility of amphetamines in weight management programs when used over the short term and carefully supervised does not produce conflict with the challenged regulation. The federal view permits, does not command, amphetamines to be used in the treatment of obesity. The Board is not by this regulation forbidding what federal law mandates be done.

The appellants also argued that the regulation conflicted with state law because the board does not have the responsibility to classify controlled substances. The court, however, found no conflict because the board was not classifying controlled substances but merely announcing its position on the use of amphetamines in treating obesity.

The contention of the appellant association of physicians that the regulation violates a patient's constitutional right of privacy is clearly without merit. There is no question but that to the extent a physician is not permitted to prescribe schedule II amphetamines as treatment for obesity, his judgment in that regard has been superseded by the Board. The same, however, is true with respect to any drug whose use is totally proscribed, such as those on schedule I. There are, no doubt, doctors who would prescribe heroin for terminal cancer patients if they were legally permitted to do so. That they are not so permitted by current law is not, however, a violation of their patient's right of privacy. The same is true with respect to the permitted uses of schedule II amphetamines. A physician's right to practice his profession, and prescribe drugs, is as subject to law as is any other profession.

The challenged regulation concerns the dispensing of controlled dangerous substances, albeit by a physician's prescription. The government's vital concern with the movement and disbursement of such narcotic and addictive substances is too clear to require citation. Although the means chosen by the Board to implement the policy expressed in N.J.S.A. 45:1–13 may be open to debate, there can be no doubt but that those means are at least reasonably related to such a purpose. That other means exist or that some would employ such other means, or that such other means would yield better results in the opinion of some, does not disrupt the reasonable relationship between regulation and legitimate governmental objective which clearly exists in this matter.

In summary, the challenged regulation represents an exercise of the Board's power to implement legislative policy described in N.J.S.A. 45:1–13, a necessary regulation not inconsistent with state or federal law, or in violation of state or federal constitutional guarantees. The regulation is reasonably related to the legitimate governmental objective of controlling the traffic in controlled dangerous substances, and the means chosen to deal with this problem, although open to debate, finds more than substantial support in the record of this appeal.

The court affirmed the lower court's decision.

Notes on *Lemmon Company v. State Board of Medical Examiners*

1. The use of amphetamines for weight loss has a long history of controversy and abuse. Amphetamines have been freely prescribed by physicians who have not performed examinations or taken medical histories. Many of the patients never even had obesity problems. The magnitude of the amphetamine abuse problem prompted the DEA to place the drugs in schedule II in the 1970s. The New Jersey Medical Board felt that even further action was necessary to stop amphetamine abuse because the risks outweighed the benefits, and thus passed the regulation. One does have to question the board's authority for the regulation. The statute relied on appears to give the board case-by-case authority to discipline individual practitioners for inappropriate prescribing and dispensing. The court felt that because the board has the authority without regulation to discipline prescribers for prescribing without good cause, it has the authority to give prescribers advance notice of what is not good cause. However, by its regulation, the board has declared that in all cases the use of amphetamines for obesity is not for a good cause. Whether this action is within the intent of the statute raises a legitimate concern. From another perspective, it is generally lawful and desirable for administrative agencies to define and give examples of acts that clarify vague terms. The court indicated that the board's approach to regulating amphetamine abuse was open to debate, but because it was reasonably related to the purpose, the court felt that the approach was justifiable.

2. This case also raises the question of just how far a board can go to prevent diversion and abuse. Could it, for example, prohibit the use of schedule II opioids for certain types of pain because certain members of the board believe other treatments are more appropriate? This action would be unlikely without substantial proof of diversion, abuse, or safety problems. Otherwise, these regulations would be invalidated on the basis of being arbitrary and capricious. The board's regulation is not at odds with the CSA. In fact, the board could classify amphetamines as schedule I if it could substantiate a significant public health threat.

3. The regulation would not conflict with the FDCA. Labeling approved by the FDA is permissive, not mandatory.

CASE 4-3	*Seeley v. State of Washington*, 940 P.2d 604 (Wash. 1997)

Issue

Whether a Washington state law restricting marijuana to schedule I, thus precluding its use for medical treatment, violates the Washington Constitution.

Overview

For years terminally ill patients have advocated that marijuana effectively controls the nausea and other side effects produced by chemotherapeutic drugs. Nonetheless, marijuana is listed as a schedule I drug under the federal CSA and under state laws. Schedule I drugs have no accepted medical use and thus cannot be prescribed or dispensed. Some states, such as California, have passed referendums allowing the use of marijuana for medical purposes. In these states, patients with a legitimate medical need, as certified by a physician, may grow marijuana for their own personal use. However, this does not change the fact that marijuana may not be prescribed, dispensed, or legally purchased.

In this case, Seeley contends that his constitutional rights are violated, in particular his right of equal protection under the law, because he is prohibited by law from being prescribed marijuana by his doctor. Seeley argues that he has a "fundamental right" to be prescribed marijuana. Plaintiffs bringing equal protection lawsuits often argue that their right allegedly being violated is not just any right, but a "fundamental right." If the court agrees, the state and federal laws in question face a much higher degree of judicial scrutiny. As you read this case, consider whether patients have a right to be prescribed and to take whatever medication they choose, and, if so, is it a "fundamental right"? Also consider these issues: What is the governmental interest in preventing terminally ill patients from obtaining marijuana? Is the governmental interest greater than the individual interest, and why? Also, evaluate the strength of the dissent's arguments discussed in the note after the case.

The Washington Supreme Court related the facts of the case as follows:

> The Respondent, Mr. Seeley, was diagnosed with chordoma, a rare form of bone cancer, in 1986. Mr. Seeley has undergone numerous surgeries including the removal of his right lung and a removal of part of the lower lobe of his left lung. Mr. Seeley also suffers from "severe Obstructive Airway Disease." Mr. Seeley's condition is diagnosed as terminal.

> Throughout his battle with cancer, Mr. Seeley has received radiation therapy and chemotherapy. Mr. Seeley was treated with various chemotherapeutic agents which commonly produce nausea and vomiting. He was treated with synthetic tetrahydro-

cannabinol (THC) (Marinol or dronabinol) and other antiemetic drugs for the nausea and vomiting, which resulted from the chemotherapy. Mr. Seeley has also smoked marijuana during chemotherapy. Mr. Seeley prefers smoking marijuana to control these side effects. Mr. Seeley states that smoking marijuana has been more effective in relieving his symptoms than other antiemetics.

The court continued its findings of fact by noting that marijuana is regulated by both the federal government and the state, each of which lists marijuana as a schedule I controlled substance. As such, marijuana cannot be legally prescribed or dispensed in Washington.

Seeley filed a lawsuit asking for a declaratory judgment that the Washington law categorizing marijuana as a schedule I controlled substance violates the constitution of the state of Washington. He also sought an order directing the board of pharmacy to reclassify marijuana so that it may be prescribed for those who have a legitimate medical need for its therapeutic effects. The county superior court granted Seeley's motion for summary judgment, finding that the placement of marijuana in schedule I violated his constitutional rights and the state appealed to the Washington Supreme Court.

The Washington Supreme Court then proceeded to examine the rationale of Seeley's arguments, noting that although he raised various constitutional issues, the one most pertinent is that his constitutional right of equal protection was violated. The Fourteenth Amendment to the U.S. Constitution provides that no state shall deny any person equal protection under the law.

> In an equal protection analysis this court must first determine the standard of review against which to test the challenged legislation. Respondent contends that the legislative decision placing marijuana in schedule I threatens a fundamental right and is therefore entitled to strict scrutiny. If governmental action threatens a "fundamental right," the classification will be upheld only if it is necessary to accomplish a compelling state interest.

> This court has held that "[t]he right to smoke marijuana is not fundamental to the American scheme of justice, it is not necessary to ordered liberty, and it is not within a zone of privacy." Other federal and state courts have agreed that possession of marijuana is not a fundamental right guaranteed by the United States Constitution.

> Here, Respondent asserts a constitutionally protected interest in having his physician prescribe marijuana, an unapproved drug which is regulated as a schedule I controlled substance, for medical treatment. In an equally compelling case, the United States Supreme Court recently held that terminally ill patients do not have a constitutionally protected right to physician assisted suicide nor did they constitute a suspect class for purposes of an equal protection analysis. Thus, it is apparent from the case law that although the Respondent is facing a terminal illness, he is not part of a suspect class nor does he have a fundamental right to have marijuana prescribed as his preferred treatment over the legitimate objections of the state.

Rejecting the strict scrutiny analysis, the court noted that the proper standard in this case is the rational basis test. Under this test, the legislation will be upheld, unless the classification created by the law is irrelevant to achieve a legitimate state interest.

> Respondent argues that (1) no rational basis exists for classifying marijuana as a schedule I controlled substance, and (2) comparable drugs such as cocaine, morphine, and methamphetamines are not similarly classified. First, we will address Respondent's contention that marijuana's placement on schedule I is irrational because it is an effective medical treatment for the nausea and vomiting associated with chemotherapy.

To support his first argument that no rational basis exists for the classification of marijuana as a schedule I drug, Seeley cited an administrative law judge (ALJ) ruling (in a hearing before the DEA) finding that marijuana has an accepted medical use and should be rescheduled. The court rejected this argument, however, because the administrator of the DEA did not even follow the ALJ's ruling. The administrator found that the evidence submitted and relied on by experts lacked scientific credibility. Furthermore, the court was provided reliable evidence that showed that currently available therapies are more effective and do not carry the same risks attributable to marijuana.

> The State maintains that placing marijuana in schedule I is rationally related to the state's dual interest in controlling potential drug abuse and assuring efficacy and safety in medicines. Respondent argues that placing marijuana in schedule I is not rationally related to the State's purpose of preventing drug abuse. Respondent maintains that placing marijuana in schedule II could not possibly contribute to the drug abuse problem because marijuana would be available only by prescription. However, the Legislature could reasonably consider marijuana's widespread availability and its pattern of abuse as requiring a different legislative response than to other substances. "It is enough that there is an evil at hand for correction, and that it might be thought that the particular legislative measure was a rational way to correct it."

Respondent Seeley introduced physicians to testify that marijuana is a safe and effective medicine for controlling the vomiting and nausea associated with cancer chemotherapy. The state countered with the testimony of physicians stating that there is no scientific basis for marijuana's safety and efficacy. On the basis of all this testimony and the history of marijuana, the court concluded:

> The challenged legislation involves conclusions concerning a myriad of complicated medical, psychological and moral issues of considerable controversy. We are not prepared on this limited record to conclude that the legislature could not reasonably conclude that marijuana should be placed in schedule I of controlled substances. It is clear not only from the record in this case but also from the long history of marijuana's treatment under the law that disagreement persists concerning the health effects of marijuana use and its effectiveness as a medicinal drug. The evidence presented by the Respondent is insufficient to convince this court that it should interfere with the broad judicially recognized prerogative of the legislature. Respondent has not shown that the legislative treatment of marijuana is "so unrelated" to the achievement of the legitimate purposes of the legislature or that "the facts have so far changed as to render the classification arbitrary and obsolete."

> Respondent also attacks the rationality of the classification scheme, arguing that it is under-inclusive. Respondent makes an equal protection challenge asserting that marijuana's classification is irrational because other more harmful substances such as cocaine, morphine, and methamphetamine are not similarly classified in schedule I and, thus, can be prescribed by a physician. Respondent also maintains that it is arbitrary to place marijuana in schedule I while classifying the synthetic form of THC, otherwise known as Marinol, in schedule II.

The court replied that to prevail in an under-inclusive claim, the plaintiff must show that the governmental choice is clearly wrong, a display of arbitrary power, not an exercise of judgment. The court continued:

> In light of this policy of legislative freedom when confronting social problems, the exclusion of other potentially more harmful drugs from schedule I does not render the scheme unconstitutional. That cocaine or morphine have adverse health effects does not mean that placing these substances in schedule I is the best means of regulating these substances, or that marijuana should be treated similarly. The fact

that cocaine, morphine, and methamphetamines have all been approved for medical use and marijuana has not is sufficient reason for treating the substances differently. Likewise, the synthesized form of THC has been approved for medical use. Marijuana, unlike synthesized THC contains over 400 different chemicals and there is no way to create a standardized dosing system because there are no chemically consistent plants. The differences between marijuana and synthesized THC, in addition to the health risks associated with inhaled marijuana, justify the Legislature's decision to treat the substances differently.

The court reversed the superior court's decision, finding against Seeley.

Notes on *Seeley v. State of Washington*

1. One of the justices in this case filed a lengthy dissent leading with a quote from a book *The Wanderer* by Joseph Sobran: "When our rulers worry about our health, we should worry about our liberty." The dissenting justice argued that the due process clause of the Fourteenth Amendment is more applicable than the equal protection clause. The due process clause mandates that no state shall "deprive any person of life, liberty, or property, without due process of law." The dissent felt that the real problem is how the government treats Mr. Seeley, not that Mr. Seeley is treated differently from others. Quoting the dissenting justice: "Equalizing injustice does not cure it."

   The dissent argued that the *Seeley* case cannot be distinguished from the U.S. Supreme Court abortion cases, which held that although the state has an important interest to preserve the life of the fetus, this interest is insufficient when measured against the liberty interests of the mother. Stated the dissent: "If the state cannot prohibit abortions consistent with due process, it can hardly constitutionally prohibit drug use as its interest to do so is arguably much less important."

   The dissent concluded by stating that the real issue should not be whether one has a fundamental right under equal protection but rather whether the state's relevant interests in intervention can be balanced against the individual's violated liberty interests. Under this balancing test, Seeley clearly should prevail because his need is personal and great, whereas the state's interest is small.

2. This case is similar to the *Rutherford* case. In both cases, the drugs are unapproved by the FDA and in both cases the plaintiffs are the terminally ill. Consider the differences in the cases and if they're important. Seeley is not asking directly that he has a right to use marijuana, but that his physician has a right to prescribe the drug for his use. Also, marijuana is a controlled substance, whereas Laetrile is not.

3. Even if Seeley won this case, his legal quest would not likely be ended. The federal government could still contend that Washington could not reclassify marijuana because to do so would conflict with federal law. Seeley would then have to argue that his rights under the U.S. Constitution have been violated.

CASE 4-4   *United States v. Little*, 59 F. Supp. 2d 177 (D. Mass. 1999)

Issue

Whether the administrative inspection warrant was properly issued, and whether the applicable standard for recordkeeping violations of the CSA is strict liability or negligence.

Overview

This case actually incorporates several issues. The defendants in this case are Little's Pharmacy and its owner, James Little. The DEA conducted an audit of the pharmacy and determined that there were significant shortages and overages of controlled substances. An audit involves examining a pharmacy's records for controlled substances received and dispensed together with inventory records and comparing the results to the stock on hand to determine whether shortages or overages exist. In this case, the audit was triggered by a tip that diversion was occurring. Because this was not a routine audit, the agent obtained an administrative inspection warrant rather than relying on a notice of inspection, which would have required Little's consent. As you read this case, consider several points: What is the probable cause requirement for an administrative inspection warrant, as opposed to a search warrant? When would a search warrant be required over an administrative inspection warrant? Should the change in the CSA penalty standard from strict liability to negligence be made retroactive? What is the difference between strict liability and negligence? Has the DEA proved recordkeeping violations exist even though all the records seized conformed with the law?

The court began its analysis by relating the facts of the case:

> In April of 1995, DEA investigator Jerry Campagna received an anonymous tip that an employee of Little's Pharmacy may have been diverting an oxycodone-based drug. On May 9, 1995, pursuant to the Controlled Substances Act, the Government submitted an application for an administrative warrant to inspect, copy, and verify the correctness of records, reports, and other documents. According to the application, Little's Pharmacy had never before been inspected to ensure its compliance with the Act.

> After the warrant was issued by this court, an administrative inspection was conducted at Little's Pharmacy on May 11, 1995, followed by a records audit. The inspection and audit uncovered inaccuracies in Little's Pharmacy's records, including shortages of five schedule II controlled substances. Those shortages included 3,084 tablets of Roxicet, 642 tablets of Methylphenidate 5 mg, 561 tablets of Methylphenidate 10 mg, 286 tablets of Percocet, and 250 tablets of Roxiprin.

In addition to the shortages, the government found several overages of schedule II substances, which could not be accounted for by the Forms 222 on file. There was also no power of attorney form on file for its pharmacist, John Fantasia. A power of attorney must be filed for individuals authorized by the pharmacy to obtain and execute order forms.

The government brought a summary judgment action against Little and Little's Pharmacy, citing several counts of CSA recordkeeping violations and contending that the CSA establishes strict liability for the violations. The defendants countered by moving for summary judgment on the basis that the government did not present sufficient evidence. They also moved to suppress the evidence obtained through the administrative warrant.

The court then provided its analysis of the issues.

> Defendants assert that all evidence seized as a result of the May 11, 1995, execution of the administrative inspection warrant should be suppressed. Defendants claim that the particularity requirements for issuance of an administrative warrant were not met and that the inspection was mere pretense for a criminal investigation.

> There appears to be no dispute that items to be inspected and seized through an administrative warrant need be stated with some degree of particularity. The mere assertion in an application for an administrative warrant that the search will be limited

to evidence deemed violative of a particular statute may be impermissibly overbroad. "Delineating the scope of a search with some care is particularly important where documents are involved." If a warrant provides "sufficient standards by which the DEA Investigator reasonably could distinguish between those documents he could inspect and those he could not, the warrant [is] sufficiently particular."

The court found that the warrant application served on Little was highly specific as to the documents sought and therefore proper.

Defendants' second line of defense against the Government's use of evidence seized as a result of the administrative warrant is that the civil investigation was a subterfuge for a criminal investigation. They argue that the Government sought an administrative warrant to avoid the more stringent Fourth Amendment probable cause requirement applicable in criminal matters.

There is no dispute that, in light of the desire to protect public safety and prevent the diversion of drugs, the probable cause requirement is comparatively lenient in the context of highly regulated pharmacies. It may be based solely on the fact that a pharmacy has not been previously inspected. Even so, the government's actual motivation to conduct its investigation is irrelevant so long as the inspector has reason to inspect pursuant to the Act, even if searching for criminal activity.

The court is unconvinced that the instant inspection was mere pretense. In short, Defendants have provided insufficient evidence in support of their claim. In fact, Defendants were ultimately charged civilly, not criminally. That fact alone demonstrates that the execution of the administrative warrant was not a subterfuge for a criminal investigation, Defendants' fears to the contrary. Accordingly, the court will recommend that Defendants' motion to suppress be denied.

After deciding that the evidence was admissible, the court then addressed the defendant's next claim that the negligence standard for recordkeeping violations should be made retroactive to this case.

At the time this case was filed in April of 1997, the Act mandated strict liability for recordkeeping violations. In addition, civil penalties could amount to as much as $25,000 for each violation. Pursuant to the October (1998) amendments, however, strict liability is no longer the substantive standard. Rather, the Government must allege and prove negligence in recordkeeping for liability to attach. In addition, the maximum fine was decreased to $10,000 per violation.

After reviewing U.S. Supreme Court decisions, the court concluded that there is a presumption against retroactivity and it should be followed in this case, especially because Congress did not specify that the amendment be retroactive. The court then proceeded to examine the government's claim for summary judgment under strict liability.

The Controlled Substances Act mandates adherence to stringent recordkeeping with regard to various regulated drugs. The law is well settled that the Act, as applied here, imposes strict liability for those who dispense drugs. What Defendants knew or should have known is immaterial.

The government then argued that because strict liability is applicable, summary judgment is unavoidable on the basis of the evidence that the defendants failed to make and maintain proper records. The defendants, however, asserted that the government cannot point to any specific records as being inaccurate because all the records collected pursuant to the warrant were accurate and proper. The defendants continued that the government can only guess that some records in general must be improper on the basis of the controlled substances shortages and overages. The court replied to the defendants' argument:

> Viewing this testimony along with Defendants' arguments in opposition to summary judgment, it is clear to the court that Defendants miss the aim of the Controlled Substances Act. A violation of the Act occurs each time the Government can prove that controlled substances are missing. Proven shortages, or overages for that matter, constitute recordkeeping violations under the statute. The Government is not required to produce documents in support when none exist. If such documents existed there would be no shortage.

The court noted that strict liability may seem harsh, especially because the controlled substances may have been stolen by an employee through no fault of the defendants. The court also noted that the timing of the investigation was unfortunate for the defendants because if the search had been a month later, the defendants would have conducted their scheduled controlled substances inventory and might have discovered the shortages. They then could have filed the appropriate theft and loss forms, correcting their records. Continued the court:

> The harsh result exemplified here may well be the reason why, in October of 1998, Congress changed the standard to be applied to one of negligence. As described, a pharmacy empowered to dispense controlled substances will now be held liable only if it knew or should have known about an illegal diversion, or inaccurate records, and chose to do nothing. As applied here, however, the Act imposes strict liability.

The court denied the defendants' motion for summary judgment and granted the government's summary judgment motion.

Notes on *United States v. Little*

1. Little challenged the validity of the application for the inspection warrant, hoping that if the warrant was ruled invalid, the evidence would be inadmissible under the exclusionary rule. However, this is a civil case, and the exclusionary rule is technically applicable to criminal cases. Even if the warrant had been invalidated, there was no guarantee that the evidence would not still be allowed by the court. Note that although the probable cause requirement for an AIW is lenient, the application must specify what is to be searched. Little also contended that because the inspection was the result of a tip, the DEA was conducting a search to determine if a crime had been committed, and therefore a search warrant should have been executed. Courts have regularly supported the legality of the use of an administrative inspection warrant, even when the search was triggered by evidence that diversion might have occurred.

2. Little argued that the negligence standard should have been made retroactive to his situation. The court even remarked that the strict liability standard applied to Little was harsh because the thefts may have been by an employee without Little's knowledge. Under strict liability, the simple fact that there were significant shortages makes Little liable. Under negligence, the government would have had to prove that a reasonable pharmacist would have detected the shortages, and that because Little did not detect them, he was negligent. This would require that the DEA introduce a lot more evidence such as how long the employee had been stealing the drugs; how much Little worked in the pharmacy; if there were any clues that thefts were occurring, such as increased ordering quantities without an attendant increase in prescription volume; and so forth.

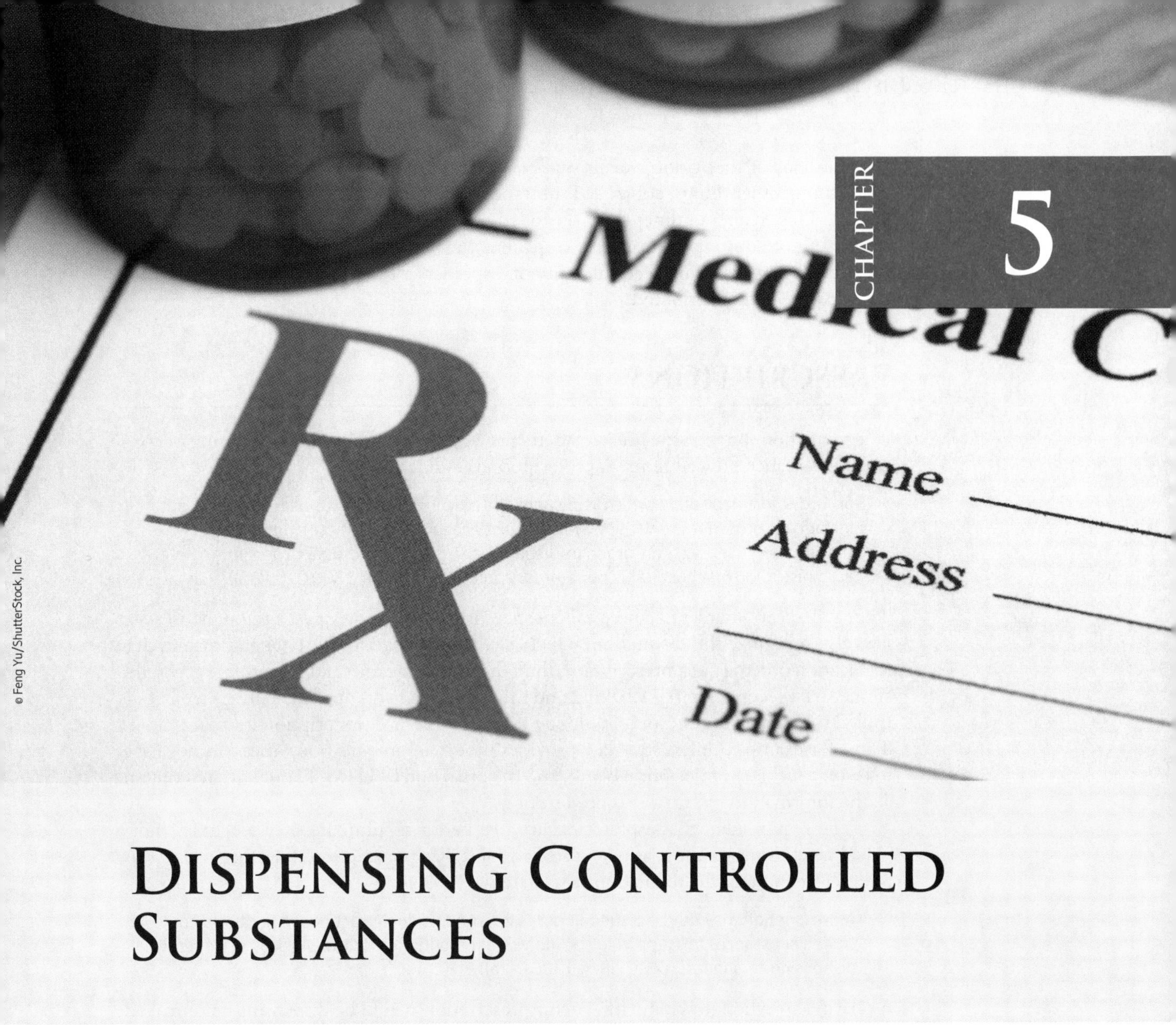

© Feng Yu/ShutterStock, Inc.

CHAPTER 5

DISPENSING CONTROLLED SUBSTANCES

CHAPTER OBJECTIVES

Upon completing this chapter, the reader will be able to:

- Understand the "legitimate medical purpose" and "corresponding responsibility" doctrine and the application to pharmacy practice.
- Identify the dispensing requirements for each schedule of controlled substances.
- Describe the function and execution procedures of Drug Enforcement Administration Order Form 222.
- Recognize the recordkeeping requirements under the Controlled Substances Act.

As guardians of the nation's drug supply, pharmacists have a responsibility to ensure that, among other things, controlled substances are not diverted outside the distribution system. This chapter outlines the Controlled Substances Act's (CSA's) requirements for dispensing of controlled substances to patients, including the documentation requirements necessary to ensure accountability of dispensers for the controlled substances they have acquired and distributed.

PRESCRIPTIONS

The regulations provide specific requirements for the prescribing and dispensing of controlled substance prescriptions. A prescription is defined as

> an order for medication which is dispensed to or for an ultimate user but does not include an order for medication which is dispensed for immediate administration to the ultimate user (e.g., an order to dispense a drug to a bed patient for immediate administration in a hospital is not a prescription). (21 C.F.R. § 1300.01(b)(35))

Thus a medication order in a hospital or other institution is not a prescription. Most state laws also recognize this distinction, which is very important for hospital pharmacies. If a medication order is not a prescription, then the pharmacy does not have to comply with all the strict recordkeeping, labeling, and other requirements applicable to either a controlled substance prescription or a noncontrolled substance prescription for that matter. Thus, for example, unless state law provides otherwise, medication orders do not have to be on a security prescription blank, and the order and label would not have to contain all the information required of a prescription.

The requirement that a prescription must be for an ultimate user precludes individual practitioners from writing controlled substance prescriptions for office use. If this is not clear enough, the regulations also state:

> A prescription may not be issued in order for an individual practitioner to obtain controlled substances for supplying the individual practitioner for the purpose of general dispensing to patients. (21 C.F.R. § 1306.04(b))

A pharmacist who knowingly fills such a prescription would be dispensing a controlled substance pursuant to an invalid prescription and would be in violation of the law.

THOSE ALLOWED TO PRESCRIBE CONTROLLED SUBSTANCES

A prescription for a controlled substance may be issued only by an individual practitioner who is both (1) authorized to prescribe controlled substances in the state in which he or she is licensed to practice and (2) registered or exempt from registration under the CSA (21 C.F.R. § 1306.03).

The definition of individual practitioners includes physicians, dentists, veterinarians, and others authorized in their appropriate jurisdiction to dispense controlled substances. The term also includes those individuals the regulations call mid-level practitioners (e.g., nurse practitioners, nurse midwives, physician assistants, pharmacists). In some states, these individuals are authorized to prescribe controlled substances. (*Note:* No state grants pharmacists true general prescriptive authority because pharmacists must be dependent on collaborative practice agreements.) Pharmacists in those states must know state law to determine which nurse practitioners and physician assistants can prescribe controlled substances and the scope of their prescriptive authority. Some states grant these practitioners the authority to prescribe only certain controlled drugs or only certain classes of controlled substances. Some states grant authority only in institutional settings and under protocol. Some states have other restrictions, and some states have none.

Although only an individual practitioner can issue a controlled substance prescription, an employee or agent of the individual practitioner may communicate it to a pharmacist (21 C.F.R. § 1306.03(b)). Furthermore, a secretary or agent may prepare the prescription for the individual practitioner's signature (21 C.F.R. § 1306.05(a)).

An individual practitioner may not delegate his or her prescriptive authority to an agent unless that agent has been granted prescriptive authority under state law. In practice, pharmacists who call for refill authorization often find it difficult to determine if the individual practitioner has actually authorized the refill. Some situations are obvious, such as when the pharmacist calls for authorization and the office nurse, without hesitation, indicates the refill is permitted. Most likely the nurse has not communicated with the prescriber, and the pharmacist has a duty to ascertain who is really authorizing the refill. Most situations are not so obvious, however. When the prescriber's agent calls the pharmacist back several minutes later to authorize the refill, for example, the pharmacist can usually assume that the individual practitioner has indeed authorized the refill. The same would apply to voice mail and fax responses from the prescriber's office.

When confronted with a suspicious controlled substance prescription, as occasionally happens, a pharmacist may try to determine whether the prescription is fraudulent by checking the Drug Enforcement Administration (DEA) registration number of the prescriber when the number is not known to the pharmacist. A DEA registration number is a nine-character number consisting of two alphabet letters followed by seven digits. Initially, registration numbers for practitioners registered as dispensers began with the letter A. After all registration numbers starting with A had been assigned, the DEA started new dispenser registration numbers with the letter B. Ultimately all B numbers were exhausted and new practitioner registrants now receive a number starting with the letter F. Registration numbers for mid-level practitioners begin with an M. Distributor registration numbers begin with a P or an R; once the R numbers are exhausted, a new initial letter will be chosen.

The second letter in the registration number is usually, but not always, the first letter of the registrant's last name. If the registrant is a business and the business name begins with a number, the second space contains a number. The next six positions represent a computer-generated number unique to each registrant. The last and ninth position is a computer-calculated check digit and a key to verifying the number.

To check the validity of a DEA registration number, a pharmacist

1. Adds the first, third, and fifth digits
2. Adds the sum of the second, fourth, and sixth digits, multiplied by 2, to the first sum
3. Determines if the right-most digit of this sum corresponds with the ninth check digit

For example, to check the validity of hypothetical registration number AN1257218 for Dr. Bill Nash, a pharmacist adds the first, third, and fifth digits:

$$1 + 5 + 2 = 8$$

Next, the second, fourth, and sixth digits are added and multiplied by 2:

$$(2 + 7 + 1) \times 2 = 20$$

The sum of 20 and 8 equals 28.

The right-most digit, 8, corresponds to the ninth digit of the registration number. Thus, the number could be valid.

In reality, many forgers are familiar with the procedure to verify a DEA registration number and can invent a number that would be plausible. Therefore, pharmacists cannot rely on this check alone to determine the validity of a controlled substance prescription.

THOSE ALLOWED TO DISPENSE CONTROLLED SUBSTANCES

Only a pharmacist who is acting in the usual course of professional practice and who either is registered individually or is employed by a registered pharmacy or registered institutional practitioner may fill a prescription for a controlled substance (21 C.F.R. § 1306.06). A pharmacist is defined as a person licensed by a state to dispense controlled substances, as well as any other person (e.g., pharmacist intern) authorized to dispense controlled substances under the supervision of a pharmacist. Whether pharmacy technicians or other ancillary personnel may engage in dispensing controlled substances under the supervision of a pharmacist depends on state law. Individual practitioners also may dispense if authorized by state law.

ISSUANCE OF PRESCRIPTIONS

All controlled substance prescriptions issued by an individual practitioner must be dated as of the date of issuance; in other words, a prescriber may not predate or postdate prescriptions. In addition to the date of issuance, all controlled substance prescriptions must contain at least the following information (21 C.F.R. § 1306.05):

- The full name and address of the patient
- The name, address, and registration number of the practitioner
- The drug name, strength, dosage form
- The number of units or volume dispensed
- Directions for use

A prescription issued pursuant to the Drug Addiction Treatment Act (DATA) must also contain the identification number of the physician or a written notice that the physician is acting in "good faith" while waiting for the identification number to be issued. A prescription written for gamma-hydroxybutyric acid must include the medical need of the patient written on the prescription. The regulation establishes a "corresponding liability" on the pharmacist to ensure that the prescription is prepared properly.

The prescriber must sign written controlled substance prescriptions on the day of issuance. When oral orders are not permitted, the prescription must be written in ink or indelible pencil, or typewritten, and manually signed by the prescriber. A computer-generated prescription that is printed out or faxed by the prescriber must be manually signed. If the pharmacist receives the prescription orally, the pharmacist may write in the name of the prescriber. Electronic controlled substance prescriptions must comply with DEA regulations summarized later in this chapter.

Although the prescriber's agent may prepare the prescriptions for the prescriber's signature, it is the responsibility of both the individual practitioner and the pharmacist to ensure that the prescriptions conform to all essential aspects of the law and regulations.

Individual practitioners exempt from registration must include on the prescriptions the registration number of the hospital or other institution at which they practice and the special internal code number assigned to them by the hospital or institution (21 C.F.R. § 1306.05(b)). Each written prescription must have the name of the physician stamped, typed, or handprinted on it, as well as the signature of the physician. Those exempt from registration because they are members of the armed services or public health service must include on each prescription their service identification number in lieu of the registration number (21 C.F.R. § 1306.05(c)).

Before filing the prescription in the pharmacy, regulation also requires the prescription to contain the written or typewritten name or initials of the pharmacist dispensing the drug (21 C.F.R. § 1304.22(c)).

Correcting a Written Controlled Substance Prescription

Occasionally, pharmacies receive controlled substance prescriptions that are incomplete or that contain errors and the question becomes whether the pharmacist can legally correct the prescription. Regarding schedule III, IV, or V prescriptions, the DEA has provided a clear answer at its website: http://www.deadiversion.usdoj.gov/faq/prescriptions.htm#rx-7. If the prescription does not contain the patient's address or contains an incorrect address, the pharmacist may add or correct the address upon verification. The pharmacist may also add or change the dosage form, drug strength, drug quantity, directions for use, or issue date after consultation with and agreement of the prescriber and after documentation on the prescription. The pharmacist is never permitted to make changes to the patient's name, controlled substance prescribed (except for generic substitution), or the prescriber's signature. Of course, a pharmacist may contact the prescriber and simply convert the written prescription to an oral one if any of this information does need to be changed or added.

Whether a pharmacist can correct a schedule II prescription has involved conflicting opinions from the DEA and has created considerable controversy. Prior to 2009, the DEA's website had provided that a pharmacist could essentially correct a schedule II prescription in the same manner as a schedule III, IV, or V prescription. However, in the preamble to a regulation enacted in November 2007 entitled "Multiple Prescriptions for Schedule II Controlled Substances" (discussed later in this chapter), the DEA stated that the "essential elements of the [schedule II] prescription written by the practitioner (such as the name of the controlled substance, strength, dosage form, and quantity prescribed) . . . may not be modified orally."

In October 2008, the DEA issued a policy statement that it recognized the conflict and instructed pharmacists to follow state regulations or policy until the DEA could resolve this issue by a regulation. Subsequently, some time in 2009 and without notice, the DEA withdrew its original policy statement (that permitted correcting schedule II prescriptions) from the website and replaced it with the statement from the preamble to the regulation stating that schedule II prescriptions may not be corrected. The health care community complained vigorously and the DEA appeared to have listened. A few months later in 2010, the DEA again reversed its position and changed its website, instructing pharmacists to follow state law or policy as to whether they can correct a schedule II prescription (available at http://www.deadiversion.usdoj.gov/faq/prescriptions.htm#rx-7). However, the DEA then proceeded to further confuse the matter by issuing a letter in late 2010 to a pharmacy audit firm stating that the pharmacist is not an agent of the prescriber for the purposes of adding the prescriber's DEA registration number on the written prescription. (Letter from Mark Caverly, Chief Liaison and Policy Section, Office of Diversion Control, to Rena Bielinski, Chief Pharmacy Officer, National Audit (Nov. 1, 2010)).

This letter raised the question of whether the DEA had again changed its mind, believing that a pharmacist is not an agent and thus cannot make any changes. The National Association of Boards of Pharmacy (NABP) then requested a clarification on DEA's policy in July 2011. In August 2011, the DEA issued a letter to NABP stating that whether it is appropriate for pharmacists to make changes in a schedule II prescription varies on a case-by-case basis; and, that a pharmacist should exercise professional judgment and knowledge of state and federal laws to make a decision. (Letter from Joseph Rannazzisi, Deputy Assistant Administrator, Office of Diversion Control, to Carmen Catizone, NABP (Aug. 24, 2011). Available at http://www.nabp.net/news/assets/DEA-missing-info-schedule-2.pdf). It thus seems at this time that pharmacists can make corrections if state law or policy allows.

PURPOSE OF A CONTROLLED SUBSTANCE PRESCRIPTION

Federal regulations provide as follows:

> A prescription for a controlled substance to be effective must be issued for a legitimate medical purpose by an individual practitioner acting in the usual course of his professional practice. The responsibility for the proper prescribing and dispensing of controlled substances is upon the prescribing practitioner, but a corresponding responsibility rests with the pharmacist who fills the prescription. An order purporting to be a prescription issued not in the usual course of professional treatment or in legitimate and authorized research is not a prescription within the meaning and intent of Section 309 of the Act (21 U.S.C. § 829) and the person knowingly filling such a purported prescription, as well as the person issuing it, shall be subject to the penalties provided for violations of the provisions of law relating to controlled substances. (21 C.F.R. § 1306.04(a))

Corresponding Responsibility Doctrine

The preceding regulation, referred to as the corresponding responsibility doctrine, clearly indicates that both the prescriber and the pharmacist are legally responsible for the proper prescribing and dispensing of controlled substances. Therefore, pharmacists must be particularly alert that the controlled substance prescriptions they receive and dispense are for a legitimate medical purpose and are issued by a lawful practitioner in the usual course of professional practice.

Defining "Knowingly"

The corresponding responsibility doctrine is not absolute because the regulation states that a violation occurs when the pharmacist "knowingly" dispenses an improper prescription. Thus, the definition of "knowingly" is critical because a pharmacist who does not know a prescription is not for a legitimate medical purpose cannot have violated the regulation. In other words, a pharmacist should not be accountable for filling an invalid prescription that the pharmacist could not have known was invalid.

In *United States v. Hayes*, 595 F.2d 258 (5th Cir. 1979), included in the case studies section of this chapter, a pharmacist challenged the constitutionality of the corresponding responsibility doctrine, contending that the doctrine imposes an unfair burden on pharmacists because they cannot prescribe and do not have the means of knowing if a prescription is really valid. The most that a pharmacist can do, argued the pharmacist, is to call the physician and seek verification of the prescription, which he did. The facts of the case indicate that the pharmacist dispensed a tremendous number of prescriptions from a single physician for massive quantities of drugs to patients who admitted selling the drugs. The court rejected the constitutional argument, essentially finding that the regulation does not impose an unattainable obligation on pharmacists. However, the court added, verification of a prescription may not in itself be enough to establish that the pharmacist has met the knowledge requirement in situations such as this where the prescriptions are obviously false. Thus, the court disagreed with the pharmacist and affirmed his conviction.

In a similar case, *United States v. Lawson*, 682 F.2d 480 (4th Cir. 1982), a physician who operated a diet clinic created medical records for fictitious patients and sold prescriptions written for Preludin and Tuinal for these fictitious patients to an obese patient. Then the patient would present the prescriptions to the defendant pharmacist, Lawson. Initially, Lawson had contacted the physician to ascertain the validity of the prescriptions, but he subsequently dispensed the prescribed drugs without question.

Lawson was charged with dispensing schedule II drugs that he knew were not for a legitimate medical purpose. He contended that he did not know the prescriptions were not for a legitimate medical purpose. The court, however, convicted Lawson, finding that he should have known for a number of reasons. First, one person was presenting a large number of prescriptions, all written by one physician. Second, the prescriptions were uniform in dosages and quantities. Third, the sudden surge in the quantity of prescriptions for the controlled substances should have been suspect. The appellate court confirmed Lawson's conviction.

The court's opinion in a California case, *Vermont & 110th Medical Arts Pharmacy v. State Board of Pharmacy*, 177 Cal. Rptr. 807 (Cal. App.2d 1981), states the pharmacist's responsibility very well. In this case, over a 45-day period the pharmacy filled 10,000 prescriptions written by a small group of physicians for four controlled substances. All together, these prescriptions accounted for 748,000 dosage units. Many of these prescriptions were filled in consecutively numbered batches for the same prescriber and for the same person with different addresses, although many of the addresses were nonexistent. Many of the names were suspect as well (e.g., Henry Ford, Fairlane Ford, Glenn Ford, Pearl Harbor). In response to the pharmacist's argument that he did not know the prescriptions were not valid, the court replied:

> The statutory scheme plainly calls upon pharmacists to use their common sense and professional judgment. When their suspicions are aroused as reasonable professional persons by either ambiguities in the prescriptions, the sheer volume of controlled substances prescribed by a single practitioner for a small number of persons or, as in this case, when the control inherent in the prescription process is blatantly mocked by its obvious abuse as a means to dispense an inordinate and incredible amount of drugs under the color and protection of the law, pharmacists are called upon to obey the law and refuse to dispense. (177 Cal. Rptr. at 810)

These cases indicate that whether a pharmacist knew that prescriptions were not for a legitimate medical purpose can be inferred from strong circumstantial evidence. Thus, for criminal purposes, "knowingly" could be defined as when a pharmacist should have known based on obvious facts but rather chose to consciously disregard the obvious. Stated another way, the pharmacist recognized the possibility of wrongdoing but consciously refused to conduct a proper investigation. A pharmacist is expected to exercise professional judgment when suspicions should arise and should take action to determine if the prescription is valid. In these situations, verification with the prescriber is a critical first step; this step may not be enough, however, when facts indicate that the pharmacist should have investigated further.

On the other hand, although pharmacists must be ever vigilant for invalid prescriptions, they also must guard against being overly suspicious. In the case of *Ryan v. Dan's Food Stores, Inc.*, 972 P.2d 395 (UT 1998), reported in the case studies section of this chapter, a pharmacist contended that he was wrongfully discharged for questioning the validity of controlled substance prescriptions. The court, however, found the discharge to be valid because the discharge was based on the pharmacist's behavior of being suspicious of most of the patients with controlled substance prescriptions and of being rude to those patients. The *Ryan* case is a good example that a pharmacist should not be suspicious of a patient unless the pharmacist has a reason to be suspicious. Without any indication to the contrary, a pharmacist should presume that a controlled substance is legitimate. The *Gordon v. Frost* case, 388 S.E.2d 362 (1989 GA), also reported in the case studies section, demonstrates the civil liability consequences of a pharmacist who was overly suspicious and "jumped to the conclusion" that a regular patient was attempting to fraudulently obtain a refill of a controlled substance prescription.

Legitimate Medical Purpose and Usual Course of Professional Practice

Only prescriptions written for a "legitimate medical purpose" in the "usual course of professional practice" are valid under the law. Although these terms are not specifically defined, at least one court has found the term to mean acting "in accordance with a standard of medical practice generally recognized and accepted in the United States" (*United States v. Moore*, 423 U.S. 122, 139 (1975)). Some examples of invalid controlled substance prescriptions not written for a legitimate medical purpose include

- Fraudulent or forged prescriptions written by persons not authorized to issue drug orders
- Prescriptions written by individual practitioners for office use
- Prescriptions written by individual practitioners:
  - For fictitious patients
  - For patients not named on the prescription
  - When the individual practitioner has not performed a good-faith medical examination
  - When there is no medical reason for the prescription
- Narcotic prescriptions written by individual practitioners to maintain an addiction or to detoxify an addict
- Prescriptions written by individual practitioners that exceed the usual course of their professional practice; for example, a dentist who prescribes a controlled drug for a patient's back pain unrelated to dental diagnosis

This list clearly demonstrates that facial validity of a prescription does not in itself make a prescription valid. A controlled substance prescription must be based on a legitimate physician–patient relationship, where the prescriber has taken a patient history, conducted an assessment, developed a treatment plan, and documented these steps. As will be discussed later in this chapter, the CSA was amended to provide that when controlled substances are dispensed via the Internet, a valid prescription requires the practitioner to have conducted at least one in-person medical evaluation of the patient. This means a good-faith examination in compliance with standards of practice. Although this amendment applies to Internet pharmacy, the requirement is no less applicable to every controlled substance prescription in any practice setting. Courts will consider if a situation violates "legitimate medical purpose" and "usual course of professional practice" on a case-by-case basis. However, cases where courts have determined that violations occurred have been based upon blatant or glaring misconduct, not merely questionable legality (*United States v. Rosen*, 582 F.2d 1032 (5th Cir. 1978)).

The DEA has published a guide, titled *A Pharmacist's Guide to Prescription Fraud*, to help pharmacists ensure that controlled substance prescriptions are being issued for a legitimate medical purpose. The guide can be found at http://www.deadiversion .usdoj.gov/pubs/brochures/pharmguide.htm (or in Appendix D of the 2010 *Pharmacist's*

Manual at http://www.deadiversion.usdoj.gov/pubs/manuals/index.html) and includes some situations that should make pharmacists suspicious, such as:

- The prescriber writes significantly larger numbers of prescription orders (or in larger quantities) compared with other practitioners in your area.
- The prescriber writes for antagonistic drugs, such as depressants and stimulants, at the same time. Drug abusers often request prescription orders for "uppers and downers" at the same time.
- Patients appear to be returning too frequently. For example, a prescription that should have lasted for a month is being refilled weekly.
- Patients appear presenting prescription orders written in the names of other people.
- A number of people appear simultaneously, or within a short time, all bearing similar prescription orders from the same practitioner.
- Numerous "strangers," people who are not regular patrons or residents of your community, suddenly show up with prescription orders from the same physician.

The guide urges pharmacists to contact the state board of pharmacy or local DEA office if they think they may have discovered a pattern of prescription abuses.

Exercise of Clinical Judgment and the Treatment of Pain

The treatment of pain with controlled substances is unquestionably a legitimate medical purpose. Pharmacists must take care that the legitimate medical purpose rule not be misapplied to determining the appropriateness of the drug therapy. In some instances controlled substances may not be the best treatment, the amount prescribed may seem excessive, or the patient may have become addicted as a result of treatment.

For example, a frequently seen patient who complains of back pain may be using opioids to relieve that pain. There are medical alternatives, some invasive and some conservative, to the use of opioids, but the patient refuses these alternatives in favor of treatment with opioids. The patient may develop dependence to these drugs but sees the dependence as the price that must be paid to avoid the alternative treatments that do not appeal to the patient. Controlled substances are not strictly necessary for this patient because alternative treatments are available. However, the patient really does suffer pain, and controlled substances are rationally related to the control of pain. Thus, although it might not be the best medical treatment, the prescribing of controlled substances for this patient is certainly both legitimate and medical. It does not matter that some physicians may treat the patient without prescribing opioids.

If the patient in this hypothetical case receives other controlled substances not just for pain but also for anxiety and insomnia, the prescribed dosages of each drug may be extremely high. Some may say that the prescriptions then become nonlegitimate. This position is not consistent with the federal framework, however. Under federal interpretations of the legitimate medical purpose rule, the objective is to prevent the diversion of medications to the illicit market without impeding the legitimate use of medications. The DEA is a law enforcement agency that does not have the expertise to make medical judgments, and there is nothing to suggest that anyone other than the patient is using the prescribed drugs or that the drugs are being used for anything other than conditions requiring the medical treatment for which they are indicated. Even though the dosages may be high and the combination risky, the use is legitimate because patients differ in their need for drugs and in their attitudes toward risk.

This is not to say that the pharmacist should not question the prescriber's choice of drug therapy when professional judgment warrants. For example, if one drug has been shown more effective than another for a particular type of pain, or the dosage selected raises significant safety or efficacy issues, the pharmacist should intervene as appropriate. Perhaps the pharmacist, in an extreme case, may make a decision not to dispense the medication. Decisions to intervene and/or not dispense, however, should be based upon patient safety, weighing all clinical factors. The decisions should not be based upon the legitimate medical purpose rule.

In response to comments and solicitations from professionals and professional organizations in the pain management sector, the DEA published a notice in September 2006 titled, "Policy Statement: Dispensing Controlled Substances for the Treatment of Pain" (70 Fed. Reg. 52716, Sept. 6, 2006; http://www.deadiversion.usdoj.gov:80/fed_regs/notices/2006/fr09062.htm). Although directed primarily at prescribers, the notice might help pharmacists better understand the position of the DEA on this subject.

Differentiating Treatment of Addiction from Treatment of Pain

Federal regulations specifically state that it is illegal to prescribe and dispense narcotic drugs for the purpose of maintaining an addiction or detoxifying an addict (21 C.F.R. § 1306.04(c)). The intent of the regulation is to ensure that addicts are treated for their addiction in registered opioid treatment programs. DATA does allow office-based practitioners to prescribe schedule III, IV, and V opioid drugs specifically approved by the FDA for the purpose of treating addicts. Thus, it may be simply stated that, absent legal exceptions (most notably DATA), it is not a legitimate use or a legitimate medical purpose of a controlled substance prescription to maintain an addiction or detoxify an addict.

The application of this principle in pharmacy practice is not often simple. For example, assume that the patient with back pain has taken the medication for several months and the pharmacist has reason to believe that the patient really does not have pain any longer. The pharmacist suspects that the patient is addicted to the drug and that is the only reason the patient is taking the drug. In this situation, the pharmacist should try to determine if the medical condition for which the drug was prescribed still exists or if the drug is being issued for the illegal purpose of maintaining a narcotic addiction. At this point, the pharmacist has a duty to contact the prescriber and inquire. If the prescriber can substantiate that the patient still has the back pain and the use of the drug is still necessary for this purpose, the pharmacist should continue to dispense the drug. The regulations support this action because they state that a physician may administer or dispense narcotic drugs to persons with intractable pain in which no relief or cure is possible or has been found after reasonable efforts (21 C.F.R. § 1306.07(c)). On the other hand, the prescriber might share the pharmacist's concern that the purpose of the prescription is really the addiction and not the pain. In this situation, the prescriber might seek to enter the patient into an opioid treatment program or, if qualified, treat the patient under the requirements of DATA.

Situations get even more complicated when a pharmacist receives an opioid prescription with directions to gradually taper down the dosage. This complex situation requires the pharmacist to differentiate addiction from dependence. Addiction is generally characterized as psychological dependence characterized by compulsive use of the drug despite harm, a loss of control, and a preoccupation with obtaining opioids. Physical dependence is a state of adaptation in which withdrawal occurs when the drug is stopped or quickly decreased. Physical dependence is normal and expected with long-term opioid use. Thus, if the purpose of the opioid prescription is to gradually withdraw the pain patient from dependence, the prescription is legitimate. If the purpose is detoxification of an addict, the prescription is not legitimate. If the patient has been a regular pain patient of the pharmacy, the pharmacist can likely presume the taper-down dosage is withdrawal from dependence. If, however, the patient is new or a stranger, the pharmacist would likely need to query the prescriber and learn more.

There are exceptions under federal law, other than DATA, that allow for the limited treatment of addicts outside of opioid treatment programs (OTPs). Under CSA regulations (21 C.F.R. § 1306.07(b)), it is permissible for the prescriber to administer from his or her office supply, but not prescribe, narcotic drugs to an addict for a maximum of 3 days for the purpose of relieving acute withdrawal symptoms while arrangements are being made for referral for treatment. Not more than 1 day's medication may be administered to the person at one time. (Note that the pharmacist may not dispense the medication pursuant to a prescription.) The regulations also permit a physician or authorized hospital staff member to administer or dispense narcotic drugs to maintain or detoxify a hospitalized patient incidental to treating a condition other than the addiction (21 C.F.R. § 1306.07(c)).

Ascertaining the Legitimacy of Opioid Prescriptions in Pain Treatment

One of the most difficult situations pharmacists encounter is when a prescriber or prescribers issue several prescriptions to chronic pain patients for very large quantities and very large doses of opioids. Large quantities and doses are sometimes necessary to treat severe chronic pain patients. Because pharmacists are held to a corresponding responsibility with the prescriber, these situations can be uncomfortable if the pharmacist fears the patient might not be a legitimate pain patient. General DEA tips on determining the validity of prescriptions were mentioned previously and should be considered. More specifically to pain treatment, pharmacists should be aware of the standards of practice for diagnosing and treating pain. One good source is the model guidelines established by the Federation of State Medical Boards (available at http://painpolicy.wisc.edu). If a pharmacist is concerned about the legitimacy of a pain patient, the pharmacist should not hesitate to contact the prescriber and ascertain if he or she is complying with practice standards. Pain management physicians should have no problem sharing medical records with the pharmacy, or developing a collaborative practice arrangement with the pharmacy.

Absent medical record documentation or a collaborative practice situation when uncertainty exists, pharmacists should consider interviewing the patient when appropriate with such questions as: What causes the pain? What past treatments has the patient attempted for the pain? What is the nature and intensity of the pain? What is the duration of the pain? What effect is the pain having on the patient's quality of life? The pharmacist should then ask the same questions of the prescriber and should receive the same answers from both the prescriber and the patient. If available, pharmacists should also utilize the state's prescription monitoring program to evaluate a chronic pain patient's behavior.

DISPENSING OF SCHEDULE II CONTROLLED SUBSTANCES

Subject to special exceptions, a pharmacist may dispense schedule II drugs only pursuant to a written prescription, signed by the individual practitioner (21 C.F.R. § 1306.11(a)). Electronic prescriptions for schedule II drugs also are permitted, as discussed later in this chapter, provided all DEA requirements are met. Schedule II prescriptions may not be refilled (21 C.F.R. § 1306.12).

State Multiple-Copy Prescription Programs

In the past some states required prescribers to issue schedule II prescriptions on multiple-copy, state-issued prescription forms. Typically, only the prescriber could request and possess these forms. When the prescriber executed a multiple-copy prescription form, generally the prescriber kept one copy, the dispensing pharmacy kept one copy, and the pharmacy sent another copy to a state office. In *Whalen v. Roe*, 429 U.S. 589 (1977), reported in the case studies section of this chapter, New York's multiple-copy law was challenged as unconstitutionally violating the patient's right of privacy. The U.S. Supreme Court upheld the law, however, finding that the law might have the intended effect of minimizing drug misuse and deterring potential violators without substantially interfering with any privacy rights.

Electronic data transmission programs (known as prescription monitoring programs (PMPs)) have generally replaced state multiple-copy prescription programs and have been implemented in most states. State PMPs generally require the electronic reporting of all controlled substance prescription information, not just schedule II prescriptions; this topic is discussed later in this chapter.

Emergency Situations

Emergency situations constitute an exception to the requirement that a pharmacist may dispense schedule II drugs only pursuant to a written (or electronic) prescription. In an emergency situation, a pharmacist may dispense a schedule II drug on the oral authorization of an individual practitioner, provided that

- The quantity prescribed and dispensed is limited only to the amount necessary to treat the patient for the emergency period.
- The prescription must be immediately reduced to writing by the pharmacist and shall contain all required information, except the signature of the prescriber.
- If the prescriber is not known to the pharmacist, the pharmacist must make a reasonable, good-faith effort to determine that the oral authorization came from a registered individual practitioner. This reasonable effort could include a call back to the prescriber using the phone number in the telephone directory, rather than the number given by the prescriber over the phone.
- Within 7 days after authorizing an emergency oral prescription, the prescriber must deliver to the dispensing pharmacist a written prescription for the emergency quantity prescribed. (*Note:* The requirement was 72 hours before March 28, 1997.) The prescription must have written on its face "Authorization for Emergency Dispensing," and the date of the oral order. The written prescription may be delivered to the pharmacist in person or by mail. If delivered by mail, it must be postmarked within the 7-day period. On receipt, the dispensing pharmacist shall attach this prescription to the oral emergency prescription previously reduced to writing. If the prescriber fails to deliver the written prescription within the 7-day period, the pharmacist must notify the nearest office of the DEA. Failure of the pharmacist to do so will void the prescription (21 C.F.R. § 1306.11(d)). (*Note:* Although the regulation specifies "oral authorization," the DEA has indicated in the *Pharmacist's Manual* that a faxed prescription from the prescriber also would be acceptable.)

An emergency situation is defined as a situation in which

- Immediate administration of the controlled substance is necessary for the proper treatment of the patient.

- No appropriate alternative treatment is available.
- It is not reasonably possible for the prescribing physician to provide a written prescription to the pharmacist before dispensing. (21 C.F.R. § 290.10)

Facsimile (Fax) Prescriptions for Schedule II Drugs

DEA regulations permit the limited use of faxed prescriptions as another exception to the requirement that pharmacists may only dispense schedule II drugs pursuant to the actual written prescription from the prescriber. In general, faxed schedule II prescriptions are permitted but only if the pharmacist receives the original written, signed prescription before the actual dispensing and the pharmacy files the original (21 C.F.R. § 1306.11(a)). (In essence, this general provision does not provide an exception for pharmacists because the original prescription is still required.) In three situations, however, the faxed prescription may serve as the original:

1. If the prescription is faxed by the practitioner or practitioner's agent to a pharmacy and is for a narcotic schedule II substance to be compounded for the direct administration to a patient by parenteral, intravenous, intramuscular, subcutaneous, or intraspinal infusion (21 C.F.R. § 1306.11(e)).
2. If the prescription faxed by the practitioner or practitioner's agent is for a schedule II substance for a resident of a long-term care facility (LTCF) (21 C.F.R. § 1306.11(f)).
3. If the prescription faxed by the practitioner or practitioner's agent is for a schedule II narcotic substance for a patient enrolled in a hospice care program certified by/or paid for by Medicare under Title XVIII, or licensed by the state. The practitioner or agent must note on the prescription that the patient is a hospice patient (21 C.F.R. § 1306.11(g)).

Note that for LTCF residents the prescription may be for any schedule II drug, in contrast to prescriptions for home care and hospice patients. Pharmacists may dispense faxed prescriptions for hospice patients regardless of whether the patient lives at home or in an institution. Allowing faxed schedule II prescriptions for home health care, LTCF, and hospice patients has somewhat eased the burden of pharmacists, who often find it impractical to obtain the original written prescription for patients in these situations.

Partial Filling of a Schedule II Prescription

If a pharmacist is "unable to supply" the full prescribed quantity of a schedule II drug, partial filling of the prescription is permissible (21 C.F.R. § 1306.13(a)). The pharmacist must make a notation of the quantity supplied on the face of the prescription, and the balance of the prescription amount must be filled within 72 hours after the partial filling. If the pharmacist is unable to fill the prescription within this time frame, the pharmacist must notify the prescriber. No further quantity may be supplied beyond 72 hours without a new prescription.

Historically, pharmacists have interpreted the phrase "unable to supply" as meaning that partial filling is permissible only if the pharmacy is out of stock. This interpretation places the pharmacist in a dilemma when the pharmacist receives a prescription for a large quantity of an opioid in a situation where validation may be necessary but not possible at the time. The pharmacist, not absolutely certain if the prescription is legitimate, must either fill the entire amount (risking possible diversion) or not dispense the prescription (resulting in the suffering of a legitimate patient). When queried about this dilemma, the DEA's chief of the liaison and policy section replied that in such situations the pharmacist could partially fill the prescription, even if the drug is in stock, while waiting for verification. The DEA official additionally stated that a pharmacist could partially fill a prescription if the prescription was for a large quantity and the patient could not afford to pay for the entire amount or did not want the entire amount for some other reason. The response was that these situations also would fit within the definition of "unable to supply" (Brushwood, 2001).

In LTCFs, or for a patient with a medical diagnosis documenting a terminal illness, schedule II prescriptions may be partially filled to allow for the dispensing of individual dosage units but for no longer than 60 days from the date of issuance (21 C.F.R. § 1306.13(b)). The total quantity of drug dispensed in all partial fillings must not exceed the quantity prescribed. If there is any question as to whether a patient may be classified as having a terminal illness, the pharmacist must contact the prescriber before partially filling the prescription. Both the pharmacist and the prescriber have a corresponding responsibility to ensure that the controlled substance is for a terminally ill patient. The pharmacist must record on the prescription whether the patient is "terminally ill" or an "LTCF patient." A prescription that is partially filled and does not contain the notation "terminally ill" or "LTCF patient" is deemed to have been filled in violation of the CSA.

For each partial filling, the pharmacist must record

- The date
- The quantity dispensed
- The remaining quantity authorized to be dispensed
- The identification of the dispensing pharmacist

This record may be kept on the back of the prescription or on any other appropriate record, including a computerized system. If a computerized system is used, it must have the capability to permit the following:

- Output of the original prescription number; date of issue; identification of the prescribing individual practitioner, the patient, the LTCF, and the medication authorized, including the dosage form strength and quantity; and a listing of partial fillings that have been dispensed under each prescription
- Immediate (real-time) updating of the prescription record each time that the prescription is partially filled (21 C.F.R. § 1306.13(c))

Multiple Schedule II Prescriptions for the Same Drug and Patient Written on the Same Day

The fact that the law prohibits the pre- or postdating of controlled substance prescriptions and the refilling of schedule II prescriptions can create hardships for patients who regularly require the dispensing of drugs in this schedule. Recognizing this, the DEA for years has permitted physicians to prepare multiple prescriptions on the same day for the same schedule II drug with written instructions that they be filled on different days. In 2003, the DEA issued a private letter to a physician confirming that this practice is permissible (letter from Patricia Good, DEA, to Howard Heit, physician, January 31, 2003). Subsequently, the DEA posted confirmation of the policy on its website, as well as on a pain management website. Then, without warning, the DEA reversed its position and issued a *Federal Register* notice to this effect in 2004 (69 Fed. Reg. 67170), causing an uproar among pain management and health care professional organizations. Nonetheless, the DEA reiterated its new position in another *Federal Register* notice in August 2005 (70 Fed. Reg. 50408), stating that this practice amounts to illegal refills.

After repeated complaints from pain specialists, in September 2006 the DEA admitted it had made the wrong decision and issued yet another reversal of opinion, proposing a new regulation on the subject (http://www.deadiversion.usdoj.gov/fed_regs/rules/2006/fr0906.htm) as well as an accompanying policy statement, "Dispensing Controlled Substances for the Treatment of Pain" (71 Fed. Reg. 52724; 71 Fed. Reg. 52715; http://www.deadiversion.usdoj.gov/fed_regs/notices/2006/fr09062.htm). (The policy statement is an attempt by the agency to clarify the legal requirements and agency policy regarding the prescribing of controlled substances for the treatment of pain.) The DEA issued the final rule in November 2007, permitting the issuance of multiple prescriptions subject to the following restrictions (72 Fed. Reg. 64921):

- Each prescription must be issued on a separate prescription blank.
- The total quantity prescribed cannot exceed a 90-day supply.
- The practitioner must determine there is a legitimate medical purpose for each prescription and be acting in the usual course of professional practice.
- The practitioner must write instructions on each prescription (other than the first) as to the earliest date on which the prescription may be dispensed.
- The practitioner concludes that the multiple prescriptions do not create an undue risk of diversion or abuse.
- The issuance of multiple prescriptions must be permissible under state law.
- The practitioner must comply fully with all other CSA and state law requirements.

DISPENSING OF SCHEDULE III, IV, AND V CONTROLLED SUBSTANCES

A pharmacist may dispense a schedule III, IV, or V prescription drug pursuant to either a written, faxed, electronic, or oral order from the individual practitioner or practitioner's agent, providing that all required information is contained on the prescription, and that electronic prescriptions conform to DEA requirements. Oral orders must be promptly reduced to writing; written and faxed prescriptions must contain the signature of the prescriber (21 C.F.R. § 1306.21(a)). Individual practitioners may administer or dispense a schedule III, IV, or V controlled substance in the course of professional practice without a prescription (21 C.F.R. § 1306.21(b)). Institutional practitioners may administer or dispense (but not prescribe) a schedule III, IV, or V controlled substance pursuant to a written, faxed, or oral prescription promptly reduced to writing by the pharmacist, as well as administer or dispense an order for medication by an individual practitioner that is to be dispensed for immediate administration to the ultimate user (21 C.F.R. § 1306.21 (c)).

Refills

No schedule III or IV prescription may be filled or refilled more than 6 months after the date of issuance of the prescription or more than five times, whichever comes first (21 C.F.R. § 1306.22). These restrictions do not apply to schedule V prescription drugs. After the expiration of the 6-month period or the fifth refill, the prescriber must authorize a new prescription. The pharmacist may telephone the prescriber for authorization and create a new prescription.

If the prescriber who issued the original prescription initially authorized fewer than five refills, that prescriber can authorize additional refills without having to issue a new prescription. In any event, the total quantity of refills authorized, including the number on the original prescription, cannot exceed five refills. A pharmacist who obtains oral authorization for additional refills must record the refill either in hard copy form or in an automated data system. The quantity of each additional refill authorized cannot exceed the quantity originally authorized on the prescription.

If an automated system is not used, every refill must be recorded either on the back of the prescription or on another document in a way that makes the information readily retrievable. The recorded information must be retrievable by prescription number and must include

- The name and dosage form of the drug
- The date refilled
- The quantity dispensed
- The initials of the dispensing pharmacist for each refill
- The initials of the pharmacist receiving the refill authorization
- The total number of refills for that prescription

If the pharmacist merely initials and dates the back of the prescription, it is deemed that the full face amount of the prescription was dispensed.

It is not advisable that pharmacists refill controlled substance prescriptions when the prescriber is not available for authorization on the expectation that the prescriber will subsequently approve the refill. This practice is illegal, unless authorized by state law, and even in states that so authorize, refills are generally confined to emergency situations where the patient's health would be jeopardized if the prescription was not refilled. In the case of *Daniel Family Pharmacy*, 1999 WL 43613 (Fed. Reg., February 3, 1999), reported in the case studies section of this chapter, a pharmacist refilled a narcotic drug prescription for an employee believing the refill would be approved by the prescriber. The prescriber, however, refused authorization, leading the pharmacist down a path of escalating illegal activities.

Electronic Refill Records

As an alternative to the method of recording refill information previously discussed, a pharmacy may use an electronic system for the storage and retrieval of refill information for schedule III and IV prescriptions (21 C.F.R. § 1306.22(f)). Such a system must provide online retrieval of the original prescription order information and the up-to-date refill history of the prescription. The pharmacist must verify and document that the refill data entered into the system are correct.

If the system provides a hard copy printout of each day's refill data, that printout must be provided to the pharmacy within 72 hours of the date on which the refill was dispensed. The printout must be verified, dated, and signed by each pharmacist who refilled the prescriptions listed on the printout. This document must be maintained in a separate file at the pharmacy for a period of 2 years from the dispensing date. In lieu of the printout, the pharmacy may maintain a bound logbook or separate file for refills in which each individual pharmacist involved in dispensing medications signs a statement verifying the prescriptions that the pharmacist refilled. The logbook also must be maintained for a period of 2 years.

All computerized systems must be able to print out any refill data that the pharmacy is responsible for maintaining. This includes, for example, a refill-by-refill audit trail of any schedule III or IV prescription. The printout must include

- The name of the prescriber
- The name and address of the patient
- The quantity dispensed on each refill
- The date of dispensing for each refill

- The name or identification code of the dispensing pharmacist
- The number of the original prescription order

If records are kept at a central location, the printout must be capable of being sent to the pharmacy within 48 hours.

Pharmacies with an automated system must have an auxiliary system for documenting refills in the event that the computerized system suffers downtime. The auxiliary system must maintain the same information as the automated system. A pharmacy must use either a manual or electronic system, but not both, to store and retrieve refill information.

Partial Filling of Schedule III, IV, or V Prescriptions

It is permissible for pharmacists to partially fill a prescription for a schedule III, IV, or V drug provided that

- The partial filling is recorded in the same manner as a refill.
- The total quantity dispensed in all partial fillings does not exceed the total quantity prescribed.
- No dispensing occurs 6 months after the date of issuance.

Labeling of Schedule II, III, IV, and V Prescriptions

A pharmacist dispensing a controlled substance must affix to the container a label that shows the date of filling if it is a schedule II drug (21 C.F.R. § 1306.14(a)). The label must show the date of the initial filling if it is for a schedule III, IV, or V drug (21 C.F.R. § 1306.24(a)). The date of initial filling should be used when dispensing refills of schedule III or IV prescriptions. Technically, because the Food, Drug, and Cosmetic Act (FDCA) specifies that the label must contain the date of filling, both dates should be on the label of a refill to comply with both laws. In addition, the regulation requires the label to include

- Pharmacy name and address
- Serial number of the prescription
- Name of the patient
- Name of the prescriber
- Directions for use and cautionary statements, if any

For schedule II, III, and IV drugs, the label should also include a cautionary statement with the following language: "Caution: Federal law prohibits the transfer of this drug to any person other than the person for whom it was prescribed" (21 C.F.R. § 290.5).

These labeling requirements do not apply if the drug is prescribed for administration to an institutionalized ultimate user (medication order) (21 C.F.R. § 1306.14(c) and 21 C.F.R. § 1306.24(c)) provided that

- If the drug is in schedule II, no more than a 7-day supply is dispensed at one time. If the drug is in schedule III, IV, or V, no more than a 34-day supply or 100 dosage units, whichever is less, is dispensed at one time.
- The drug is not in the possession of the ultimate user before the administration.
- The institution maintains appropriate safeguards and records regarding the proper administration, control, dispensing, and storage of the drug.
- The system used by the pharmacist in filling the prescription is adequate to identify the supplier, the product, and the patient, and to state the directions for use and cautionary statements.

REMS FOR LONG-ACTING AND EXTENDED-RELEASE OPIOIDS AND TRANSMUCOSAL IMMEDIATE RELEASE FENTANYL PRODUCTS

The FDA published a risk evaluation and mitigation strategy for specific long-acting and extended-release opioid products. Effective in March 2012, the FDA added a REMS specifically for transmucosal immediate-release fentanyl (TIRF) products. Called the TIRFREMS Access Program, it is a single, shared system REMS for the entire class of TIRF products (http://www.fda.gov/Drugs/DrugSafety/InformationbyDrugClass/ucm284717.htm). The TIRFREMS creates a restricted distribution program for these TIRF products aimed at reducing the risk of misuse, abuse, addiction, and overdose associated with them. Those who prescribe TIRF products in outpatient settings must review the education program, complete a knowledge assessment, and complete an enrollment form. The same requirement applies for both community and inpatient pharmacies that dispense TIRF products. Information about enrollment is available at http://www.tirfremsaccess.com.

ELECTRONIC TRANSMISSION PRESCRIPTIONS

After years of waiting and anticipation by practitioners, in 2010 the DEA authorized the electronic transmission of controlled substance prescriptions. (Proposed regulations were issued in June 2008 (73 Fed. Reg. 36721) and interim final regulations (IFR) on March 31, 2010 (75 Fed. Reg. 16236).) The IFR permits the e-prescribing and dispensing of controlled substances in schedules II–V.

The DEA structured the regulations to accomplish two purposes: (1) security, such that only authorized persons have access to the electronic system, and that only the authorized persons are actually using the system; and (2) accountability, such that a prescription cannot be repudiated and that violators of the law can be readily identified.

Prescriber Requirements

To ensure that only authorized persons have access to an e-prescribing system, the regulations require that prescribers must undergo identity proofing, either in person or remotely, with a federally authorized entity. Once identity is proven, the prescriber is provided an authentication credential or a digital certificate.

To sign and transmit e-prescriptions the prescriber must use a two-factor authentication method. The prescriber must choose two of three factors for this purpose, which act as a digital signature. These factors include: (1) something you know, such as a password or PIN number; or (2) something you have, a hard token separate from the computer such as a personal digital assistant (PDA), cell phone, or flash drive; or (3) something you are (biometrics).

An agent of the prescriber may enter the appropriate prescription information into the system for later approval and authentication by the prescriber. However, an agent cannot have access to the two-factor authentication to sign the prescriptions. The prescription ultimately transmitted to the pharmacy must contain all of the information required on paper prescriptions.

Pharmacy Requirements

When the electronic prescription is transmitted to the pharmacy, the first recipient of the e-prescription (either the pharmacy or its application service provider [ASP] if it uses one) must digitally sign, and the pharmacy must archive the e-prescription. If a prescription transmission fails, the prescriber may write a copy of the transmitted prescription and sign it. The copy must indicate that it was originally transmitted to a specific pharmacy and that the transmission failed. The pharmacy must check to ensure that the e-prescription was not received or dispensed before it dispenses the paper prescription. Similarly, if a pharmacist receives a paper or oral prescription indicating that it was originally transmitted electronically to another pharmacy, the pharmacist must check with that pharmacy to determine whether the e-prescription was received. If it was received but not dispensed, the pharmacy that received it must void it. If the original e-prescription was dispensed, the pharmacy with the paper prescription must void it.

A pharmacy may make changes to the electronic prescription after receipt in the same manner that it may make changes to paper controlled substance prescriptions. The pharmacy must maintain a daily internal audit trail that compiles a list of auditable events (those that indicate a potential security problem). Pharmacies must back up all electronic prescription records daily and they must be kept for 2 years. Electronic prescriptions may be electronically transferred between pharmacies subject to the same requirements as if the transfer was by paper or oral. More information on the e-prescription requirements are available at http://www.deadiversion.usdoj.gov/ecomm/e_rx/index.html#faq.

Audit or Certification Requirements

The DEA has strongly emphasized that both the prescriber's and the pharmacy's application systems must either be approved by a third-party audit conducted by a qualified person or verified and certified by a certifying organization whose process has been approved by the DEA (76 Fed. Reg. 64813, available at http://www.gpo.gov/fdsys/pkg/FR-2011-10-19/pdf/2011-26738.pdf). All certifying organizations with an approved certification process are posted on the DEA's website: http://www.deadiversion.usdoj.gov, under electronic prescriptions. E-prescriptions may not be transmitted, received, or dispensed unless the application systems meet all DEA requirements. Thus, if doubts exist, the pharmacy should request proof from the prescriber that its system has been properly audited or certified.

TRANSFERRING OF PRESCRIPTION INFORMATION

Pharmacies may transfer information between themselves for refill purposes for schedule III, IV, and V prescriptions on a one-time basis only, if state law allows. Regulations enacted March 28, 1997, however, allow pharmacies electronically sharing a real-time, online database to transfer back and forth up to the maximum refills permitted by law and the prescriber's authorization. A transfer can take place only by means of direct communication between two licensed pharmacists (21 C.F.R. § 1306.25).

The transferring pharmacist must

- Write "void" on the face of the invalidated prescription
- Record on the back of the invalidated prescription the name, address, and DEA registration number of the pharmacy to which the prescription was transferred, as well as the name of the pharmacist receiving the information
- Record the date of the transfer and the name of the pharmacist transferring the information

The pharmacist receiving the information must

- Write "transfer" on the face of the transferred prescription
- Reduce to writing all information required on a schedule III, IV, or V prescription, including
  - The date of issuance of the original prescription
  - The original number of refills authorized
  - The date of original dispensing
  - The number of refills remaining and the date(s) and locations of previous refill(s)
  - The transferring pharmacy's name, address, and DEA number, and the prescription number
  - The name of the transferor pharmacist
  - The pharmacy's name, address, DEA number, and prescription number from which the prescription was originally filled

Both the original and the transferred prescription must be kept for 2 years from the date of the last refill.

RETURN OF CONTROLLED SUBSTANCES TO PHARMACY FOR DISPOSAL

The DEA has determined that the CSA does not permit the return of controlled substances by a nonregistrant (e.g., patients, long-term care facilities) to a pharmacy for disposal (General Questions & Answers: http://www.deadiversion.usdoj.gov/faq/general .htm). The basis for the DEA's opinion is that the law does not expressly permit this practice. A regulation provides that a nonregistrant wishing to dispose of a controlled substance must submit to the DEA a letter including the name and address of the person; the name and quantity of the drug to be disposed; how the person obtained the drug, if known; and the name, address, and registration number, if known, of the person who possessed the drug prior to the applicant (21 C.F.R. §1307.21(a)(2)). The DEA took enforcement action against a Washington State pharmacy for accepting unit dose packaging returns for schedule III and IV drugs from a LTCF, even though state law and Medicaid allowed for such returns. Surprisingly, the DEA served the pharmacy with an order for immediate suspension of the pharmacy's registration on the basis that the pharmacy's acts pose an imminent danger to the public. The pharmacy immediately sought a restraining order against the DEA. The court, finding no evidence to support the DEA's contention, granted the pharmacy the restraining order (*Bates Drug Stores, Inc. v. Holder*, 2011 WL 1750066 (E.D.Wash., May 06, 2011)).

The action by the DEA against the Washington pharmacy is inconsistent with other developments by the agency and by Congress. The agency has recognized that its strict position on returns to a pharmacy conflict with its primary concern of reducing diversion and abuse, as well as the concerns of many in society who want safe and responsible options for the disposal of controlled substances. To these ends, the agency issued an advance notice of rulemaking in January 2009, seeking comments from stakeholders as to what should be included in a regulation allowing ultimate users and long-term care facilities to dispose of controlled substances (74 Fed. Reg. 3480). Subsequently, the DEA held a series of national take-back programs in 2010, 2011, and 2012 through local law enforcement agencies to facilitate the disposal of prescription drugs.

It was Congress, however, that proposed a real remedy to the problem by passing the Secure and Responsible Drug Disposal Act of 2010 (P.L. 111-273). This law permits an ultimate user (i.e., patient) who has lawfully obtained a controlled substance to deliver it to another person for disposal, if the person receiving the controlled substance is authorized to engage in disposal and the disposal takes place pursuant to regulations to be issued by the DEA. The law also directs the DEA to develop regulations authorizing long-term care facilities to dispose of controlled substances on behalf of their residents. The DEA has yet to issue regulations.

Separately, the White House Office of National Drug Control Policy (ONDCP) and FDA have partnered to offer guidelines to consumers for disposing of medications (http://www.fda.gov/forconsumers/consumerupdates/ucm101653.htm).

CENTRAL FILLING OF PRESCRIPTIONS

A central fill pharmacy is one that fills prescriptions for retail pharmacies pursuant to a contractual agreement or common ownership. When a retail pharmacy receives a prescription and then sends it to a second pharmacy to prepare and deliver back to the first pharmacy for dispensing to the patient, the second pharmacy is engaging in a "central fill activity." Retail pharmacy conceived of central fill pharmacies in the late 1990s as a means to assist in handling increased volumes of prescriptions. A central fill pharmacy provides pharmacists the opportunity to increase the efficiency of resources, frees pharmacists' time for patient care activities, reduces dispensing errors, and reduces patient wait time. Most state boards of pharmacy have enthusiastically embraced central fill pharmacies, and many states have enacted laws to enable such operations.

The DEA, however, did not originally recognize central fill pharmacies, and thus the central filling of controlled substance prescriptions was not legal. In order to rectify this situation, the DEA proposed regulations in 2001 (66 Fed. Reg. 46567, Sept. 6, 2001), to allow the central filling of controlled substances, and finalized the regulations on June 24, 2003 (68 Fed. Reg. 37405, 21 C.F.R. parts 1300, 1304, 1305, and 1306). Pursuant to the final regulations, central fill pharmacies may be registered as pharmacies, as long as state law authorizes this activity. Any person wishing to register as a central fill pharmacy and dispense controlled substances must do so the same as any pharmacy. A central fill pharmacy must be staffed by a licensed pharmacist and may fill both new and refill prescriptions. Any prescription dispensed by the central fill pharmacy must be transported to the retail pharmacy that initially received the prescription, which would then deliver it to the patient. The label of the dispensed drug must contain a unique identifier (i.e., the central fill pharmacy's DEA registration number), indicating that the prescription was filled at the central fill pharmacy (21 C.F.R. § 1306.24(b)). A central fill pharmacy cannot accept a prescription directly from a patient or individual practitioner or deliver a prescription directly to the patient or individual practitioner. Both the pharmacist at the central fill pharmacy and the pharmacist who ultimately dispenses the prescription to the patient are bound by the corresponding responsibility doctrine (21 C.F.R. § 1306.05(f)).

A central fill pharmacy must have a contractual arrangement with the retail pharmacies for which it provides services, keep a list of those pharmacies, and verify the DEA registration of those pharmacies (21 C.F.R. §1304.05). A retail pharmacy similarly must keep a list of the central fill pharmacies with which it contracts and verify their DEA registration. The information at both pharmacies must be available to the DEA upon request.

A retail pharmacy may contract with a central fill pharmacy in another state providing that both states allow this activity. A retail pharmacy may, as a coincidental activity, operate also as a central fill pharmacy without maintaining a separate registration, inventories, or records.

The retail pharmacy must write the words "CENTRAL FILL" on the original paper prescription (21 C.F.R. § 1306.15; § 1306.27). The retail pharmacy may then transmit the prescription to the central fill pharmacy in two ways. First, the controlled substance prescription (including schedule II prescriptions) may be faxed. The retail pharmacy must maintain the original hard copy and the central fill pharmacy must maintain the faxed prescription. Second, the prescription information may be transmitted electronically. The DEA has determined that there appears little risk of diversion in this situation and thus does not require specific security standards for transmission. Of course, both pharmacies must keep all records related to the prescriptions transmitted and comply with all federal and state patient confidentiality and recordkeeping requirements.

INTERNET PHARMACY PRESCRIPTIONS

There are generally three types of Internet pharmacies. One type is operated by legitimate pharmacies that require a valid prescription from a community prescriber before they will dispense the medications. Generally, these are brick-and-mortar or mail-order pharmacies that have created websites where patients can request refills online and where prescribers can phone or fax new prescriptions for patients. These pharmacies are generally legal and the DEA is not concerned with this type of pharmacy.

The other two types of Internet pharmacies are often termed "rogue pharmacies." Under the more blatant type of rogue Internet pharmacy, the patient transmits a request for particular prescription medications and the Web business mails the drugs to the patient without a prescription. In the second type of rogue operation, patients also transmit requests for particular prescription medications. However, the patients are required to complete an online survey asking some basic questions such as weight, sex, if they have high blood pressure, and the like. This survey is electronically routed to a physician who has contracted with the Internet operation and usually resides in a different state from the patient. The physician reviews the survey and issues a prescription to a contracting pharmacy. The pharmacy often is a community state-licensed pharmacy in a different state than the prescriber. The pharmacy then dispenses and mails the prescription medication to the patient, who generally lives in yet a different state.

The FDA, DEA, most state boards of pharmacy, and most pharmacy organizations consider rogue pharmacy operations illegal because there is no valid physician–patient relationship because the physician never personally sees the patient. A prescription issued in such a situation, although perhaps facially valid, is not a legal prescription.

Unfortunately, it required the highly publicized overdose death of an 18-year-old Californian, who had ordered hydrocodone from an online pharmacy to treat his back pain, to trigger a federal law in 2008 to regulate these rogue pharmacies. The law, known as the Ryan Haight Online Pharmacy Consumer Protection Act of 2008 (P.L. 110-425), and the accompanying DEA regulations (74 Fed. Reg. 15596 (April 6, 2009)), amend the CSA to define a valid prescription as one that has been issued for a legitimate medical purpose by a practitioner who has conducted at least one in-person medical evaluation of the patient. The Haight Act and regulations also provide in part that online pharmacies must do the following:

- Obtain a DEA modification of registration permitting it to operate.
- Notify the DEA and state pharmacy boards of intent to dispense through the Internet 30 days before activity commences.
- Display on the website a declaration of compliance with the law and regulations.
- Complete information about the pharmacy, including its name and address as it appears on the DEA certificate, telephone number, email address, the name of the pharmacist in charge, professional degree, state of licensure, and telephone number, and so on.
- Include this statement on the website: "This online pharmacy will only dispense a controlled substance to a person who has a valid prescription issued for

a legitimate medical purpose based upon a medical relationship with a prescribing practitioner. This includes at least one prior in-person medical evaluation or medical evaluation via telemedicine in accordance with applicable requirements of section 309."

- Report on a monthly basis all controlled substances dispensed, if they dispense 100 or more controlled substance prescriptions or 5,000 total dosage units in a month.

The law imposes criminal penalties for any person that knowingly or intentionally violates the law. Unfortunately, the law applies only to controlled substances (although there is a bill before Congress to apply it to all prescription drugs (Online Pharmacy Safety Act, S. 2002)). Thus, it is left to the states to regulate these rogue pharmacies for dispensing noncontrolled substances. Although some states have enacted specific laws directed at Internet prescribing and dispensing, others must struggle with regulating the practice by applying more general laws and regulations that were enacted long before anyone anticipated the Internet. Any pharmacy invited to dispense prescriptions for an Internet business should be suspicious and seek legal advice. State boards of pharmacy have stepped up enforcement. As an example, the California Board of Pharmacy since 2009 has assessed $600 million in fines against pharmacies and pharmacists for dispensing invalid Internet prescriptions.

STATE ELECTRONIC PRESCRIPTION MONITORING PROGRAMS (PMPS)

Most states have implemented electronic prescription monitoring programs (PMPs) (see http://www.deadiversion.usdoj.gov/faq/rx_monitor.htm). Although the details of a PMP may vary from state to state, typically the program requires pharmacists and prescribers to electronically transmit to the state a record of each controlled substance prescription dispensed. (Some states only require the reporting of C–II and C–III prescriptions.) PMPs allow investigators to obtain pharmacy data from multiple locations without actually having to visit each pharmacy. States review the data generated through a PMP to determine if diversion or abuse exists and can track patients, physicians, and pharmacies. Thus, PMPs can identify such situations as patients shopping multiple prescribers or multiple pharmacies. Most states allow treating health care professionals to request patient-specific information from the PMP upon request. Some states also authorize the state agency responsible for the PMP to proactively notify health care professionals when data indicate that a patient may be engaged in possible diversion or abuse.

Congress recognizes the importance of PMPs. In 2002, Congress authorized a federal grant program through the Department of Justice enabling states to apply for and receive funding to develop a new PMP or enhance an existing PMP. In 2005, Congress passed the National All Schedules Prescription Electronic Reporting Act (NASPER) (P.L. 109-60; 42 U.S.C.A. § 280g-3), which also provides grant funding to states to develop or enhance PMPs. States that receive funding must agree to meet specified standards; share controlled substance data with other states; collect specified prescription information from pharmacies for schedule II, III, and IV drugs; and allow prescribers and dispensers access to patient records to determine therapeutic duplication and whether diversion, abuse, or fraud might exist.

A weakness of state PMP programs had been that the data in one state were unavailable to another state. This obviously presents monitoring problems when patients cross state lines. In response, the National Association of Boards of Pharmacy (NABP) established in 2011 a nationwide platform to facilitate the transmission of PMP data across state lines called NABP PMP InterConnect (http://www.nabp.net/programs/pmp-interconnect/nabp-pmp-interconnect). A number of states now participate in the system.

Long-Term Care (LTC) Pharmacy

Prescription medications for LTCF residents are generally dispensed by community pharmacies pursuant to prescription orders from a prescriber. LTCFs usually store the medications for the residents and LTCF staff administers the medications to the residents. The dispensing and storage of controlled substances in long-term care facilities causes the DEA many special considerations and concerns, especially because these facilities are not DEA registrants. One concern is the amount of controlled substances stored at LTCFs. The DEA prefers that pharmacies that dispense to LTCF residents dispense as minimal quantity of controlled substances as possible. Excess supply of controlled substances is particularly troublesome for the DEA because it currently prohibits an LTCF, as a nonregistrant, from distributing the drugs back to the dispensing pharmacy, or anywhere off site, even for destruction. (Disposal of controlled substances is discussed later in this chapter in the section titled Recordkeeping.) This is one reason why the agency allows up to 60 days for the partial filling of schedule II drugs. Another means by which the stock of controlled substances in LTCFs can be reduced is by the use of automated dispensing systems, as described next.

Automated Dispensing Systems

The DEA issued a final regulation in May 2005 allowing retail pharmacies to install automated dispensing systems (ADSs) in long-term care facilities provided that state law also permits (70 Fed. Reg. 25462, May 13, 2005). An ADS is defined as "a mechanical system that performs operations or activities, other than compounding or administration, relative to the storage, packaging, counting, labeling, and dispensing of medications, and which collects, controls, and maintains all transaction information." Thus, the pharmacy stores drugs in the ADS and controls the machine remotely. Authorized LTCF staff is allowed access to the ADS contents, which are dispensed on a single-dose basis at the time of administration pursuant to a prescription. The drugs in the ADS are pharmacy stock until dispensed.

The intent of the ADS regulations is to reduce accumulated stocks of excess controlled substances. Excess stock results because pharmacies may supply several days' quantities of drugs to patients who ultimately do not take all the medications because of death, discharge, or a change of drugs. ADSs allow the dispensing of single dosage units of the drug, thus reducing the problem of excess stock and disposal. Retail pharmacies that install an ADS must maintain a separate DEA registration at the LTCF location.

LTCF Nurses as Agents of the Prescriber

It is a common scenario in LTC pharmacy, and authorized by many states, for a prescriber to communicate a drug order for a patient to a LTCF nurse and for that nurse to then communicate the order to the pharmacy. For example, a terminally ill LTCF resident might relate to a nurse that he is in severe pain. The nurse contacts the prescriber who tells the nurse to phone the pharmacy with an order for Vicodin (a schedule III opioid). The issue here is whether the nurse can lawfully be the agent of the prescriber and communicate the order to the pharmacy. In 1995, the DEA commented that a prescriber could designate, in writing, a responsible person at an LTCF to act as an agent. In a *Federal Register* posting in 2001 the DEA changed its position, stating that no agency relationship exists between an LTCF nurse and a physician. A pharmacist may only fill the order as issued by the prescriber and communicated by the prescriber or the prescriber's agent (66 Fed. Reg. 20833).

In 2009, the DEA began enforcing its position, causing several complaints regarding the DEA's policy. These complaints led to a Senate Special Committee on Aging session in March 2010 (http://www.gpo.gov/fdsys/pkg/CHRG-111shrg57545/pdf/CHRG-111shrg57545.pdf) and an article in the *New York Times* highlighting the adverse consequences of the DEA's position for nursing home residents (http://www.nytimes.com/2010/10/03/us/03rules.html). Perhaps these events prompted the DEA to amend its position. In October 2010, the agency issued a policy notice that it will recognize an agency relationship between a prescriber and an LTCF or hospice employee provided there is a formal, written, and witnessed agreement between them (75 Fed. Reg. 61613). An example of such an agreement is included in the *Federal Register* notice. The notice lists the limited acts that an agent may perform as follows:

- Preparing a written prescription for the signature of the practitioner
- Conveying orally to a pharmacy prescription orders from a practitioner for drugs in schedules III through V (but not for schedule II drugs, even in an emergency)
- Transmitting a fax prescription from the prescriber, including schedule II prescriptions

Dispensing from LTCF Emergency Kits

The DEA permits pharmacies to place sealed "emergency kits'" in LTCFs (45 Fed. Reg. 24128, April 9, 1980), which are routinely stocked with commonly dispensed prescription drugs, including controlled substances. The kits are considered extensions of the pharmacy and the pharmacy is responsible for the proper control and accountability of the kit. It has been a common practice for the LTCF nurse to contact the prescriber on behalf of a resident in an emergency and for the prescriber to instruct the nurse to administer a controlled substance to the patient from the kit. The nurse would then subsequently notify the pharmacy, which would replace the medication in the kit and reseal it. Although many states permit this procedure, the DEA again does not recognize a nurse as an agent for this purpose, even with a formal, written agreement (75 Fed. Reg. 37463, June 2010; http://www.deadiversion.usdoj.gov/faq/general.htm#lt-2). Thus, the prescriber must issue a prescription to the pharmacy and the pharmacist must authorize the nurse to dispense the medication from the kit.

© Stockbyte/Thinkstock

STUDY SCENARIOS AND QUESTIONS

1. Alex Swanson is a pharmacist in a modern chain pharmacy located in a new strip mall in a trendy suburb of a major metropolitan area. Alex got a telephone call one day from a nearby community pharmacist who is part of a "hot line" to alert area pharmacists about suspicious prescriptions. The message is that a 30-year-old black male is attempting to pass a prescription for Demerol, and the prescription appears very worn, as if many people have handled it. The pharmacist tells Alex, "The best thing to do is just say you're out of the drug. There's no sense in asking for trouble." Just as Alex hangs up the telephone, he sees a black male standing at the counter. Sure enough, he has a prescription

for Demerol 50 mg, #50, with directions for one tab every 4 hours for pain. The name of the patient on the prescription is John Smith. The paper on which the order is written is a bit frayed on the edges. Alex feels that the prescription looks authentic. It is from the major teaching hospital downtown and is written by a doctor that Alex has heard of. Alex calls the hospital, using the telephone number listed in the phone book. He is referred to the hematology department, where he finally locates a resident who knows the prescriber and the patient. The prescriber is out. The resident assures Alex that the prescription is valid. Alex fills the prescription. Two weeks later Alex is visited by the local police, who tell him that the prescription he filled was a photocopy. The person who presented the prescription was not the patient but a friend of the patient. The Demerol tablets Alex dispensed were sold on the playground of the local junior high school. List three factors that suggest Alex might not have met his responsibility. List three factors that suggest Alex might have met his responsibility. Can you conclude that Alex "knowingly" dispensed the invalid prescription? Is race a factor in this incident? Why or why not?

2. Mary Lee is a terminally ill patient in chronic, severe pain. Her physician has elected to aggressively treat her pain with oxycodone and other schedule II drugs for breakthrough pain. Mary gets her prescriptions filled at LessPay Pharmacy. Tom Tam, a pharmacist at LessPay, knows Mary's condition but became concerned after he noticed that every month her dosages kept increasing considerably to the point that her prescriptions were for a few hundred tablets at a time. Tom became convinced that Mary was addicted to the drug and concerned that diversion was occurring because of the large number of tablets. Tom called the physician with his concerns. The physician reacted angrily and told Tom that whether Mary is addicted or not is irrelevant and none of his business and that her treatment is appropriate. To suggest diversion, the physician added, was absurd, and he abruptly hung up on Tom. When Mary came to the pharmacy a few days later with new prescriptions for even greater quantities of opioids, Tom told her that he could not fill the prescriptions any longer. Are Tom's concerns and actions justified under the corresponding responsibility doctrine? In other words, should addiction and diversion be a concern in this case? What would you do if you were Tom and had Mary for a patient? Would it matter in your actions if Mary did not have a terminal illness but did have chronic, severe pain?

3. Tammy is a nurse at a skilled nursing facility. One of the residents, Ben, has been experiencing increasing pain as the result of a condition he was diagnosed with a couple of months ago by his physician. Until now an NSAID had controlled Ben's pain. Tammy called the physician, who told her that he would like to now have Ben put on morphine. He instructed the nurse to order from the pharmacy 15-mg tablets, #50, with the directions of one every 6 hours. The nurse phoned the order in to the pharmacy. Is the oral order of the nurse legal under federal law? Is this an emergency situation? If not, how should the prescription order have been transmitted to the pharmacy?

4. A patient presented a prescription to the pharmacy for Oxycontin 10 mg, #60, 1 tablet bid. The patient had no insurance and told the pharmacist that she could only afford to pay for 20 tablets presently but would come back in 5 or 6 days with enough money to pay for the balance. What should the pharmacist do in this situation? Is this a valid reason for a partial fill? Does the balance of the prescription have to be dispensed to the patient within a certain time? What is in the best interest of the patient?

5. Mary, a patient at Primrose Pharmacy, requested a refill of her Valium prescription on June 12. The prescription was issued on April 15 and written for one refill, which she received on May 10. Sally, the pharmacist at Primrose, called the prescriber's office for refill authorization. The physician spoke directly to Sally and authorized five refills. How should Sally handle this authorization? Should she document the authorization on the existing prescription or make a new prescription? Explain.

6. A patient asked the pharmacist at Redwing Pharmacy if she could get her Valium prescription transferred to Redwing from Bluewing Pharmacy, which was in another part of town. The pharmacist said that she would find out. After contacting Bluewing, the pharmacist discovered that the prescription had three refills remaining. Detail the recordkeeping requirements for transferring the Valium prescription from Bluewing to Redwing. What if Redwing and Bluewing were part of the same chain and shared common electronic files? How would this change the recordkeeping requirements?

RECORDKEEPING

The CSA requires that every registrant keep a "complete and accurate record" of all controlled substances (§§ 827(a) and (b)). Three types of records are involved:

1. Records of inventory
2. Records of drugs received
3. Records of drugs dispersed

As part of a controlled substance inspection or audit, inspectors typically examine the pharmacy's records of those substances received and subsequently dispersed (by prescription or otherwise) for a particular period of time. The pharmacy's beginning inventory of controlled substances, plus its purchases during the period, minus the drugs dispersed during the period should equal the inventory of controlled substances on hand.

THE IMPORTANCE OF ADEQUATE RECORDKEEPING

Pharmacists cannot take the recordkeeping requirements of the CSA lightly. Negligent recordkeeping violates the act and may result in fines of up to $10,000 per offense. Intentional recordkeeping violations can result in up to 1 year imprisonment plus a fine. In an October 21, 2005, news release, the DEA announced that King Soopers, City Market, and the parent company, Kroger, agreed to pay a record $7 million settlement for recordkeeping violations (http://www.thekrogerco.com/corpnews/corpnewsinfo_pressreleases_10212005b.htm). According to the DEA, its audits revealed a pattern of noncompliance with recordkeeping requirements at the company's pharmacies.

Moreover, discrepancies in records can lead to charges that controlled substances were illegally diverted, whether in fact diversion occurred or not. Conviction of illegal drug diversion—in essence, drug trafficking—carries more severe penalties. In *United States v. Bycer*, 593 F.2d 549 (3rd Cir. 1979), Bycer, a pharmacist, was the manager of a drugstore whose records failed to account for approximately 100,000 tablets of various controlled substances. The government charged Bycer with improper recordkeeping and illegal distribution of controlled substances. The government had no direct evidence that Bycer had been illegally distributing the drugs but rather inferred it from the pharmacist's records. The court, however, was not convinced that the government's evidence supported a diversion charge. It noted that there is a difference between inferring illegal diversions by nonregistrants and inferring illegal diversions by a registrant, as in this case, who was legally in possession of controlled substances. The court noted that six other pharmacists in the pharmacy had access to the controlled substances and that any one of them could have diverted the drugs. It further noted that Bycer's father, who had been the manager of the pharmacy, had been seriously ill and had died during the period in question, requiring that Bycer be frequently absent from the pharmacy. The pharmacist was acquitted on all counts of illegal distribution but found guilty of improper recordkeeping.

GENERAL RECORDKEEPING REQUIREMENTS

Regulations establish procedures for the general maintenance of records and inventories (21 C.F.R. §§ 1304.04 and 1304.22). Controlled substances records must be kept for at least 2 years at the place of registration. In practice, it is wise to keep records for longer than 2 years because of concern over state statutes of limitations and other state laws.

Registrants (e.g., chain pharmacies) may maintain certain types of records, such as financial and shipping records (e.g., invoices, packing slips), at a central location rather than the registered location if they notify the DEA (21 C.F.R. § 1304.04 (a)–(e)). The notification must include:

- The nature of the records to be kept centrally
- The exact location where the records will be kept
- The registrant's name, address, DEA number, and type of DEA registration
- Whether the central records will be maintained in manual or computer-readable form

Centralized records are subject to these conditions:

- Executed order forms and inventory records cannot be maintained centrally but rather must be maintained at each registered location.
- If the records are kept on microfilm, on computer media, or in any form that requires the use of special equipment to read the records, the registrant must provide access to such equipment together with the records. If any code system is used, other than for pricing, the registrant must provide the key to the code.
- The registrant agrees to deliver all or any part of the records to the registered location within 2 business days on receipt of a written request from the DEA for the records or, alternatively, to allow authorized DEA employees to inspect the records at the centralized location without a warrant of any kind.
- In the event that the registrant refuses to comply with any of these procedures, the special agent in charge may cancel any central recordkeeping authorization without a hearing.

Registrants who wish to use central recordkeeping must notify the DEA in writing by registered or certified mail. The registrant may engage in central recordkeeping 14 days after the DEA receives notification, unless the DEA denies permission. It is not necessary to notify the DEA or obtain central recordkeeping approval to maintain records on an in-house computer system.

Records (including inventory records) of all schedule I and II controlled substances must be maintained separately from all other pharmacy records (21 C.F.R. § 1304.04(h)(l)). Records of controlled substances in schedules III, IV, and V need not be maintained separately, provided that they are readily retrievable from other records. For electronic records, this means that the system can separate the records in a reasonable time. For hard-copy records, *readily retrievable* means that the schedule III, IV, and V items are marked in such a manner as to visually distinguish them from other items.

INVENTORY RECORDS

Before a pharmacy begins business, an initial inventory must be conducted. The inventory must "contain a complete and accurate record of all controlled substances on hand on the date the inventory is taken" (21 C.F.R. § 1304.11(a) and (b)). Controlled substances are considered to be "on hand" when they are in the possession of or under the control of the registrant. Thus, substances returned by a customer, substances ordered by a customer but not yet invoiced, and substances stored at a warehouse for the registrant are "on hand." Registrants must maintain and keep at each registered location a separate inventory.

Every 2 years after the date on which the initial inventory was taken, the registrant must take a new inventory (21 C.F.R. § 1304.11(c)). The biennial inventory date may be taken on any date that is within 2 years of the previous biennial inventory date.

The inventory may be taken either at the beginning of the business day or at the close of business. The records must be maintained at the registered location in written, typewritten, or printed form. If taken by use of an oral recording device, the inventory must be promptly transcribed (21 C.F.R. § 1304.11(a)).

When a drug is newly scheduled by the DEA, the registrant must take an inventory of that drug on the effective date of scheduling (21 C.F.R § 1304.11(d)). Thereafter, the drug must be included in each inventory made by the registrant. Notices of new schedulings appear in the *Federal Register* and in many professional publications, and it is the responsibility of registrants to watch for this information.

If a substance is listed in schedules I or II, the registrant must make an exact count or measure of that substance for the inventory. If a substance is listed in schedules III, IV, or V, an estimated count or measure is generally permissible. If its container holds more than 1,000 tablets or capsules, however, an exact count is required (21 C.F.R. § 1304.11(e)(3)). The inventory record for each controlled substance must also include the name of the substance, dosage form, strength, number of units or volume in each container, and number of containers (21 C.F.R. § 1304.11(e)).

RECORDS OF RECEIPT

Invoices are acceptable records of receipt for schedule III, IV, and V substances; the official federal order form, DEA Form 222, is acceptable for schedule I and II substances. When a pharmacist receives an order from the supplier, the date of receipt must be written on the enclosed invoice or DEA Form 222, and these records must be filed appropriately. Because schedule III, IV, and V records must be readily retrievable, if the invoice lists both noncontrolled and controlled substances interchangeably, the controlled substances must be identified in some manner (e.g., marked with a red asterisk or underlined in red) (21 C.F.R. § 1300.01(b)(38)). Records of receipt must contain the following (21 C.F.R. § 1304.22(c)):

- The name of the substance
- The dosage form
- The strength of the substance
- The number of dosage units or volume in the container
- The number of commercial containers received
- The date of receipt
- The name, address, and registration number of the supplier

RECORDS OF DISPERSAL

Any records that document the removal of drugs from the pharmacy are records of dispersal. They include prescriptions, record books, DEA Form 222, invoices, institutional records (e.g., medication orders), records of disposal, and records of theft or loss.

Prescriptions

The term *prescription* is defined as "an order for medication which is dispensed to or for an ultimate user" (21 C.F.R. § 1300.01(b)(35)). The regulations are confusing as to how a pharmacy may file paper prescriptions for controlled substances. In one place it provides that paper prescriptions for schedule II drugs must be maintained in a separate file (21 C.F.R. § 1304.04(h)(2)–(4)). Later the regulation provides they can be filed with schedule III, IV, and V paper prescriptions (21 C.F.R. § 1304.04(h)(4)). To avoid controversy, a pharmacy should follow the 2010 DEA *Pharmacist's Manual* that specifies two options:

1. In three separate files: One file for schedule II drug prescriptions; a second file for the prescriptions of schedule III, IV, and V drugs; and a third file for noncontrolled drug prescriptions.
2. In two separate files: One file for schedule II drug prescriptions, and a second file for schedule III, IV, and V prescriptions, together with all prescriptions for noncontrolled drugs.

If using filing method 2, all schedule III, IV, and V prescriptions must be stamped with the letter "C" in red ink, not less than 1 inch high, in the lower right-hand corner of the prescription. The red "C" requirement is waived, however, if the pharmacy uses an electronic recordkeeping system for prescriptions that permits identification by prescription number and retrieval of original documents by the prescriber's name, patient's name, drug dispensed, and date filled.

Nonprescription Schedule V Sales

Many schedule V drugs, such as codeine cough syrups and antidiarrheals, are not legend drugs. In some states, these drugs may be dispensed and sold without a prescription, provided that these requirements are met (21 C.F.R. § 1306.26):

- The dispensing is done only by a pharmacist. (The term pharmacist also includes other persons authorized to dispense by state law under the direct supervision of a pharmacist, such as an intern.) Nonpharmacist employees are not allowed to dispense even under the supervision of a pharmacist. After the pharmacist has fulfilled his or her professional and legal responsibilities, a nonpharmacist employee may perform the actual sale transaction.
- No more than 240 ml (8 oz) or 48 dosage units of any controlled substance that contains opium, nor more than 120 ml (4 oz) or 24 dosage units of any other controlled substance, may be dispensed at retail to the same purchaser in any given 48-hour period.
- The purchaser is at least 18 years of age.
- The pharmacist requires every purchaser not personally known to furnish suitable identification (including proof of age, where appropriate).
- The pharmacist maintains a bound record book, which contains the name and address of the purchaser, the name and quantity of controlled substance purchased, the date of each purchase, and the name or initials of the pharmacist who dispensed the substance.
- Federal, state, or local law does not require a prescription to dispense the controlled substance.

Distributions from a Pharmacy to Another Practitioner

The sale or transfer by a pharmacy of a schedule III, IV, or V drug to another registrant (e.g., pharmacy, individual practitioner) must be recorded by means of an invoice (a prescription may not legally be used for this purpose) that contains all required information (21 C.F.R. § 1307.11) including the following:

- The name of the substance
- The dosage form
- The strength of the substance
- The number of dosage units or volume in the container

- The number of commercial containers distributed
- The date distributed
- The name, address, and registration number of the person to whom the containers were distributed

If the drug is a schedule II drug, the purchaser must execute a DEA Form 222. The same requirements apply to the return of controlled substances to the supplier. The total number of dosage units distributed to another registrant must not exceed 5 percent of the total units of controlled substances distributed and dispensed in 1 year, or the pharmacy may be required to register as a distributor (21 C.F.R. § 1307.11(a)(4)).

Institutional Medication Records

In hospitals and other institutional settings, individual practitioners order controlled substances for administration to inpatients. This information is entered in the patient's hospital chart, and the order for medication is sent to the hospital pharmacy, which then dispenses the medication. The amount of medication dispensed is usually small, ranging anywhere from one dose to a supply for 3 or 4 days. The medication is kept under the control of those at the nursing station, not the patient, and administered by nurses.

These orders (called medication or chart orders) for inpatients are not prescriptions under the CSA, and thus need not conform to all the requirements of a prescription record (e.g., packaging and labeling requirements). Nonetheless, medication orders for controlled substances must contain the minimum information necessary to provide an acceptable record for drug dispersal and must be readily retrievable. Because medication orders kept as part of a patient's chart are not likely to be considered readily retrievable, the institution should maintain these controlled substance orders separately or have the capability of electronic retrieval of the required information. In addition to the medication order, the institution should maintain some type of record system to account for the actual administration of the drug. (The form this information is recorded on often is called a medication administration sheet or profile sheet.)

Orders for take-home medications for a discharged patient must normally be dispensed only pursuant to prescriptions (not medication orders). Because these medications are not for immediate administration and will be in the control of the patient, prescription recordkeeping requirements are applicable.

Disposal or Destruction of Controlled Substances

DEA regulations provide that any registrant wishing to dispose of a controlled substance may ask the DEA for the authority to do so, as well as for instructions on the appropriate procedure (21 C.F.R. § 1307.21). The request should be made on DEA Form 41, which is available online at the DEA's website. The form may be completed interactively online and printed by the applicant, or the blank form may be printed and completed manually. The form requires the registrant to list the name of the drug, the number of containers, and the content of each container to be disposed of or destroyed.

The regulations state that the DEA will then instruct the registrant as to which of four courses of action to take to dispose of the drug (21 C.F.R. §1307.21(b)):

1. By transfer to a registrant authorized to possess the substance
2. By delivery to a DEA agent or the nearest DEA field office serving the registrant's area
3. By destruction in the presence of a DEA agent or other authorized person
4. By any other means authorized by the DEA

If a registrant, such as a hospital or clinic, is required to dispose of controlled substances regularly, the DEA may authorize the registrant to dispose of them without prior approval in each instance (21 C.F.R. §1307.21(c)). The registrant must keep records of these disposals and file periodic reports to the DEA. The DEA may place conditions on the disposals, such as the method and frequency.

The DEA's *Pharmacist's Manual* (2010) provides that a pharmacy may transfer the controlled substances to a DEA-registered reverse distributor. If C-II drugs are transferred, the reverse distributor must issue a DEA Form 222 or electronic equivalent to the pharmacy. For other scheduled drugs, the pharmacy must keep a record of the distribution with all required information. The reverse distributor who will destroy the drugs is responsible for submitting the DEA Form 41. The form should not be used to record the transfer of the drugs between the pharmacy and reverse distributor disposing of the drugs.

Records of Theft or Loss

A registrant must notify the nearest DEA office in writing of the "theft or significant loss of any controlled substances within one day of discovery " and submit DEA Form 106 (21 C.F.R. § 1301.76(b)). In addition, the registrant should also notify local law enforcement and most likely is required by state law to notify the board of pharmacy. In an effort to clarify what is meant by "significant loss," the DEA amended the regulation in 2005 (70 Fed. Reg. 47094) and added a list of factors to be considered when determining whether the loss is significant. These factors include the quantity lost in relation to the type of business, the specific drugs lost or stolen, whether the loss can be attributed to individuals or unique activities, whether the losses are random or fit a pattern, and local trends and other indicators of diversion. The DEA commented that the registrant shoulders the burden of responsibility as to whether a loss is significant and, if the registrant is in doubt, it is better to err on the side of caution and report the loss.

The loss of a small quantity of controlled substances repeated over time may indicate a significant loss that must be reported. Breakage or spillage of controlled substances does not constitute a loss but rather becomes a disposal issue and must be reported on DEA Form 41.

When all or part of a shipment of controlled substances fails to arrive at the purchaser's address, the supplier is responsible for reporting the loss to the DEA. The purchaser is responsible for reporting loss after signing for or taking custody of a shipment.

DEA Form 106 was modified by the DEA in October of 2008 and is available online at the DEA's website. The form may be completed interactively online and printed by the applicant, or the blank form may be printed and completed manually. As required on the form, the registrant must specify the date of the theft or loss (or when discovered if not known); the name and phone number of the local police department, if notified; the type of theft that occurred; the symbols, identifiers, or cost code used by the pharmacy in marking the containers (if any); and a list of the controlled substances missing, including NDC number, dosage strength, form, and quantity.

A national pharmacy chain discovered that a nonpharmacist employee had been stealing controlled substances over a several month period. The chain fired the employee but failed to report the theft to the DEA, resulting in a regulatory action by the DEA against the chain. The chain ultimately settled the case by paying a fine of $150,000.

RECORDS REQUIRED OF INDIVIDUAL PRACTITIONERS

Recordkeeping requirements for individual practitioners differ from those for pharmacies. Under the statute (21 U.S.C. §§ 827(c)(1)(A) and (B)) and the regulations (21 C.F.R. § 1304.03(b)–(d)), individual practitioners must keep records of the controlled substances that they dispense but not of the controlled substances that they prescribe—unless they prescribe these substances in the course of maintenance or detoxification treatment of an individual patient. This provision is intended to apply to physicians who dispense the prescription medications they prescribe (as an alternative to using a pharmacy). Individual practitioners need not keep records of the controlled substances administered either, unless the individual practitioner regularly engages in the dispensing or administering of controlled substances and charges patients, either separately or with other professional services. Records must be kept of controlled substances administered in the course of maintenance or detoxification treatment of an individual. Individual practitioners may also administer or dispense a controlled substance in the course of professional practice without a prescription (21 C.F.R. § 1306.21(b)).

Not requiring individual practitioners to keep records of the controlled substances that they administer without charge to the patient is a significant loophole in the CSA. Practitioners who have been suspected of illegal diversion of controlled substances and whose records could not account for the missing substances have successfully asserted this as a defense. Several states have enacted laws or regulations requiring individual practitioners to account for all controlled substances dispensed or administered, regardless of the circumstances.

DRUG ENFORCEMENT ADMINISTRATION ORDER FORM 222

Section 828 of the CSA provides that it is unlawful for any person to distribute a controlled substance in schedule I or II to another except pursuant to a written form issued by the attorney general. This written form is known as DEA Form 222 (see **Figure 5-1**).

See Reverse of PURCHASER'S Copy for Instructions			No order form may be issued for Schedule I and II substances unless a completed application form has been received, (21 CFR 1305.04).				**OMB APPROVAL No. 1117-0010**		
TO: *(Name of Supplier)* Wholesale Drugs, Inc.				STREET ADDRESS 538 Distribution Street					
CITY and STATE Anywhere, USA			DATE 6/6/00		TO BE FILLED IN BY SUPPLIER SUPPLIERS DEA REGISTRATION No.				

LINE No.	No. of Packages	Size of Package	Name of Item	National Drug Code	Packages Shipped	Date Shipped
			TO BE FILLED IN BY PURCHASER			
1	3	100	Methylphenidate HCL, 5mg tabs			
2	2	100	Oxycodone APAP caps, 5/500			
3	2	100	Secobarbitol caps, 100mg			
4						
5						
6						
7						
8						
9						
10						

◄ LAST LINE COMPLETED *(MUST BE 10 OR LESS)* | SIGNATURE OF PURCHASER OR ATTORNEY OR AGENT

Date Issued 11/15/99	DEA Registration No. BR1234567	Name and Address of Registrant Richard's Pharmacy 419 Main Street Anywhere, USA
Schedules 2, 2N, 3, 3N, 4, and 5		
Registered as a Retail Pharmacy	No. of this Order Form 841266854	

DEA Form -222 (Oct. 1992)	**U.S. OFFICIAL ORDER FORMS - SCHEDULES I & II** DRUG ENFORCEMENT ADMINISTRATION SUPPLIER'S Copy 1	74325420

FIGURE 5-1 Sample DEA Order Form 222.

Source: U.S. Department of Justice, Drug Enforcement Administration

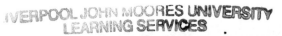

The DEA has stated that if a drug is listed as schedule II by state law, but not federal law, and the state requires distribution pursuant to the Form 222, it does not violate federal law to execute the form.

Only registrants are entitled to obtain copies of Form 222 from the DEA (21 C.F.R. §§ 1305.04 and 1305.05). To obtain the forms initially, the registrant must submit an order form requisition. This procedure is part of the application for registration. When the applicant is approved for registration, the order forms are supplied to the registrant. To obtain subsequent forms, the registrant requests them in writing from the nearest DEA domestic field office.

Each request for order forms must show the name, address, and registration number of the registrant, and the number of envelopes of order forms desired. The requisition must be signed and dated either by the same person who signed the most recent application for registration or reregistration or by a person authorized to obtain and execute order forms through a power of attorney.

Order forms are issued in mailing envelopes that contain seven forms. Each form contains an original, duplicate, and triplicate copy, respectively titled Copy 1, Copy 2, and Copy 3. The registrant's business activity determines the number of forms that the registrant may obtain; however, the DEA has stated that it will only provide a maximum of six books at one time. A registrant who needs more order forms must contact the DEA and show a reasonable need.

The order forms are serially numbered and issued with the name, address, and registration number of the registrant; the authorized activity; and the schedules that the registrant is authorized to handle. The registrant may not correct or change any information or errors but rather must contact the DEA should corrections or changes be necessary.

EXECUTION OF ORDER FORM 222

The purchaser must prepare and execute all three copies of each form simultaneously (21 C.F.R. § 1305.06), using either typewriter, pen, or indelible pencil. Only schedule I or II drugs may be ordered on these forms. There are 10 numbered lines on each order form, and only one item can be entered on each line. An item is one or more commercial containers of the same substance in the same finished form and in the same quantity (e.g., Demerol, 50-mg tablets, #100). Multiple units of the same item may be ordered on the same line (e.g., five bottles of Demerol, 50-mg tablets, #100). The number of the last line completed must be noted on each form in the appropriate place. If one order form is insufficient to include all the items needed, an additional form must be used.

Order forms for etorphine hydrochloride and diprenorphine must contain only orders for these substances. For each item, the form must show the name of the substance ordered, the finished form (e.g., tablets), the number of units or volume in each container (e.g., #100), and the number of commercial containers ordered. The national drug code number of the drug is optional, especially because the pharmacist may not know which brand of the controlled substance ordered will be sent by a supplier. The supplier is not precluded by DEA policy from substituting identical products in packaging sizes different from those ordered, provided the quantity received does not exceed the quantity ordered. The supplier must enter the NDC number of the drug product shipped.

The purchaser must include on the form the name and address of the supplier to whom the order is being sent. Each order form must be signed and dated by an authorized person. If someone other than the purchaser is signing the order form, the purchaser's name must also appear in the signature space.

The purchaser submits Copy 1 and Copy 2 of the order form to the supplier and retains Copy 3 for the purchaser's own files. The supplier records on the first and second copies the number of containers furnished on each item and the date on which the containers were shipped to the purchaser. If the order cannot be filled in its entirety, the supplier may fill the order in part and supply the balance within 60 days of the date on the order form. After 60 days from the date of execution by the purchaser, the order form becomes invalid. The supplier retains Copy 1 for the supplier's files and forwards Copy 2 to the DEA.

On receiving the order from the supplier, the purchaser must record in the appropriate column on Copy 3 the number of containers received of each item and the date received. It is crucial that the purchaser complete this requirement. Failure to do so could result in a substantial penalty and lead to an extensive controlled substance audit.

A supplier is unlikely to accept an order form that is not complete, legible, properly prepared, or endorsed (21 C.F.R. § 1305.11). Moreover, the supplier will not accept any form that shows any alteration, erasure, or changes. If the purchaser makes an error, it is necessary to void and file all three copies of the form. If the supplier cannot fill the order because the order form was illegible, incomplete, altered, or erased—or for any other reason—the supplier should return Copy 1 and Copy 2 to the purchaser with a statement that explains why the order was not filled. The purchaser must attach the two copies of the order and the statement to Copy 3 and file them appropriately (21 C.F.R. § 1305.11).

PROPOSED SINGLE COPY FORM 222

The DEA has proposed converting the triplicate DEA Form 222 into a single-sheet tamper-resistant form (72 Fed. Reg. 66118 (Nov. 2007). The forms would no longer be produced in books of seven order forms, and the number of forms a registrant can receive would depend upon its business activity. Using the single-sheet form, the purchaser would send the original completed form to the supplier after making and retaining a copy. The supplier would then send the original completed form to the DEA after making and retaining a copy. The DEA contends the single-sheet form will allow for improved security features including a special embedded watermark with the Agency's emblem and having the word "copy" appear on a photocopy. In essence, with the single-sheet form, the DEA is shifting the burden of making copies to the purchaser and supplier.

ELECTRONIC DEA ORDER SYSTEM (CSOS)

In response to E-Sign, the DEA issued a notice of proposed regulations in 2003 to provide an electronic equivalent to Form 222 (68 Fed. Reg. 38558 (June 27, 2003)) and published the final regulations in 2005 (70 Fed. Reg. 16901). A registrant may use either the electronic order system or DEA Form 222. An important difference between the two, however, is that the electronic system allows the registrant to order controlled substances not in schedule I or II and noncontrolled substances. In order to use the electronic system, called the Controlled Substance Ordering System (CSOS), the registrant or individual granted a power of attorney must apply for a digital certificate for signing the order and submit proof of identity. A digital certificate is required for each location with a DEA registration. In other words, a digital certificate could not centrally serve multiple locations. One registered location could have more than one certificate if the registrant has granted a power of attorney to others (see the next section) to order the substances. A registrant must appoint a CSOS coordinator to serve as the recognized agent to manage digital certificates. More information regarding a CSOS certificate can be accessed at http://www.deaecom.gov.

A supplier may refuse to accept any electronic order for any reason and must notify the purchaser and provide a statement. The purchaser must then electronically link the statement of nonacceptance to the original order. A defective order cannot be corrected and the purchaser must issue a new order. If an unfilled electronic order is lost, the purchaser must provide the supplier a signed statement including the unique tracking number and date of the lost order, and state that the goods were not received. If the purchaser issues a new order, it must electronically link the electronic record of the second order with a copy of the statement with the record of the first order and retain them.

POWER OF ATTORNEY

Because the person who signed the most recent registration or reregistration is not always available when the pharmacy needs to order forms or schedule II drugs, the person who signed (or is authorized to sign) the registration or reregistration may sign a power of attorney (POA) authorizing a designated individual to obtain and execute order forms (see **Figure 5-2**) (21 C.F.R. § 1305.07). This POA must be made for each individual for whom the pharmacy wants to have order authority, filed with the executed order forms, and made available for inspection with the order form records. The individuals granted the power of attorney are not required to be licensees nor located at the registered location. The person granting the power of attorney may revoke it at any time.

POWER OF ATTORNEY FOR DEA ORDER FORMS

_____ (Name of registrant)

_____ (Address of registrant)

_____ (DEA registration number)

I, _____ (name of person granting power), the undersigned, who is authorized to sign the current application for registration of the above-named registrant under the Controlled Substances Act or Controlled Substances Import and Export Act, have made, constituted, and appointed and by these presents, do make, constitute, and appoint _____ (name of attorney- in-fact), my true and lawful attorney for me in my name, place, and stead, to execute applications for books of official order forms and to sign such order forms in requisition for Schedule I and II controlled substances, in accordance with section 308 of the Controlled Substances Act (21 U.S.C. § 828) and Part 305 of Title 21 of the Code of Federal Regulations. I hereby ratify and confirm all that said attorney shall lawfully do or cause to be done by virtue hereof.

_____

(Signature of person granting power)

I, _____ (name of attorney- in-fact),hereby affirm that I am the person named hereinas attorney-in -fact and that the signature affixed hereto is my signature.

_____

(Signature of attorney-in-fact)

Witnesses:

1. _____

2. _____

Signed and dated on the ____ day of _____ , 20 ___ , at _____

NOTICE OF REVOCATION

The foregoing power of attorney is hereby revoked by the undersigned, who is authorized to sign the current application for registration of the above-named registrant under the Controlled Substances Act or the Controlled Substances Import and Export Act. Written notice of this revocation has been given to the attorney-in-fact _____ this same day.

_____

(Signature of person revoking power)

Witnesses:

1. _____

2. _____

Signed and dated on the ____ day of _____ , 20 ___ , at _____

FIGURE 5-2 Power of Attorney and Notice of Revocation.

Source: U.S. Department of Justice, Drug Enforcement Administration

DISTRIBUTIONS OF SCHEDULE I AND II DRUGS BETWEEN REGISTRANTS

The order form must be used whenever one registrant distributes a schedule I or II drug to another. For example, Pharmacy A has a prescription for a schedule II drug but has none left in stock. Pharmacy B is willing to sell the drug to Pharmacy A. As the purchaser, Pharmacy A executes an order form, keeps Copy 3, and sends Copy 1 and Copy 2 to Pharmacy B. Pharmacy B keeps Copy 1 and sends Copy 2 to the DEA. If Pharmacy B discontinues business, Pharmacy A follows the same procedure to purchase its schedule I and II drugs. Similarly, the order forms must be executed if Pharmacy B transfers its schedule I and II drugs as part of a transfer of business to the buyer.

An individual practitioner who wishes to purchase a schedule I or II drug from a pharmacy for office use must execute an order form as the purchaser and keep Copy 3. The pharmacy, as the supplier, completes the information necessary on Copy 1 and Copy 2, keeps Copy 1, and mails Copy 2 to the DEA. The individual practitioner may not legally write a prescription to obtain the drugs for office use.

If a pharmacy wishes to return schedule I or II drugs to a wholesaler or manufacturer, the pharmacy becomes a supplier. The pharmacy must ask the wholesaler or manufacturer to send an order form, in which case it will send the first two copies of the order form. The pharmacy will record the proper information on the order form, keep Copy 1, and submit Copy 2 to the DEA.

Only schedule I and II controlled substances may be transferred by means of the order form. The transfer of schedule III, IV, and V controlled substances must be recorded by means of an invoice or similar type of record.

LOST OR STOLEN ORDER FORMS

If an unfilled order form is lost in the course of transmission, the purchaser must execute another, together with a statement noting the serial number of the lost form, the date of the lost form, and the fact that the substances ordered were not received (21 C.F.R. § 1305.12). Copy 3 of the second order form, Copy 3 of the lost order form, and the statement must be retained together. The purchaser must send a copy of the statement to the supplier with Copy 1 and Copy 2 of the second order form. If the supplier ultimately receives the first order form, the supplier must mark on its face "not accepted" and return Copy 1 and Copy 2 to the purchaser, who must attach it to Copy 3 and the statement.

If any used or unused order forms are stolen from or lost by the purchaser or supplier other than in the course of transmission, the purchaser or supplier must immediately notify the DEA and provide the serial number of each missing form. If an entire book of forms is lost or stolen from the pharmacy and the serial numbers are not known, the pharmacy must report the date or approximate date of issuance. If any unused forms are subsequently found, the DEA must be notified immediately.

PRESERVATION OF FORMS

Under the CSA, the executed order forms must be maintained separately from all other records and retained by the purchaser and supplier for a period of 2 years (21 C.F.R. § 1305.13). State laws may require that these records be retained for longer than 2 years, however. The purchaser must keep Copy 3 of the executed form at the registered location printed on the order form.

© Stockbyte/Thinkstock

STUDY SCENARIOS AND QUESTIONS

1. DEA agents entered a pharmacy, presented an administrative inspection warrant, and announced they required access to all schedule II records for the past 2 years. What specific records would the agents need? Assume that the agents determined that significant shortages in schedule II drugs exist. Describe how the agents could use records to arrive at that conclusion.
2. You are a pharmacist at SlowGo Pharmacy. The manager noted some outdated bottles of controlled substances for which the pharmacy would not get credit if returned. He instructs you to pour them into the toilet and flush them away. Under the CSA, what should you do?
3. Sally's Pharmacy did not have enough oxycodone in stock to complete a prescription, and partially filling it was not an option. The pharmacist at Sally's called Tim's Pharmacy to ask if the pharmacy could sell the necessary quantity to Sally's. The pharmacist at Tim's said they had enough to sell. Describe the recordkeeping requirements for this transfer to take place.

REFERENCE

U.S. Drug Enforcement Administration Diversion Control Program website: http://www.deadiversion.usdoj.gov

BIBLIOGRAPHY

Abood, R. R. Pharmacists correcting schedule II prescriptions: DEA flip-flops continue. *Journal of Pain and Palliative Care Pharmacotherapy* 24, no. 4 (2010): 393–396.

American Pharmacists Association. Legislative and Regulatory Updates. Available at: http://www.pharmacist.com

American Society for Pharmacy Law. Available at: http://www.aspl.org

Brody, R. Is the DEA on your case? *American Druggist* 203, no. 6 (1991): 27.

Brushwood, D. B. What can you do about forged prescriptions? *U.S. Pharmacist* 11 (1986): 24.

Brushwood, D. B. Reinterpreting "unable to supply." *National Association of Board of Pharmacy Newsletter* 30 (2001): 82–83.

Drug Enforcement Agency (DEA). *Pharmacist's Manual: An Informational Outline of the Controlled Substances Act of 1970*, 2010. Available at: http://www.deadiversion.usdoj.gov/pubs/manuals/index.html

Drug Enforcement Agency (DEA). *Pharmacist's Guide to Prescription Fraud*, 2000. Available at: http://www.deadiversion.usdoj.gov/pubs/brochures/pharmguide.htm

Joranson, D. E., and A. M. Gilson. Policy issues and imperatives in the use of opioids to treat pain in substance abusers. *American Journal of Law, Medicine and Ethics* 22 (1994): 215–223.

Martino, A. M. In search of a new ethic for treating patients with chronic pain: What can medical boards do? *American Journal of Law, Medicine and Ethics* 26 (1998): 332–349.

Milenkovich, N. Controlled substances, LTC nurses, and verbal drug orders. *Drug Topics* (July 15, 2010). Available at: http://drugtopics.modernmedicine.com/drugtopics/Long-Term+Care/Controlled-substances-LTC-nurses-and-verbal-drug-o/ArticleStandard/Article/detail/678155

National Community Pharmacists Association (NCPA). *Governmental Affairs/Legal Proceedings*. Available at: http://www.ncpanet.org

Uelmen, F. G., and V. G. Haddox. *Drug Abuse and the Law*. St. Paul, MN: West Publishing Co., 1974.

Vivian, J. C., and D. B. Brushwood. Monitoring prescriptions for legitimacy. *American Pharmacy* NS31 (1991): 640.

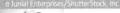

CASE STUDIES

| CASE 5-1 | *United States v. Hayes*, 595 F.2d 258 (5th Cir. 1979) |

Issue

Whether the corresponding responsibility doctrine is unconstitutionally vague.

Overview

Section 841 (the criminal provision of the CSA) applies to registrants of the CSA when they dispense outside the scope of their practice. In this case the pharmacist, Hayes, has been charged with dispensing invalid prescriptions in violation of the corresponding responsibility doctrine. The government contends that Hayes should be charged under section 841 because he knew the prescriptions were not for a legitimate medical purpose. Hayes insists that only the physician can be liable under section 841 because a pharmacist cannot know whether the prescriptions are written for a legitimate medical purpose or not. As you read this case, consider: When should a pharmacist be charged under section 841, rather than section 842, which normally applies to registrants and carries lesser penalties? Is the corresponding responsibility doctrine unfair to pharmacists? Also, does the pharmacist's argument that the corresponding responsibility doctrine is unconstitutionally vague for pharmacists have some merit? What does the corresponding responsibility doctrine really mean to a busy pharmacist? Will pharmacists be liable per se for prescriptions issued for other than legitimate medical purposes?

The court began by addressing the facts of the case:

> Hayes, a registered pharmacist, was convicted under 21 U.S.C. § 841(a) (1) and 21 C.F.R. 1306.04(a) for dispensing Dilaudid and Preludin (schedule II) prescriptions that he knew bore false names or were not issued in the usual course of professional practice. Hayes asserts that the statute and accompanying regulation are unconstitutionally vague and that there was insufficient evidence to support the convictions.

> The court noted that section 841(a) provides in part that it is unlawful for any person to knowingly or intentionally manufacture, distribute, or dispense a controlled substance. Section 1306.04(a) provides that a prescription for a controlled substance must be for a legitimate medical purpose by an individual practitioner acting in the usual course of his or her professional practice and that there is a corresponding responsibility of the pharmacist with the physician to ensure proper prescribing and dispensing.

The court then applied its analysis of the law to this case.

> The purpose of the regulation is to define the circumstances in which a physician or pharmacist who is registered to dispense controlled substances may nevertheless be held to have violated the proscription against manufacturing, distributing, or dispensing a controlled substance contained in 21 U.S.C. § 841. In *U.S. v. Moore*, 423 U.S. 122, 96 S. Ct. 335, 46L.Ed.2d 333 (1975), the Supreme Court concluded that a doctor may be convicted for violations of § 841 when he dispenses controlled substances "outside the usual course of professional practice." A registered doctor or pharmacist is exempted from § 841's proscription only when he acts in the normal course of his professional activities.

> In *U.S. v. Collier*, 478 F.2d 268 (CA5, 1973), this court rejected a physician's vagueness challenge to § 841 and accompanying regulations. The *Collier* court decided

that a doctor's judgment whether a patient needs a schedule II drug is also a routine judgment and that a criminal standard that only makes unlawful the prescribing of drugs outside the course of professional practice is not unconstitutionally vague.

We turn then to application of statute, regulations, and case law to pharmacists. We need none of these to tell us that pharmacists usually are engaged in dispensing drugs on the basis of prescriptions issued by doctors. The regulation, 21 C.F.R. § 1306.04(a), teaches us that under some circumstances a purported prescription is not a prescription at all for purposes of the statute.

(A)n order purporting to be a prescription issued not in the usual course of professional treatment or in legitimate and authorized research is not a prescription within the meaning and intent of Section 309 of the Act (21 U.S.C. § 829) and the person knowingly filling such a purported prescription, as well as the person issuing it, shall be subject to the penalties provided for violations of the provisions of law relating to controlled substances.

Thus, a pharmacist may not fill a written order from a practitioner, appearing on its face to be a prescription, if he knows the practitioner issued it in other than the usual course of medical treatment. The regulation gives "fair notice that certain conduct is proscribed."

Hayes contends that the regulation is unconstitutionally vague because of the language immediately preceding the foregoing, stating that "(t)he responsibility for the proper prescribing and dispensing of controlled substances is upon the prescribing practitioner, but a corresponding responsibility rests with the pharmacist who fills the prescription." A pharmacist, he argues, cannot have a "corresponding responsibility" to that of a practitioner because he cannot prescribe at all but only dispense; an attempt by regulation to impose on him the obligations of a prescriber must, therefore, be ineffectual. From this predicate he urges that the physician cases must be distinguished as applied to him; that is, a practitioner may be held criminally liable for prescribing outside the course of his professional practice, but a pharmacist may not be criminally liable based upon a "corresponding responsibility" because he cannot have responsibility as a prescriber nor does he have any reasonable means to fulfill a duty of establishing that the practitioner prescriber who issued the order did so in the usual course of medical treatment. He points out that the most the pharmacist can do to verify the bona fides of a prescription is to check with the issuing practitioner; anything more would require him to examine the patient, which he is neither qualified nor legally permitted to do.

Verification by the issuing practitioner on request of the pharmacist is evidence that the pharmacist lacks knowledge that the prescription was issued outside the scope of professional practice. But it is not an insurance policy against a fact finder's concluding that the pharmacist had the requisite knowledge despite a purported but false verification. The pharmacist is not required to have a "corresponding responsibility" to practice medicine. What is required of him is the responsibility not to fill an order that purports to be a prescription but is not a prescription within the meaning of the statute because he knows that the issuing practitioner issued it outside the scope of medical practice.

This court said in *Collier* that "Congress did not intend for doctors to become drug 'pushers.'" Nor do we think that Congress intended to allow pharmacists to aid doctors in becoming pushers. When a pharmacist fills a prescription that he knows is not a prescription within the meaning of the regulations he is subject to the penalties of § 841.

The court lastly turned to Hayes's contention that the evidence against him was insufficient. The court, however, considered the argument "almost frivolous." Hayes dispensed a tremendous number of prescriptions from a single physician who was continually under the influence of alcohol. The volume of drugs was massive. For example, Hayes filled 34 prescriptions for Dilaudid for one customer in 1 month, representing 3,400 tablets. He dispensed 101 prescriptions for Dilaudid and 137 for Preludin to another patient the next month, who admitted selling the drugs on the street. Hayes even had a supply of the physician's prescription forms that he would give to customers to fill out and have signed by the physician. On the basis of this evidence, the appellate court stated that the jury was justified in finding that Hayes knew that the prescriptions were not for a legitimate medical purpose.

The court affirmed the decision of the trial court.

Notes on *United States v. Hayes*

1. This case demonstrates that a pharmacist who knows or should have known that a prescription was not written for a legitimate medical purpose can be criminally liable under the corresponding responsibility doctrine. Knowledge or intent can be proved by circumstantial evidence that would lead a court to believe that a pharmacist failed to exercise good faith.

2. Hayes argued that a pharmacist cannot have a corresponding responsibility to the prescriber because the pharmacist does not generally have knowledge of the relationship between the prescriber and the patient. Rather, said Hayes, the most a pharmacist can do is to verify the prescription with the prescriber. There is some validity to Hayes's argument. Although pharmacists must exercise vigilance when dispensing controlled substances, they cannot ensure that every prescription will be legitimate. Pharmacists cannot be faulted for dispensing an invalid prescription when they have no way of suspecting the prescription. Similarly, pharmacists cannot be faulted for dispensing an invalid prescription even if they have suspicions, and if in good faith, they allay those suspicions by calling the prescriber and by talking to the patient. As the court pointed out, however, verification is not an insurance policy when the verification is a sham.

3. The fact that a pharmacist conformed to the letter of the law did not protect him or her from liability when he or she violated the spirit or intent of the law. In *Sloman v. Iowa Board of Pharmacy Examiners*, No. 88-709, Sup. Ct. Iowa (May 17, 1989), a pharmacist had his license suspended for selling schedule V cough syrups without a legitimate medical purpose, even though he conformed to the over-the-counter recordkeeping and quantity of sale restrictions for schedule V nonlegend products. The court found that the evidence showed the pharmacist indiscriminately sold the products over long periods of time to the same patients without exercising good professional judgment as to the purpose of their use. Thus, the court concluded, the board was justified in its determination that the sales were not for a legitimate medical use.

CASE 5-2   *Ryan v. Dan's Food Stores, Inc.*, 972 P.2d 395 (UT 1998)

Issue

Whether a pharmacist was wrongfully discharged for advancing public policy by questioning the validity of controlled substance prescriptions.

Overview

The pharmacist in this case was an employee at will, which means that he was not subject to an employment contract and as such could be terminated for any reason or no reason at all. Despite this broad authority of an employer over an at-will employee, however, an employer cannot generally terminate an at-will employee on the basis of conduct that furthers a clear and substantial public policy. For example, assume an employer orders a pharmacist to violate a state law or regulation (e.g., refill a prescription without authorization). If the pharmacist refuses and is terminated, the pharmacist may be able to successfully establish wrongful discharge if it can be proven that the law or regulation furthers public policy. The pharmacist in this case contends he was discharged for adhering to the corresponding responsibility mandates of the federal CSA. In fact, it would appear that the pharmacist distrusted nearly every controlled substance prescription and treated patients with these prescriptions very poorly. As you read this case, consider: Why was the pharmacist really terminated? Should the public policy aspect of the corresponding responsibility doctrine even have been an issue? What public policy action did the court believe the regulation established? Can pharmacists be too zealous in scrutinizing controlled substance prescriptions? Should pharmacists be suspicious of every controlled substance prescription? Would it be legal to terminate a pharmacist on the basis of verifying controlled substance prescriptions if the pharmacist was also rude to patients?

The court began with the facts of the case:

> Ryan began employment with Dan's (Dan's Food Stores) as a part-time pharmacist in 1992. In September of 1993, Ryan met with Ted D. Gardiner, president of Dan's, to interview for a full-time pharmacy position. During this meeting, Ryan told Gardiner that his previous employer, Harmon's, had fired him from one of its pharmacies; Ryan also told Gardiner that he believed Harmon's fired him because he reported that another Harmon's employee was taking narcotics from the pharmacy. In response, Gardiner stated, "I've got no problem with that. . . . I'll never reprimand a pharmacist for following the law. . . . That's one thing I demand of all my pharmacists that work for me, that they do everything by the book." Following this meeting, Gardiner made Ryan a full-time pharmacist at Dan's Sandy, Utah, store.

During the next 18 months many customers complained about the way Ryan treated them, saying he was rude or treated them poorly. Several complaints were also received when Ryan was part-time as well. The pharmacy management of Dan's repeatedly counseled and warned Ryan about the complaints and his treatment of customers. Ryan indicated he would try to change. Meanwhile, he received commendations from Gardiner and law enforcement officers on his thoroughness in detecting fraudulent prescriptions. The customer complaints continued and the pharmacy supervisor for Dan's asked Gardiner for permission to terminate Ryan, which Gardiner granted, and Ryan was terminated on April 26.

Ryan filed an action in state court alleging wrongful termination on the basis of two claims: breach of an implied contract and violation of public policy. The trial court awarded Dan's summary judgment on both claims and Ryan appealed to the Utah Supreme Court.

The court then applied its analysis to the facts of the case.

As to Ryan's first claim, the court concluded that Ryan was an employee at will and as such there is a legal presumption that Dan's could fire Ryan for any reason or no reason. Ryan's second claim if proven, however, that he was terminated in violation of public policy, would rebut the presumption that his discharge was lawful. Therefore, the court proceeded to address the issue of whether Ryan's discharge violated public policy.

> Ryan claims that Dan's violated a clear and substantial public policy by terminating him for questioning the validity of customers' prescriptions as required and allowed

by federal law. Utah law has recognized that a public policy limitation applies to all employment arrangements. That is, all employers have a duty not to terminate any employee, "whether the employee is at will or protected by an express or implied employment contract," in violation of a clear and substantial public policy.

To make out a prima facie case of wrongful discharge, an employee must show (i) that his employer terminated him; (ii) that a clear and substantial public policy existed; (iii) that the employee's conduct brought the policy into play; and (iv) that the discharge and the conduct bringing the policy into play are causally connected.

The court quickly disposed of the first element because it was undisputed that Ryan was terminated. As to the second element, the court noted that a public policy is clear if plainly defined by law, constitutional standards, or judicial decisions. A public policy is substantial if it is of overarching importance to the public and of such public interest as to warrant being beyond the reach of contract.

Ryan argued that he was following clear and substantial public policy set out in 21 C.F.R. § 1306.04, which provides that there is a corresponding responsibility with the pharmacist to ensure that a prescription for a controlled substance is issued for a legitimate medical purpose by an individual practitioner acting in the usual course of professional practice.

Ryan argues that this section "clearly requires him to check on prescriptions that he believes are unusual under the broad definition of 'usual course'" and that "it is the policy of the state of Utah to require licensed pharmacists to check on the validity of prescriptions to determine if those prescriptions are not in the ordinary course of treatment." We disagree.

Section 1306.04 does contain a clear and substantial public policy, but it is a narrow one, one which only prohibits pharmacists from knowingly filling an improper prescription. Violation of Section 1306.04 "require[s] a willful violation." Section 1306.04 does not mandate or even authorize a pharmacist to question every prescription or to conduct an investigation to determine whether an otherwise facially valid prescription has been issued other than in the "usual course" of the doctor's practice. But when faced with a prescription that is irregular on its face "no date, no physician signature, an obviously toxic dose" Section 1306.04 requires further inquiry. However, after inquiring and obtaining the necessary information, a pharmacist cannot use Section 1306.04 as a basis to refuse to fill a prescription. Therefore, Section 1306.04 does not set forth the public policy Ryan suggests: it does not establish a policy requiring pharmacists to verify prescriptions.

The court then turned its attention to the third element, whether Ryan's conduct of questioning prescriptions furthers the public policy of Section 1306.04's prohibition against knowingly filling improper prescriptions or general public policy encouraging citizens to report violations of criminal law. The court noted that some conduct almost always furthers public policy, such as refusing to violate a law. Other conduct, such as Ryan's, is not so clear. The court noted that Ryan's conduct could fall into three types: (1) questioning prescriptions that Section 1306.04 does not require him to question; (2) questioning prescriptions it does require him to question; and (3) contacting public authorities of suspected criminal conduct.

Because the latter two actions do involve a clear and substantial public policy, the court turned to the fourth element: whether his discharge and the conduct furthering public policy are causally connected. If Ryan can show that the policy-related conduct was the cause of his discharge, Dan's must offer a legitimate reason for discharging him. If Dan's can establish a legitimate reason, Ryan must then show that his policy-related conduct was a substantial factor in the termination.

Ryan has not even shown that his contacting the public authorities was a cause of his termination. Although the record established that Ryan, in fact, contacted the police, it shows no evidence that his termination had anything to do with his contacting any public authority.

On the other hand, the record does establish that Ryan's questioning of prescriptions as required by Section 1306.04 could have been a cause of his termination. The employee separation report Dan's completed indicates Ryan's questioning could have been a cause in Dan's motivation for terminating him. The report stated in part:

> On several occasions Jim has questioned regular customers' doctors' decisions on medication, specifically painkillers (Jim has a genuine concern about prescription drug abuse and on several occasions has caught forged prescriptions). He, however, has also angered several customers by questioning their prescriptions or telling them we were out of stock to avoid filling the script.

Even if Ryan could show that the policy-related conduct was a cause of the termination, Dan's has already articulated a legitimate reason for termination. Dan's has produced relevant and admissible evidence showing that it terminated Ryan because of his history of customer complaints and repeated warnings to him about improving his treatment of customers. Accordingly, Ryan must prove by a preponderance of the evidence that the policy-related conduct was a substantial factor in his termination. Determining whether an employee's engaging in protected conduct was a substantial factor in motivating an employer to discharge the employee is an inquiry that defies precise definition. However, we need not attempt to articulate today a standard to use in this determination because the facts in this case, as a matter of law, could not support the conclusion that Ryan's engaging in protected conduct was a substantial factor in Dan's deciding to terminate him.

The court affirmed the decision of the trial court, that Dan's did not terminate Ryan in violation of public policy.

Notes on *Ryan v. Dan's Food Stores, Inc.*

1. A concurring justice believed that the majority's extensive analysis of the public policy question was not only unnecessary but unwise. This justice believed that the facts clearly showed that Ryan was terminated for rudeness and poor treatment, not because he verified prescriptions. Do you agree?
2. There are pharmacists in practice who strongly believe that Ryan's approach to controlled substance dispensing is right. They consider that stopping illegal diversion is a higher calling than patient care. These pharmacists are suspicious that every controlled substance prescription might be for an invalid purpose. Some even think that controlled substance prescriptions for valid purposes are wrong because noncontrolled drugs could be used. These pharmacists do a disservice to patients and to pharmacy. Pharmacists must always exercise professional judgment and be vigilant against illegal prescriptions, but these efforts must be transparent to patients. Patients should not be made to feel guilty or receive rude treatment because they are receiving controlled substances.
3. This case establishes that even if Ryan had proven he was discharged for verifying prescriptions, his discharge might still be valid because he was also fired because of his rude treatment of patients. If the employer can establish that there was a legitimate reason for the discharge, then the employee must counter by proving that the action involving public policy was the substantial reason he was fired. Because the court construed the public policy aspect of the regulation very

narrowly (not requiring verification of every prescription), Ryan's burden of proof would have been difficult.

| CASE 5-3 | *Gordon v. Frost*, 388 S.E.2d 362 (1989 GA) |

Issue

Whether a pharmacy and pharmacists are liable for intentional infliction of emotional distress for having a patient arrested on the mistaken belief that the patient was attempting to fraudulently obtain a controlled substance.

Overview

This case demonstrates the adverse consequences that result when a pharmacist over-zealously applies the corresponding responsibility doctrine without bothering to determine the facts. It also shows how important communication and the need to exercise common sense are in a pharmacy. As you read this case, consider how you would have handled this situation. Should the pharmacist have been liable to the plaintiff? Did the pharmacist harbor some prejudice against the patient that may have affected her actions? Should pharmacists second-guess physicians in their selection of controlled substances? Was communication among pharmacy personnel a problem, and how could it be improved?

The court began by describing the facts of the case:

The plaintiff, Mrs. Gordon, telephoned Treasure Drug store for a refill of a Fiorinal No. 3 prescription that had been prescribed for her migraine headaches. Mrs. Gordon was well known to the pharmacists because she had been a patient of the pharmacy for more than 4 years, during which time she had had several different prescriptions filled and refilled. An intern at the pharmacy answered and Mrs. Gordon stated: "I am calling to renew a prescription for Gail Gordon." The intern asked for the name of the drug, the name of the physician, and additional information.

The intern then asked for the doctor's DEA number. Mrs. Gordon answered that she did not know the number and that the intern could call the physician's office to get it. The intern replied that the prescription could not be refilled without the DEA number and then put Mrs. Gordon on hold while she got Frost, the pharmacist, to take over the call. Frost reiterated on the phone that she could not fill the prescription without the DEA number, and Mrs. Gordon told Frost to call the physician's office for the number. Frost told Mrs. Gordon she was very busy but would try.

> Apparently believing that the caller requesting Fiorinal was a representative from Mrs. Gordon's physician's office, Frost called the doctor's office to inquire about the prescription but everyone at the office was out to lunch.

> Approximately 2 hours later, Mrs. Gordon called the pharmacy, identified herself and asked whether or not her prescription was ready. She was told that it would be ready in a couple of minutes, by the time of her arrival. In the meantime, Frost spoke with the prescribing physician's office and learned that no one from the office had recently prescribed Fiorinal No. 3 with Codeine for Mrs. Gordon. Frost did not inquire further as to whether or not the doctor would have permitted the prescription, did not check the store computer to see the status of the Fiorinal prescription, and did not call Mrs. Gordon to attempt to clarify the situation. Mrs. Gordon's physician did not believe Mrs. Gordon abused the prescribed medications and probably would have refilled the Fiorinal prescription.

After learning that the initial call had not come from the doctor's office, Frost reached the conclusion that Mrs. Gordon was attempting to fraudulently acquire the prescription. Consequently, Frost called the DEA to report her suspicion. The DEA told Frost they would send someone to take care of the situation and instructed her to try to keep Mrs. Gordon at the store.

Mrs. Gordon, after being arrested in the store, became shocked, upset, and hysterical. She was then taken to jail, fingerprinted, photographed, handcuffed, and held for several hours.

Eventually the charges against Mrs. Gordon were dismissed and she sued the pharmacy, pharmacist Frost, and the pharmacy manager alleging intentional infliction of emotional distress, malicious prosecution, false imprisonment, negligence, and loss of consortium. The trial court directed a verdict in favor of the manager on all causes of action and directed a verdict for the remaining defendants on the false imprisonment and negligence counts. The jury found in favor of the defendants on the cause of action for malicious prosecution but in favor of the plaintiffs on their claims of intentional infliction of emotional distress and loss of consortium. The jury returned a verdict for Mrs. Gordon for $200,000 general damages and for Mr. Gordon in the amount of $20,000.

The defendants then moved for a judgment notwithstanding the verdict (NOV) and/or a new trial. The trial court granted the motion for judgment NOV and denied the motion for new trial. The plaintiffs appealed the judgment NOV.

The appellate court began its analysis by noting that a judgment NOV is proper only where "there is no conflict in the evidence as to any material issue. . . ." In applying this standard, the court stated, it must view the evidence in a light most favorable to the party securing the jury's verdict.

The tort of intentional infliction of emotional distress is recognized in this state, where the "defendant's actions were so terrifying or insulting as naturally to humiliate, embarrass, or frighten the plaintiff." Claims for intentional infliction of emotional distress have been upheld by this court when the threats on which those claims were based were outrageous and egregious. [T]he conduct . . . must be of such serious import as to naturally give rise to such intense feelings of humiliation, embarrassment, fright or extreme outrage as to cause severe emotional distress.

Some claims as a matter of law do not rise to the requisite level of outrageousness and egregiousness. Others raise circumstances which properly put the issue before a jury. Once the evidence shows that reasonable persons might find the presence of extreme or outrageous conduct, the jury must find the facts and make its own characterization. This is a case of the latter class.

Evidence of a defendant's malicious purpose or of a defendant's wanton disregard of a plaintiff's rights may be considered in evaluating whether or not the objected to behavior can reasonably be characterized as outrageous or egregious. "Comment f, 46(1) of the Restatement (Second) states that the extreme and outrageous character of the conduct may arise from the actor's knowledge that the other is peculiarly susceptible to emotional distress by reason of some physical or mental condition or peculiarity. The conduct may become heartless, flagrant, and outrageous when the actor proceeds in the face of such knowledge, where it would not be so if he did not know." Moreover, the existence of a special relationship in which one person has control over another . . . may produce a character of outrageousness that otherwise might not exist. [Cit.] . . . [However,] "major outrage in the language or conduct complained of is essential to the tort."

There was a relationship of professional trust of several years duration between Mrs. Gordon and pharmacist Frost. Frost was in a position of control over Gordon's health and welfare to the extent of properly dispensing needed medications, and as the evidence demonstrated, on occasion making other health recommendations, i.e., advising a nonprescription remedy. Moreover, Frost's position put her in the particular posture of familiarity with Mrs. Gordon's physical and/or emotional state by her ready and continuing access to the lengthy computerized documentation of Mrs. Gordon's prescribed medication in addition to personal exchanges and encounters with the customer relative to her health needs.

The court concluded that Frost's actions could be considered by the jury as evidence of malicious or wanton disregard. Because of this evidence, the trial court was not authorized to grant a judgment NOV. Therefore the court reversed the judgment NOV and found for the plaintiffs.

Notes on *Gordon v. Frost*

1. Some days before this event occurred, Frost had remarked to the intern that Mrs. Gordon was a hypochondriac because she took a lot of medication. The court considered this as evidence that Frost perceived Mrs. Gordon as having emotional problems and thus should have realized her susceptibility to emotional distress. It would probably be more accurate to surmise that because Frost viewed Gordon as a hypochondriac, she probably prejudged Mrs. Gordon as a prescription drug abuser, which then colored her judgment and actions.

2. This case is a classic example of an overzealous pharmacist making prejudicial assumptions based on miscommunication that patients who take several medications are likely drug diverters. Suspecting a well-known patient of phoning in a fraudulent prescription without thoroughly confirming those suspicions is inexcusable behavior and arguably unprofessional conduct. Every pharmacy should have written protocols about how pharmacists should handle suspicious prescriptions, which would prevent situations like this from ever happening.

3. This case does raise a significant issue, however: Should a pharmacist regard a prescription as not for a legitimate medical purpose when the pharmacist thinks the patient is a hypochondriac, not really requiring the controlled substance for treatment? If there is a legitimate physician–patient relationship and the drug is prescribed in good faith to treat the patient, it is not the pharmacist's role under normal circumstances to second-guess the physician. The fact that the pharmacist believes a noncontrolled drug or no drug would be more appropriate would not be a sufficient basis in which to conclude the use is not legitimate. Of course a pharmacist must exercise professional judgment for every prescription, and if the concern warrants, the pharmacist should contact the prescriber to discuss the situation.

CASE 5-4   *Daniel Family Pharmacy*, 1999 WL 43613 (Fed. Reg.) (February 3, 1999)

Issue

Whether it would be inconsistent with public interest to allow a pharmacy to retain its DEA registration after its owner was found guilty in federal court for illegally distributing Vicodin.

Overview

This is an administrative hearing before the DEA, not a court case. The pharmacist in this case initially meant well by refilling a narcotic prescription for an employee that he was certain would be authorized. The prescriber, however, refused authorization, and what transpired after the refill could be described as a criminal nightmare for the pharmacist. In this hearing, the DEA is attempting to determine whether the pharmacy should retain its DEA registration after the owner was convicted of a controlled substance felony. The case was first argued before an administrative law judge (ALJ). After the ALJ rendered her opinion, the case was referred to the deputy administrator of the DEA for either approval or disapproval. The following decision then is from the perspective of the deputy administrator reviewing the ALJ. Despite the fact that the government established a prima facie case that the pharmacy's registration be terminated, the ALJ found in favor of the pharmacy, and the deputy administrator agreed with the decision. As you read this case, ask yourself: Would you refill a prescription for a controlled substance on the expectation of subsequent authorization by the prescriber? (Defend both sides of this issue.) If you were the ALJ, would you have decided for the pharmacy; why or why not? Should deep remorse be a defense? Should the fact that the pharmacist has obeyed the law since the illegal activities occurred be a defense? Does this decision send a positive or negative message to pharmacists about the consequences of their actions and why?

The facts of this hearing can be summarized as follows:

George Daniel, a pharmacist, owns and manages Daniel Pharmacy. In 1989, Daniel's delivery person injured his back in an accident and was prescribed Vicodin. The prescription was regularly refilled with prescriber authorization until sometime in 1991. At that time, the employee requested another refill, but no refills remained. Nonetheless, Daniel refilled the prescription believing that the prescriber would subsequently authorize it, but the prescriber refused. Although Daniel stated that this upset him, he later refilled the prescription again a month later for the employee. When Daniel then said he would not refill the prescription again, the employee threatened to report the illegal refills to authorities, so Daniel continued refilling the Vicodin. In 1993, the employee, cooperating with law enforcement officials, obtained Vicodin without a prescription from Daniel on two separate occasions. A search warrant was then executed by authorities and Daniel cooperated, consenting to the search of his residence as well. The audit showed substantial shortages of several controlled substances to which Daniel stated he had no knowledge. It was then determined that the employee and a pharmacy technician had been stealing controlled substances from Daniel for some time.

In 1993, Daniel was indicted in U.S. district court and pled guilty to two felony counts of illegally distributing the Vicodin. He was sentenced to 2 years probation, fined, and ordered to perform community service. In 1996, the Illinois Department of Public Regulation (IDPR) suspended his pharmacist license for 6 months, placed him on probation for 4 years and 6 months, and placed his pharmacy's license on probation for 5 years. His registration to dispense controlled substances was not affected, except that he was ordered to maintain a perpetual inventory of schedule II drugs.

In 1996 the DEA began hearings to determine whether to revoke Daniel's DEA Certificate of Registration. At the hearing, Daniel testified that he had implemented new security measures, and a controlled substances inventory confirmed there were only minor discrepancies. Daniel presented other testimony as to why his registration should not be revoked including that unlike the chain pharmacies in the area, he offered drive-up window service, compounding, delivery service, after-hours service, and charge accounts. A member of the Illinois Board of Pharmacy testified that if Daniel's registration was revoked, the pharmacy would close because of the importance of controlled substances to the business. He also expressed concern that losing independent pharmacies would affect small towns. Daniel also introduced letters attesting that he was well regarded in the community.

After stating the facts, the deputy administrator noted the applicable statutes.

Pursuant to 21 U.S.C. 824(a)(2), the Deputy Administrator may revoke a DEA Certificate of Registration upon a finding that the registrant "has been convicted of a felony . . . relating to any substance defined . . . as a controlled substance. . . ." In addition, pursuant to 21 U.S.C. 823(f) and 824(a)(4), the Deputy Administrator may revoke a DEA Certificate of Registration and deny any application for such registration, if he determines that the continued registration would be inconsistent with the public interest. Section 823(f) requires that the following factors be considered:

(1) The recommendation of the appropriate state licensing board or professional disciplinary authority.
(2) The applicant's experience in dispensing, or conducting research with respect to controlled substances.
(3) The applicant's conviction record under federal or state laws relating to the manufacture, distribution, or dispensing of controlled substances.
(4) Compliance with applicable state, federal, or local laws relating to controlled substances.
(5) Such other conduct which may threaten the public health or safety.

These factors are to be considered in the disjunctive; the Deputy Administrator may rely on any one or a combination of factors and may give each factor the weight he deems appropriate in determining whether a registration should be revoked or an application for registration be denied.

Daniel argued that revocation pursuant to section 824(a)(2) is not appropriate because he is not the registrant; the pharmacy is the registrant. The deputy administrator, however, noted that the DEA has consistently held that the law applies to the owner, officer, or any employee with responsibility over controlled substances.

Nonetheless, the government decided to proceed against Daniel on the basis of section 823(f). On this basis, the deputy administrator analyzed each of the five factors under the statute. Starting with factor three, he determined that Daniel's criminal conviction and conduct directly relates to whether continuing the registration would be inconsistent with the public interest. Therefore, he proceeded to apply the other four factors of section 823(f) to determine the public interest issue.

Starting with factor one, the deputy administrator noted that the state board of pharmacy made no recommendation, except for requiring Daniel to maintain a perpetual inventory of his schedule II drugs.

As to factors two and four, it is undisputed that Mr. Daniel dispensed Vicodin and other controlled substances without a prescription in violation of 21 U.S.C. 841(a)(1). The Deputy Administrator finds that Mr. Daniel's explanation that he was being threatened by the cooperating individual does not justify or excuse his behavior. First, Mr. Daniel himself admitted that initially he did not take the cooperating individual's threats seriously. Second, the other pharmacist at Respondent testified that Mr. Daniel did not appear nervous or upset when he observed Mr. Daniel with the cooperating individual. Finally, if in fact Mr. Daniel felt threatened by the cooperating individual he should have reported it to the proper authorities rather than continuing to unlawfully dispense controlled substances to him for over a year.

In addition, the significant shortages revealed by the audits indicate that Respondent did not maintain complete and accurate records of its handling of controlled substances as required by 21 U.S.C. 827. While there is some evidence that controlled substances were being stolen from Respondent, this does not minimize Respondent's responsibility for the shortages. It is quite disturbing that Mr. Daniel did not detect that over 17,000 dosage units were missing from Respondent in less than a 1 year period.

As a DEA registrant, Respondent must ensure that controlled substances are properly dispensed. Respondent clearly abrogated this responsibility.

Judge Bittner concluded that the Government made a prima facie case for revoking Respondent's DEA Certificate of Registration. However, she recommended that Respondent should nonetheless be permitted to remain registered. While expressing extreme concern regarding Mr. Daniel's "egregious abuse of his responsibilities as a pharmacist and as a DEA registrant," Judge Bittner also found that "Mr. Daniel seemed genuinely remorseful and that . . . he now understands the enormity of his misconduct." Judge Bittner recommended that Respondent's continued registration be subject to the conditions that:

(1) Respondent maintain a perpetual inventory of all controlled substances for at least 3 years following issuance of a final order in this proceeding;
(2) Respondent verify the perpetual inventory by a physical count, reduced to writing, of all controlled substances for each calendar quarter of that 3-year period;
(3) Respondent submit the perpetual inventory and quarterly verification to the Special Agent in Charge of the DEA field office having jurisdiction over Respondent; and
(4) Respondent consent to undergo unannounced inspections by DEA diversion investigators, without an administrative inspection warrant.

The Government filed exceptions to Judge Bittner's recommended decision objecting to the continuation of Respondent's registration on the sole basis that George Daniel appears remorseful. The Government argued that Mr. Daniel was remorseful to the extent that he got caught and that his DEA registration is now threatened with revocation; that Mr. Daniel refused to take any responsibility for the shortages; and that Mr. Daniel's contention that he was threatened into unlawfully dispensing controlled substances is hard to believe.

The Deputy Administrator is deeply concerned by the egregious conduct of Respondent and Mr. Daniel. Mr. Daniel actively diverted controlled substances by dispensing them without a prescription and allowed additional significant diversion to occur as evidenced by the shortages revealed during the audits. However, the Deputy Administrator notes that this conduct occurred in January 1993. Had this case been adjudicated at that time, or even right after his criminal conviction in October 1994, the Deputy Administrator would have revoked Respondent's DEA Certificate of Registration. But, in the subsequent 6 years, Respondent has maintained its DEA registration and available evidence indicates that it has acted in a responsible manner as demonstrated by the January 1997 state inspection which revealed only minor violations. In addition, the Deputy Administrator concurs with Judge Bittner's conclusion that Mr. Daniel has exhibited remorse for his actions, and finds it significant that Respondent is the only pharmacy in the area that performs prescription compounding. Therefore, the Deputy Administrator concludes that it would not be in the public interest to revoke Respondent's registration at this time. This decision however, should in no way be interpreted as an endorsement of the past illegal behavior of Mr. Daniel and Respondent. Mr. Daniel's remorse and the fact that available evidence indicates that the pharmacy has acted responsibly in the past 6 years provide adequate assurance that the prior illegal activity at Respondent will not be repeated.

The Deputy Administrator therefore agreed with the ALJ that Daniel should retain the registration, subject to the restrictions placed on Daniel by the ALJ.

Notes on *Daniel Family Pharmacy*

1. The government elected to proceed against Daniel under section 823(f) rather than section 824(a)(2). Section 824(a)(2) would have allowed the DEA to revoke

Daniel's registration simply on the basis of his felony conviction. It seems, then, that the DEA was being kind. In fact, section 823(f) states that the government may deny an application for registration on the basis of a finding that granting the registration would be inconsistent with the public interest. Section 824, on the other hand, provides for revocation or suspension of registrations already granted. Section 824(a)(4), however, states that the registration can be revoked or suspended if the registrant has committed acts under section 823 that would be inconsistent with public interest. One could contend that section 823 should not be invoked when the pharmacist's action clearly falls under section 824(a)(2), although this issue did not trouble the parties involved.

2. This case indicates that in a registration revocation hearing, the objective is not to punish but to ascertain whether continuing registration would be inconsistent with the public interest. The DEA believed that Daniel's deep remorse plus the fact that he has been a model pharmacist for the past 6 years does not make him a risk to the public interest. However, how do you measure remorse? Does this case send a message that a pharmacist can violate the CSA, show remorse (the right amount), and retain the registration? The case also seems to say that it is in the pharmacist's best interest to delay the DEA hearing as long as possible so the pharmacist can demonstrate good behavior. In facts of the case not mentioned earlier, it was stated that Daniel supplied not only Vicodin to the employee but also Tussionex, Dilaudid, and morphine. Yet this fact never was mentioned in the decision of the case. Would this fact make a difference in how you would decide this case?

3. This case should not be used as a reason why a controlled substance prescription should never be refilled without authorization when authorization cannot be obtained at the time. The decision should be made on the basis of professional judgment. In fact, some state laws specifically allow pharmacists to refill controlled substances without authorization in very narrow circumstances, such as emergencies. The problem in this case for Daniel was not the unauthorized refill but what transpired after the refill.

CASE 5-5   *Whalen v. Roe*, 429 U.S. 589 (1977)

Issue

Whether New York's schedule II triplicate prescription law unconstitutionally interfered with a patient's right to privacy and a physician's right to practice medicine.

Overview

About six or seven states require that schedule II drugs be prescribed pursuant to triplicate prescription forms. The states passed these laws in an attempt to better control the illegal diversion of schedule II drugs by physicians and pharmacists. These prescription forms are issued by the state to prescribers. The pharmacy sends one copy of the prescription to the state, thus raising the issues of patient privacy and confidentiality, which *Whalen* addresses. With the computer technology available today, multiple copy prescription programs will ultimately be phased out in favor of direct electronic submission of data from the pharmacy to the state. Some states now require that pharmacies transmit all controlled substance prescription information electronically. Thus, the threat to patient privacy and confidentiality is much greater today than it was when *Whalen* was decided. As you read this case, consider whether controlled substance data reporting systems should be implemented in all states. Does a reporting system negatively deter physicians from prescribing schedule II drugs when they are necessary, such as in pain management? Does a reporting system really invade a patient's right to privacy? When can a state go too far in collecting information?

The U.S. Supreme Court first related the facts of the case as summarized here:

> In response to concern that certain drugs were being illegally diverted, New York passed a law in 1972 requiring that schedule II drugs be written on triplicate prescription forms. One copy is retained by the prescriber, one copy by the dispensing pharmacy, and the third copy filed with the state health department. The health department then enters the data into computer records. The law required that the records be destroyed after 5 years, prohibited the public disclosure of patients' identities, and limited the access of the records to certain employees of the Department of Health and investigatory personnel.

> A group of patients receiving controlled substances and physicians brought this action challenging the constitutionality of the patient identification requirements of the law. The patients offered proof that some persons in need of treatment with schedule II drugs declined treatment because of their fear that the misuse of the computerized data will cause them to be stigmatized as "drug addicts." A three-judge district court enjoined the enforcement of the law, finding that "the doctor–patient relationship is one of the zones of privacy accorded constitutional protection" and that the Act's patient identification provisions invaded that zone with "a needlessly broad sweep" because the appellant had been unable to demonstrate the necessity for those requirements. The state appealed to the U.S. Supreme Court.

The Supreme Court began its analysis of the case by noting that, although the state could not prove the necessity for the triplicate law, this would not invalidate the law as the district court had held.

> State legislation which has some effect on individual liberty or privacy may not be held unconstitutional simply because a court finds it unnecessary, in whole or in part. For we have frequently recognized that individual States have broad latitude in experimenting with possible solutions to problems of vital local concern.

> The New York statute challenged in this case represents a considered attempt to deal with such a problem. It is manifestly the product of an orderly and rational legislative decision. It was recommended by a specially appointed commission which held extensive hearings on the proposed legislation, and drew on experience with similar programs in other States. There surely was nothing unreasonable in the assumption that the patient identification requirement might aid in the enforcement of laws designed to minimize the misuse of dangerous drugs. For the requirement could reasonably be expected to have a deterrent effect on potential violators as well as to aid in the detection or investigation of specific instances of apparent abuse. At the very least, it would seem clear that the State's vital interest in controlling the distribution of dangerous drugs would support a decision to experiment with new techniques for control.

The Court then addressed the issue of whether the law invaded a constitutionally protected "zone of privacy." If it did, then the state indeed must show necessity for the law, and because it could not, the law would be unconstitutional. (The Supreme Court has determined in other cases that the Constitution affords persons a right of privacy in such personal areas as procreation and contraception.)

> The cases sometimes characterized as protecting "privacy" have in fact involved at least two different kinds of interests. One is the individual interest in avoiding disclosure of personal matters, and another is the interest in independence in making certain kinds of important decisions. Appellees argue that both of these interests are

impaired by this statute. The mere existence in readily available form of the information about patients' use of schedule II drugs creates a genuine concern that the information will become publicly known and that it will adversely affect their reputations. This concern makes some patients reluctant to use, and some doctors reluctant to prescribe, such drugs even when their use is medically indicated. It follows, they argue, that the making of decisions about matters vital to the care of their health is inevitably affected by the statute. Thus, the statute threatens to impair both their interest in the nondisclosure of private information and also their interest in making important decisions independently.

We are persuaded, however, that the New York program does not, on its face, pose a sufficiently grievous threat to either interest to establish a constitutional violation.

In response to the appellees' fear concerning the public disclosure of information, the Court remarked that the security provisions in the law were sufficient and that the appellees offered no proof to the contrary. The Court then proceeded to find that no evidence was presented that suggested that an invasion of patient privacy had or might occur. Rather, the Court found that the appellees were only relying upon the "clearly articulated fears" of patients. Disclosures of patients' records, noted the Court, could only be made if the law was violated.

Even without public disclosure, it is, of course, true that private information must be disclosed to the authorized employees of the New York Department of Health. Such disclosures, however, are not significantly different from those that were required under the prior law. Nor are they meaningfully distinguishable from a host of other unpleasant invasions of privacy that are associated with many facets of health care. Unquestionably, some individuals' concern for their own privacy may lead them to avoid or to postpone needed medical attention. Nevertheless, disclosures of private medical information to doctors, to hospital personnel, to insurance companies, and to public health agencies are often an essential part of modern medical practice even when the disclosure may reflect unfavorably on the character of the patient. Requiring such disclosures to representatives of the State having responsibility for the health of the community does not automatically amount to an impermissible invasion of privacy.

Nor can it be said that any individual has been deprived of the right to decide independently, with the advice of his physician, to acquire and to use needed medication. Although the State no doubt could prohibit entirely the use of particular schedule II drugs, it has not done so. This case is therefore unlike those in which the Court held that a total prohibition of certain conduct was an impermissible deprivation of liberty. Nor does the State require access to these drugs to be conditioned on the consent of any state official or other third party. Within dosage limits which appellees do not challenge, the decision to prescribe, or to use, is left entirely to the physician and the patient.

The Court thus concluded that the law does not threaten either the reputation or the independence of patients for whom schedule II drugs are prescribed sufficiently to violate any right or liberty under the Fourteenth Amendment.

The appellee doctors argue separately that the statute impairs their right to practice medicine free of unwarranted state interference. If the doctors' claim has any reference to the impact of the 1972 statute on their own procedures, it is clearly frivolous. For even the prior statute required the doctor to prepare a written prescription identifying the name and address of the patient and the dosage of the prescribed drug. To the extent that their claim has reference to the possibility that the patients' concern about disclosure may induce them to refuse needed medication, the doctors' claim is derivative from, and therefore no stronger than, the patients'. Our rejection of their claim therefore disposes of the doctors' as well.

A final word about issues we have not decided. We are not unaware of the threat to privacy implicit in the accumulation of vast amounts of personal information in computerized data banks or other massive government files. The collection of taxes, the distribution of welfare and social security benefits, the supervision of public health, the direction of our Armed Forces, and the enforcement of the criminal laws all require the orderly preservation of great quantities of information, much of which is personal in character and potentially embarrassing or harmful if disclosed. The right to collect and use such data for public purposes is typically accompanied by a concomitant statutory or regulatory duty to avoid unwarranted disclosures. Recognizing that in some circumstances that duty arguably has its roots in the Constitution, nevertheless New York's statutory scheme, and its implementing administrative procedures, evidence a proper concern with, and protection of, the individual's interest in privacy. We therefore need not, and do not, decide any question which might be presented by the unwarranted disclosure of accumulated private data whether intentional or unintentional or by a system that did not contain comparable security provisions. We simply hold that this record does not establish an invasion of any right or liberty protected by the Fourteenth Amendment.

The Court reversed the decision of the court of appeals, finding for the state.

Notes on *Whalen v. Roe*

1. This case demonstrates that a state can invade an individual's privacy as long as it is not a serious invasion. (In fact, virtually every law invades personal freedom in some manner.) If the invasion is serious or substantial, however, the state must show necessity for its action, meaning here that the triplicate program would have to be determined to be indispensable to the state's efforts to control drug abuse. Obviously, then, the question becomes: When is the privacy invasion serious enough to warrant a showing of necessity? Justice Brennan, in concurring with the majority, noted his concern of central computer storage of data and stated: "The central storage and easy accessibility of computerized data vastly increase the potential for abuse of that information, and I am not prepared to say that future developments will not demonstrate the necessity of some curb on such technology."

2. Justice Brennan's comment warrants consideration. Today's technology allows states to require pharmacists to submit electronically not only all controlled substance data but also all prescription data. Such is the case currently with Medicaid retrospective drug utilization review programs. Pain management experts, especially, fear extensive reporting laws could unduly burden or frighten prescribers from legitimately using opioids in the management of pain. The Court in *Whalen* stated that New York's statute was constitutional because it contained adequate safeguards against unwarranted disclosures. It also believed that the law's effect of deterring patients from filling schedule II prescriptions was minimal. Thus, until data collection laws overreach to significantly threaten confidentiality without adequate safeguards, and unduly deter patients from treatment, they will likely be upheld by the courts. It would appear the better battleground for confidentiality and privacy issues is in the legislature.

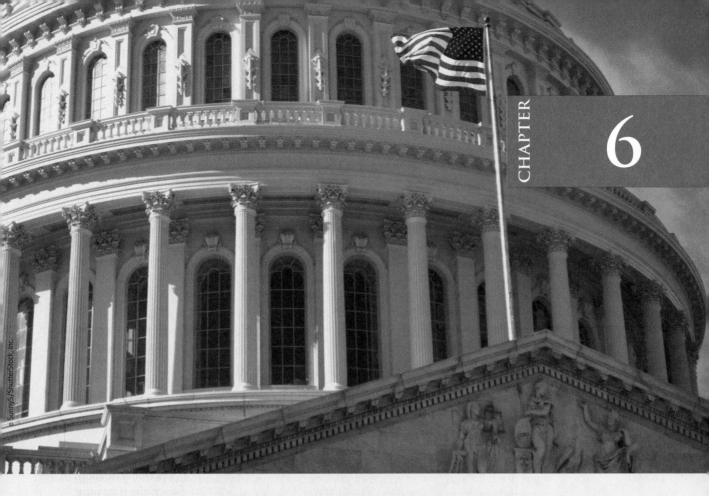

FEDERAL REGULATION OF PHARMACY PRACTICE

CHAPTER OBJECTIVES

Upon completing this chapter, the reader will be able to:

▶ Understand the provisions and requirements established by the Omnibus Budget Reconciliation Act of 1990 (OBRA '90).

▶ Describe the requirements of the Health Insurance Portability and Accountability Act of 1996 (HIPAA).

▶ Identify the basic drug and pharmacy-related provisions of Medicare.

▶ Identify the basic drug and pharmacy-related provisions of Medicaid.

▶ Recognize the application of the Medicare/Medicaid fraud and abuse laws.

▶ Describe the application of the Sherman Antitrust Act to pharmacy practice.

▶ Describe the application of the Robinson-Patman Act to pharmacy practice.

State governments regulate pharmacists and pharmacies by licensing them. State governments ensure that pharmacists are competent and that pharmacies are appropriately managed to protect the public health. The federal government regulates drug products that are distributed and monitored by state-licensed pharmacists in state-licensed pharmacies. Indirectly, however, the federal regulation of drugs also regulates pharmacists and pharmacies because the drug product is so significantly interwoven into pharmacy practice. The U.S. Congress and federal administrative agencies derive their authority to regulate drug distribution from the Interstate Commerce Clause of the Constitution. The courts have liberally interpreted this clause on several occasions to give Congress considerable power to regulate commerce among the states.

THE OMNIBUS BUDGET RECONCILIATION ACT OF 1990

Federal laws such as the Food, Drug, and Cosmetic Act (FDCA) and the Controlled Substances Act (CSA) create for pharmacists an important set of responsibilities related to the integrity of drug distribution to patients. By establishing rules that affect the drug product, these laws indirectly regulate those who handle medications. Yet, until 1990, federal law had not dealt directly with practice standards for pharmacists. The Omnibus Budget Reconciliation Act of 1990 (P.L. 101-508, commonly referred to as OBRA '90) took a giant leap beyond the rules about drug products set out in the FDCA and the CSA. OBRA '90 mandates changes in the way that pharmacy is actually practiced. OBRA '90 recognizes a public expectation of pharmacists that goes beyond oversight of drug distribution to include the detection and resolution of problems with drug therapy.

Before the passage of OBRA '90, state legislatures, administrative agencies, and courts of law had imposed a variety of requirements on pharmacists. However, none of the efforts that preceded OBRA '90 were as comprehensive as this federal legislation. Although the ideas in OBRA '90 are not new, the uniform application of them throughout the states marks an unprecedented expansion of pharmacy practice standards. Thus, OBRA '90 is perhaps the most important pharmacy-related law of all time, and it merits special attention.

OBRA '90 is a massive law that deals with many issues related to government funding. Only a small part of OBRA '90 deals with pharmacy practice, but that small part has a profound effect. The establishment of a federal policy requiring drug use review (DUR) to ensure that drug therapy is as safe and effective as possible is a monumental step in the direction of expanded responsibility for pharmacists. Unlike any federal or state legislation that preceded it, OBRA '90 places public trust in the pharmacist's ability to make decisions that improve the quality of drug therapy and increase the likelihood of good outcomes.

The primary goal of OBRA '90 is to save money. The U.S. Congress recognized that, as a major payer for health care in the United States, it has the responsibility to ensure that taxpayer dollars are spent properly. Evidently believing that improving the quality of drug therapy could reduce the costs of health care, Congress sought to ensure that patients who need drugs get them, that patients who do not need drugs do not get them, and that patients use drugs as effectively and as safely as possible. Increased quality and reduced cost are by no means mutually exclusive objectives of federal legislation.

Background

OBRA '90 was not the first piece of congressional legislation to require that pharmacists review prescribed drug therapy. In 1988, Congress passed the Medicare Catastrophic Coverage Act, which introduced the concept of DUR to improve drug therapy and reduce its costs (P.L. 100-360, 102 Stat. 683 (1988)). The law was repealed in 1989 for economic and financing reasons unrelated to the pharmacist's DUR, but many of its basic tenets have been incorporated into OBRA '90 and expanded. In addition, the Health Care Financing Administration (HCFA), now the Centers for Medicare & Medicaid Services (CMS), in 1990 promulgated regulations that expand the pharmacist's functions in optimizing drug therapy for patients in long-term care facilities.

The U.S. Congress turned to the pharmacy profession for help in solving a national problem. Healthcare costs are excessive, and outcomes of therapy are not as good as they should be. Pharmacy has adopted a "pharmacist care" (originally called "pharmaceutical care") model of practice in which pharmacists accept responsibility for producing good therapeutic outcomes and improving a patient's quality of life. In simple terms, OBRA '90 has taken the goal that pharmacy developed for itself and has made it a national policy.

The establishment of a national policy regarding pharmacy practice standards requires an indirect approach because only the states, not the federal government, can regulate professional practice. Therefore, the federal government has proclaimed that, as a condition of participation in Medicaid, states must establish expanded standards of practice for pharmacists. Technically, this condition does not require that pharmacists take any action; it requires only that states take action. Furthermore, states do not really have to establish the standards, although they cannot continue receiving federal funds for Medicaid if they fail to meet this condition. As a practical matter, of course, this is a professional practice requirement at the federal level because no state can afford not to meet the condition.

Some states have chosen to have the state board of pharmacy promulgate regulations imposing the expanded requirements for pharmacists, whereas other states have left that responsibility to the state Medicaid agency; a few states have established pharmacy practice standards through their legislatures. Depending on the way in which the state acts to fulfill the federal requirement, DUR requirements may appear to apply only to Medicaid prescriptions or they may expressly apply to all prescriptions. Such a distinction is probably meaningless, however. No profession, including pharmacy, has standards of practice that change according to the person being served at the time. The net result of the OBRA '90 mandate is that it elevates the standard of care owed by pharmacists to all patients.

Basic Framework of OBRA '90

OBRA '90 contains a number of significant provisions, but most involve one of three major areas:

1. Rebates
2. Demonstration projects
3. DUR

The parts of the law dealing with rebates and demonstration projects are significant for pharmacy because they can help provide funds for the reimbursement of pharmacists under state Medicaid programs or justify payments to pharmacists for the provision of cognitive services to patients. However, it is the DUR provisions that most directly relate to the everyday practice of pharmacy.

Rebates

The rebate provision of OBRA '90 not only is an important expression of public policy, but also stimulates revenue for state Medicaid programs. Essentially, it requires manufacturers to provide pharmaceuticals to Medicaid at their "best price," the lowest price at which they sell the product to any customer (42 U.S.C. § 1396r-8(a)). This is accomplished by requiring that the manufacturer pay to each state Medicaid agency the difference between the average manufacturer's price and the "best price." The average manufacturer's price is the price that wholesalers pay to the manufacturer for drugs distributed to the retail pharmacy class of trade, after deducting customary prompt pay discounts. For example, if a manufacturer's best price for a product is $20 per 100 capsules, and the average manufacturer's price is $30 per 100 capsules, then a rebate of $10 per 100 capsules is owed to Medicaid. The formulas for calculating the amount of the rebate are complex, but the basic concept is quite simple. Medicaid no longer pays top dollar for pharmaceuticals, and other drug purchasers, such as hospitals and health maintenance organizations, benefit from preferential prices.

Demonstration Projects

The goal of the demonstration projects funded by OBRA '90 is to determine through scientific studies whether the outcomes of patient care improve and the costs decrease when pharmacists are paid to provide DUR services to patients, whether a drug is dispensed or not. The demonstration projects also address the efficiency and cost effectiveness of online computerized DUR and the cost effectiveness of face-to-face consultation. If the results of the demonstration projects show that pharmacists can provide cost-effective services, it is highly likely that government agencies and other payers for pharmaceutical services will increase the compensation that they provide for pharmacists.

Drug Use Review

The rebate and the demonstration project provisions of OBRA '90 deal primarily with healthcare financing. The DUR provisions, on the other hand, deal primarily with healthcare outcomes. The DUR process has three parts:

1. Retrospective review
2. Educational programs
3. Prospective review

The three functions are all elements of a continuous quality improvement cycle. They are all ongoing, they are necessarily interrelated, and they are of equal importance in DUR.

Retrospective Review

A DUR board that is composed of both physicians and pharmacists oversees the retrospective review (42 U.S.C. § 1396r-8(g)(2)(B)). The DUR board performs many activities, but perhaps its most important function is to review data concerning the use of medications over a particular period of time and compare those data with criteria for medication use previously developed by the DUR board. In other words, the DUR board recognizes "ideal" drug therapy and determines whether actual medication use (as evidenced by the data reviewed) conforms to the ideal. During this process, the DUR board will undoubtedly discover that there is room for improvement in the way in which medications are being used. For example, some patients may be receiving duplicative therapy, taking drugs together that have a negative effect on each other, or continuing drug therapy for too long or too short a duration. After identifying areas for improvement, the DUR board may recommend that educational programs be conducted.

Educational Programs

Physicians, pharmacists, or both can be the target of educational programs (42 U.S.C. § 1396r-8(g)(2)(D)). These programs can be face-to-face visits by an expert who calls on a physician or pharmacist; they can be symposia attended by professionals involved with medication use; or they can be written materials delivered to the healthcare professional. The goal of the educational programs is to improve the way that medications are used. This is not unlike the goal of most current continuing education programs for pharmacists and physicians, except that the identification of actual problems through a review of medication-use data prompts the educational programs recommended by the DUR board. These programs should be more effective than current continuing education programs because they address solutions to real problems.

Prospective Review

Through prospective DUR, pharmacists have an opportunity to consider prescribed drug therapy and apply what they know about proper medication use (some of which they have probably learned through educational programs). Prospective DUR generates new data concerning the dispensing of medications, and these data represent the most up-to-date patterns of actual medication use. The DUR board can examine these new data and determine which old problems with drug therapy have been eliminated or diminished and whether new problems have become evident. The DUR process then continues through its three-step cycle. Theoretically, if the DUR board carried out the review cycle enough times, the drug use system could reach a state of perfection, and no additional efforts would be necessary. With new drugs, new patients, new pharmacists, and new physicians entering the system on a regular basis, however, the reality is that DUR will never stop; there will always be room for improvement.

COMPONENTS OF PROSPECTIVE DRUG USE REVIEW

Under OBRA '90, prospective DUR requires the active resolution of problems through a comprehensive review of a patient's prescription order at the point of dispensing. The pharmacist evaluates the appropriateness of medication prescribed for the patient within the context of other information that is known about the patient. Prospective DUR has three components under the OBRA '90 mandate:

1. A screen of prescriptions before dispensing
2. Patient counseling by the pharmacist
3. Pharmacist documentation of relevant information

Pharmacists are required to find out necessary information about patients and their medications before dispensing occurs. In addition, pharmacists can empower patients and their caregivers through patient counseling so the patients and their caregivers can improve compliance with therapeutic regimens, avoid medication errors, and ultimately increase the probability of success with their drug therapy.

Screening Prescriptions

In the screening function that OBRA '90 requires, pharmacists must detect "potential" problems. Specifically, OBRA '90 states:

> The state plan shall provide for a review of drug therapy before each prescription is filled or delivered to an individual receiving benefits under this subchapter, typically at the point-of-sale or point of distribution. The review shall include screening for potential drug therapy problems due to therapeutic duplication, drug-disease contraindications, drug-drug interactions (including serious interactions with nonprescription or over-the-counter drugs), incorrect drug dosage or duration of treatment, drug-allergy interactions and clinical abuse/misuse. (42 U.S.C. § 1396r-8(g)(2)(A)(i))

Particularly noteworthy is the language indicating that the review shall "include" screening. Other activities required to perform prospective DUR go beyond screening. For example, because it makes little sense to conduct a screen of prescribed drug therapy and do nothing with the results of the screen, some action (e.g., notifying the prescriber and requesting clarification; discussing the matter with the patient) should be taken when a problem is detected.

Although computer programs can greatly assist the pharmacist in meeting the screening requirements, OBRA '90 is not about computers; it is about professional people and their acceptance of responsibility for the outcome of a patient's drug therapy. Professional judgment is required to determine whether, for a particular patient at a particular time, there is a possible problem with the way in which a medication has been prescribed.

Counseling Patients

Some potential problems with drug therapy cannot be resolved before dispensing. Even the best screen of potential problems and appropriate action to resolve them cannot remove all the inherent risks in medication use. Therefore, OBRA '90 requires a pharmacist to offer to counsel patients or their caregivers so they can prevent potential problems or can manage problems that arise after the product has been dispensed and the therapy has begun.

Patient Counseling Standards

Pharmacists must "offer to discuss" with each patient or caregiver matters that in the pharmacist's professional judgment are significant, including

- The name and description of the medication
- The dosage form, dosage, route of administration, and duration of drug therapy
- Special directions and precautions for preparation, administration, and use by the patient
- Common severe side effects, adverse effects, or interactions and therapeutic contraindications that may be encountered, including ways to prevent them and the action required if they do occur
- Techniques for self-monitoring drug therapy
- Proper storage
- Prescription refill information
- Action to be taken in the event of a missed dose (42 U.S.C. § 1396r-8(g)(2)(A)(ii)(I))

The deference to professional judgment in the patient counseling requirement means that pharmacists should rely on their training and experience to determine what information is relevant for a particular patient. The goal of OBRA '90 is not for all patients to receive the same information about a drug, but for each patient to receive the information about a drug that is particularly relevant to that patient's circumstances. Furthermore, "professional judgment" does not mean business judgment. Deciding not to counsel a patient or to reduce the length of a counseling session because it is inconvenient or difficult for the pharmacist is not consistent with the purpose of OBRA '90. A pharmacist should withhold information from a patient only when it is in the patient's best interest not to receive the information, not when it is in the pharmacist's best interest to withhold the information.

The phrase "common severe side effect" can be interpreted in various ways. It could be argued that only for extremely serious illnesses does the Food and Drug Administration (FDA) approve drugs with side effects that are both common and severe. Congress probably did not intend that patients be counseled only under those rare circumstances, however. Rather, the intent of Congress appears to be that pharmacists discuss with patients those side effects that are common (of high probability) or severe (of high magnitude), as well as those that are both common and severe. As a result, standards may vary in different states. For example, some states require patient counseling for new prescriptions only, whereas others require counseling for refills as well.

Even a superficial reading of the OBRA '90 legislation discloses that there really is no explicit patient counseling requirement. Instead, the legislation requires the pharmacist make an offer to discuss medications with patients. Some states have permitted a non-pharmacist to make this offer, whereas others require that the pharmacist make the offer personally. In all states, a pharmacist must do the actual counseling. If it is not practicable to counsel in person, such as a mail order prescription, the pharmacy must provide access for counseling by means of a telephone service that is toll-free for long-distance calls.

Waiver of Counseling

The pharmacist's duty to counsel under OBRA '90 and under the rules implemented by states pursuant to the mandate of OBRA '90 is for the benefit of patients. If patients prefer not to be counseled, then they have a right to refuse counseling. Specifically, OBRA '90 states:

> Nothing in this clause shall be construed as requiring a pharmacist to provide consultation when an individual receiving benefits under this subchapter or caregiver of such individual refuses such consultation. (42 U.S.C. § 1396r-8(g)(2)(A)(ii)(II))

Although patients can waive the right to be counseled about drug therapy, the law contemplates an informed right. If a clerk or other personnel asks, "You don't want to wait 45 minutes to be counseled by the pharmacist, do you?" and the patient or caregiver answers, "No," this is not the type of informed refusal that Congress anticipated. Even asking the question in a completely neutral and uninviting tone (e.g., "Do you want to be counseled?") can lead to a refusal by a patient who would really like to be counseled if the patient understood what was being offered. A refusal can be considered effective only if the patient truly understood the offer and really did not want the counseling. A patient who refuses counseling because the pharmacist or someone else in the pharmacy made it clear that the pharmacist really does not want to be bothered with counseling has not received the benefit of the services that OBRA '90 intends.

Just as some pharmacists now ask patients who refuse child safety closures on prescription containers to put their refusal in writing, it may be prudent for a pharmacist to obtain a written waiver of the right to be counseled. It is much more important that the waiver be informed and voluntary, however, than that the waiver be put in writing. If a pharmacist has maintained a logbook or other written record in which most notations show refusals to be counseled, the pharmacist has made a record of his or her own lack of compliance with the OBRA '90 mandate. The waiver of the right to be counseled should be the exception to the rule. Those pharmacists who permit the exception to become the rule will discover that they have created legal difficulties for themselves.

Documenting Information

OBRA '90 requires pharmacists to maintain a written record that contains information about patients and the pharmacists' impressions of the patients' drug therapy. OBRA '90 provides:

> A reasonable effort must be made by the pharmacist to obtain, record, and maintain at least the following information regarding individuals receiving benefits under this subchapter:
>
> **(aa)** Name, address, telephone number, date of birth (or age), and gender.
> **(bb)** Individual history where significant, including disease state or states, known allergies and drug reactions, and a comprehensive list of medications and relevant devices.
> **(cc)** Pharmacist comments relevant to the individual's drug therapy. (42 U.S.C. § 1396r-8(g)(2)(A)(ii)(II))

The "reasonable effort" that pharmacists must make to record information about patients, including their comments relevant to a patient's drug therapy, would be deemed reasonable only if an impartial observer can review the documentation in a pharmacy and understand what has occurred in the past. It should be possible to tell from the documentation what a pharmacist discovered about a patient, what the pharmacist told the patient, and what the pharmacist thought about the patient's drug therapy at the time of dispensing. The documentation should:

- Serve as a reminder to the pharmacist (because nobody's memory is perfect)
- Provide a reference for other pharmacists in the same pharmacy
- Contain information for surveyors who need to record what was done and connect that action with an outcome if possible
- Show enforcement officials that the OBRA '90 requirements are being met

© Stockbyte/Thinkstock

STUDY SCENARIO AND QUESTIONS

Jack is the V.P. for Pharmacy Services for a drugstore chain whose pharmacies are extremely busy. Some of the chain pharmacies and pharmacists have been fined for not counseling and not following other OBRA '90 requirements. As a result, Jack sent out instructions to all pharmacies that for every new prescription, a clerk or technician must ask the patient if he or she would like counseling. If the patient does want counseling, the clerk must tell the patient that because the pharmacists are very busy, it could be a 10- to 15-minute wait. If the patient then declines counseling, the clerk must have the patient sign a waiver of counseling. Clerks are instructed to give to patients information forms to be completed, asking for demographic characteristics and significant medical and drug information.

1. In what ways has Jack complied with the requirements of OBRA '90? In what ways has Jack failed to comply with the requirements of OBRA '90?
2. If you were an employee of one of Jack's pharmacies, what further changes would you recommend to bring Jack's pharmacies into compliance with the language and intent of OBRA '90?

HEALTH INSURANCE PORTABILITY AND ACCOUNTABILITY ACT OF 1996

Congress's enactment of the Health Insurance Portability and Accountability Act of 1996 (HIPAA) significantly affected pharmacy practice and the entire healthcare system (P.L. No. 104-191, 110 Stat. 1936 (1996)). HIPAA is a sweeping, complex law with the overall goal of improving the efficiency and effectiveness of the healthcare system. Among other things, the law seeks to improve the portability and continuity of health insurance coverage and to prohibit discrimination in health coverage. Of greatest interest to pharmacists, HIPAA also regulates the privacy and security of health information, and authorizes the Department of Health and Human Services (HHS) to enact regulations to this effect. Public concern over the use, efficiency, security, and abuse of electronic records provided the catalyst for the development of patient health information requirements.

HIPAA targets four aspects of health information: (1) transaction and code sets, (2) national provider identities, (3) security, and (4) privacy. HHS has enacted final regulations for all four of these areas. In February 2003, the agency enacted final regulations addressing electronic data transaction and code sets (68 Fed. Reg. 8381). These regulations provide for uniform standards in the electronic transmission of claims and data with the intent of improving efficiency and lowering costs. HHS established final regulations for national provider identities in January 2004 (69 Fed. Reg. 3434). The regulations took effect May 23, 2005, at which time health care providers could begin applying for a national provider identifier (NPI) number. All health care providers covered by HIPAA had to receive and use the NPI by the compliance date of May 23, 2007. Prior to the NPI requirement a provider may have had a different identification number for each plan in which the provider participated. The intent of requiring only one NPI for each provider is uniformity, administrative simplicity, and cost.

The final security regulations, enacted in February 2003, seek to protect the confidentiality, integrity, and availability of electronic health information (68 Fed. Reg. 8334). They establish requirements that covered entities (those entities to whom the regulations apply) must implement to protect the information from unauthorized access, alteration, deletion, and transmission. Physical, technical, and organizational procedure safeguards must be established. Entities are free to develop their own security measures by written policies and procedures, as long as they achieve the objectives and standards contained in the regulations.

In contrast to the security requirements, the privacy regulation standards are concerned with the patient's rights and how and when the patient's information may be used (67 Fed. Reg. 53182). The privacy regulations, which took effect April 14, 2003, generally represent the greatest concern to practicing pharmacists and their staff, and are the subject of most of the remainder of the HIPAA discussion. The intent of the HIPAA privacy discussion in this chapter is to provide a general overview. Readers requiring more information are urged to go to the HHS and Office of Civil Rights (OCR) websites, where they can access guidance documents and answers to frequently asked questions. (See http://www.hhs.gov/ocr/privacy.)

EXAMPLES OF PRIVACY ABUSES

Prior to HIPAA, numerous abuses of patient health information were reported. For example:

- A chain pharmacy sold its used computers to the public complete with patient prescription and patient profile databases still intact.

- A retiring physician sold his patients' medical records to a business, which then resold the records back to the patients.
- The 13-year-old daughter of a hospital employee obtained a list of hospital patients' names and phone numbers from the hospital and as a joke called patients and told them they had HIV.
- Drug manufacturers commonly obtained from pharmacies lists of patients taking certain prescription medications and then would send those patients letters urging them to ask their physician to change them to another medication.
- Laboratories commonly sold patient lab results to drug companies, which would then use the information to target patients to promote their medication.
- Employers would access individuals' medical information and use it to determine whether to hire or fire employees.

These represent only a few examples of patient privacy abuse. Prior to HIPAA, no federal regulation of the privacy of patient health information existed. Moreover, state laws in many instances were inadequate to protect patients against these abuses. HIPAA requirements establish national uniformity and preempt state laws that are less strict.

WHO MUST COMPLY WITH HIPAA

Called "covered entities" under the privacy rule, health plans, health care clearinghouses, and health care providers that conduct financial or administrative transactions electronically must comply. The regulations ordinarily apply to the entire covered entity; however, a company may exempt certain non–health care parts of its operation, such as a grocery store that contains a pharmacy.

PROTECTED HEALTH INFORMATION

Information covered under HIPAA is called protected health information (PHI). Originally the government intended to include only electronic information, but ultimately extended the definition of PHI to include all forms of health information that (1) relate to past, present, or future physical or mental health; the provision of care; or payment for care; and (2) identify the patient or could reasonably be expected to identify the patient.

Obviously, in a pharmacy this would include any prescription or other health information, including payment records for tax purposes or otherwise.

NOTICE PROVISION

A pharmacy must provide a "Notice of Privacy Practices" to each patient containing several items of information including

- How the pharmacy intends to use and disclose the information
- Descriptions of the legal duties of the pharmacy to protect the confidentiality of PHI
- A statement of the patient's rights and a brief explanation of how the patient may exercise those rights
- A statement that patients may complain to the pharmacy or HHS and that explains the method for filing a complaint
- A person in the company whom a patient may contact with privacy concerns, including the person's name or title and telephone number

The notice must be provided on the day the pharmacy first provides service in paper form, unless the patient consents to electronic transmission. The notice must also be posted in a prominent and visible location and made available upon request to any person, whether the person is a patient or not. If the pharmacy has a website, the notice must be posted on the site.

ACKNOWLEDGMENT OF NOTICE

A pharmacy must make a good-faith effort to distribute the notice to patients and obtain a written acknowledgment of receipt. Only one signed acknowledgment is required for each patient, meaning an acknowledgment is not required every time a prescription is dispensed. A pharmacy may not refuse treatment to a patient who refuses to sign the acknowledgment. The written acknowledgment can occur by several means, including having the patient sign or initial a tear-off form on the notice or by having the patient sign a logbook.

If the patient does not personally pick up the prescription, the pharmacy could mail the notice to the patient with an acknowledgment form that the patient could sign and return. Alternately, the pharmacy could attempt to obtain the acknowledgment electronically. If the patient does not return the acknowledgment, the pharmacist should attempt again. Failure to receive an acknowledgment is not a violation because the pharmacy need only make a good-faith effort; however, the effort should be documented. The patient's personal representative (someone authorized by state law to act for a patient, such as the parent of a minor child, a legal guardian, or someone with a power of attorney) may sign the acknowledgment for the patient. Although friends and relatives may pick up a prescription for a patient as an agent of the patient, they may not sign the acknowledgment unless they are also personal representatives of the patient.

USE AND DISCLOSURE OF PHI

The privacy rule allows pharmacies to use and disclose PHI for treatment, payment, and operations (TPO). Treatment includes providing, coordinating, or managing the health care of the patient. In pharmacies, this includes dispensing medications, counseling patients, maintaining patient profiles, and consulting with the patient's other health care providers. Importantly, the pharmacist may disclose PHI with the patient's primary care physician or nurse practitioner, as well as any other health care professionals involved in treating the patient. Payment activities include submitting claims for reimbursement, determining patient eligibility and extent of coverage, and sending bills to patients. Operations encompass those activities necessary to operate a pharmacy such as quality assessment, fraud detection, audits, certifications, and business management.

Pharmacists, of course, may always provide complete disclosure of PHI to the patient, and in fact the regulations require the pharmacist to do so if the patient requests. Pharmacies may charge a reasonable, cost-based fee for providing patients a copy of their records. Disclosure may also be made to the patient's personal representative, or agent, such as a friend, relative, roommate, or neighbor. In the case of an agent, the pharmacist should exercise professional judgment to determine if it would really be in the patient's best interests to provide disclosure. This puts the pharmacist in somewhat of a dilemma, especially in mandatory consultation states such as California, because state regulation requires the pharmacist to counsel the patient or the patient's agent if present. Regardless of the counseling requirements, it would be best not to counsel the patient's agent unless professional judgment clearly warrants, and instead, send a notice for the patient to call for counseling.

Accounting for Disclosures

Under the initial HIPAA law and regulations, patients had a right to request and receive an accounting of disclosures of PHI made by a covered entity in the 6 years prior to the date of the request. That right did not extend to disclosure for treatment, payment, and health care operations because covered entities commonly make these disclosures several times a day and tracking them would be unduly burdensome. However, a 2009 law called the Health Information Technology for Economic and Clinical Health (HITECH), which is part of the American Recovery and Reinvestment Act (ARRA) (P.L. 111-5), made an important change. Under HITECH if a covered entity utilizes an electronic health record (EHR), the entity will be required to account for all disclosures, including disclosures of TPO, within 3 years prior to the date of the request. Pharmacy organizations are very concerned that this new HITECH requirement will unduly burden pharmacies since pharmacies make several disclosures daily when claims processing is considered, and have requested to HHS that exceptions be made for pharmacy.

HITECH contains another disclosure-related requirement problem for pharmacies. Patients may request that their PHI not be disclosed to a health plan if the purpose is for payment or operations and pertains to an item or service for which the patient has paid out of pocket in full. Pharmacy claims submitted to health plans, however, include PHI related to treatment, payment, and operations, and it might be very difficult to extract this information. Not including all this information might also violate the contract between the pharmacy and the health plan.

Minimum Necessary Requirement

A pharmacy may only disclose the minimum amount of PHI necessary to accomplish the objective. For example, if a claims processor needs more information in order to process a claim, the pharmacy may provide only that information and no more. Exceptions to the "minimum necessary requirement" include

- Communications to the patient
- Communications regarding the treatment of the patient with other providers involved in the treatment
- When authorized by the patient
- When required by HHS for compliance and enforcement purposes
- When required by law

In all of these situations, the pharmacist may provide complete disclosure of PHI. Prior to HITECH, HIPAA contained no definition of minimum necessary. HITECH changed this and limits the covered entities' discretion for determining what constitutes minimum necessary to, if possible, a "limited data set." A limited data set is PHI that excludes direct identifiers of the patient, such as name, address, phone numbers, and social security number. If restricting the PHI to a limited data set is not possible, the pharmacy may include direct identifiers to the minimum amount necessary to achieve the intended purpose. The pharmacy must be prepared, however, to justify why the request or disclosure was not limited to the limited data set.

Incidental Use and Disclosure

It is virtually inevitable that no matter how careful a pharmacy is about protecting PHI, the information will inadvertently be used or disclosed in an unintended manner. For example, while counseling a patient, another patient may overhear the conversation. Pharmacies are not liable for these incidental uses and disclosures provided they have applied "reasonable safeguards" to protect the PHI. Pharmacies are not expected to make structural modifications, such as building a soundproof room for counseling. Pharmacists, however, are expected to exercise professional judgment and common sense. Reasonable safeguards for counseling would indicate that the counseling be conducted in a location as far away from other patients as possible. If other patients are nearby, they should be asked to stand back a few feet and the pharmacist should speak softly while counseling.

The OCR has specifically stated that under the incidental use and disclosure policy, no violation occurs when the pharmacy calls out the name of the patient who is waiting for a prescription, nor would it be a violation if another patient incidentally hears the pharmacist speaking to a technician or another pharmacist about a prescription. Pharmacists may also leave messages on the patient's answering machine, although it would be wise to say as little as possible.

De-identification of PHI

Information from which all individual identifying factors have been removed, termed de-identification, is not PHI and thus not subject to HIPAA. Pharmacists and pharmacy students when using patient information for educational and other non-TPO purposes should take care to de-identify the information. The following 18 items are considered identifiable:

1. Names
2. Geographic subdivisions such as street address, city, county, and zip code
3. All dates: birth, admission, discharge, death, ages over 89 (may aggregate to category, e.g., age 90 and over)
4. Telephone numbers
5. Fax numbers
6. Electronic mail addresses
7. Social Security numbers
8. Medical record numbers
9. Health plan beneficiary numbers
10. Account numbers
11. Certificate/license numbers
12. Vehicle identifiers and serial numbers, license plate numbers
13. Device identifiers and serial numbers
14. Web universal resource locators (URLs)
15. Internet protocol (IP) address numbers
16. Biometric identifiers (finger and voice prints)
17. Full-face photographic images and comparable images
18. Any other unique identifying numbers, characteristics, or codes

Considerations for Pharmacy Students in Early and Advanced Experiences

Pharmacy students often monitor assigned patients and give case presentations. Unless the patient gives specific authorization, all patient identification information should be removed. In institutional settings, pharmacy students should refrain from discussing patients in public places such as on elevators, in hallways, and in the cafeteria. Patient charts or other PHI should not be left where others can read them, and this includes computer screens. If a computer is shared with others, protect files containing PHI from access. In community settings, apply essentially the same rules. In addition, do not discuss a patient's medications with pharmacy staff such that other patients can overhear, and do not counsel patients in store aisles about OTC drugs when other people can overhear.

Other Permissible Use and Disclosure of PHI

As discussed, a pharmacy may not use or disclose PHI except for TPO purposes, or to the patient or the patient's personal representative or agent. In addition, the privacy regulations allow the pharmacy to disclose PHI for governmental-type reasons, including

- Public health activities (e.g., to authorized health officers)
- Judicial and administrative proceedings (requests should be made pursuant to a court or administrative order, or subpoena)
- Law enforcement purposes (e.g., to law enforcement officers in certain circumstances)
- Serious threats to health or safety (e.g., in suspected cases of abuse, neglect, or endangerment)
- As required by law

In these and related situations, the pharmacist should always contact the privacy officer and an attorney before releasing information.

Breach of PHI

HIPAA privacy laws and regulations failed to address the issue of breaches of PHI. HITECH does so and requires HHS to issue interim final regulations requiring covered entities to provide notification when unsecured PHI is breached. HHS complied by issuing interim final breach notification regulations in August of 2009 (74 Fed. Reg. 42740). The regulations apply to HIPAA covered entities, including pharmacies, and their business associates. Importantly, the law and regulations apply only to unsecured PHI, defined as PHI that is not secured through the use of technology or methodology as approved by HHS. All unsecured PHI in all forms, including electronic, paper, or oral, are subject to the regulations. Pharmacies must confirm with their intellectual technology vendor whether the pharmacy's PHI is secured or not.

A breach is defined as "the acquisition, access, use, or disclosure" of PHI in an unpermitted manner that compromises the security or privacy of the PHI. The regulations provide exceptions including (1) when the acquisition, access, use or disclosure is unintentional and in good faith and does not result in further use or disclosure; (2) when the unauthorized person to whom the PHI has been disclosed would not reasonably have been able to retain it; and (3) when the disclosure is inadvertent between two authorized individuals at the same facility if the information is not further used or disclosed. Thus, the first step a pharmacy must take is to determine whether a breach occurred. The second step requires that the pharmacy determine whether the breach "poses a significant risk of financial, reputational, or other harm to the individual." If there is no significant risk of harm, the pharmacy need not act upon the breach. If a pharmacy determines that a breach has occurred and poses a significant risk of harm, it must notify the affected individual(s) by first-class mail (or electronically if the individual has agreed) within 60 days after the breach was discovered. The regulation contains the elements that must be included in the notification.

As an example: Assume that a pharmacy employee places patient A's medication in a bag for patient B and places patient B's medication in a bag for patient A. Patient A is given the bag and starts to walk away from the pharmacy when the error is discovered. If the pharmacy personnel can determine that patient A could not have read or retained the information, then this situation would most likely not be a breach pursuant to the exception. If, however, patients A and B were each given the wrong bags and each patient later discovered the error and returned the medications, most likely this should be considered a breach. Notification would be required to patients A and B. If the pharmacy does not have sufficient contact information for either patient, the regulation allows for substitute notice. The regulations specify what constitutes substitute notice depending upon whether less than 10 or more than 10 individuals are affected. If more than 500 individuals are affected, the pharmacy must also notify the media within 60 days after discovery and must notify HHS immediately.

Disposal of PHI

Because of incidents involving improper disposal of PHI, such as CVS pharmacy disposing of PHI in dumpsters resulting in a $2.5 million fine, OCR posted FAQs (frequently asked questions) about the disposal of PHI in February 2009 (http://www .hhs.gov/ocr/privacy/hipaa/enforcement). The document emphasizes that covered entities must implement reasonable safeguards to protect PHI that is disposed, including the training of workforce members who dispose of PHI. Although the regulations do not require a particular disposal method, simply abandoning PHI or disposing of it in dumpsters accessible to the public without rendering the PHI unreadable and unable to be reconstructed is definitely not permitted. Covered entities must develop and implement reasonable policies and procedures for disposal. Examples provided in the FAQ include shredding or burning paper records; placing labeled prescription containers in opaque bags in a secure area to be picked up by a disposal vendor; and clearing, purging, or destroying electronic media. Although it is preferable to hire a business associate to ultimately dispose of PHI, it is not required.

PATIENT AUTHORIZATIONS AND MARKETING

Most any use of PHI for other than TPO or as described in the previous section requires written patient authorization. The most notable examples include using PHI for marketing purposes or for employment or insurance determinations. Authorizations must be detailed and customized for the particular use or disclosure intended, contain an expiration date, and be signed by the patient. A patient may not be denied treatment for refusing to sign an authorization.

The regulation defines marketing as "to make a communication about a product or service that encourages recipients of the communication to purchase or use the product or service. . . ." This is a broad definition subject to varying interpretations and considerable confusion, but some direction is possible. It would clearly be a marketing activity to provide any PHI to another company, such as a pharmaceutical manufacturer, so it can promote its products to those patients. It would also likely constitute marketing for a pharmacy to mail advertising notices for specific diabetic products to its diabetic patients identified through its prescription database. The pharmacy has used PHI most likely for marketing purposes and thus must get a signed authorization from the patient before doing so.

Exceptions to marketing include communications about general health issues. If, in the previous example, the pharmacist used PHI to identify diabetic patients to send them general information regarding the treatment of diabetes and wellness activities, this would not be marketing. Other exceptions to marketing include communications made

- Face to face
- For case management or care coordination

- To direct or recommend alternative treatment, therapies, health care providers, or settings of care
- About the services offered by the pharmacy or a health plan

Under these exceptions, as applied to the diabetic patient example, it would be permissible without patient authorization to promote the diabetic products to a diabetic patient who is present at the pharmacy. It would also be permissible for a pharmacy to mail to its diabetic patients general information about diabetes treatment, alternative treatments, and wellness activities. The pharmacy could also mail information to diabetic patients about its diabetic disease state management or training programs.

Concern existed initially as to whether refill reminder programs constituted marketing; however, the OCR has specifically stated these are treatment activities and permissible. When OCR enacted the privacy regulations in 2003 it had indicated that recommending alternative medications to patients does not fall under marketing, even if paid by a pharmaceutical manufacturer or prescription benefit manager to do so. Being paid to initiate a medication alternative, however, may now be considered illegal under HITECH, which provides that payment in exchange for making a communication is prohibited unless the communication describes only a drug or biologic that is currently being prescribed. The practice of being paid to communicate medication alternatives also raises other legal issues, especially under consumer fraud and antikickback statutes.

BUSINESS ASSOCIATES

Pharmacies do business with outside entities in which the sharing of PHI is necessary. A few examples include businesses that engage in claims processing, data processing, software developing, quality assurance analysis, billing services, and refill reminder services. The regulations term these outside businesses as business associates. The pharmacy must have a business associate contract with the entity in order to share PHI, and all PHI is subject to the minimum necessary requirement. Prior to HITECH, the privacy and security responsibilities of a business associate were defined by the contract with the covered entity. Thus, if the business associate violated any privacy and security requirements, it was liable to the covered entity under breach of contract. Under HITECH, business associates are now directly responsible and accountable to maintain and protect PHI in the same manner as covered entities and are subject to HIPAA enforcement authority.

TRAINING PROGRAMS

All pharmacies must train all members of its pharmacy department workforce about its HIPAA policies and procedures within a reasonable time after being hired. The pharmacy must provide additional training if it makes a material change in its policies and procedures. HHS estimates that workers should receive on average one hour of training. The pharmacy must document that each worker has completed training. The training requirement creates a hardship for pharmacy students in early experiential and clerkship programs. They will have to complete a training program for each covered entity at which they work. Moreover, the pharmacy school itself should provide a training program that each student should complete. As if this is not enough, the students must complete training programs at the pharmacies where they intern.

POLICIES AND PROCEDURES

Pharmacies must develop policies and procedures to implement the HIPAA privacy standards. This includes identifying a privacy officer to oversee the pharmacy's privacy compliance program and enumerating the privacy officer's responsibilities. The policies and procedures must provide for the imposition of sanctions against any worker who violates the privacy rules or the pharmacy's policies and procedures.

PENALTIES

Penalties for violating HIPAA can be severe and were made even more so under the 2009 HITECH law. Unintentional violations can result in fines of $100 per violation, up to $25,000 per person for all violations in a calendar year. Violations due to reasonable cause and not willful neglect can result in fines of $1,000 per occurrence, but not more than $50,000 for all violations in a calendar year. Willful neglect violations that are corrected within 30 days can result in fines of $10,000 with an annual cap of $250,000. Fines for willful neglect violations not corrected within 30 days can be up to $50,000 per violation with an annual cap of $1,500,000. Violations that are intentional or that involve fraud are subject to more severe penalties including prison. HITECH now allows state attorneys general in addition to HHS to bring civil actions in federal court to enforce HIPAA.

HEALTH INFORMATION TECHNOLOGY INFRASTRUCTURE

Health information technology (HIT) is generally considered the critical element in improving the quality and efficiency of the nation's health care system. Although adoption of electronic record systems has increased at larger health care facilities, many heath care professionals and facilities have yet to convert. Cost appears the most significant barrier. HITECH, in addition to strengthening the privacy and security requirements of HIPAA, appropriates almost $20 billion to develop a nationwide HIT infrastructure. The objectives of establishing the HIT infrastructure are to protect the privacy of PHI, reduce medical errors, reduce costs by improving administrative efficiency, improve coordination among health care providers, and improve the provision of public health services and emergency response systems. Prescribers and hospitals (not pharmacies) will receive financial incentives to adopt electronic medical record technology.

The law expands and adds funding to the Office of the National Coordinator for HIT (ONCHIT), which oversees the HIT infrastructure. ONCHIT, within the Department of HHS, is responsible for developing HIT standards and regulations in conjunction with HHS and two appointed committees, the HIT Policy Committee and the HIT Standards Committee. ONCHIT and HHS are also responsible for developing and regulating national and regional HIT research centers and for providing grant funding to educational institutions (including pharmacy schools) to incorporate HIT into clinical education and to develop medical informatics education programs.

© Stockbyte/Thinkstock

STUDY SCENARIO AND QUESTIONS

Sue is the privacy officer for a chain pharmacy and responsible for HIPAA compliance. Top management has told Sue that they do not want to be caught with any HIPAA violations or to be subject to any HIPAA complaints. In keeping with this philosophy, Sue has developed an extensive list of rules with which each pharmacy and its staff are expected to comply. Some of these rules include:

    a. Only the patient may sign the acknowledgment of the privacy notice.
    b. At least 90 percent of each pharmacy's patients must have signed an acknowledgment.

c. Patients may not be called by name to pick up their prescriptions.
d. The pharmacist shall not counsel anyone other than the patient, unless the patient provides written authorization.
e. No counseling may occur unless it is absolutely certain that other patients will not hear the counseling.
f. No information will be shared with the patient's physicians unless the patient provides written authorization.
g. No information will be shared with other pharmacies where the patient does business unless the patient provides written authorization.
h. No information will be shared with a patient's agents, relatives, or friends without written patient authorization.
i. No refill reminder information may be sent to patients without written patient authorization.

1. Which of the preceding rules go beyond the intent of HIPAA? Why?
2. How should these rules be rewritten, or should they?

MEDICARE

Enacted in 1965, Medicare represents the federal government's effort to reduce economic barriers to health care for the elderly. Medicare is title XVIII of the Social Security Act of 1935 (42 U.S.C. §§ 1395 and 1396; 42 C.F.R. § 405.1 et seq.). It provides for federal health insurance for those who are 65 years of age or older; with a permanent disability; having end-stage renal disease; or exposed to environmental health hazards. Medicare and Medicaid are administered by the Centers for Medicare & Medicaid Services (CMS), formerly the Health Care Financing Administration (HCFA).

The law has four components. Part A provides hospitalization insurance without any monthly premium to eligible beneficiaries, such as workers and their dependents who receive Social Security checks or railroad retirement checks. Part B insures beneficiaries for outpatient medical services. Part C at a minimum combines the benefits offered under original Medicare (Parts A and B). Part C is called Medicare Advantage, and gives beneficiaries the option to choose a managed care plan. Part D is the prescription drug benefit added in 2003 and fully implemented in 2006; it is discussed in the following section.

Most beneficiaries pay a monthly premium for Part B or C and Part D and may elect not to have this coverage. In addition to hospitalization costs, including drugs administered in the hospital, Part A covers certain skilled nursing facility stays, home health visits, and hospice care. Part B partially covers outpatient diagnostic services, such as x-ray studies and laboratory tests; outpatient hospital, physical, and speech therapy; some colostomy supplies; rental and purchase of medical appliances and equipment; and certain ambulance services. Part B also includes prescription drugs that the patient cannot self-administer and that are furnished by the physician or hospital outpatient department as incidental to the physician's professional service and not charged for separately. Coverage also includes durable medical equipment, certain vaccines, and diabetic supplies.

MEDICARE PART D

On December 8, 2003, President Bush signed into law the Medicare Prescription Drug, Improvement, and Modernization Act of 2003 (MMA), known as Medicare Part D, the most significant and at the time controversial change in the Medicare program since its inception in 1965. Subsequently, CMS issued final regulations clarifying and explaining the law (70 Fed. Reg. 13397 (March 21, 2005)). Initially the program allowed Medicare beneficiaries the option of purchasing drug discount cards, until full program benefits commenced in 2006.

Eligible beneficiaries choose and receive prescription drug benefits from among a multitude of private plans approved by CMS, either as stand-alone plans or as a component of a Part C plan. These private plans negotiate directly with pharmaceutical manufacturers to obtain lower prices. Patients initially choosing a plan or considering changing plans can access the CMS website for assistance in finding the plan that best fits their specific needs (https://www.medicare.gov/find-a-plan/questions/home.aspx). It is important that patients reevaluate and compare their plan to other plans annually because plans continually change their cost-sharing and formulary structures, and a patient's needs can change. CMS rates plans on the basis of their quality and performance, including such criteria as customer service, complaints, drug pricing, patient safety, and member experience.

Enrollment Periods

Eligible beneficiaries must initially choose a plan during a 7-month period starting 3 months prior to the month of their 65th birthday and ending 3 months after the month of their 65th birthday. Failure to choose a plan during that eligibility period may result in a higher monthly premium (assessed at 1 percent per month for every month enrollment is delayed) should they choose a plan later. One exception, however, is that beneficiaries may remain in their current plan if it provides coverage at least as good as a standard Part D plan, called "creditable coverage." In this situation no premium penalty will be assessed if they remain in such a plan. Once enrolled in a Part D plan, most beneficiaries are locked into that plan until the next annual open enrollment period. However, if CMS has rated a plan with five stars, the beneficiary can make a one-time change to that plan at any time during the year. The open enrollment period for 2013 is from October 15 to December 7. Plans must accept all eligible enrollees who reside in their service area.

Beneficiary Cost

Premiums are determined by each plan and range from $15 to $132 per month, averaging $30 in 2012, according to CMS. In addition to a monthly premium, MMA establishes standard beneficiary costs, meaning that Part D plans cannot require enrollees to pay more than these standard costs. Under the standard cost plan for 2013, beneficiaries pay a maximum annual deductible of $325 and 25 percent coinsurance for drug expenditures between $325 and $2,970. Once $2,970 in total (patient + plan) drug costs are incurred, the benefit then enters the third phase known as the coverage gap, also called the "doughnut hole." The beneficiary will remain in the coverage gap until $6,733.75 of total drug cost is reached. This equates to $4,750 in true out-of-pocket (TrOOP) expenses (excluding premiums). After $4,750 in TrOOP expenditures, under what is known as "catastrophic" coverage, the beneficiary will then pay the greater of a 5 percent copayment, or $2.65 for formulary-covered generic drugs or $6.60 for covered brand drugs. Individual plans have the flexibility to vary from the standard benefit cost plan, for example, entirely eliminating the deductible and coverage gap if they choose. Plans cannot require beneficiaries pay amounts above the $325 maximum deductible or $4,750 TrOOP maximum before catastrophic coverage commences.

Under the Patient Protection and Affordable Care Act of 2010, the "doughnut hole" will be gradually reduced through the Medicare Coverage Gap Discount Program. The first step in the closing of the doughnut hole coverage gap was the issuance of a one-time

$250 rebate check to people who reached the coverage gap in 2010. Starting in 2011, beneficiaries receive a 50 percent discount on "applicable" drugs at the point of sale and a 7 percent discount for all other covered drugs while they are in the gap. "Applicable" drugs are those approved by the FDA under NDAs (not ANDAs) and that are covered by a signed discount agreement between the manufacturer and CMS. Over the next several years, prescription drug coverage will continue to increase for all covered drugs in the gap until at the conclusion of the Coverage Gap Discount Program beneficiaries will pay only 25 percent of the costs of drugs in the gap.

Low-income beneficiaries, depending upon the percentage of their income compared to the federal poverty levels (FPLs), will pay less than other beneficiaries do; often no premium or deductible and a fixed copayment amount based upon whether the dispensed drug product is generic or brand. Pharmacies may waive or reduce the costs to low-income beneficiaries, provided they do so in an unadvertised and nonroutine manner, and only after determining that the beneficiary qualifies as low-income or that the pharmacy is unable to collect the amount owed by the beneficiary after reasonable effort.

Covered Drugs and Plan Formularies

Part D covers prescription drugs used for medically accepted indications, and also includes biological products, insulin, and medical supplies associated with administering insulin such as syringes, needles, alcohol swabs, and the like. Certain classes of prescription drugs are specifically excluded from coverage, including

- Weight loss or weight gain drugs
- Fertility drugs
- Erectile dysfunction drugs
- Cosmetic or hair growth drugs
- Cough and cold drugs used to treat symptoms
- Vitamins and minerals (except prenatal vitamins and fluoride preparations)
- Outpatient drugs for which the manufacturer requires testing or monitoring

Barbiturates and benzodiazepine drugs were also on the excluded list; however, a law passed in 2008, the Medicare Improvements for Patients and Providers Act (MIPPA) (P.L. 110-275), removes barbiturates and benzodiazepine drugs from the excluded list effective January 1, 2013. Barbiturates, to be covered, must be used for the indications of epilepsy, cancer, or a chronic mental health disorder. Part D plans may cover these excluded drugs as a supplemental benefit subject to certain restrictions.

Part D plans may use drug formularies that incorporate drug tiers with variable copays, drug utilization review, prior authorization, generic substitution, and other tools. If a plan uses a formulary, it must have a pharmacy and therapeutics (P&T) committee to develop and review the formulary on the basis of scientific evidence and standards of practice. The majority of the committee must be composed of practicing physicians or pharmacists and must include at least one of each. The pharmacists and physicians must have expertise in the care of the elderly and disabled and no conflict of interest.

Generally, the formulary must include all therapeutic categories and classes of drugs as determined by model United States Pharmacopeia (USP) guidelines. However, the formulary only needs to include at least two drugs in each class. Exceptions where all drugs must be covered include

- Antidepressants
- Antipsychotics
- Anticonvulsants

- Antiretrovirals
- Antineoplastics
- Immunosuppressants

MIPAA authorizes CMS to require the inclusion of additional categories and classes of drugs where all drugs must be covered, provided that two criteria are met: that restricted access to the drug or class would have major life threatening consequences for individuals with the disease being treated, and that there is a significant clinical need for these individuals to have access to multiple drugs within the category or class because of unique chemical and pharmacological effects of the drugs (interim final rule 74 Fed. Reg. 2881 (JA 16, 2009)). CMS is required to review formularies to ensure that beneficiaries have access to a broad range of appropriate drugs and that the formulary does not discriminate or discourage enrollment of particular groups.

Plans may not change therapeutic categories and classes in the formulary other than at the beginning of the year, except as necessary to include new drugs or new therapeutic uses. If a plan makes any change in the formulary such as additions or deletions, it must notify CMS within 30 days of the P&T committee's decision. Plans must provide at least a 60-day advance notice to prescribers, pharmacies, beneficiaries, and other affected parties prior to removing a drug from the formulary or changing the status of a drug. If the plan formulary does not include a particular drug, a beneficiary may appeal for an exception if the beneficiary's prescriber determines that the nonformulary drug is medically necessary.

Pharmacy Access

Unless granted a waiver, Part D plans must ensure that beneficiaries have convenient access to a network of pharmacies. The law requires that at least 90 percent of beneficiaries in urban areas live within 2 miles of a retail pharmacy participating in the plan; that 90 percent of beneficiaries in suburban areas live within 5 miles; and that 70 percent of beneficiaries in rural areas live within 15 miles of a participating pharmacy. Plans may use mail order pharmacies, but cannot use them to replace the previously stated access requirements. Traditionally, beneficiaries have often received drugs from mail order pharmacies at lower prices than community pharmacies because plans have favored mail order pharmacies by allowing them to dispense 90-day supplies for one copayment. Community pharmacies have usually been limited to dispensing 30-day supplies. In order to level the playing field and prevent plans from steering beneficiaries to mail order, the law requires that beneficiaries may receive the same supply of drugs at either the community or mail order pharmacy. The beneficiary is, however, responsible for any resulting differential copayment. Plans must provide provisions for beneficiaries to receive prescriptions outside the network when necessary, such as when the beneficiary has a medical emergency while on vacation.

The law creates a federal "any willing provider" requirement, meaning that a Part D plan must permit any pharmacy to participate in the plan that meets the terms and conditions of the plan. This provision was an important concern of pharmacists, who for years have pursued legislation at the state level to allow all pharmacies to participate in third-party plans.

Electronic Prescribing (E-prescribing)

Electronic prescribing has proven effective in reducing medication errors and reducing health care costs, so the law provides for the development of national e-prescribing standards, and mandates that plans support e-prescribing by 2009. Subsequently, CMS published regulations establishing the foundation standards for e-prescribing in 2005 (70 Fed. Reg. 67568), followed by an interim final regulation in 2006, which updated one of the foundation standards (71 Fed. Reg. 36020). The Agency issued a final rule in 2008, specifying and requiring specific uniform standards for communicating formulary and benefits information to prescribers, exchanging medication histories of patients, expressing patient instructions for taking medications, communicating fill status notification, and communicating prior authorizations (73 Fed. Reg. 18918).

The e-prescribing provision preempts any state law or regulation that restricts the ability of prescribers to electronically transmit Medicare prescriptions. E-prescribing participation by prescribers and pharmacies is voluntary. However, in order to encourage e-prescribing, MIPPA of 2008 permits the payment of bonuses to prescribers to e-prescribe starting in 2009 and ending in 2012. At that time prescribers who do not e-prescribe might face penalties. However, this issue became confusing when CMS enacted somewhat different e-prescribing rules for another program, the Medicare Electronic Health Record (EHR) Incentive Program (75 Fed. Reg. 44314, July 28, 2010). As a result, CMS issued a final rule to better align the two programs (76 Fed. Reg. 54953, Sept. 6, 2011). Among other things the rule establishes two hardship exemptions from the 2012 payment penalties: one for practices in rural areas without sufficient high-speed Internet access; and the other for practices in an area without sufficient available pharmacies to engage in e-prescribing. E-prescribing requirements were further revised in May 2012 to achieve consistency with HIPAA transaction standards (77 Fed. Reg. 29002, May 16, 2012).

Pharmacy Reimbursement

Reimbursement for a Part D prescription, both the cost of the product and the dispensing fee, is negotiated by each plan with its network pharmacies. Dispensing fees are based on the costs associated with transferring the prescription from the pharmacy to the beneficiary, but do not include costs associated with medication therapy management (MTM; discussed in the following section). Each plan determines the dispensing fee, not CMS. The pharmacy must inform beneficiaries of any price differential between a covered Part D drug and the lowest-priced generic version of that drug available under the plan at the pharmacy. Addressing pharmacy concerns that plans were not paying claims promptly, MIPAA required that by 2010 plans must pay pharmacy claims within 14 days of electronic submission or within 30 days for claims submitted by other means. MIPAA also requires plans to update their drug cost database weekly to reflect accurate market prices and requires the plans to disclose the sources they used for the updates.

Printed Notice Required When Prescription Claims Not Covered

Beginning May 1, 2012, each Part D plan sponsor must have a system that transmits instructions to the pharmacy to provide to the enrollee a printed notice when a prescription cannot be covered at the point of sale (76 Fed. Reg. 21432, April 15, 2011). The printed notice must inform the enrollee how to request a coverage determination by contacting the toll-free number of the plan. Prior to May 1, 2012, the pharmacy was allowed to post the notice for patients to read rather than providing the printed notice.

Medication Therapy Management

The law requires plans to provide coverage for disease management programs, termed medication therapy management (MTM) programs. Pharmacists may receive fees for providing MTM services to those patients with multiple chronic diseases who take multiple covered drugs and who will likely exceed annual drug costs as determined by HHS. The law defines the MTM benefit as drug therapy management designed to assure that covered drugs are appropriately used to optimize therapeutic outcomes and reduce adverse events. A plan's MTM services must be developed jointly by pharmacists and physicians, and fees to pharmacists and others must take into account the resources used and time required. MTM services should include performing patient health assessments, formulating prescription drug treatment plans, managing high cost specialty medications, evaluating and monitoring patient response to drug therapy, providing education and training, and similar type services.

CMS's 2010 Final Call Letter to Part D plan providers to provide bids contained some enhanced requirements for MTM services. The plan must use an opt-out method only for targeted beneficiaries and must target beneficiaries at least quarterly. Plans may not require more than three chronic diseases to qualify for MTM and must target at least four of seven listed core chronic conditions (hypertension, heart failure, diabetes, dyslipidemia, respiratory disease, bone disease/arthritis, and mental health). In addition, plans may not require that the beneficiary be on more than eight drugs as the minimum number of drugs taken to qualify for MTM. Plans also must offer a minimum level of MTM services for beneficiaries, including an annual comprehensive medication review and person-to-person consultations.

Plan and Provider Marketing Limitations

MIPPA addressed concerns that some plans have been engaged in questionable marketing activities, including using illegal and coercive tactics to enroll beneficiaries. Beginning January 1, 2009, MIPAA prohibits plans from unsolicited direct contact of prospective enrollees, including door-to-door and outbound telemarketing; selling non–health-related products such as life insurance during marketing activities; providing meals at promotional events; marketing in a health care setting, such as a pharmacy, except when conducted in a common area; and at educational events.

Pharmacies can inform patients of the plans in which they participate and distribute plan marketing materials and enrollment applications. They can also display brochures and posters about particular plans, provided they include all plans in which they participate. Printed information from plans can be provided to patients provided there is no ranking or highlighting of specific plans and that plan promotional materials are CMS-approved. New plan affiliations can be announced to patients by direct mail or e-mail one time, after which any communications must include all affiliated plans. Pharmacies may distribute CMS-approved plan finder information and any information from the CMS website (http://www.cms.gov) and the Medicare website (http://www.medicare.gov). Importantly, pharmacies cannot direct, urge, or steer patients to a particular plan. They also may not compare different plan benefits unless created by CMS. Pharmacies also may not collect or accept Medicare enrollment applications and may not accept compensation for conducting enrollment or marketing activities.

Fraud and Abuse

Any false claims submitted for drugs dispensed under Part D will be considered a violation of the federal fraud and abuse statute discussed later in this chapter. The law and regulations require that plan sponsors must have a "comprehensive fraud and abuse plan to detect, correct and prevent Fraud, Waste and Abuse." CMS has interpreted this to mean that both plans and providers must have policies and procedures in place to identify and address fraud, waste, and abuse. (See the CMS policy manual published in 2006

at http://www.cms.gov/Medicare/Prescription-Drug-Coverage/PrescriptionDrugCov
Contra/index.html?redirect=/PrescriptionDrugCovContra/12_PartDManuals.asp).
The 2010 Affordable Care Act (ACA) and the CMS regulations enacted pursuant to the
act signal the government's intensified efforts to control fraud, waste, and abuse (76 Fed.
Reg. 5862, Febr. 2, 2011). Pharmacies must certify that the data they submit are true,
accurate, and complete, and must keep records for 10 years. As a check, the guidance
requires sponsors to audit providers and further requires sponsors to ensure that pharmacies and their employees undergo training regarding avoiding and reporting fraud,
waste, and abuse. In addition, pharmacies must check employees against an exclusion list
of persons issued by the Office of the Inspector General (OIG). If the pharmacy uses a
relief service, CMS recommends that the pharmacy obtain certification from the service
that the individuals are not on the list. In May 2012, OIG issued a report indicating that
more than 26,000 participating pharmacies had questionable billing practices suggesting incidents of fraud and abuse (http://oig.hhs.gov/oei/reports/oei-02-09-00600.asp).
Among other recommendations in the report, OIG suggested that CMS strengthen its
pharmacy audits and oversight program.

Durable Medical Equipment, Prosthetics, Orthotics, and Supplies (DMEPOS)

The MMA not only affects pharmacies dispensing Medicare prescriptions, but also
those supplying medical equipment, prosthetics, orthotics, and supplies (DMEPOS).
(Complete information on this issue can be obtained from the CMS website http://
www.cms.hhs.gov/Medicareprovidersupenroll). The MMA mandates HHS to establish
and implement quality standards for DMEPOS suppliers. In order for suppliers to prove
to HHS that they are in compliance with the standards, they must be accredited by an
HHS recognized independent accrediting agency. Originally it was believed that pharmacies would be exempt from the accreditation requirements since most other health
care professions are exempt, but such was not the case. The MMA also mandates that a
competitive bidding program replace the fee schedule payment methodology previously
in place, with the intent of lowering costs for beneficiaries and the Medicare program.
As a result, CMS now awards contracts to suppliers who offer the best bid price. (CMS
passed final regulations for competitive bidding in April 2007 (72 Fed. Reg. 17992).)
In addition to obtaining accreditation and submitting bids, suppliers must also post a
surety bond of $50,000 per location. Pharmacy organizations generally opposed being
included in the accreditation and competitive bidding requirements and managed to
have a provision included in MIPPA to delay the competitive bidding program until
2011. Pursuant to the ACA, an accreditation exemption is available to pharmacies that
meet several criteria including that the total billings of the pharmacy for DMEPOS are
less than 5 percent of total pharmacy sales for the previous 3 years. (See the DMEPOS
Fact Sheet at http://www.cms.gov/MLNProducts/downloads/DMEPOS_Pharm_Fact
Sheet_ICN905711.pdf.) The ACA also authorizes the secretary to establish an alternative accreditation requirement for pharmacies if the secretary determines this would be
more appropriate.

MEDICARE AND THE REGULATION OF HOSPITAL PHARMACY

Hospitals that wish to admit Medicare patients must comply with certain federal
requirements called the Medicare conditions for participation (42 C.F.R. § 482). Those
conditions of participation most directly applicable to pharmaceutical services require
that a hospital have a pharmacy directed by a registered pharmacist or a drug storage area
under competent supervision. The medical staff is generally responsible for developing

policies and procedures that minimize drug errors, although the staff may delegate this function to the hospital's organized pharmaceutical service. The effect of these basic requirements is to establish a firm mandate for organized pharmacy services under a pharmacist's supervision (42 C.F.R. § 482.25).

The importance of having a pharmacy directed by a pharmacist was underscored in *Sullivan v. Sisters of St. Francis of Texas*, 374 S.W.2d 294 (Tex. Civ. App. 1963), a case brought against a hospital on behalf of a child who died after receiving fluid extract of ipecac instead of syrup of ipecac. (The fluid extract is approximately 17 times more potent than the syrup, and emetine, the active ingredient of both, is cardiotoxic.) In treating the child for the ingestion of a poison, the hospital's emergency department personnel had ordered "ipecac." A nurse who did not know the difference between fluid extract of ipecac and syrup of ipecac retrieved it from the pharmacy. When asked whether she recognized the difference between the two products, the nurse said, "Well, I don't know. I couldn't—I am not a pharmacist, and I wouldn't know." The court ruled in favor of the child's parents and the estate in the lawsuit against the hospital.

Under the Medicare conditions of participation, the pharmacy or drug storage area must be administered in accordance with accepted professional principles. Thus, the hospital must employ a full-time, part-time, or consultant pharmacist to supervise and coordinate the pharmacy department activities. Adequate personnel must be employed and accurate records must be maintained (42 C.F.R. § 482.25(a)).

The conditions of participation further specify that all services must be delivered in accordance with standards of practice and relevant laws (42 C.F.R. § 482.25(b)).

- A pharmacist must supervise the compounding, packaging, and dispensing of drugs.
- Drugs and biologicals must be kept in a locked storage area.
- Outdated products must be made unavailable for patient use by placing them in a special area where a pharmacist cannot retrieve them when processing an order.
- When a pharmacist is not available, only personnel designated by the medical staff and pharmaceutical service may remove drugs from the pharmacy. There must be a stop-order policy for drugs that are prescribed without a specified duration of therapy.
- Drug administration errors, adverse drug reactions, and incompatibilities must be reported immediately to the attending physician and, if appropriate, to the hospital-wide quality assurance program.
- Abuses and losses of controlled substances must be reported.
- Information relating to all aspects of drug therapy must be available to the professional staff.
- A formulary system must be established by the medical staff to ensure the availability of quality pharmaceuticals at reasonable cost.

Most modern pharmacy departments provide services that vastly expand on these basic requirements. Nevertheless, it is important to be aware of these requirements because they describe the backbone of legally mandated institutional pharmaceutical services.

FDA Regulation of Pharmacy in Hospitals

Just as with community pharmacy practice, the FDA has established several rules that indirectly apply to hospital pharmacy practice by virtue of regulating drug products. These FDA rules complement the Medicare conditions of participation.

The modern hospital pharmacy engages in drug packaging and compounding in much the same way that pharmaceutical manufacturers do, but the U.S. Congress has chosen to exempt hospital pharmacies from the close regulation to which drug manufacturers are subjected. The FDA follows this lead by focusing on the mass commercial distribution of drugs rather than on professional practice within hospital pharmacies. Many drug compounding and repackaging activities that would be heavily regulated if performed by manufacturers are not regulated by the FDA if performed by hospital pharmacists. This policy was affirmed in *United States v. Baxter Healthcare Corporation*, 901 F.2d 1401 (7th Cir. 1990), in which the court upheld FDA action against regional compounding centers that were reconstituting drugs (in a way similar to that of most hospitals) on a massive scale. The court noted that hospital pharmacies are exempted from rules that apply to regional compounding centers. Of course, there are some FDA requirements that hospital pharmacies must meet.

The FDA has issued guidelines on the proper labeling of unit-dose drugs. Many unit-dose containers are quite small, and the FDA recognizes that it may not be possible to include all the recommended information. Although the inclusion of this information is not a formal requirement, the prudent hospital pharmacist will seriously consider the FDA's advice.

DEA Regulation of Pharmacy in Hospitals

One might expect that the Drug Enforcement Administration (DEA) might have rules at the federal level that would be directed specifically at hospital-pharmacy practice. However, the reality is that the hospital pharmacy is less regulated at the federal level than is the community pharmacy practice. The numerous and complex requirements for labeling and recordkeeping of controlled substances ordered pursuant to a prescription do not apply to a controlled substance ordered pursuant to a hospital drug order because under federal law the term "prescription" does not include an order to dispense a drug to an inpatient for immediate administration (21 C.F.R. § 1306.02(f)). The word "immediate" in this instance does not mean that the intent must be to administer the drug within the next several seconds; rather, the intent must be that the patient will receive the drug while the patient is hospitalized. The effect of this regulatory approach is to exempt controlled substances ordered for inpatients from requirements (e.g., the form and content of a prescription or the required information on the label of a vial of dispensed controlled substance medication) that are not useful in the institutional environment.

MEDICAID

The most significant Medicaid requirements applicable to pharmacy practice are those found in the OBRA '90 provisions. However, there are other Medicaid provisions that are directly relevant to pharmacy practice because they relate to reimbursement for the products pharmacists provide to patients. Title XIX of the Social Security Act of 1935, Medicaid (42 U.S.C. § 1396 et seq.), provides for the health care costs of certain categories of indigents, including

- The blind
- The disabled
- The aged
- Members of families with dependent children

Eligibility is determined by an individual's income and assets. Some patients (called dual-eligible) are eligible for both Medicare and Medicaid. Prescription drug benefits for dual-eligible patients are covered by Medicare Part D rather than Medicaid.

Although administered by each state, the Medicaid program is subject to federal approval and federal regulation under the authority of CMS. The state's program is jointly funded, with the federal government reimbursing the state government for a certain percentage of its Medicaid expenditures. Medicaid covers all or part of several services, including

- Inpatient and outpatient hospitalization
- Laboratory and x-ray studies
- Care in a skilled nursing facility
- Physician care
- Home health care
- Dental care
- Nursing care
- Optometry
- Outpatient prescription drugs

PRESCRIPTION DRUG COVERAGE

Medicaid provides prescription drug coverage as an optional service. Each state may or may not provide this coverage; all states currently choose to provide it. In the mid-1970s, the federal government became concerned about the rising costs of the Medicaid drug program. The government believed that the amount reimbursed to pharmacies by many state Medicaid agencies was too high. In an effort to correct this perceived problem, contain costs, encourage the use of generic drugs, and establish a more uniform drug benefit program in each state, the government established the maximum allowable cost for drugs (MAC) program in 1975 (42 C.F.R. part 19). The original MAC program was modified in 1987 (42 C.F.R. parts 430 and 447). Under the 1987 law, a pharmacist's reimbursement varies according to whether the drug is a multiple-source drug for which CMS has established a specific upper limit (called the federal upper limit (FUL)) or another drug. A multiple-source drug is one that is produced and marketed by more than one manufacturer, for example amoxicillin.

Reimbursement for Multiple-Source Drugs

CMS has identified certain commonly used multiple-source drugs. The agency publishes a list of these drugs with the FUL price for each drug and the source for the FUL. A pharmacy that dispenses a drug on the FUL list is usually reimbursed by the state for the listed price of the drug, plus a reasonable dispensing fee. (The dispensing fee is determined by each state.)

The FUL reimbursement scheme was conceived in response to pharmacist complaints about the original MAC list of drugs, which was similar to the FUL list. Pharmacists complained that some of the reimbursement prices specified by CMS on the MAC list were so low that they could not even purchase the drug at that price. When pharmacists asked CMS to justify such prices, the agency often was evasive.

In an effort to address these concerns, the regulations specified that the reimbursement price for FUL drugs must be equal to 150 percent of the published price for the least costly therapeutic equivalent (42 C.F.R. § 447.332(b)). The published price is the average wholesale price (AWP) of the drug. AWP is the manufacturer's suggested price for wholesalers to sell to pharmacies. In reality the AWP is often greatly inflated compared to the actual acquisition cost of pharmacies. A report of the Office of Inspector General (OIG) in June 2005 found that FUL amounts were five times higher than the average manufacturer's price (AMP) (DHHS Office of Inspector General, 2005). The AMP is defined as the average price paid by a wholesaler to a manufacturer for the retail class of trade based upon sales records.

As a result of the problems associated with AWP, the Deficit Reduction Act (DRA) (P.L. 109-171) of 2005 authorized CMS to base the calculation of FUL prices on AMP. CMS subsequently published a final regulation that as of October 1, 2007 it would base FUL at 250 percent of AMP (72 Fed. Reg. 39142, July 17, 2007). The agency estimated that basing the FUL on AMP rather than AWP would save the federal government and the states $8.4 billion over the next 5 years. The new basis for calculating FUL, however, caused great alarm in pharmacy. A report from the General Accounting Office (GAO) dated December 22, 2006, but released in late January 2007, appeared to justify the alarm (http://www.gao.gov/new.items/d0669r.pdf). The report notes that basing the FUL on AMP would, on average, result in pharmacy reimbursements 36 percent below average retail pharmacy acquisition costs.

These concerns caused pharmacy organizations to launch legal and legislative efforts to block the impending CMS regulation. The National Community Pharmacists Association and National Association of Chain Drug Stores obtained a federal court injunction in November of 2007, preventing the implementation of the CMS regulation (*NACDS & NCPA v. U.S. DHHS et al.*, Case: 1:07-cv-02017 (U.S.D.C. D.C. Nov. 2007)). The pharmacy organizations criticized the regulation on four grounds:

- Misrepresenting the intent of the DRA and contravening the definition of AMP in the Social Security Act
- Including mail-order pharmacies and PBMs within the definition of retail class of trade, arguing that including these entities would result in lower AMP determinations
- Not including a provision to ensure that the FUL price is actually available in a particular state
- Not limiting FUL calculations to therapeutically equivalent drug products as the law required

Awarding the injunction, the court agreed that the plaintiffs likely would succeed on the merits of their claims and that implementation of the regulation would put pharmacies out of business. In partial response to the injunction, CMS issued a final rule in October 2008 revising its definition of multiple source drugs, changing the definition of a drug from one sold or marketed in the United States to one sold or marketed in the state (73 Fed. Reg. 58491). The rule, however, places the burden on the state or pharmacy to prove that the FUL price is not available nationally. Meanwhile, pharmacy scored a legislative victory to accompany its judicial success. The Medicare Improvements for Patients and Providers Act of 2008 (MIPPA) delayed implementation of the AMP regulation until October 1, 2009. Nonetheless, the AMP regulation would not have gone into effect on October 1 because the regulation was still subject to the injunction.

Subsequently, the ACA revised the FUL limit at no less than 175 percent of the weighted average of the most recently reported AMPs for therapeutically equivalent drug products available for purchase by retail pharmacies on a nationwide basis. The ACA also revised the definitions of AMP and multiple source drugs and replaced the contentious "retail pharmacy class of trade" with "retail community pharmacy." Ultimately, in November 2010, CMS decided to withdraw from the 2007 final regulation its determination of AMP, its calculation for upper limits for multiple source drugs, and its definition of multiple source drug (75 Fed. Reg. 69591, November 15, 2010). Between the summer of 2011 and the spring of 2012, CMS issued draft proposals for calculating FUL prices (http://medicaid.gov/Medicaid-CHIP-Program-Information/By-Topics/Benefits/Prescription-Drugs/Federal-Upper-Limits-.html). The proposed regulation released in February 2012 (77 Fed. Reg. 5318, Febr. 2, 2012) defines "retail community pharmacy" as not including mail-order pharmacies, LTCF pharmacies, or hospital pharmacies.

Regardless of whether the FUL price is determined by AWP or AMP, it must be based on quantities of 100 tablets or capsules, or, if the drug is liquid or is not commonly available in quantities of 100, it must be based on the quantity that is commonly provided by pharmacists. Moreover, the agency must specify the compendia source for its price basis for each drug (e.g., Medi-Span, Blue Book, Red Book). A drug cannot be placed on the FUL list unless it has been evaluated by the FDA as therapeutically equivalent in the Approved Drug Products with Therapeutic Equivalence Evaluations (Orange Book) and has been listed by at least two suppliers. (*Note:* Prior to the DRA amendments, the law required that there must be three therapeutically equivalent drug products on the market.)

Under the original MAC program the state had little flexibility with respect to the reimbursement of individual multiple-source drugs. If the MAC list specified that a pharmacy be reimbursed 3.2 cents per capsule for a particular multiple-source drug, the state had to reimburse the pharmacy at that rate, regardless of the fact that no generic was available at that price. The FUL program grants the state much more flexibility. The regulations specify that, in the aggregate, the state agency must not exceed its payment levels (42 C.F.R. § 447.333(b)). Thus, the state can override the FUL list and reimburse pharmacies for more than the FUL price for a particular drug or drugs as long as it compensates by reducing the reimbursement price for another drug or drugs. In other words, if at the end of the year the state has not reimbursed pharmacies more than it would have had it followed the list exactly, the state would be in compliance with the regulations. Because of this flexibility, many states have developed their own MAC list programs that include more drugs at lower reimbursement prices to pharmacies than the FUL list.

Reimbursement for Other Drugs

If a drug is not on the FUL list, or if it is on the FUL list but is one for which the prescriber has requested the brand-name product, the regulations specify that the pharmacy is to be reimbursed the lower of (1) the estimated acquisition cost (EAC) of the drug, plus a reasonable dispensing fee; or (2) the provider's usual and customary charges to the general public (42 C.F.R. § 447.331(b)). Under the "lower of" provision, a pharmacy that regularly sells certain competitive drugs at low prices to non-Medicaid patients must honor these prices to Medicaid as well. Pharmacies have been subject to disciplinary actions and substantial fines for violating this provision. The EAC is the state Medicaid agency's best estimate of what pharmacists pay for the drug.

For the pharmacy to be reimbursed for the EAC of a brand-name product rather than the FUL amount, the prescriber must certify in the prescriber's own handwriting that the specific brand is "medically necessary" for a particular recipient. The regulations allow the state Medicaid agency to decide what certification form and procedure are used; however, a check-off box on a form is not acceptable (42 C.F.R. § 447.331(c)). Notations such as "brand necessary" on the prescription form are allowable.

Estimated Acquisition Cost and Average Wholesale Price

For several years, most state Medicaid agencies traditionally have defined the EAC of a drug product as the average wholesale price (AWP), an estimated price established by the manufacturer for its product, but not actually the average price wholesalers charge pharmacy customers. For years, CMS disapproved of this interpretation of the EAC, contending that AWPs are in excess of pharmacies' actual acquisition costs. In fact, the agency threatened to force states to reimburse pharmacies on the basis of actual acquisition cost in 1975, but withdrew after deciding that determining the actual acquisition cost would be too expensive.

In 1984, the U.S. Office of the Inspector General published a report finding that 99.6 percent of purchases by pharmacies fall 15.93 percent below the AWP. The report recommended that CMS prohibit the use of AWP as the EAC. CMS complied by seeking a requirement that states reduce AWP by 10.5 percent, but national pharmacy organizations blocked this proposal. Finally, CMS issued a memo to the states saying that they could not rely on AWP as the EAC without evidence showing that it was the closest estimate. Nonetheless, some states continued to define the EAC as such, although many began defining the EAC as a discounted AWP.

Proving that it meant what it said, CMS disapproved Louisiana's Medicaid plan on the basis that the state defined the EAC as AWP, and Louisiana sued in *Louisiana v. U.S. Department of Health and Human Services*, 905 F.2d 877 (5th Cir. 1990). Louisiana argued that federal law does not prohibit reimbursing pharmacists at a rate based on AWP, and CMS was attempting to change federal law. The court disagreed, stating that CMS is not prohibiting the use of AWP, but only saying that this price is not the closest estimate of the price that pharmacists are paying for the drugs. Louisiana further contended that consideration of its reimbursement plan for pharmacists as a whole would reveal that the state's method actually reduced payments by 9.36 percent below AWP. The court acknowledged that this may be so, but held that it does not excuse the state from complying with the requirement that the EAC must be the state's closest estimate, and AWP is clearly not. After its victory in Louisiana, CMS would not approve any state plan that reimbursed pharmacies at AWP.

Following the government's lead, private third-party programs also no longer reimburse pharmacists at the full AWP. AWP as a basis for any pricing may disappear; not just because the price bears little relevance to actual cost, but because of lawsuits against drug manufacturers establishing that artificially inflated AWP prices provide an opportunity for pharmacy benefit managers (and dispensing pharmacies) to bill higher prices for prescriptions, thus allowing them greater profits at the expense of government and private third-party plans as well as patients (*In re Pharmaceutical Industry Average Wholesale Price Litigation*, 2009 WL 3019691, C.A.1 (Mass., Sept. 23, 2009)).

Perhaps the most significant assault against AWP was a lawsuit against First DataBank (FTB) and McKesson because they conspired to inflate AWP prices by using a markup of 1.25 percent over WAC instead of the 1.2 percent figure historically used for AWP (*New England Carpenters Health Benefits Fund v. First DataBank, Inc.*, 244 F.R.D. 79 (D. Mass. 2007)). The court approved a settlement in this case in 2009 (*New England Carpenters Health Benefits Fund v. First DataBank, Inc.*, 602 F.Supp.2d 277 (D. Mass. (2009)). Under the settlement, FTB agreed to apply the 1.2 factor to about 1,400 drug products that had been fraudulently increased. In actuality, on September 26, 2009, FTB rolled back the AWP to 1.2 percent for 28,000 drug products and announced that it would discontinue publishing AWP prices within 2 years. McKesson ultimately settled for $350 million. The settlement affects pharmacies in that third-party plan reimbursements for thousands of drug products have been potentially reduced by 5 percent. This prompted NACDS to bring an unsuccessful lawsuit, opposing the settlement on the basis that the pharmacies were innocent bystanders that would be adversely affected by the settlement (*National Association of Chain Drug Stores v. New England Carpenters Health Benefits Fund*, . . . F.3d . . ., 2009 WL 2824867 (C.A.1 (Mass.) 2009)). Meanwhile, a group of third-party payors not only do not believe that pharmacies are innocent but also believe they conspired with FTB and McKesson to fraudulently inflate AWP prices and thus initiated a class action lawsuit in June 2009 against nine Northern California retail pharmacy chains (*Skilstaf Inc. v. CVS Caremark Corp et al.*, 3:2009cv02514 (CA.N.D, June 5, 2009)).

On September 30, 2011, CMS announced that it was proposing a new pricing benchmark to assist states in determining the EAC (76 Fed. Reg. 60845, September 30, 2011). The new pricing benchmark will replace EAC with AAC. The AAC will likely be an average determined by states providing supporting data that could include, but are not limited to, a national survey of actual pharmacy acquisition costs (77 Fed. Reg. 5318, February 2, 2012).

Litigation Over State Medicaid Cuts

Faced with large deficit budgets, some state legislators have enacted legislation to cut the reimbursement of Medicaid providers, including pharmacies, resulting in lawsuits by the providers. In California, for example, the State legislature voted to reduce Medicaid payments to pharmacies and other health care providers by 10 percent in 2008. Pharmacies, pharmacy organizations, and other health care providers sued the State to enjoin the cuts. The plaintiffs would not likely have standing to bring action on the basis of financial injury to themselves. So instead, the plaintiffs raised the issue that the State's action violated the federal Medicaid Act and thus the cuts are preempted under the Supremacy Clause of the U.S. Constitution. The plaintiffs based their legal claim on the contention that the cuts would cause irreparable harm to Medi-Cal (the name of California's Medicaid program) beneficiaries, and that the State did not analyze whether the cuts would be consistent with efficiency economy, quality of care, and beneficiary access to providers as required under federal law. The Ninth Circuit Court of Appeals found that that the plaintiffs had standing to bring this issue and awarded the injunction on the basis that the plaintiffs demonstrated a likelihood of success on the merits of their argument (*Independent Living Center of Southern California, Inc. v. Maxwell-Jolly*, 572 F.3d 644 (C.A.9 (Cal.), 2009)). The California legislature then sought a 5 percent reduction, but this action also was enjoined by the court of appeals on the same basis that the state did not evaluate whether the reduced payments would comply with federal Medicaid law (*Independent Living Center of Southern California, Inc. v. Maxwell-Jolly*, 2009 WL 2430939 (C.A.9 (Cal.), 2009)). On appeal to the U.S. Supreme Court, the Court declined to decide whether the plaintiffs could proceed under the Supremacy Clause (*Douglas v. Independent Living Center of Southern California, Inc.*, 132 S.Ct. 1204 (Febr. 22, 2012)). Instead, the Court remanded to the Ninth Circuit to reconsider whether the case should proceed under the Supremacy Clause or the Administrative Procedures Act, after CMS made a decision to approve California's reductions.

Litigation Over Medicaid Dispensing Fees

Pharmacists have not only contested the amount reimbursed under Medicaid for a drug's acquisition cost, but also challenged the adequacy of the dispensing fees. State Medicaid agencies determine the dispensing fees paid to pharmacies, which leads to considerable variation in the amount of the fees from one state to another.

In *Pennsylvania Pharmaceutical Association v. Department of Public Welfare*, 542 F. Supp. 1349 (W.D. Pa. 1982), a group of pharmacists and Medicaid recipients contended that the dispensing fee and reimbursement costs paid to participating pharmacies were so low as to violate state and federal Medicaid requirements. When the lawsuit was brought, federal regulations provided that the state pay pharmacies a dispensing fee calculated on the basis of a statewide survey of the cost to dispense prescriptions. The plaintiffs argued that the state failed to conduct the pharmacy surveys in order to obtain the dispensing cost data and that, if the state had done so, it would have found the dispensing fee to be less than the cost to dispense. The court held, however, that the regulation imposed no duty on the state to conduct the surveys. Moreover, stated the court, the intent of the surveys was to determine maximum reimbursements, which the state was not required to pay.

The plaintiffs also argued that the low reimbursement schedule discouraged many pharmacies from participating in the program, thus denying Medicaid recipients adequate access as required by law. (Medicaid law requires that the fees to providers be high enough to ensure that an adequate number of providers participate in the state Medicaid program to serve recipients.) The court responded that Congress enacted Medicaid to provide health care for the poor and aged, not to subsidize or benefit health care providers. The state has no duty to guarantee that providers receive a profit. "If a provider finds participation in the program unprofitable, he should withdraw from the program" (542 F. Supp. at 1356).

The 1987 regulations eliminated the provision that states conduct periodic cost surveys. This elimination was hardly a substantial change, in view of the *Pennsylvania* decision and the fact that pharmacies were reimbursed inadequately even in many of the states that did perform the surveys. In *Massachusetts Pharmaceutical Association v. Rate Setting Commission*, 438 N.E.2d 1072 (Mass. 1982), the court held that, as long as the agency did not act arbitrarily and capriciously, the adequacy of the reimbursement rate could not be challenged. These decisions were typical of pharmacists' lack of success in challenging reimbursement rates.

Tamper Resistant Prescription Pads

In 2007 Congress passed the U.S. Troop Readiness, Veterans' Care, Katrina Recovery, and Iraq Accountability Appropriations Act that surprisingly included a provision that written (not including electronic, oral, or fax) prescriptions must be executed on a tamper resistant pad. The requirement was to go into effect on October 1, 2007, but pharmacy and physician organizations vehemently protested that they could not comply by that date, and Congress extended the deadline to October 1, 2008. To be considered tamper resistant the prescription form must contain one or more industry-recognized features designed to prevent:

- Unauthorized copying of a completed or blank prescription pad
- Erasure or modification of information written on the prescription pad by the prescriber
- The use of counterfeit prescription pads in order to be considered tamper resistant by a state

Emergency fills are permitted as long as a prescriber provides a verbal, faxed, electronic, or compliant written prescription within 72 hours.

MEDICARE/MEDICAID FRAUD AND ABUSE STATUTE

When providing products and services to Medicare or Medicaid patients, pharmacists should be aware of the Medicare and Medicaid fraud and abuse statute (42 U.S.C. § 1320a-7b), especially since the Part D program requires pharmacies to have a comprehensive program to prevent and correct waste, fraud, and abuse. The fraud and abuse statute prohibits knowingly making a false statement of a material fact in any application for a benefit or payment. Some examples include billing for nonexistent prescriptions, billing for the brand drug when a generic was dispensed, billing for prescriptions that are filled but never picked up, splitting prescriptions in order to receive additional dispensing fees, and inappropriate use of dispense-as-written codes.

The law also contains an antikickback provision. As amended over the years to its current form, the antikickback provision prohibits anyone from knowingly and willfully soliciting, receiving, offering, or paying any remuneration in exchange for inducing referrals or for furnishing any goods or services paid for by Medicare or Medicaid. Violation of the fraud and abuse statute will constitute a felony punishable by a maximum fine of $25,000 per violation, 5 years imprisonment, or both. Each prescription claim for reimbursement that is illegally submitted to Medicare or Medicaid would be considered as a separate false claim. Thus, 100 prescriptions deemed as false claims could result in a fine of $2.5 million. Violators also will likely be expelled from the Medicare and Medicaid programs as well as face civil penalties to HHS. The agency within HHS charged with enforcing this aspect of the fraud and abuse statute is the Office of Inspector General (OIG).

SAFE HARBOR REGULATIONS

In 1991, after considerable public controversy and commentary, the Department of Health and Human Services promulgated final regulations to give health care providers better guidance as to the types of investments and business arrangements that are safe from the antifraud statute (42 C.F.R. § 1001.952). Commonly called the safe harbor regulations, they describe 11 broad areas, and the criteria for each that must be followed if an activity is to be protected. The safe harbors are quite narrow in scope and exclude many common business practices. Some of the 11 areas covered by the regulations include

- Investment interests
- Space and equipment rental
- Referral services
- Warranties
- Discounts

If a particular business practice does not fall into a safe harbor, the practice may be

- Clearly legal because it does not intend to induce referrals
- Clearly illegal in violation of the antikickback statute
- Unclear but containing risk because it may violate the statute in a nonobvious or less serious manner

CMS created another safe harbor in 2006 by allowing pharmacies, physicians, certain other health care providers, and health plans to receive and give free hardware and software to enable e-prescribing and e-records (71 Fed. Reg. 45109). This safe harbor fits with the federal government's other efforts to encourage e-prescribing and e-records as discussed earlier.

OIG COMPLIANCE GUIDANCE

In 2003, the OIG issued a voluntary compliance guidance, "OIG Compliance Program Guidance for Pharmaceutical Manufacturers" (68 Fed. Reg. 23731, May 5, 2003), to help manufacturers better understand what activities might violate the fraud and abuse laws. The OIG commented that manufacturer-funded educational programs that induce health care providers to generate business for the manufacturer might violate the anti-kickback statute. The guidance also discusses how educational grants and research funding by manufacturers to health care providers might run afoul of the law. The guidance noted that manufacturers should scrutinize the legitimacy of their relationships with providers whereby remunerative relationships, such as gifts, dinners, entertainment, and personal services, could influence the provider to prescribe or dispense the manufacturers' products. Manufacturers may offer discounts, but only if they are properly disclosed and accurately reported.

The guidance also commented that switching arrangements, in which the manufacturer pays a provider to change the patient from a competing product to the manufacturer's product, are highly suspect. One such example occurred in 1995 when a drug manufacturer offered pharmacies a $30 "consultation fee" for switching a patient from a competitor's product to its product. To obtain the fee, the pharmacy had to contact the prescriber for authorization to switch the product and counsel the patient about the switch. As applied to Medicaid patients, the government viewed this practice as a violation of the antikickback law because it involved a payment in order to induce the furnishing of a drug product, and it forced the manufacturer to discontinue the practice.

In addition to the antikickback statute, the False Claims Act (31 U.S.C. §§ 3729–3733) prohibits a person from knowingly presenting a false or fraudulent claim for payment or approval. It also prohibits knowingly making or using a false record or statement to get a false claim paid or approved.

PHYSICIAN ANTI-SELF-REFERRAL LAW (THE STARK LAW)

Congress passed another law in 1989 (amended in 1993) with the same objective as the antikickback statute, titled the Ethics in Patient Referrals Act (EPRA) (P.L. 101-239; 103-66). This law, however, is much more commonly known as the Stark Law, for its sponsor, California Congressman Pete Stark. The Stark law aims to prevent overuse of health care services and reduce costs to Medicare and Medicaid. More particularly the law is directed at physicians and rises out of concern that some physicians were taking financial advantage by directing patients to health care service providers, such as laboratories, in which they had a financial relationship. Having this type of financial incentive can induce some physicians to overuse health services resulting in fraud, waste, and abuse.

The Stark law with all its regulations is quite complex, but in general it prohibits a physician (also including dentists, podiatrists, optometrists, and chiropractors) from referring Medicare or Medicaid patients to certain entities in which the physician, or an immediate family member, has a financial relationship. If a financial relationship does exist, unless an exception applies (and there are many), the physician cannot legally refer patients to the entity for the following types of services:

- Clinical laboratory services
- Radiology services, for example MRIs, CAT scans, and ultrasound
- Radiation therapy services and supplies
- Physical and occupational therapy services
- Durable medical equipment and supplies
- Parenteral and enteral nutrients, equipment, and supplies
- Prosthetics, orthotics, prosthetic devices, and supplies
- Outpatient prescription drugs
- Home health services
- Inpatient and outpatient hospital services

Violations of the Stark law can result in significant fines and exclusion from the Medicare and Medicaid programs. Unlike the antikickback statute, the government does not have to prove the defendant acted knowingly and willfully. Merely making a prohibited referral, even without intent, is a violation of the law. Intentional violations of the Stark law most likely would also violate the fraud and abuse and antikickback laws.

© Stockbyte/Thinkstock

STUDY SCENARIOS AND QUESTIONS

1. A Medicare-eligible patient of a pharmacy is considering switching from an employer-sponsored plan to a particular Part D plan in which her friends have enrolled. She has several questions for the pharmacist. How should the pharmacist answer each of the following questions?
   a. "Can I join the Part D plan at any time during the year?"
   b. "I heard I might have to pay a penalty because I was eligible to join a Part D plan a year ago. Is that true?"
   c. "Will the Part D plan cover all my drug expenditures?"
   d. "One of the drugs I currently get is Valium. Will it be covered?"
   e. "Will the Part D plan cover my antidepressant medications, and if it does, could it decide to drop coverage after I join?"
   f. "Can you provide me with 90-day coverage of my medications the same as the mail order plan?"
2. Bob's Pharmacy has several Medicaid patients. Bob likes Medicaid prescriptions because his profit margin is higher than for some private plans. Some of the physicians tend to write the Medicaid prescriptions for brand-name drugs. Bob will write "medically necessary" on these prescriptions so he can get reimbursed the EAC rather than the FUL price. Bob is part of a buying cooperative that sends him different brands of generic drugs nearly every month. Because the generic equivalents are all about the same price to Bob, he cannot see changing the NDC numbers in the computer all the time. Therefore, Bob often will dispense a generic drug but submit a claim to Medicaid with an NDC number other than the one dispensed. Several Medicaid patients do not pick up the prescriptions that are phoned in to Bob. Bob submits the claim when he fills the prescription but does not always remember to notify Medicaid when the prescription is not picked up.

   List three potential Medicaid violations that exist and explain why they are violations. Why might it cause the state and the manufacturers problems if Bob uses the wrong NDC number for his claims, even if his cost is the same for the drug dispensed and the drug whose NDC number he used?

FEDERAL REGULATION OF LONG-TERM CARE

Pharmaceutical (pharmacist) care in long-term care facilities traditionally has presented regulatory challenges that reflect issues from both institutional and community pharmacy practice. Because the residents in long-term care facilities are not, strictly speaking, ambulatory patients, they can be thought of as institutionalized patients. On the other hand, most providers of pharmacy products and services to long-term care facilities have been community pharmacies for which the patients in long-term care facilities have seemed little different from those patients who live at home. A specialty area of practice in consulting and nursing home pharmacy has evolved over the past two decades so the trend is in the direction of recognizing a hybrid type of pharmacy practice, combining some aspects of institutional practice with other aspects derived from community pharmacy. To a large degree, it has been government regulation that has driven this development of a specialized pharmacy practice; thus it is important for pharmacists to understand the specific legal rules that have an impact on the provision of pharmacist care in the long-term care environment.

THE TREND TOWARD LONG-TERM CARE

The American public is aging, and geriatric patients traditionally use more drugs than do younger patients. In addition, the health care system has discovered a critical integrated role for facilities that do not provide the intense level of care that hospitals provide but still can provide care of a kind that many patients need and cannot get at home. It should come as no surprise that there are a large number of patients in long-term care facilities who require specialized pharmacist care services. Because most long-term care facilities participate in government programs that cover the costs for residents in the facilities, government standards are important in determining the level of care that patients will receive. This high level of government oversight is at least as stringent for pharmacy as it is for any other service; thus, pharmacists are particularly attentive to the requirements that the law establishes for pharmacist care services in long-term care facilities.

At one time, terminology was important as a way to distinguish the classes of facilities at which a patient might reside over the long term. Technically, a skilled nursing facility (SNF) is a nursing home that is recognized for reimbursement under both Medicaid and Medicare. An intermediate care facility (ICF) is a nursing home that is recognized only under Medicaid. An SNF provides a level of care that is higher than the care available at an ICF. Because the regulations for an SNF and an ICF are now the same, however, the distinction is unimportant for a discussion of pharmacist care services. Therefore, this section uses the generic term long-term care facility (LTCF).

The many complex issues surrounding rights and responsibilities in long-term care have been extensively addressed by federal regulations. Federal legislation in OBRA '87 and the modifications contained in OBRA '90 prompted CMS regulations. These exhaustive regulations should be referenced by anyone who attempts to devote time to the practice of pharmacy in an LTCF. They are so extensive that they occupy the field and set the standard for long-term care insofar as patient-care matters are concerned. Any questions that may remain after reading the specific regulations are probably answered in CMS's published guidance to surveyors of LTCFs. Issues related to the furnishing and dispensing of controlled substances to LTCFs are addressed in Chapter 5.

SELF-ADMINISTRATION OF DRUGS

For each resident, a comprehensive care plan must be developed. This plan must be prepared by an interdisciplinary team that includes the attending physician, a registered nurse with responsibility for the patient, and other appropriate staff from disciplines as determined by the resident's needs. Individual residents of LTCFs may self-medicate if the interdisciplinary team has determined that this practice is safe. The interdisciplinary team must also determine who will be responsible for storage and documentation of the administration of drugs, as well as the location of the drug administration (e.g., resident's room, nurse's station, activities room). The decision that a resident has the ability to self-administer medications is subject to periodic reevaluation on the basis of changes in the resident's status. If a resident chooses to self-administer drugs, this decision should be made at least by the time the care plan is completed and always within 7 days after completion of a comprehensive assessment. Medication errors occurring with residents who self-administer drugs should not be counted in the facility's medication error rate but should call into question the judgment made by the facility in allowing self-administration for those residents (42 C.F.R. § 483.10(n)).

Unnecessary Drugs

Each resident's drug therapy must be free from unnecessary drugs. An unnecessary drug is any drug when used

- In excessive dose (including duplicative therapy)
- For excessive duration
- Without adequate monitoring
- Without adequate indications for its use
- In the presence of adverse consequences that indicate the dose should be reduced or discontinued
- Any combination of these reasons

On the basis of a comprehensive assessment of a resident, the facility must ensure that residents who have not used antipsychotic drugs are not given these drugs unless antipsychotic drug therapy is necessary to treat a specific condition as diagnosed and documented in the clinical record. Residents who use antipsychotic drugs must receive gradual dose reductions and behavioral interventions, unless clinically contraindicated, in an effort to discontinue these drugs (42 C.F.R. § 483.25(l)).

Fourteen-Day Dispensing Cycle

The ACA mandates CMS to consider alternative dispensing strategies for LTCFs to reduce medication waste. In response, CMS promulgated a final regulation requiring that pharmacies may not dispense more than a 14-day cycle of medications beginning January 1, 2013 (76 Fed. Reg. 21432, April 15, 2011). Originally, CMS considered requiring pharmacies to dispense in 7-day or less increments, but ultimately modified the proposal based upon concerns from stakeholders. CMS noted, however, that nothing precludes LTCFs and pharmacies from selecting 7-day or less methodologies, or Part D sponsors from incentivizing the adoption of more efficient dispensing techniques. Drugs exempt from the 14-day requirement include antimicrobials, those where FDA approved labeling require them to be dispensed in the original packaging, and drugs whose packaging helps patients comply with the prescribed regimen.

Medication Errors

Each facility must ensure that it is free of medication error rates of 5 percent or greater and that residents are free of any significant medication errors. A medication error means a discrepancy between what the physician ordered and what is observed of an individual or several different individuals administering drugs to residents in the facility. A medication error rate is determined by calculating the percentage of errors. The numerator is the total number of errors that were observed, both significant and insignificant. The denominator is called opportunities for error, and includes all the doses observed being administered plus the doses ordered but not administered. The relative significance of medication errors is a matter of professional judgment in light of the following three factors:

1. The resident's condition
2. The drug category
3. The frequency of error (42 C.F.R. § 483.25(m))

PHARMACY SERVICES

A long-term care facility must provide pharmaceutical services (including procedures that ensure the accurate acquiring, receiving, dispensing, and administering of all drugs and biologicals) to meet the needs of each resident. The facility may either do this itself or enter into an agreement with a pharmacy to provide pharmacy services. The facility is responsible for ensuring that pharmacy services are provided in a "timely manner." If the failure to provide a prescribed drug in a timely manner causes the resident discomfort or endangers the resident's health and safety, then this requirement has not been met (42 C.F.R. § 483.60).

SERVICE CONSULTATION

The facility must employ or obtain the services of a pharmacist who provides consultation on all aspects of the provision of pharmacy services in the facility. The pharmacist-consultant must establish a system of records of receipt and disposition of all controlled substances in sufficient detail to enable an accurate reconciliation. A facility can use existing documentation such as a medication administration record to meet the requirement for records of disposition. The pharmacist-consultant must determine that drug records are in order and that an account of all controlled substances is maintained and periodically reconciled. Reconciliations should be done monthly; if they reveal shortages, the pharmacist and the director of nursing should consider initiating more frequent reconciliations. Federal regulations do not prohibit shortages of controlled substances, only that a record be kept and that it be periodically reconciled. If the evidence shows that all controlled drugs are not accounted for, then federal surveyors will refer the matter to the state nursing home licensure authority or the state board of pharmacy (42 C.F.R. § 483.60(b)).

DRUG REGIMEN REVIEW (CONSULTANT PHARMACIST)

Each resident's drug regimen must be reviewed at least once a month by a consultant pharmacist. It may be necessary to review more frequently, perhaps every week, depending on the resident's condition and the drugs that the resident is using. The pharmacist must report any irregularities to the attending physician and the director of nursing, and these reports must be acted on. The director of nursing and the attending physician are not required to agree with the pharmacist's report, nor are they required to provide a rationale for their acceptance or rejection of the report. They must, however, act on the report. This may be accomplished in many ways. For example, they may specifically indicate acceptance or rejection of the report, or they may simply sign their names to it. Although it is not specifically required, facilities are encouraged to provide the medical director with a copy of drug regimen review reports and to involve the medical director in reports that have not been acted on (42 C.F.R. § 483.60(d)).

In 2011, CMS proposed to mandate that consultant pharmacists must be independent from the LTCF pharmacy and drug manufacturers or distributors to avoid conflicts of interest. However, CMS has instead proposed, at least for the present, that the LTCF industry voluntarily adopt specific changes to avoid overprescribing (77 Fed. Reg. 22072, April 12, 2012). Those voluntary changes proposed by CMS include separate contracting for LTCF consultation services from dispensing and other pharmacy services; payment by the LTCF at a fair market rate for the consultant pharmacist's services; and disclosure by the consultant pharmacist to the LTCF of any potential conflicts of interest.

LABELING OF DRUGS AND BIOLOGICALS

Drugs and biologicals used in an LTCF must be labeled in accordance with currently accepted professional principles, and this must include the appropriate accessory and cautionary instructions and the expiration date when applicable. When applicable means that the expiration date must be on the labels of drugs used in LTCFs unless state law stipulates otherwise. These requirements are imposed on the facility, even though pharmacists will be immediately responsible for accomplishing specific tasks. The critical elements of the drug label in an LTCF are the name of the drug and its strength. The names of the resident and the physician do not have to be on the label of the package, but they must be identified with the package in such a manner as to ensure that the drug is administered to the right person (42 C.F.R. § 483.60(d)).

STORAGE OF DRUGS AND BIOLOGICALS

In accordance with state and federal laws, long-term care facilities must store all drugs and biologicals in locked compartments under proper temperature controls and permit only authorized personnel to have access to the keys. Compartments in the context of this rule include, but are not limited to, drawers, cabinets, rooms, refrigerators, carts, and boxes. The provisions for authorized personnel to have access to keys must be determined by the facility management in accordance with federal, state, and local laws, as well as facility practices. The phrase "separately locked" means that the key to the separately locked schedule II drugs is not the same key that is used to gain access to the nonschedule II drugs. The facility must provide separately locked, permanently affixed compartments for storage of controlled substances listed in schedule II, except when the facility uses a unit-dose distribution system in which the quantity stored is minimal and a missing dose can be readily detected (42 C.F.R. § 483.60(e)).

FEDERAL ANTITRUST LAWS

Federal antitrust laws have assumed a significant role as the provision of pharmacy goods and services has become intensely competitive, with the major emphasis on cost containment. A myriad of individuals and business entities compete vigorously for the revenue that comes from providing pharmacy goods and services including:

- Manufacturers
- Wholesalers
- Hospitals

- Health maintenance organizations (HMOs)
- Preferred provider organizations (PPOs)
- Pharmacies
- Prescribers

The addition of employers, insurance companies, and managed health care plans into this competitive mix—with their goal of controlling costs—results in some interesting and unique marketplace dynamics and the potential for unfair competition.

The business of pharmacy has both struggled and thrived in this system and has been the subject of (and will continue to be the subject of) important antitrust litigation. This chapter focuses on two of the most important antitrust laws: the Sherman Antitrust Act and the Robinson-Patman Act.

The Sherman Antitrust Act

Passed in 1890, the Sherman Antitrust Act contains two sections. Section 1 of the act (15 U.S.C. § 1) makes unlawful every contract, combination, or conspiracy in restraint of trade. Section 2 of the act (15 U.S.C. § 2) prohibits monopolies, attempts to monopolize, or conspiracies to monopolize. The purpose of the Sherman Antitrust Act is not to protect competitors but rather to protect competition. As one court stated, "In an openly competitive market, the inefficient fail; in a noncompetitive system, the efficient are precluded from competing" (*Klamath-Lake Pharmaceutical Association v. Klamath Medical Service Bureau*, 701 F.2d 1276, 1292 (9th Cir. 1983)). Because the Sherman Antitrust Act is designed to facilitate a competitive market, it does not protect businesses from failing as a result of intense competition.

Concerted Activity

Congress enacted Section 1 of the Sherman Antitrust Act to prevent individual competitors from entering into agreements that would reduce competition and thereby adversely affect the consumer's welfare. Read literally, Section 1 seems to preclude any contract or combination because every contract in some way restrains trade. Courts, however, invalidate only unreasonable restraints on competition.

Competitors can violate Section 1 of the act only if there is an agreement, formal or informal, between them; a single competitor cannot violate Section 1. Thus, although it may violate Section 1 for two or more independent pharmacies to agree to reject a third-party prescription plan, it is permissible for each pharmacy independently to reject that third-party plan. Similarly, it is not illegal under Section 1 for a chain pharmacy to reject a third-party plan, even if it owns hundreds of pharmacies, because the chain is considered one legal entity.

The fact that no concerted activity exists does not mean that a business cannot unfairly affect competition. Section 2 of the act places limitations on individual businesses that constitute monopolies. Although just being a monopoly is not illegal, it is illegal for a business to exploit its monopoly power for the purpose of harming competition rather than for legitimate business purposes.

Market Power

Crucial to almost any antitrust case is the market power of the defendant. If the defendant does not possess adequate market power, the plaintiff is not likely to have the grounds for an antitrust action. In general terms, market power is the amount of business that the defendant controls of all the available business in the geographic area. In legal terms, market power is the ability of a business to raise prices above those that would be charged in a competitive market or the ability to exclude competition. Conduct that may be unreasonably anticompetitive or restrictive in one market may have little effect in another. For example, in a geographic area with only one hospital, the joint venture of the hospital and a community pharmacy to create a durable medical equipment (DME) business could adversely affect other equipment suppliers who rely on the hospital's referred patients. The same joint venture in an area with several hospitals and DME businesses would likely have little impact on competition.

A crucial question is, "At what percentage of the market does a defendant possess market power?" For example, if a third-party prescription program represents 20 percent of the prescription business to all the pharmacies in the area, is this sufficient market power to trigger an antitrust problem? The only answer possible is that there is no magic percentage. A 10 percent market share may be market power in one situation, whereas a 20 percent market share may not be in another. The threshold for market power depends on the facts of each situation.

Monopoly Power

A related question is, "At what percentage of the market does a business have monopoly power?" Again, each situation must be analyzed separately. Generally speaking, a market share of more than 40 percent may raise monopoly concerns.

Rule of Reason and Per Se Rule

In deciding whether an activity violates the Sherman Act, courts often apply one of two types of analyses: the rule of reason or the per se rule. Under the rule-of-reason analysis, a court determines whether the defendant's activity is reasonable by balancing the procompetitive and anticompetitive effects of the activity. The court considers the purpose, nature, duration, effect, and justification of the activity, as well as the market power of the entities involved. Essentially, the court attempts to determine whether the net effect of the defendant's action is to promote competition or suppress it.

The courts have traditionally classified certain types of activities to be unreasonably anticompetitive. If a defendant's activity falls under one of these classifications, the court will usually invalidate the activity without the need to hear additional evidence and regardless of any justification by the defendant. This approach is called the per se rule. Often, courts are reluctant to apply the per se rule to novel health care arrangements, however, because these arrangements do not easily fit into the traditional types of activities previously ruled as per se violations, such as price fixing and boycotting. Pharmacists must be careful not to engage in any activity the courts have classified as a per se violation.

Types of Per Se Violations

Price Fixing

An explicit or implicit agreement among competitors to affect price or the allocation of services is price fixing. For example, assume that a city has five competing pharmacies that are each enjoying a reasonable profit. The pharmacy owners and managers hold a meeting and decide not to underprice each other, thus preserving each pharmacy's healthy share of the market. This is price fixing, a per se violation of the Sherman Act. This concerted activity by the pharmacies in effect deprives the consumer of competition that would probably result in lower prices or better services. Moreover, if these five competitors could conspire to fix prices, they could also conspire to make it difficult for other competitors to start pharmacies in the community, further depriving the consumer of the benefits of competition.

Associations of competitors must be careful not to engage in price fixing activities as well because they represent a collective group of competitors. In *Northern California Pharmaceutical Association v. United States*, 306 F.2d 379 (9th Cir. 1962), cert. denied, 83 S. Ct. 119 (1962), the court found that the Northern California Pharmaceutical Association had engaged in price fixing by publishing a suggested price schedule for prescription drug prices and distributing it to its members. Both the association and members who participated in the price schedule were held liable.

The *Northern California* case and related case law must not be interpreted to mean that pharmacy associations cannot distribute economic information to educate their members. Associations may lawfully disseminate such information as cost-to-dispense data to members and third-party administrators, for example. Associations may even discuss reimbursement and similar issues with third-party administrators, provided that they do not enter any agreements on behalf of their members or threaten the third-party plan with price fixing or a boycott.

Boycotting

Closely related to price fixing is the issue of boycotting, an agreement among competitors not to deal with another party. Boycotting often occurs innocently when one pharmacist owner or manager asks other pharmacy owners whether they plan to accept or reject a particular third-party prescription program. The group may then decide to stick together and reject the third-party plan unless its reimbursement level is raised. Regardless of the intent or frustrations of the pharmacists involved, this activity is a per se violation of the Sherman Antitrust Act.

Tying Arrangements

Conditioning the purchase of one product on the purchase of another is a tying arrangement. Only when the seller can force the buyer to purchase the tied product is such an arrangement illegal, however. For example, it is not normally illegal for a pharmacy to require a customer to buy a toothbrush with every tube of toothpaste purchased. Customers who do not wish to purchase the two products together can simply go to another store and purchase the items separately.

Many pharmacists first became familiar with the issue of tying arrangements in 1990 when Sandoz Pharmaceuticals introduced its antischizophrenia drug clozapine (Clozaril). Sandoz restricted the distribution of the drug to those pharmacies that could provide blood monitoring under the Clozaril Patient Management System. As a result, several states brought antitrust suits against Sandoz on the ground that the company was illegally tying the sale of the drug to the sale of an exclusively licensed blood-monitoring program. Because Sandoz had the patent on Clozaril, a buyer did not have the option of buying clozapine from another seller. Sandoz denied that its activity violated the law but nonetheless agreed to no longer specify that a particular blood-monitoring program be implemented in conjunction with the sale of its drug. The company subsequently entered into a consent agreement with the Federal Trade Commission (FTC) and settled the lawsuits brought by the states.

The Clozaril case differs from classic tying arrangements in that it has quality of care and public health ramifications. Most likely, it will not be the last case of its type. Other manufacturers will undoubtedly seek to restrict the distribution, control the administration, and require the provision of additional services for certain drugs. In light of the

Clozaril example, however, they would be wise if they did not benefit from any of the additional required services unless absolutely necessary.

Third-Party Prescription Programs

Nationwide, pharmacists became quite upset with third-party prescription plans, especially over the inadequacy of reimbursement. Frustrated that the Sherman Act prohibited pharmacists from collectively negotiating with third-party plans for better dispensing fees, pharmacists attempted to enforce the Sherman Act against the plans. In the landmark case of *Group Life and Health Insurance Co. v. Royal Drug Co.*, 440 U.S. 205 (1979), a group of independent pharmacists in San Antonio, Texas, contended that the fixed dispensing fee offered pharmacies by the plans in the pharmacy agreements constituted price fixing and, thus, violated Section 1 of the Sherman Antitrust Act. Before the court could address the antitrust issue, however, it had to determine whether the defendant was exempt from the Sherman Antitrust Act under the exemption granted to the business of insurance by the McCarran-Ferguson Act. The U.S. Supreme Court found for the pharmacists, holding that the pharmacy agreements are not the business of insurance because they are not part of determining risk.

The Supreme Court decision meant that the case could go back through the federal court system to resolve the antitrust issues. On these grounds, the pharmacists were not so successful (*Royal Drug Co. v. Group Life and Health Insurance Co.*, 737 F.2d 1433 (5th Cir. 1984)). The pharmacists contended that Group Life's action of offering all pharmacies a fixed professional fee constituted price fixing and, in particular, resale price maintenance. A manufacturer's refusal to sell its product to a retailer unless the retailer agrees to sell the product at or above a certain price set by the manufacturer (resale price maintenance) is per se illegal because it deprives the consumer of price competition among retailers.

The court disagreed with the analogy, finding that the challenged arrangement did not resemble resale price maintenance agreements closely enough to apply the per se rule. In the court's opinion, there was no resale transaction in which to maintain a price. Rather, said the court, the pharmacy agreements are "merely arrangements for the purchase of goods and services by Blue Shield" (737 F.2d at 1438). The court emphasized that, in its view, the third-party plan is the purchaser, not the enrollees; therefore, this is simply a contractual arrangement in which the purchaser has a right to bargain for the best deal possible.

Although the court closed the door to a per se invalidation of the activity, it did not at this point find that the defendant's activity was legal. Rather, the court sought to apply a rule-of-reason analysis and balance all the evidence to determine if the activity was procompetitive or anticompetitive. The pharmacists, however, had rested their entire case on the per se argument and had no evidence to present to the court that would indicate anticompetitive effect. Thus, the court found in favor of the third-party plan.

The *Royal Drug* decision on the antitrust issues was consistent with federal court decisions in other districts on the same issues, such as *Medical Arts Pharmacy of Stanford, Inc. v. Blue Cross and Blue Shield of Connecticut, Inc.*, 518 F. Supp. 1100 (D. Conn. 1981), and *Sausalito Pharmacy, Inc. v. Blue Shield of California*, 677 F.2d 47 (9th Cir. 1982). In each of these decisions, the court refused to invalidate the third-party plan's activity as a per se violation of the Sherman Antitrust Act. In both cases, the pharmacists failed to present evidence to substantiate anticompetitive effect. Since these decisions, pharmacists have not again attempted to establish in court that the plans are anticompetitive.

Prescription Benefit Managers

Prescription Benefit Managers (PBMs), as the name indicates, are companies that contract with health plans to manage the prescription benefit component of the plan; with the primary objective of lowering costs for the plan. PBMs generally attempt to accomplish this objective by performing several activities such as negotiating discounts with drug manufacturers, developing drug formularies typically favoring generic drugs, contracting with community pharmacy providers, processing claims from pharmacies, engaging in prospective and retrospective drug utilization review, and dispensing to patients through their own mail-order facilities. PBMs have always been controversial among pharmacists, but have become even more so because of ownership and integration issues that have occurred since the 1990s. Drug manufacturers, such as Lilly and Merck, first acquired large PBMs, raising antitrust concerns that PBM formularies would favor the drug manufacturer's products. Ultimately, the drug companies divested the PBMs; however, now some chain pharmacies have merged with PBMs, raising antitrust and unfair competition concerns. Of particular concern is that a PBM could steer patients to the affiliated chain pharmacy either directly or indirectly. For example, the PBM could use its database to determine that a patient is using multiple pharmacies and provide this information to the affiliate chain pharmacy, which in turn could attempt to induce the patient to shop at only the chain pharmacy.

Pharmacists have also accused PBMs of a lack of transparency because they share very little financial data with plans, pharmacies, and beneficiaries. This lack of transparency results in the public not knowing the extent of the rebates and discounts that PBMs receive from drug manufacturers and whether any of that is actually passed on to reduce health care costs. Lack of transparency conceals some important information including whether a PBM has a contract to favor a particular manufacturer's product, even though it might be more costly than a competitor's; and what price the health plan pays to the PBM for the prescription versus what the PBM pays the pharmacy for the prescription. Bills have been introduced in Congress and legislation has been passed in some states to require more transparency from PBMs.

Exclusive Contracts

In an exclusive contract, a seller agrees to sell its product or service only to a particular buyer. Pharmacies may use exclusive contracts in several ways. A pharmacy may contract with a manufacturer (e.g., cosmetics, cards, candy) to be the only retailer in the area to sell that manufacturer's products. A pharmacy may contract with a long-term care facility to be its only supplier of medications and health supplies. A pharmacy may contract with a third-party plan to be the only supplier of prescription medications for the plan's patients.

Exclusive contracts are generally legal. Antitrust problems may arise, however, if an exclusive contract unreasonably restrains competition. Often, the market share of the contracting parties is the determining factor. For example, an exclusive contract between a third-party plan that represents 60 percent of all the prescription business in a particular area and one pharmacy could force many of the other pharmacies in the area out of business, ultimately restraining the competition for pharmacy goods and services.

Joint Ventures

The antitrust implications of joint ventures are analogous in many respects to those associated with exclusive contracts. A joint venture occurs when two or more independent entities integrate into a new organization for the purpose of increasing business or entering a new market. Joint ventures are generally legal, unless the market share of the new organization unreasonably harms competition.

In *Key Enterprises of Delaware, Inc. v. Venice Hospital*, 919 F.2d 1550 (11th Cir. 1990), the court held that the joint venture of a hospital and a DME supplier violated both Section 1 and Section 2 of the Sherman Act. The defendant hospital wished to diversify into the DME business. At that time, it enjoyed 80 percent of the patient admissions to the hospitals in the area, and its equipment referral patients represented more than 46 percent of the total market. The hospital entered into a joint venture with the codefendant, Medicare Patient Aid Centers (MPAC), after which MPAC captured 85 percent of the hospital's DME referrals. The plaintiff, a competitor of MPAC, watched its business slip from 72.8 percent of the market before the joint venture to 30 percent after the venture. In contrast, MPAC's market share went from 9 percent before the joint venture to 61 percent after the joint venture.

The court found that the defendants violated the Sherman Antitrust Act because of the unreasonable nature of their business behavior. For example:

- The defendants entered into a reciprocal agreement with the area home health care nurses whereby the nurses would recommend MPAC in exchange for hospital privileges.
- The hospital had refused to allow vendors of DME access to the hospital in the past, although it changed that policy after the joint venture by allowing access only to MPAC.
- An employee of MPAC was allowed to represent him- or herself as having a position with the hospital and engage in discharge counseling.
- The reason that MPAC sought the joint venture was to exclude competitors.
- The hospital had different rules regarding physician standing orders for home health care nurses than for DME vendors for no reason. (Physicians were allowed to make standing orders indicating a preference for a home health agency, but not for DME providers, where they had to indicate this preference on each patient's chart.)
- The hospital and MPAC used a default rule whereby, if the patient did not choose an equipment supplier, MPAC was automatically selected for the patient.
- The hospital used its monopoly power in acute care to leverage itself into the DME market with the intent of avoiding competition.

The defendants contended that the patients had the freedom to choose any vendor they wished, to which the court replied:

> However, a patient's freedom to choose under these circumstances may be illusory. The evidence presented in this case shows that patients rarely have preference for a DME vendor. The patients know very little about the equipment or the companies that rent the equipment. Thus, they are very susceptible to recommendations made by anyone who appears knowledgeable on the subject. It therefore becomes very easy to channel patient choice by limiting the patient's exposure to competition. (919 F.2d at 1557)

Venice Hospital raises the important point that consumers really are not knowledgeable about many health care goods and services, and they must rely heavily on professional advice. The decision in this case sends a warning that health care providers must exercise caution when referring patients to affiliated businesses. Hospitals in particular should

- Advise the patient in writing of all providers in the community
- Require hospital employees to answer all questions about competitors objectively

- If a no solicitation rule is in effect, make sure that it was in effect before the hospital started its affiliate business and make sure that the rule applies to everyone
- Not pressure employees to recommend the hospital's affiliate
- Not have a default rule that patients without preference automatically are sent to the hospital's affiliate

Preferred Provider Organizations

As both private and government third-party programs have increased their market share, participation in these programs has become vital to the survival of many pharmacies. Increasingly, however, third-party prescription programs entered into exclusive contracts with pharmacies, selected on a bid basis. Independents and smaller chain pharmacies often are not even allowed to bid because they do not offer the number of outlets that a single large chain offers. In an effort to compete for third-party contracts, community pharmacies started what became known as pharmaceutical services administrative organizations (PSAOs) that are analogous to preferred provider organizations (PPOs). A typical PSAO contracts with several pharmacies to represent them in third-party program bidding and negotiating. In effect, the PSAO unites several pharmacies under one administrative roof. To attract third-party contracts, most PSAOs offer several services (e.g., delivery service, 24-hour on-call emergency prescription services), which each pharmacy member must agree to provide.

Because they represent a group of competitors, PSAOs and PPOs must be structured carefully to avoid antitrust problems. In *Arizona v. Maricopa County Medical Society*, 457 U.S. 332 (1982), a medical care foundation composed of several physicians set maximum fees for services. The physician members agreed to accept those fees for patients insured under third-party plans that contracted with the foundation. Although the fees were less than the physicians' normal charges, the U.S. Supreme Court invalidated the foundation's fee schedule. To the Supreme Court, this practice was simply price fixing. The court stated that if providers were allowed to agree to set lower fees one day, then nothing would prevent them from setting higher fees the next day.

The *Maricopa* decision means that a PSAO should not establish dispensing fees to offer third-party plans. Rather, a PSAO should invite the third-party plan to submit a reimbursement proposal. Each member pharmacy of the PSAO must unilaterally decide whether to accept or reject the plan's proposal. The U.S. Department of Justice has taken the position that the *Maricopa* decision should not be interpreted as an absolute ban on the use of fee schedules. If the fee schedules are procompetitive, necessary to enhance the bargaining power of the PSAO, and unlikely to dampen price competition, they may be allowed, provided that the PSAO does not represent a large market share. No health care providers, however, should consider establishing a fee schedule without legal counsel.

To reduce antitrust risks even further, the PSAO should be open to any pharmacy that wishes to join it. Each pharmacy member should be allowed to participate in other PSAOs and in other third-party plans that have not contracted with the PSAO in question. All precautions must be taken to ensure that the PSAO is procompetitive for the patient, not simply a means to obtain higher fees for pharmacies.

Purchasing Cooperatives

To obtain a better price from sellers, some competitors may form a cooperative to pool their purchasing power. Hospitals have purchased pharmaceuticals through buying groups for several years, but community pharmacies have become significantly involved in purchasing co-ops more recently. Participation in a purchasing co-op is often the only way that many pharmacies can compete. The courts generally regard co-ops favorably because they usually result in lower prices for consumers. In fact, co-ops received an endorsement from the U.S. Supreme Court in *Northwest Wholesale Stationers, Inc. v. Pacific Stationery and Printing Co.*, 472 U.S. 284 (1985), when the court noted that "cooperative arrangements would seem to be designed to increase economic efficiency and render markets more, rather than less, competitive" (472 U.S. at 295–296).

Although the courts will generally approve of the procompetitive nature of purchasing cooperatives, co-ops must be alert to potential antitrust problems. In Northwest, the Court was quick to point out that, if a cooperative has market power or exclusive access to an element—essential to effective competition, the effect could be anticompetitive. Thus, a co-op could violate the Sherman Antitrust Act if it expelled a member to prevent the member from competing with the other co-op members and that member had no access to another purchasing cooperative. Also, problems could arise if a purchasing cooperative that represented a significant market share for competing sellers exclusively contracted with a seller. Similarly, co-ops with market power should be cautious about refusing to purchase particular products or refusing to do business with particular sellers because these activities could be construed as boycotts. In most markets, however, a co-op does not have the type of market power necessary to present anticompetitive problems.

Efforts to Influence Government Action

Individual and collective efforts to influence government action are immune from antitrust liability. This immunity is called the Noerr-Pennington doctrine, a name taken from the two U.S. Supreme Court decisions that created the doctrine (*Eastern Railroad Presidents Conference v. Noerr Motor Freight*, 365 U.S. 127 (1961), and *United Mine Workers v. Pennington*, 381 U.S. 657 (1965)). Based on the First Amendment, the doctrine protects efforts to induce legislative, judicial, or administrative action. Under the doctrine, pharmacists and pharmacy organizations, for example, can collectively lobby a state legislature or state Medicaid agency to convince it to offer a higher dispensing fee for Medicaid prescriptions.

THE ROBINSON-PATMAN ACT

In 1936, Congress passed the Robinson-Patman Act (15 U.S.C. § 13), which makes it unlawful for sellers to discriminate in price between purchasers of like products when the effect of the discrimination may substantially injure competition, unless the discrimination is cost justified. Savings to the manufacturer through economies of manufacture, sale, or delivery (e.g., large-quantity purchases) may justify such a price difference between buyers. An injured competitor has a cause for action against both the seller who discriminated and the buyer who knowingly purchased the products at the discriminatory price. The act was passed in an effort to protect independently owned grocery stores against unfair purchasing practices by chain operations.

Pharmaceutical manufacturers have long sold their pharmaceutical products at different prices to different buyers (often termed preferential or differential pricing). Hospitals, HMOs, and other institutional buyers have traditionally purchased pharmaceuticals at much lower prices than have independent and chain pharmacies, often because of strong buying co-ops, nonprofit status, and restrictive formularies. The legality of manufacturer pricing practices falls under the Robinson-Patman Act.

Competing Buyers and Injury to Competition

The Robinson–Patman Act applies only if the price discrimination occurs between competing buyers; otherwise, there can be no injury to competition. For example, if pharmacy X in Chicago receives a much better price for drugs than does pharmacy Y in Chicago for the same drugs with no cost justification, pharmacy Y has no cause of action unless X and Y are competitors. If the two pharmacies are not in the same trade area, there is no injury to competition.

Similarly, a community pharmacy that pays more for drugs than a nearby hospital pays for the same drugs that it purchases for inpatient use has no cause of action against the hospital because it does not compete with the hospital for inpatients. If the hospital were to dispense these drugs to nonpatients, however, the situation could be different. Buyers performing different functional activities cannot be competitors; thus, a wholesaler may legally obtain lower prices from a manufacturer than a retailer because the wholesaler and retailer do not compete.

Proving injury to competition is not easy. A plaintiff must show that the discriminatory prices received by the competitor caused the plaintiff to suffer injury in the form of diverted sales and declining profits, usually because the competitor is able to offer lower prices to customers. The plaintiff can demonstrate injury by introducing into evidence the financial records of both the plaintiff and the competitor and manufacturer. It also is admissible to have witnesses testify that they ceased shopping at the plaintiff's pharmacy and began shopping at the defendant's pharmacy because of the lower prices offered by the competitor.

Nonprofit Institutions Act

In 1938, Congress established a major exemption to the Robinson–Patman Act, called the Nonprofit Institutions Act. This act (15 U.S.C. § 13(c)) exempts nonprofit schools, colleges, universities, public libraries, churches, and charitable institutions from the Robinson–Patman Act when the purchases are for their "own use."

"Own Use" Doctrine

In the landmark case of *Abbott Laboratories v. Portland Retail Druggists Association, Inc.*, 425 U.S. 1 (1976), the U.S. Supreme Court defined the "own use" doctrine and listed permissible and impermissible activities by a nonprofit hospital pharmacy under the doctrine. The Portland Retail Druggists Association brought the lawsuit against 12 drug manufacturers on the basis that the manufacturers sold their products to the nonprofit hospitals in the area at prices lower than those at which they sold their products to member pharmacies, and that the hospitals then dispensed those drug products in outpatient settings in direct competition with association members, thus violating the Robinson–Patman act. The manufacturers countered the association's arguments by claiming that their sales to the nonprofit hospitals were exempt from the Robinson–Patman Act under the Nonprofit Institutions Act.

In its analysis, the Court noted that the concept of a nonprofit hospital's activity has vastly changed since the Nonprofit Institutions Act was enacted in 1938. Hospitals have assumed a larger community role and have become centers for the delivery of health care. In light of this development, the Court stated that the exemption under the Nonprofit Institutions Act should not be expanded to whatever venture the hospital chooses but should instead be limited. Defining "own use" in this context, the Court stated that "own use" is "what reasonably may be regarded as use by the hospital in the sense that such use is a part of and promotes the hospital's intended institutional operation in the care of persons who are its patients" (425 U.S. at 14).

The Court then scrutinized various activities by a hospital and found permissible activities under the "own use" doctrine to include the sale of drugs to

- Inpatients, emergency room patients, and outpatients (defined as patients, other than inpatients or emergency room patients, who receive treatment or consultation on the premises) for use on hospital premises
- Inpatients or emergency room patients on discharge and for personal use away from the premises
- Outpatients for personal use away from the premises
- Hospital employees and their dependents, students at the hospital and their dependents, and medical staff of the hospital and their dependents, all for their own personal use

Regarding the listing of take-home prescriptions as a permissible activity, the Court held that the prescription must be for a "limited and reasonable time, as a continuation of, or supplement to, the treatment that was administered at the hospital" (425 U.S. at 15).

Impermissible activities include the sale of these drugs to

- Former patients obtaining refills
- Medical staff for resale in their practice
- Walk-in customers who have no connection with the hospital

To apply the "own use" doctrine to walk-in patients, remarked the Court, "would make the commercially advantaged hospital pharmacy just another community drug store open to all comers for prescription services and devastatingly positioned with respect to competing commercial pharmacies."

The defendants contended that the task of distinguishing exempt from nonexempt dispensations would require a burdensome segregation of drugs and accounting. The Court believed that their concern was overstated, finding at least two alternatives available. First, the hospital pharmacy need not engage in any impermissible activity. Second, the hospital pharmacy could establish a recordkeeping procedure that segregates the exempt use from the nonexempt use. The Court also noted that manufacturers may rely on certifications from their hospital customers that the hospitals are dispensing the products appropriately, but the manufacturers must assume the burden of obtaining the certifications.

When a hospital engages in an impermissible activity, it has not necessarily violated the Robinson-Patman Act. The hospital has simply lost its "own use" exemption and can now be scrutinized under the act. A plaintiff must still establish that competitive injury occurred.

Aftermath of the *Portland* Decision

The *Portland* decision was followed by *Jefferson County Pharmaceutical Association, Inc. v. Abbott Laboratories*, 460 U.S. 150 (1983). In *Jefferson County*, the U.S. Supreme Court held that the sale of pharmaceutical products to state and local government hospitals for resale in competition with community pharmacies is not exempt from the Robinson-Patman Act. This decision, although analogous to *Portland*, did not involve the Nonprofit Institutions Act. In *Jefferson County*, the Court stated that dispensations pursuant to traditional government functions would be exempt, but failed to define what constitutes traditional government functions.

In *De Modena v. Kaiser Foundation Health Plan, Inc.*, 743 F.2d 1388 (9th Cir. 1984), which did involve the Nonprofit Institutions Act, the court found that the HMO is a charitable nonprofit institution under the act, that sales to its enrollees constituted "own use," and, thus, that the sales are exempt from the Robinson-Patman Act. Critics of *De Modena* argue that the decision ignores the reality that HMOs such as Kaiser compete directly with community pharmacies that are members of other managed health care plans. Allowing Kaiser to receive preferential drug prices allows the HMO to offer enrollees lower prices and premiums than community pharmacies can offer, thus enticing patients to enroll in Kaiser.

The *Portland* and *De Modena* decisions leave unanswered several important questions about the scope of the "own use" doctrine. For example, "At what point in time does the dispensation of products by a hospital to a home health care patient who was an inpatient of the hospital exceed the 'own use' doctrine? What is a reasonable amount for a take-home medication, especially because some hospitals supply a patient with antibiotics and other medications be administered parenterally over a period of several months?" Courts will likely be called on to answer these questions in the future.

Meeting Competition Defense

For both the seller and the buyer, a defense to an alleged violation of the Robinson-Patman Act is the meeting competition provision in the act. Under this clause, price discrimination is justified if the price is established in good faith to meet the equally low price of a competitor. For example, manufacturer X and manufacturer Y each sell ibuprofen. Manufacturer X in good faith believes that manufacturer Y is going to offer ibuprofen to hospital A for $20 per bottle. Because hospital A is a large account that X does not wish to lose, X offers its ibuprofen for $20, even though it was originally going to set its price at $30. In fact, Y sets its price at $30 and X receives the contract. Meanwhile, X continues to sell its ibuprofen to hospital A's competitor hospitals for $30. Regardless that the transaction may result in competitive injury to the other hospitals, X and A have a legal defense, assuming the transaction was in good faith.

Brand-Name Prescription Drugs Antitrust Litigation

Although chain pharmacies and independent pharmacies through purchasing cooperatives have been able to negotiate low prices for generic drugs, they have had little success securing lower prices for brand-name drugs. On the other hand, manufacturers commonly negotiate the price of brand-name drugs with hospital pharmacies, HMOs, mail-order pharmacies, and others. The manufacturers contend they must offer discounts to these buyers because they utilize restrictive formularies and can determine which drugs they will prescribe and dispense. These buyers have the power to exclude a manufacturer's product if they do not receive favorable prices. Retail pharmacies, argue the manufacturers, do not have this power and do not affect market share (meaning they cannot increase or decrease the amount of product sold). Thus, there is no reason to negotiate with them.

After years and years of complaining about this situation, thousands of independent and chain pharmacies launched several class action lawsuits across the country in the early 1990s against most of the brand-name drug manufacturers, contending violations of both the Sherman and Robinson-Patman Acts. Several of the lawsuits were consolidated and proceeded on the basis that the manufacturers conspired to refuse to make lower prices available to retail pharmacies. The manufacturers asked for summary judgment but were denied (*In re Brand Name Prescription Drugs Antitrust Litigation*, April 14,

1996, WL 167350 (N.D.Ill.)). As a result, several manufacturers offered to settle and the settlement was accepted by the court (*In re Brand Name Prescription Drugs Antitrust Litigation*, June 24, 1996, WL 351180 (N.D.Ill.)).

Several other pharmacies refused the settlement and proceeded forward, attempting to prove a conspiracy on the part of the manufacturers. The court, however, found the pharmacies' evidence of a conspiracy inconclusive and awarded summary judgment for the manufacturers (*In re Brand Name Prescription Drugs Antitrust Litigation*, Feb. 10, 2000, WL 204064 (N.D.Ill.)). This decision has not ended the legal actions, however. Many pharmacy plaintiffs have continued litigation, on the basis of both the Robinson-Patman Act and the Sherman Antitrust Act (*In re Brand Name Prescription Drugs Antitrust Litigation*, 264 F.Supp.2d 1372 (N.D.Ill. 2003)).

MISCELLANEOUS FEDERAL LAWS RELATED TO PHARMACY PRACTICE

340B DRUGS

In 1992, section 602 of the Veterans Health Care Act (P.L. 102-585) enacted section 340B of the Public Health Service Act, requiring that drug manufacturers provide outpatient drugs at special reduced prices to designated covered entities serving underserved and uninsured populations. This became known as the 340B program. Covered entities entitled to participate in the 340B program include certain federally qualified health centers (such as Migrant Health Centers, Health Care for the Homeless, Office of Tribal Programs, or urban Indian organizations); family planning projects; state-operated AIDS Drug Assistance Programs and similar types of clinics, facilities and hospitals; and most recently children's hospitals (74 Fed. Reg. 45206, Sept. 1, 2009). A covered entity may contract directly with a manufacturer or wholesaler and receive 340B prices.

Many covered entities, however, do not wish to inventory and dispense drugs and may instead contract with a pharmacy to inventory and dispense the drugs. Under the contract with the pharmacy, the covered entity owns the inventory, but the drugs are delivered directly to the pharmacy. Pursuant to prescription, the pharmacy dispenses the drugs to beneficiaries of the covered entity and receives a dispensing fee. Pharmacies do not need to maintain a separate physical inventory of the 340B drugs, since inventories can be separated virtually by means of software management. Federal law makes it illegal for the covered entity or pharmacy to dispense or sell a 340B drug other than to a 340B beneficiary. Some states have added that doing so constitutes unprofessional conduct.

THE PATIENT SAFETY AND QUALITY IMPROVEMENT ACT OF 2005 (PSQIA)

In 1999 the Institute of Medicine released the results of two studies indicating that tens of thousands of Americans die each year from preventable medical errors. A subsequent IOM report in 2006 indicated that 1.5 million preventable adverse drug events occur each year. These reports combined with several others over the past few years have focused public concern on adverse medical and drug related events and have attracted the attention of Congress. Congress recognizes that incident reporting systems that include documenting and investigating errors are critical to the quality improvement of health care systems and to improving patient safety. Congress is also aware that health care providers historically have been reluctant to report and record medical and drug errors because of fear of civil liability, damage to reputation, and punitive actions by employers. As a result, Congress passed the Patient Safety and Quality Improvement Act of 2005 (PSQIA) (P.L. 109-424; regulations at 73 Fed. Reg. 70732, Nov. 2008).

PSQIA, also known as the Patient Safety Act, creates a voluntary program through which health care providers, including pharmacies, can share information related to patient safety events (called patient safety work product (PSWP)), with patient safety organizations (PSOs). Under the act, PSWP is privileged and confidential and not discoverable by plaintiff's attorneys. The hope is that the PSOs, by gathering and analyzing the data submitted to them, will be able to identify patterns of failures and propose measures to eliminate patient safety risks. Every PSO must be certified by HHS, and the regulations detail what types of organizations can become a certified PSO and the requirements that they must meet. A pharmacy with its own quality improvement program would not be considered a PSO unless it became certified with HHS.

Federal Trade Commission "Red Flag Rules"

In November 2007 the FTC issued a final rule (72 Fed. Reg. 63718) effective November 1, 2009, to implement a federal law passed in 2003 called the Fair and Accurate Credit Transactions Act. The law and the regulations require financial institutions and creditors to develop prevention programs that identify relevant patterns, practices, and specific activities that are "red flags" for identity theft. The law and regulations include a pharmacy if it extends credit or bills, for example billing for medication therapy management and long-term care pharmacy consulting fees. Accepting credit cards does not make a business a creditor. The regulations do not require a particular compliance program and each pharmacy is free to develop its own to educate consumers and provide training for employees regarding identity theft. The FTC provides guidance documents at its website (http://www.ftc.gov). Some red flags the FTC has listed include suspicious identification documents presented by consumers; information from the consumer that does not match what the provider has on file; suspicious activity such as mail returned as undeliverable even though the patient shows up; and notices from victims of identity theft, law enforcement, or insurers suggesting possible identity theft. Pending legislation in Congress would exempt health care practices, including pharmacies, with fewer than 20 employees.

Flexible Spending and Health Savings Account Debit Cards

Many employers offer health insurance plans allowing employees to withhold a certain amount of their salary pretax to pay for health care–related expenses. These funds are placed into a Flexible Spending Account (FSA) or into a Health Savings Account (HSA). When the employee makes a purchase of a qualified health care–related product or service the employee is reimbursed from the account. To get reimbursed, the employee can submit receipts to the health plan or present a debit card to the health care provider that enables point-of-sale deductions from the employee's FSA or HSA. Pharmacies that accept these debit card transactions for FSAs or HSAs must use an inventory information approval system (IIAS). Pharmacies must receive certification, in part to ensure that they can identify products that are qualified for the medical expense deduction. As of January 1, 2011, distributions from an FSA will only be allowed for OTC drugs if they are sold pursuant to a prescription.

© Stockbyte/Thinkstock

STUDY SCENARIOS AND QUESTIONS

1. The State Pharmaceutical Association is having its annual meeting. Many pharmacists are concerned about a major prescription drug benefit plan that has announced it will now significantly lower its reimbursement to pharmacies from AWP less 15 percent to AWP less 25 percent, and lower the dispensing fee to $1.25 from $2.50. Some pharmacists at the meeting are talking about the need to develop revenue sources other than from dispensing the drug. This would include an array of pharmacist care services, including disease state management. The pharmacists propose to bill patients directly for these services because, as they see it, the days of survival based upon dispensing prescriptions appear to be over. At a morning session three speakers, all of whom are members of the association, described innovative practices in which they provide services not associated with the distribution of the drug product, and how they are paid for those services. They urged the pharmacists present to engage in these services. They also added that the pharmacists should look closely at the third-party contract being currently proposed and whether they can profit if they accept it. The executive director of the association is concerned that some members of the organization might decide to reject the contract, giving the appearance that the pharmacists are working in concert to reject or boycott the contract. At the end of the morning session he cautions everyone attending not to discuss with each other the terms of the contract. He says, "If you even mention the contract and its terms to each other in the bathroom, that is a violation of the antitrust laws."

   a. Is the executive director correct in his interpretation of antitrust law? Why or why not? Have the speakers violated the law by mentioning the contract?

   b. Is it a violation of antitrust law for the speakers to discuss the pharmacist care services they provide and to tell the pharmacist audience how much they charge for those services? Why or why not?

   c. If a competitor calls your pharmacy and asks you to price a prescription, and you do so, would it be a violation of antitrust law if that person turned out to be a competitor of yours who used the information to price her prescription the same as you? Why or why not?

2. Dyer Chain Drugs owns 500 pharmacies. Dyer figures that because of its size it should be able to negotiate good prices from suppliers on drug products. Dyer, however, finds that most of the companies that make single source drugs still on patent refuse to negotiate. Generic drug manufacturers are willing to negotiate, however. One generic manufacturer, Genericide, informs Dyer that if the chain agrees to use all its drug products exclusively, it will give Dyer a 50 percent better price than it currently gives any of Dyer's competitors. Dyer agrees and signs a 2-year contract with Genericide.

   a. Explain whether it is legal for the single source drug manufacturers to refuse to negotiate with Dyer. Under what circumstances would these manufacturers be interested in negotiating with Dyer?

   b. Explain whether it is legal for Genericide to offer Dyer a 50 percent better price than it offers to competitors.

   c. Is the exclusive contract Dyer signs with Genericide to use all of its products and use only its products lawful? Why or why not?

REFERENCES

Centers for Medicare & Medicaid Services: http://www.cms.hhs.gov

U.S. Department of Health and Human Services, Office for Civil Rights—HIPAA: http://www.hhs.gov/ocr/hipaa

BIBLIOGRAPHY

Abood, R. OBRA '90: Implementation and enforcement. *U.S. Pharmacist* 18, Supp. (1993): 1–16.

American Pharmaceutical Association. *Survey of State Compliance with OBRA '90's Patient Counseling Law.* Washington, DC: Author, 1993.

American Pharmacists Association. Legislative and Regulatory Updates. Available at: http://www.pharmacist.com

American Society for Pharmacy Law. Available at: http://www.aspl.org

Bishop, S. K., and S. C. Winckler. Implementing HIPAA privacy regulations in pharmacy practice. *Journal of the American Pharmaceutical Association* 42, no. 6 (2002): 836–846.

Brushwood, D., et al. OBRA '90: What it means to your practice. *U.S. Pharmacist* 17, Suppl. (1992): 1–12.

Curtis, F. R., P. Lettrich, and K. A. Fairman. What is the price benchmark to replace average wholesale price (AWP)? *Journal of Managed Care Pharmacy* 16, no. 7 (2010): 492–501.

Department of Health and Human Services, Office of Inspector General. Comparison of Medicaid federal upper limit amounts to average manufacturer prices, June 2005. Available at: http://oig.hhs.gov/oei/reports/oei-03-05-00110.pdf

Department of Health and Human Services, Office of Inspector General. Replacing average wholesale price: Medicaid drug payment policy, July 2011. Available at: http://oig.hhs.gov/oei/reports/oei-03-11-00060.asp

Hatoum, H., et al. OBRA '90: Patient counseling—enhancing patient outcomes. *U.S. Pharmacist* 18, Suppl., (1993): 1–12.

Holleran, M. The Pharmaceutical Access and Prudent Purchasing Act of 1990: Federal law shifts the duty to warn from the physician to the pharmacist. *Akron Law Review* 26 (1993): 77.

Huang, S. The Omnibus Reconciliation Act of 1990: Redefining pharmacists' legal responsibilities. *American Journal of Law and Medicine* 24 (1998): 417–442.

National Community Pharmacists Association. *Governmental Affairs/Legal Proceedings.* Available at: http://www.ncpanet.org

Palumbo, F. Drug use review under OBRA '90. *U.S. Pharmacist* 18, Suppl. (1993): 1–12.

© Junial Enterprises/ShutterStock, Inc.

CASE STUDIES

CASE 6-1   *American Pharmaceutical Association v. Weinberger*, 377 F. Supp. 824 (D.D.C. 1974)

Issue

Whether the FDA has the authority to restrict the distribution of pharmaceutical products to hospital pharmacies, and prevent their distribution through community pharmacies for the purpose of preventing drug diversion.

Overview

Pharmacists have for years coped with the reality that many of the drugs they dispense are both useful as medications and also dangerous substances that are subject to abuse. Regulatory agencies have attempted to limit the diversion of medicinally useful controlled substances so they always will be kept within the narrow confines of the health care system and not used for illegal purposes. Caught at the interface of health care regulation and drug abuse regulation, pharmacists have at times been subject to new rules that stretch the traditional understanding of the role of law. In this case, a new approach to regulation is being attempted—the restriction of the drug methadone to some hospital pharmacies only. This is a novel approach to regulation because traditionally it has not been considered appropriate for federal regulatory authorities to decide what pharmacies may dispense a drug, although they may impose restrictions on how the drug is to be dispensed from any pharmacy that dispenses it.

Challenging this restriction, the professional society for pharmacists questioned whether the FDA had legal authority to restrict drug distribution in this way. The agency attempted to justify this novel approach by referring to traditional authority, and the result was not supportive of the agency's action.

As you read this case, ask yourself whether there might be good reasons to restrict drug distribution to particular pharmacies—but also ask yourself whether there is legal precedent for such restrictions. No matter how good an idea might be (and this is in no way an assertion that restricted distribution is a good idea), there must be legal authority for implementation of the idea. The FDA is restricted in what it does by the statutes it enforces. Drug regulation, the authorized activity of the agency, cannot be extended to direct regulation of practice, even if public policy would suggest that such an extension might be a positive move to protect the public health. The protection of the public health through the regulation of professional practice is a matter of state regulation.

The court opinion began by describing the controversy at issue:

> This is an action for judicial review of a regulation of the Food and Drug Administration (FDA) which restricts the distribution of methadone to certain specified outlets as set forth in the regulation. In effect, it prohibits virtually all licensed pharmacies from dispensing this drug when lawfully prescribed by a physician, despite the fact that methadone was invented and was first used as a safe, useful, and effective agent in the treatment of severe pain and for antitussive purposes. Decision is not made easier by the fact that in recent years methadone has become a widely known maintenance agent in the treatment of heroin addicts and there is evidence of serious abuses in the distribution of this drug. In their efforts to control improper distribution of methadone, there are strong public policy arguments on the side of defendants.

With this language, the court notes the difficulty of resolving a conflict on the basis of the traditional dual challenges for regulators (i.e., to ensure availability of useful medications for those who would suffer from being denied them and to prevent inappropriate access to abusable drugs by those who would use them inappropriately). The court then gets to the heart of the matter.

> The challenged regulation, while ruling out most so-called community pharmacies in the dispensing of methadone for any purpose, still permits approved hospital pharmacies to dispense methadone for analgesic and antitussive purposes. Stripped of the rhetoric, which abounds in the papers before us, this appears to be the basis of plaintiffs' complaint. Whether the FDA has the authority to enact the challenged regulation depends on the interplay and connection between two complementary but distinct statutes, the Food, Drug and Cosmetic Act of 1938 and the Comprehensive Drug Abuse Prevention and Control Act of 1970 and the respective roles assigned by Congress to the agencies which administer these Acts.

After thoroughly discussing the purpose of the FDCA, as well as the purpose of the Comprehensive Drug Abuse Prevention and Control Act (commonly known as the CSA), the court issued its ruling based on congressional intent.

> The Court concludes that Congress intended to create two complementary institutional checks on the production and marketing of new drugs. At the production or pre-marketing stage, the FDA is given the primary responsibility in determining which new drugs should be permitted to enter the flow of commerce. The Commissioner must approve or deny every NDA, or he may determine that a particular new drug qualifies for IND status in order to permit additional experimentation. When an IND exemption is approved, the Commissioner may, of course, severely restrict the distribution of the exempted drug to bona fide researchers and clinicians. But once a drug is cleared for marketing by way of a NDA-approval, for whatever uses the Commissioner deems appropriate, the question of permissible distribution of the drug,

when that drug is a controlled substance, is one clearly within the jurisdiction of the Justice Department. The diversion of the particular drug to a use not approved by the Commissioner would be grounds for revocation of the offending distributor's registration. FDA attempts to accomplish peremptorily by way of its challenged regulation, that which could only be accomplished, according to the scheme of the Controlled Substances Act, by way of show-cause proceedings initiated by the Attorney General, i.e., revoking the authority of otherwise duly-registered distributors with respect to the drug methadone. To allow the challenged portions of the methadone regulations to stand, therefore, would be to abrogate the collective judgment of Congress with regard to the appropriate means of controlling unlawful drug diversion.

Notes on *American Pharmaceutical Association v. Weinberger*

1. In this case, the court relies heavily on its interpretation of the enabling legislation for the FDA and not at all on questioning the advisability of that legislation. Whether it is a good or bad thing to restrict drug distribution to some small group of pharmacies is a matter for the U.S. Congress to resolve. It would be unlikely that the Congress would enact legislation to authorize such restrictions because wholesale restrictions of pharmacy practice are not a matter with which the Congress usually involves itself. Congress enables the FDA to regulate drug products but not to regulate the practice of pharmacy.

2. The authority the FDA has been granted to regulate drugs is pretty much an all-or-nothing type of authority. If the agency believes that a product is unsafe, the agency must withdraw or withhold approval of the NDA for that product. Of course, the agency may require labeling that informs users of the product that certain risks exist, but restricted distribution is too direct a control of risk. Product users, including health care professionals and patients, are free to make their own decisions about product use on the basis of product labeling. This absence of authority to make restrictions on distribution does not apply during the IND phase of drug distribution. The IND is an exemption from the prohibition on distribution of an unapproved new drug in interstate commerce. During the clinical trial phases of drug use, under an IND exemption, the FDA is fully authorized to restrict distribution to particular institutions. The agency routinely does make such restrictions.

3. The U.S. Attorney General, acting to enforce rules of the DEA, could restrict distribution of controlled substances by determining, on the basis of the evidence, that a particular pharmacy had violated the law and no longer deserved to be permitted to distribute controlled substances. However, according to this case, a general determination that any community pharmacy could divert controlled substances does not serve as adequate foundation for a conclusion that any particular pharmacy would divert controlled substances. Under the CSA, the DEA is limited to enforcement of the law after an actual violation of the law. Restricted distribution, based on the hypothetical possibility that the law might be broken, does not support restricted distribution.

CASE 6-2 | *Horner v. Spalitto*, 1 S.W.3d 519 (Mo. App. 1999)

Issue

Whether the OBRA '90 standards for drug use review and patient counseling are the standard of care for pharmacists in a professional malpractice case.

Overview

When OBRA '90 was passed by the U.S. Congress, expanding the standards of practice for pharmacists to include screening of prescriptions for potential problems and an offer to discuss medications with patients, a trend toward recognition of a standard in this area was already well underway. However, it was unclear whether the OBRA '90 rules would be adopted by state courts as the standard of practice for pharmacists. If that were to occur, it would bring to the process of standards setting a uniformity that had previously not existed. It would show that times had changed and that pharmacy practice standards had changed with the times.

Yet, there was concern among some that the legal standards applicable to pharmacists not lead the profession, but instead that they follow advances in practice. It might be considered unfair to compare pharmacists with a standard that just recently was adopted and that they did not know existed when they provided products and services to their patients. During the early 1990s, many cases brought against pharmacists alleging harm caused by the failure to do DUR or by the failure to counsel were based on incidents that occurred before the enactment of OBRA '90, and there was understandable reluctance to apply to these cases a set of rules that did not even exist when the incident occurred.

As you read this case, note the discussion of the earlier case that the court refers to as the *Kampe* case (*Kampe v. Howard Stark Professional Pharmacy, Inc.*, 841 S.W.2d 233 (Mo. App.1992)). In the *Kampe* case, the court had decided that the defendant pharmacist had no responsibility to the patient other than to accurately process a prescription order, no matter how inappropriate that order might be and no matter how easily the pharmacist might have been able to remedy the inappropriateness of it. Pay attention to the court's criticism of the earlier *Kampe* case, and notice how the federally inspired OBRA '90 standards are used to support the adoption of a new approach to pharmacist responsibility. Ask yourself whether the change in law documented in this case was because of the federal standard, or whether the change would have occurred even if the federal standard had not been established.

The court opinion began by describing the events that led to the lawsuit:

> This case requires us to revisit the issue of what conduct is required of a pharmacist in fulfilling his professional duties. The pharmacist in this case, Peter Spalitto, was an employee and son of a pharmacy owner, Anthony Spalitto, and filled two prescriptions for Franklin Horner 6 days before Horner died of an apparent drug overdose. One of the prescriptions prescribed a strong hypnotic drug at a rate of three times the normal dose.

> Horner's children and mother sued Anthony Spalitto for wrongfully causing Horner's death by acting through his employees and agents to fill prescriptions negligently at Spalitto's pharmacy in Kansas City. The circuit court granted judgment for Spalitto on the ground that Peter Spalitto's only obligation was to fill the prescriptions accurately, which Horner's family concedes that he did.

> Peter Spalitto was the pharmacist on duty at Anthony Spalitto's pharmacy on September 21, 1994, and filled two prescriptions presented by Horner. One of them was for 50, 750 mg doses of Placidyl, a strong hypnotic drug. The prescribing physician instructed on the prescription that Horner was to take one dose every 8 hours. The other was for 50, 10 mg doses of Diazepam, a central nervous system depressant, and it instructed Horner to take one dose every 8 hours. Before filling the prescriptions, Spalitto consulted *Facts and Comparisons*, an authoritative pharmacy manual, which indicated that the normal dose for Placidyl was one 500 mg dose or one 750 mg dose before bedtime. The manual also warned that the drug's effects were enhanced when it was combined with other central nervous system drugs, such as Diazepam.

Concerned about the physician's ordering such a high dose of Placidyl, Peter Spalitto telephoned the prescribing doctor's office. He said that someone in the physician's office told him that the prescription was "okay" because Horner "needed to be sedated throughout the day." Peter Spalitto filled the two prescriptions.

Six days later, on September 27, 1994, Franklin Horner was found dead. Bonita J. Peterson, MD, opined after an autopsy "that [Horner's] death resulted from adverse effects of multiple medications (drugs), especially Placidyl (etchlorvynol), which was near the toxic range."

The court then considered previous case law, criticizing the *Kampe* case that had been decided several years before by the same court. Because the *Kampe* case had been decided by the same appellate court as was considering this case, it was not binding precedent, and the court was free to rule that changed circumstances could lead to changed legal responsibilities.

Kampe ruled that a pharmacist fulfills his professional duties when he accurately fills a prescription—that he has no duty to warn or to monitor. This miscomprehended duty. Duty is an obligation imposed by law to conform to a standard of conduct toward another to protect others against unreasonable, foreseeable risks. In other words, Anthony Spalitto's duty was to exercise the care and prudence that a reasonably careful and prudent pharmacist would exercise in the same or similar circumstances—that is, his duty was to endeavor to minimize the risks of harm to Horner and others which a reasonably careful and prudent pharmacist would foresee.

Kampe wrongly held that, as a matter of law, a pharmacist's duty will never extend beyond accurately filling a prescription. This may be a pharmacist's only duty in particular cases, but in other cases, a pharmacist's education and expertise will require that he or she do more to help protect their patrons from risks which pharmacists can reasonably foresee. We must leave to a fact-finder what this duty requires of a pharmacist in a particular case. We can say at this point only that a pharmacist, as is the case with every other professional, must exercise the care and prudence which a reasonably careful and prudent pharmacist would exercise.

To hold as *Kampe* did would denigrate the expertise which a pharmacist's education provides concerning drugs and their therapeutic use. The *Kampe* holding also failed to comprehend the role a pharmacist must play in making the valuable, but highly dangerous, service of drug therapy as safe and reliable as it can be.

The court then turned to the OBRA '90 mandate as a justification for imposing new rules for pharmacist liability. The court cited the state regulation in Missouri that had been adopted for pharmacists on the basis of the federal mandate of OBRA '90.

In 1990, the federal government enacted the Omnibus Budget Reconciliation Act which required states to establish standards for pharmacist counseling of pharmacy customers or their caregivers. In fulfillment of that mandate, the Board of Pharmacy promulgated a regulation, which says:

(1) Upon receipt of a prescription drug order and following review of the available patient information, a pharmacist or his/her designee shall personally offer to discuss matters which will enhance or optimize drug therapy with each patient or caregiver of each patient. Counseling shall be conducted by the pharmacist or pharmacy extern under the pharmacist's immediate supervision to allow the patient to safely and appropriately utilize the medication so that maximum therapeutic outcomes can be obtained. . . . The elements of counseling shall include matters which the pharmacist deems significant in the exercise of his/her professional judgment and is consistent with applicable state laws.

(2) Pharmacies shall maintain appropriate patient information to facilitate counseling. This may include, but shall not be limited to, the patient's name, address, telephone number, age, gender, clinical information, disease states, allergies, and a listing of other drugs prescribed.

Under this regulation, a pharmacist is obligated to offer to discuss with each customer or their caregiver information about the safe and appropriate use of the medication based on the pharmacist's review of available patient information.

The regulation was not the only reason for adopting a new approach to pharmacists' legal responsibilities. The court also cited policy reasons in support of the change.

Pharmacists have the training and skills to recognize when a prescription dose is outside a normal range. They are in the best position to contact the prescribing physician, to alert the physician about the dose and any contraindications relating to other prescriptions the customer may be taking as identified by the pharmacy records, and to verify that the physician intended such a dose for a particular patient. We do not perceive that this type of risk management unduly interferes with the physician-patient relationship. Instead, it should increase the overall quality of health care. The physician still is responsible for assessing what medication is appropriate for a patient's condition, but the pharmacist may be in the best position to determine how the medication should be taken to maximize the therapeutic benefit to that patient, to communicate that information to the customer or his physician, and to answer any of the customer's questions regarding consumption of the medication.

We reject the suggestion in *Kampe* that the only functions which a pharmacist must perform to fulfill his duty is to dispense drugs according to a physician's prescription.

The court found for the plaintiff, reversing the lower court's decision and remanding to the lower court for further proceedings.

Notes on *Horner v. Spalitto*

1. Although state law determines pharmacist responsibilities under malpractice liability, the standard of care to which pharmacists are held may be influenced by federal mandates. In this case, the court referred to the federal mandate of OBRA '90 as a basis for rejecting the rationale from previous case law. The previous ruling from the *Kampe* case had not acknowledged the expanded responsibilities of pharmacists. By recognizing the influence of OBRA '90, the court used that federal policy to justify changing the applicable standard of care for pharmacists under state law.

2. This case is the first state case to recognize that rules adopted by state regulatory agencies, under the OBRA '90 mandate, expand expectations of pharmacists who have been alleged to have caused harm to patients by failing to prevent problems with drug therapy. Before this case, no state court had fully acknowledged the influence of the OBRA '90 standards. Whether this approach of using the OBRA '90 standards as the basis of increased expectations for pharmacists becomes a firm trend remains to be seen. State courts considering malpractice claims against pharmacists are not obligated to recognize standards that are derived from federal law, but they may do so if they wish.

3. In this case, the component of the OBRA '90 standards that was used to recognize an expanded pharmacist standard of care was the "offer to discuss" requirement. Another requirement of OBRA '90, which could be even more litigation significant, is the requirement that pharmacists detect and resolve potential problems with drug therapy before dispensing medications to patients. This "ProDUR"

responsibility of the pharmacist cannot be waived by the patient, thus it is mandatory of pharmacists if it has been included in state law.

CASE 6-3	*Van Iperen v. Van Bramer*, 392 N.W.2d 480 (Iowa 1986)

Issue

Whether the accreditation standards of the Joint Commission on Accreditation of Hospitals (JCAH; now the Joint Commission on Accreditation of Healthcare Organizations [Joint Commission]) establish a standard of care for hospital pharmacy services.

Overview

To ensure that the provision of care in institutional settings is standardized from one place to another, an organization known as the JCAH was created. This organization developed accreditation standards and permitted hospitals to become accredited by JCAH if the hospitals met the standards. Site visits by inspectors are designed to ensure that what was said to exist on paper does in fact exist in practice. The organization changed its name in the late 1980s to the Joint Commission on Accreditation of Healthcare Organizations (now The Joint Commission) after changes in health care provision caused some services to move out of hospitals and into other institutional settings.

Federal guidelines for reimbursement to health care organizations, under federal programs, generally require either that federal standards be adhered to or that Joint Commission accreditation be acquired by the institution seeking federal reimbursement. Thus, the Joint Commission has become a quasi-legal agency as a result of its standards having been incorporated into federal guidelines. Many hospitals choose Joint Commission accreditation as their ticket to federal program reimbursement, thus the standards of the Joint Commission are federally inspired standards.

As you read this case, reflect on how the Joint Commission standards are proposed for use by the plaintiff. Ask yourself whether the Joint Commission standards are really standards in the sense that the principles they describe are generally recognized as appropriate by all health care providers and the services they require are generally available at all hospitals. Are all standards uniformly agreed to by those who practice in the regulated field? Are some standards actually goals to aspire to rather than uniformly recognized duties?

The court began by describing the nature of the action brought by the plaintiff:

For many years prior to 1981, plaintiff had suffered from Crohn's disease, a chronic illness which results in serious damage to the victim's intestinal tract. In plaintiff's case, the damage was sufficiently serious that all of his large intestine and much of his small intestine had been surgically removed by June 1981. An ileostomy procedure allowed the remaining small intestine to drain into a bag outside the plaintiff's body. A segment of intestine approximately five inches in length remained attached to his rectal cavity. This was not connected to any other body organ and was sutured closed on the interior end.

When plaintiff was admitted to St. Luke's Regional Medical Center on June 1, 1981, an infection had developed in the area where this 5-inch segment of intestine pressed against the bladder wall. An opening or "fistula" in the bladder wall had developed and had contaminated the normally sterile environment within the bladder. Two prior efforts to surgically correct the fistula had been unsuccessful.

At the time of the June hospitalization, plaintiff was attended by defendants Van Bramer and Oei. Dr. Van Bramer, a specialist in internal medicine and a certified diplomat of the American Board of Internal Medicine, was in charge of plaintiff's course of treatment. Dr. Oei is certified in nephrology, a subspecialty of internal medicine relating to kidney disease. He was consulted with regard to a recommended course of drug therapy for plaintiff's bladder infection. Dr. Van Bramer identified two separate ways of dealing with the bladder infection. One alternative was to attempt again to surgically close the fistula. Such surgery involved risks of damage to the bladder wall and permanent sterility. The second alternative involved daily application of a bacteria-killing rectal flush or rinse using a liquid solution of antibiotics injected through the rectal cavity into the 5-inch intestinal segment adjacent to the infected bladder wall. Plaintiff, in consultation with defendant Van Bramer, elected to forgo surgery and engage in the rectal flush program.

A solution of Neomycin and Kanamycin was prepared by defendant Oei as the antibiotic compound to be employed in plaintiff's treatment. This compound was considered by him to be a relatively dilute concentration of those drugs. The solution was prepared by mixing one gram of Neomycin and one gram of Kanamycin with 50 cubic centimeters of saline solution. Twenty to 25 cubic centimeters of this solution was to be administered directly into the area of the fistula.

Commencing on June 18, the prescribed rectal flush solution was administered two or three times daily. Its effect on plaintiff's bladder infection was monitored by Dr. Oei. Urinalysis indicated that the infection subsided after initiation of this treatment. Upon discharge from the hospital on July 2, plaintiff was directed to continue application of the rectal flush solution at home twice daily. Dr. Van Bramer continued to monitor his progress.

The patient continued to be hospitalized on several occasions for the treatment of his underlying condition. Unfortunately, during one of these hospitalizations, an adverse effect from his medication was discovered.

During the October 29 hospitalization, plaintiff complained of ringing in his ears. Dr. Van Bramer believed this was due to the dehydration and electrolyte imbalance. This symptom subsided when plaintiff was given fluids intravenously. On November 14, 1981, plaintiff was hospitalized again for dehydration and electrolyte imbalance. At this time, his hospital record notes that it [has become] apparent that the Kanamycin, Neomycin rectal installations that we are using to sterilize his fistula have gradually affected his hearing. He began having bells and ringings, so we did a hearing test and the high frequencies have dropped off so prior to getting into trouble we are going to stop those.

Although use of the Neomycin and Kanamycin solution was discontinued in accordance with the foregoing directive, plaintiff's hearing loss worsened. By the time of trial, he was unable to discern sound levels below the intensity of a chain saw.

The court reviewed claims made against the physicians for medical malpractice and affirmed verdicts in favor of both physicians, whom the court ruled had not committed malpractice in the care they provided. In effect, the court ruled that the adverse effect the plaintiff suffered was unfortunate but unpreventable by the physicians. This ruling left open the possibility that the adverse effect may have been preventable by the hospital, if it had provided pharmacokinetic monitoring services.

The claim against the hospital alleged that the hospital had not provided a service that it was required to provide under the JCAH standards to which it had agreed to adhere. These standards are technically voluntary standards that a hospital would agree to follow to receive funds under certain federal programs. However, the plaintiff contended that by having agreed to follow the standards, the hospital had elevated the expectations of it and that those expectations would have to be met to avoid malpractice liability.

Plaintiff also contends the trial court erred in directing a verdict in favor of the defendant St. Luke's Regional Medical Center at the conclusion of plaintiff's evidence. It bases this contention on the accreditation standards of the Joint Commission on the Accreditation of Hospitals which require that, within the limits of available resources, a hospital should provide drug monitoring services through its hospital pharmacy which include:

(1) The maintenance of a medication record or drug profile for each patient, which is based on available drug history and current therapy and includes the name, age, and weight of the patient, the current diagnosis(es), the current drug therapy, any drug allergies or sensitivities, and other pertinent information relating to the patient's drug regimen. . .

(2) A review of the patient's drug regimen for any potential interactions, interferences or incompatibilities, prior to dispensing drugs to the patient. Such irregularities must be resolved promptly with the prescribing practitioner, and, when appropriate, with notification of the nursing service and administration.

The plaintiff pointed squarely at the pharmacy department as being the deficient department in the hospital, according to the JCAH accreditation standards.

Plaintiff urges that the hospital's procedures were deficient and not in accordance with its accreditation standards because it had established no formal procedures for implementing the responsibilities of the hospital pharmacy to make independent evaluations of proposed drug therapy and to communicate recommendations to the patient and his doctors.

The court concluded that the JCAH standards were not necessarily the standard of care. This holding was consistent with the rationale of an earlier case, *Menzel v. Morse*, 362 N.W.2d 465 (IA 1985), which had held the accreditation standards to be some evidence of the standard of care but not to be the beginning and ending of the standard of care issue.

We do not believe the scope and application of the written accreditation standards upon which plaintiff relies are sufficiently clear that these documents are self-authenticating with respect to the required standard of care. Although we suggested in *Menzel v. Morse* that hospital accreditation standards provide some evidence of the proper standard of care, the evidence presented in the present case is insufficient, without additional reliable interpretative data, to generate a jury issue on the claim made against the defendant hospital. We hold that the district court did not err in directing a verdict in favor of that defendant.

Notes on *Van Iperen v. Van Bramer*

1. In this case, the court did not say that accreditation standards are irrelevant to the standard of care for malpractice. The court said that Joint Commission accreditation standards are some evidence of the standard of care, but that by themselves, they are not the standard of care. The same could be said of clinical practice guidelines, which have become commonplace in managed care organizations. Clinical practice guidelines for many disease states were developed by the federal Agency for Health Care Policy and Research (now known as the Agency for Healthcare Research and Quality). These clinical practice guidelines have taken on a status similar to that of the Joint Commission accreditation standards; they are some evidence of the malpractice standard of care, but they do not by themselves define the standard of care. Federal agencies can influence professional standards in this way, although they cannot establish professional standards.

2. The court said that the Joint Commission standards were not self-authenticating; that they required additional, reliable interpretive data. The court was concerned that the standards for pharmacy services were not really standards but instead were goals to which to aspire. All professions need aspirations. It would be poor public policy to not encourage standards that would advance a profession, but it would be unfair to hold a profession accountable for the failure to meet standards that were really aspirational and not obligatory.

3. The influence of federal rules on professional standards often comes through conditions of participation. The federal government provides funding for Medicare, Medicaid, and other health care programs. Federal agencies that administer these programs can impose conditions on the receipt of federal funds by health care providers. Although technically health care providers are free to decline participation in the federally funded programs and not meet the standards, often the reality is that such a decision means going out of business.

CASE 6-4   *Harder v. F. C. Clinton, Inc.*, 948 P.2d 298 (Okla. 1997)

Issue

Whether a nursing home could be held liable to a resident for adverse effects caused by the administration to the resident of a drug that had not been ordered for the resident.

Overview

Nursing home residents are among the most vulnerable persons to whom health care services are provided. There is ample documentation of overmedication, undermedication, and mismedication of nursing home residents. For this reason, federal guidelines have been developed to protect nursing home residents from inappropriate drug therapy. Pharmacists are instrumental in the implementation of these regulations at the nursing home. By conducting drug regimen review (DRR) and other important activities, pharmacists help ensure that nursing home residents receive the high-quality care they deserve.

As you read this case, note the allegation that the plaintiff, who was a nursing home resident, had an adverse effect from the administration of a medication that had not been ordered for her. The nursing home claimed no knowledge of how this could have occurred. Ask yourself, as you read this case, how else the resident could have received this medication other than from a nursing home employee in the nursing home. The court uses a legal theory to shift the burden of proof from the nursing home resident to the nursing home, requiring that the nursing home exculpate itself from legal responsibility. The legal theory is known as *res ipsa loquitur* (the thing speaks for itself). In other words, the court says that the administration of an inappropriate medication in a nursing home speaks enough about the care being provided there and the plaintiff need not present extensive evidence of negligence beyond the fact of this inappropriate medication administration. Reflect on the facts of this case and consider what a pharmacist consultant might be able to do to prevent this sort of error from happening in the future. How should a pharmacist consultant document errors of this kind when they occur? How can a pharmacist consultant help ensure the quality of medication use in a facility in which the consultant visits only occasionally and at which the pharmacist consultant has only the power to make recommendations?

The court first described the medication error that led to this lawsuit:

Ethel Kayser [Kayser] was admitted on July 14, 1992, to the Heritage Care Center [Heritage, Center, or nursing home]. On the evening of September 30, 1992, she was transferred to the Clinton Regional Hospital after ingesting an overdose of Tolbutamide, a diabetic medication. There she was diagnosed as having a hypoglycemic coma caused by the lowering of her blood sugar from ingestion of the medication. An intravenous device was inserted in the dorsum area of her right foot to treat the coma. Gangrene later developed in the same foot, which eventually required an above-the-knee amputation.

The court then described the history of the lawsuit, in which the plaintiff had not prevailed because of the refusal of the lower courts to permit the use of the *res ipsa loquitur* theory of liability. Whether the thing speaks for itself is a decision to be made by the judge and jury, but the judge must permit the jury to hear the arguments for this type of liability; otherwise, the jury cannot consider the theory.

Minnie Harder [Harder], Kayser's sister, brought a suit against the nursing home, as Kayser's guardian, for harm caused to Kayser by an overdose of the wrong prescription administered to her while she was in the Center's care and custody. At the close of Harder's case, which followed a *res ipsa loquitur* pattern of proof, the trial court directed a verdict for the nursing home. The trial court ruled that Harder's evidence fell short of establishing a negligence claim because her proof failed to show all the requisite foundational elements for *res ipsa loquitur*. The Court of Civil Appeals affirmed.

The court described how a thing may come to speak for itself, particularly when the thing is a medication error in a nursing home.

Res ipsa loquitur is a pattern of proof which may be followed when an injury is alleged to have been negligently inflicted and the harm is shown not to occur in the usual course of everyday conduct unless a person who controls the instrumentality likely to have produced that harm fails to exercise due care to prevent its occurrence. The purpose of the *res ipsa loquitur* evidentiary rule is to aid a plaintiff in making out a prima facie case of negligence in circumstances when direct proof of why the harm happened is beyond the power or knowledge of the plaintiff. Once the foundation facts for *res ipsa loquitur* are established, negligence may be inferred from the injurious occurrence without the aid of circumstances pointing to the responsible cause.

Jackie Dixon, a licensed practicing nurse (and a medication clerk at the Center), testified that residents' prescription drugs are stored at the nurse's station. She gave a detailed account of the method used for dispensing prescribed medication to the residents. Heritage residents have no access to prescription drugs except when they are administered to them by authorized personnel—a registered or licensed practicing nurse or a certified medication aide. When medication is to be administered, the correct dosage is removed from the storage site and placed in a cart that is pushed down the halls. The nurse (or certified medication aide) removes the medication from its container, places it in a cup, and then serves it to the resident. The cart is kept locked while the nurse or aide is administering the medication. Dr. Hays—Kayser's family physician since 1973 (as well as Heritage's medical director)—testified that the administration of the wrong prescription drug in an amount that would cause harm is below the applicable standard of care.

Janis Raab, the nursing home administrator, testified that Kayser was at the nursing home on September 30, 1992, the day she ingested an overdose of Tolbutamide. She stated that Heritage was on that day responsible for Kayser's care. This includes the supervision and administration of prescribed medication. Dr. Hays gave testimony that the Mayo Clinic report indicates the drug Kayser ingested on September 30,

1992, was Tolbutamide (also known as Orinase), a prescription for diabetes. Although Dr. Hays had not ordered any diabetes medication for Kayser since her admittance to Heritage in July 1992, he had in 1987 given her a prescription for Tolinase, a different hypoglycemic medication for a mild, adult-onset diabetic condition.

The September 29, 1992, "nurses notes" indicate that when Kayser had complained of pain, she was given a placebo injection of sterile water. Later that day she received some Tylenol tablets. She was given another placebo injection for pain on September 30. That evening she was transferred to the Clinton Regional Hospital and admitted there while in an unconscious state. Dr. Hays, who attended her in the emergency room, diagnosed the condition as hypoglycemia. While she was hospitalized there, an intravenous device was inserted in the top of her right foot to treat the coma. She was later transferred to Presbyterian Hospital, where she showed signs of ecchymosis on top of the right foot. This condition ultimately developed into gangrene and required an above-the-knee amputation of her right leg. Kayser's medical records at Heritage did not indicate that she had exhibited any hypoglycemia symptoms until the evening of September 30.

According to Dr. Ellis' review of the medical records, Kayser ingested the medication while a resident at the home. Dr. Davis, the endocrinologist who treated Kayser at Presbyterian Hospital, opined that Kayser must have ingested a large dosage of Tolbutamide because 72 hours later it was still in her system.

The court concluded that a nursing home resident will not be administered an incorrect medication unless there has been negligence of some sort. In this type of case, the medication error does speak for itself.

In light of the circumstances that surround the injurious event, it seems reasonably clear that Kayser's ingestion of a Tolbutamide overdose would not have taken place in the absence of negligence by the nursing home's responsible staff. The record shows that Kayser had not been prescribed any diabetes medication while a resident at Heritage and that she had never been prescribed that type of hypoglycemic drug. It is uncontradicted that Kayser was at the nursing home when she ingested the prescribed medication. There is no direct evidence that anyone else supplied to her the harm-dealing dosage or that the substance in question was kept in her room (or elsewhere within her control). Neither is there indication that any other cause contributed to the coma. According to Jackie Dixon, a LPN at the Center, the nursing home is responsible for the administration of medication to its residents. As Dr. Hays testified, the administration of the wrong medication in an amount so excessive as to harm a resident would be below the applicable professional standard of care.

The dismissal of the case brought against the nursing home was reversed. The Supreme Court of Oklahoma concluded that the lower courts had made a mistake in refusing to permit the *res ipsa loquitur* theory to be considered by the jury.

In sum, Harder's evidence laid before the trial court the requisite *res ipsa* foundation facts from which the trier may infer that the injury—from an overdose of the wrong prescription—was one that would not ordinarily occur in the course of controlled supervision and administration of prescribed medicine in the absence of negligence on the Center's part. Because nothing in the record irrefutably negates any of the critical elements for application of *res ipsa loquitur*, Harder clearly met her probative initiative by establishing the necessary components for invoking the rule. The responsibility for producing proof that would rebut the inferences favorable to Harder's legal position thus came to be shifted to the defendant. The plaintiff was clearly entitled to have her case go to the jury—under the aid of a *res ipsa* instruction—for resolution of the disputed issues.

Notes on *Harder v. F. C. Clinton, Inc.*

1. Pharmacists who are nursing home consultants have important responsibilities under federal guidelines. These responsibilities include assisting in the development of systems to recognize and absorb medication errors. A pharmacist who is not present at all times in a facility is challenged to control what happens in the facility. The best way to approach facility improvements is to design systems that will function well when one is not present to oversee what is being done. A consultant pharmacist may not be able to assist on a day-to-day or hour-to-hour basis with patient care, but the consultant pharmacist can help develop systems that will improve every minute of care provision.

2. It makes little sense to establish a good system of medication use and then not use that system. The best way to ensure that appropriate systems are actually being used is to require documentation of what is done in the provision of patient care and then review that documentation on a regular basis. Medication errors and other problems can be seen within documentation and need not be seen when they are done. To the extent the documentation suggests that a problem may have occurred but does not fully confirm that there was a problem, indicator development and use may be helpful as a way to conclude that the thing speaks for itself and to require that explanations be provided regarding why something apparently inappropriate happened.

3. Consultant pharmacists who follow the federal mandate for drug regimen review and for professional service to nursing homes sometimes feel frustrated and irrelevant because they cannot control what happens in the nursing home they serve. This is an understandable feeling, but it is important not to discount the power of persuasion. It may be that pharmacists cannot require that changes occur, but they can suggest the need for changes and provide evidence of the reasonableness of the suggested changes. In the face of such evidence, many changes can happen, even in institutions that are not initially receptive to new ideas.

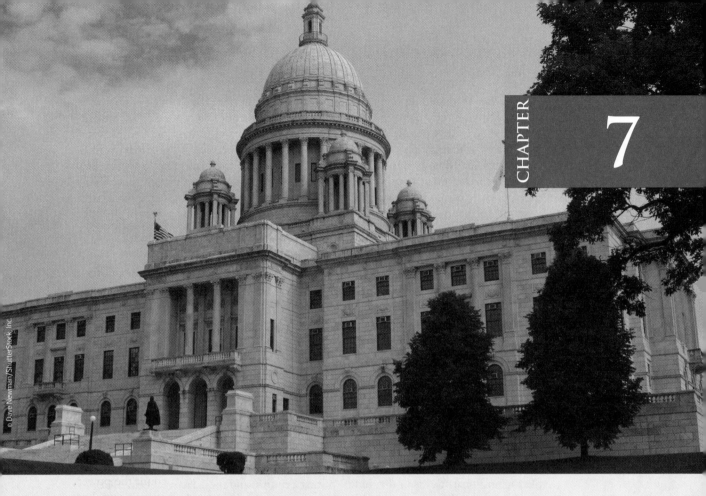

7

STATE REGULATION OF PHARMACY PRACTICE

CHAPTER OBJECTIVES

Upon completing this chapter, the reader will be able to:

▸ Identify the advantages and disadvantages of government regulation of professional practice.

▸ Describe the purpose of a state board of pharmacy.

▸ Recognize the functions of a state board of pharmacy.

▸ Discuss the grounds for disciplinary action against a licensed pharmacist.

▸ Describe the process through which disciplinary action is taken against a licensed pharmacist.

▸ Describe state regulation of institutional pharmacy practice.

▸ Discuss state regulation of third-party prescription programs.

▸ Describe the movement toward regulating for outcomes.

As discussed throughout previous chapters, the states regulate the practice of pharmacy directly through their police powers and the Tenth Amendment to the U.S. Constitution. The collection of state laws and regulations directed at pharmacies and pharmacists in a particular state is often called the pharmacy practice act. All pharmacists must have a thorough knowledge of the pharmacy practice act of each state in which they are licensed. Although state practice acts have many similarities, they also have many differences. It would be impossible in this book to attempt to discuss individual state laws and regulations. The intent of this chapter is to provide an overview of the state regulation of pharmacy practice so one can better understand the pharmacy practice act in a particular state.

SELF-REGULATION IN PHARMACY

American pharmacists purposely chose to become self-regulating health care professionals rather than externally regulated retail merchants. This conscious choice occurred during the last half of the nineteenth century, a time during which pharmacy emerged from other retailing activities as a significant component of the developing health care system. With most retail products, the tradition had been caveat emptor (let the buyer beware). However, pharmaceuticals sold at retail were among the first products in this country to which a new tradition of caveat vendor (let the seller beware) became applicable. Rules were developed to regulate the retail sale of pharmaceuticals. Many of these rules dealt with the sale of poisons and the requirement for appropriate labeling of such products, as well as records of those to whom they were sold. There were early lawsuits filed against pharmacists in the middle of that century, and these lawsuits held pharmacists liable for negligence in supplying the wrong medication to patients or for adulterating compounded products provided to patients. The notion that a provider of products could be liable for negligence was a new concept in the law, and it is no coincidence that it developed, at least in part, as the result of concern over the harm that could occur from the inappropriate use of pharmaceuticals.

By the beginning of the twentieth century, pharmacists had organized themselves and had developed clear systems of self-governance. This was an important development because it provided a framework for the organization and enforcement of federal drug laws that were soon to come. Had this state-level system of professional regulation not existed, federal authorities might well have sought far more extensive control over the practice of pharmacy. Lawyer-pharmacist James Hartley Beal and other pharmacy leaders were instrumental in the development of pharmacy as a self-regulated profession.

APPROACHES TO REGULATION

Varying countries use different approaches to regulation. In some countries, any drug can be purchased without a prescription, and anyone can be a pharmacist. Because there have been no widespread reports of mass deaths from adverse drug reactions in those countries, the open market system apparently works well there.

However, every country seems to aspire to the approach used by the United States and other developed countries. In most developed countries, licensed physicians prescribe medications, licensed pharmacists dispense them, and there are strict controls on who may be a physician or pharmacist. A lack of resources or some other practical barrier, rather than a lack of agreement with the underlying policies, is generally the reason that a country has not adopted this approach.

In the United States, it was only during the last part of the nineteenth century that states began to regulate professional practice through licensure. It was not until 1938 that pharmaceutical manufacturers were permitted to label their drugs for purchase only pursuant to a prescription. The formal classification of certain drugs as prescription only (i.e., limited to distribution by pharmacists on authority of a physician's prescription) took effect relatively recently—in 1952. Thus, the use of licensure to control drug distribution does not have a long history.

Nevertheless, licensure appears to be a cornerstone of U.S. commerce, at least insofar as professional expertise is concerned. Unlike certification, which officially recognizes particular individuals as qualified but allows those not certified to offer the same services, licensure permits only those officially recognized as qualified to provide the service.

REASONS TO REGULATE PROFESSIONS

The justification generally given to require licensure for health care providers is that people without specific training cannot distinguish between qualified and unqualified providers, and people who need health care must be protected from unqualified providers. With regard to pharmacists, the objectives of licensure are threefold:

1. To increase the quality of health care
2. To reduce the cost of health care
3. To inhibit the criminal abuse of drugs

In theory, the licensure of pharmacists increases the quality of health care because patients receive the correct medication and a qualified person monitors their drug therapy. Licensure reduces cost because pharmacists ensure that patients who do not need a medication do not receive one and that patients who do need a medication receive the least expensive of the appropriate and available alternatives. The goal of inhibiting criminal abuse is met by establishing a closed system of distribution for abusable drugs and permitting only licensed health care personnel to distribute drugs to patients.

DIFFERING PERSPECTIVES ON REGULATION

It is possible to argue that licensure may not be necessary to ensure the quality of health care. Well-informed patients may be just as capable as licensed professionals of ensuring that they use correct and appropriate medications. Better general education of the public may promote effective drug therapy just as well as does professional licensure. In addition, a requirement for licensure tends to favor traditional approaches to therapy, to the exclusion of avant-garde or unusual modes of treatment that may be appropriate for some patients. In some ways, it could be argued that licensure may protect the professions more than it protects the public.

In regard to the goal of reducing the cost of health care, pharmacist licensure also is subject to challenge. There is certainly the potential for a licensed professional to protect a patient or whoever is responsible for paying the cost of the patient's health care from paying for unnecessary procedures and products. For example, pharmacists have the authority to dispense cost-saving generic drug products under many circumstances. They can advise against the use of a product when it is not necessary; they can prevent patients from using drugs that have not been prescribed for them. On the other hand, the monopolistic nature of licensing can increase costs. Whether the increase in costs brought about by the monopoly is offset by the decrease in inefficient drug use brought about by professional oversight, the benefit of licensure is certainly subject to question.

Some regulators may view the restriction of access to controlled substances as the most important goal of pharmacist licensure. As custodians of the nation's medicinal drugs of abuse, pharmacists have a vital role to play in the "War on Drugs." Perhaps ominously for pharmacy, the criminalization of abusable drug possession is the subject of constant criticism and reassessment. Current drug abuse policy is at best only marginally effective, and there are frequent calls for abandonment of the policy that criminalizes drug abuse. If the policy was changed, the pharmacist's role in drug distribution could be diminished. Nonetheless, the decriminalization of drug abuse would require a significant shift in social policy.

STATE BOARDS OF PHARMACY

State laws regulating the practice of pharmacy, often termed pharmacy practice acts, provide for an administrative agency, the state board of pharmacy. The purpose of the board is to protect the public health, safety, and welfare. Although some pharmacists may believe that the board of pharmacy acts against the interests of the pharmacy profession, they must remember that the board of pharmacy protects the public, not the profession. In fact, boards of pharmacy are sometimes called "watchdogs" for the consumer.

The national organization that brings individual state boards of pharmacy together is the National Association of Boards of Pharmacy (NABP) (http://www.nabp.net). The NABP oversees the administration of a standardized examination that states use to evaluate the competency of applicants for pharmacy licensure. In addition, the NABP serves as a forum for the development of professional policies and standards. It also develops model legislation and regulations for use by member boards, supervises licensure transfer between states, and facilitates communication between states regarding pharmacist disciplinary actions.

Most members of the board of pharmacy are practicing pharmacists. Boards of pharmacy often have consumer members and may have members representing another health care profession. Appointment to the board of pharmacy is political, with members usually appointed directly by the governor.

Traditionally, the pharmacists on state boards of pharmacy had been independent community practitioners; often, they had been pharmacy owners. Chain pharmacists, hospital pharmacists, and others who did not own independent pharmacies had been underrepresented on the board. One chain pharmacy, Rite Aid Corporation, challenged the composition of the New Jersey Board of Pharmacy in *Rite Aid Corp. v. Board of Pharmacy*, 421 F. Supp. 1161 (D.N.J. 1976). All five pharmacists on the New Jersey board at that time were independent practitioners. Rite Aid contended that the statute allowing for the appointment of board members was unconstitutional because the statute did not specifically provide that a chain pharmacist be included on the board. Rite Aid also argued that the process for selecting board members was unconstitutional because it was biased toward the selection of independent pharmacists. The court rejected both of these arguments, finding that the statute did not prohibit chain pharmacists from being on the board and that there was no evidence of bias in the selection of board members.

In an effort to become more representative of the entire spectrum of pharmacy practice, most state boards of pharmacy have attempted to ensure the inclusion of at least one chain pharmacist and one hospital pharmacist on the board. Some states require by law the inclusion of pharmacists from different practice settings.

LICENSING

Perhaps the most important function of the state board of pharmacy is the granting of licenses to pharmacists and to pharmacies. Through this function, the state board of pharmacy ensures the competence of the individuals who practice pharmacy and the appropriateness of the physical facilities and business organizations within which they practice. Although this may change as a result of the Omnibus Budget Reconciliation Act of 1990 (OBRA '90), the current approach to licensure heavily emphasizes structure and process factors, with little attention to the outcomes of drug therapy.

LICENSING OF PHARMACISTS

The requirements of licensure for pharmacists vary somewhat from state to state, but most states require that applicants to practice pharmacy meet five criteria:

1. Graduation from pharmacy school
2. Completion of specified internship requirements
3. Attainment of a specified age
4. A passing score on the licensure examination
5. Demonstration of good moral character

Generally, a pharmacist applicant must have graduated from an accredited school or college of pharmacy or the equivalent of an accredited school or college. The American Council on Pharmaceutical Education (ACPE) accredits pharmacy schools within the United States. The NABP administers an examination called the Foreign Pharmacy Graduate Equivalency Examination, which allows state boards of pharmacy to assess whether a foreign pharmacy school graduate's education is equivalent to a U.S. pharmacy school graduate's education. On the basis of the results of this examination, a state board may permit the candidate to take the state board licensure examination, or it may require additional course work before permitting the candidate to take the examination.

Citizenship can no longer be a requirement for licensure as a pharmacist in the United States for permanent residents. The 1975 case of *Wong v. Hohnstrom*, 405 F. Supp. 727 (D. Minn. 1975), involved a challenge to a Minnesota statute that required U.S. citizenship for licensure as a pharmacist. An applicant for licensure who was not a U.S. citizen but was otherwise qualified to become a licensed pharmacist had been turned down because of citizenship. The court held that the Minnesota statute was unconstitutional, however, and enjoined the state board of pharmacy from enforcing it. Nonetheless, a state may be able to deny licensure to a nonpermanent resident of the United States under its citizenship requirement (*Van Staden v. Martin*, 664 F.3d 56 (C.A.5 La. 2011)).

In all states, the written test required for licensure is the North American Pharmacy Licensure Examination (NAPLEX). In addition, states administer an examination on state and federal laws, either one developed specifically by that state or the Multistate Pharmacy Jurisprudence Exam (MPJE) administered under the auspices of the NABP. Some states include other examinations such as a practical demonstration of ability, an oral patient consultation examination, or an interview.

Pharmacists who are already licensed in one state might not be required to take the state board of pharmacy examination to become licensed in another state. State boards of pharmacy will grant licensure through a process known as license transfer. The qualifications of an applicant for licensure transfer are reviewed by the NABP, and a license can be granted in a second state based on license by examination in the first state.

Transfer of licensure is not automatic. In *Sobel v. Board of Pharmacy*, 882 P.2d 606 (Or. Ct. App. 1994), the Oregon Board of Pharmacy denied a pharmacy license to an applicant who sought to transfer his license from Texas to Oregon, and the denial was upheld on appeal. The Oregon board had determined that the applicant committed fraud in his application for transfer. Although the applicant indicated on his application that he had not been subjected to discipline in any other state, investigators for the Oregon board determined that the applicant had been disciplined in Texas. A state may not grant a pharmacist license to a pharmacist who is under discipline in another state.

Applicants for licensure generally are required to report prosecutions, convictions, illegal drug use, and in some cases even arrests. A state board will evaluate the applicant's record to determine if the applicant lacks good moral character. The fact that an applicant might have been tried for a criminal violation and exonerated does not preclude a board from considering the event and using it as evidence of a lack of good moral character together with other facts (*In the Matter of the Application of W.D.P.*, 91 P.3d 1078 (HI 2004)).

Pharmacists must renew their licenses periodically. Generally, they need only to pay a fee and, in most states, complete a specified number of continuing education credits. Although there has been some discussion of imposing requirements for demonstrated competence to be relicensed, there is currently no such requirement. The NABP does provide a means for pharmacists to assess their knowledge base by completing a voluntary, nonpunitive multiple-choice examination called Pharmacist Self-Assessment Mechanism (PSAM) available at the NABP website.

Proposed National Licensure

A controversial proposal has been advanced for national licensure of pharmacists. The disaster of Hurricane Katrina fueled the proposal when out-of-state pharmacists were needed to assist in Louisiana. Nursing started a form of national licensure program in 1999 that has proved successful. National licensure for pharmacists is based upon several compelling points:

- All applicants for licensure must pass the same examination, NAPLEX.
- Reciprocity and license transfer is centralized through the NABP's Electronic Licensure Transfer Program.
- Many pharmacists work for corporations that do business in several states.
- Technological advances, including the Internet and telepharmacy, transcend physical borders.
- The federal government continues to expand its involvement in health care, in some cases preempting state laws in the process.
- National licensure might help alleviate pharmacist shortages and facilitate disaster relief.

Those in favor of national licensure do not necessarily envision licensure at the federal level but rather some type of multistate licensure program. Opponents to changing existing state licensure contend, among other arguments, that the current system efficiently permits reciprocity, that state boards cannot afford the loss of licensure revenue, and that pharmacists need to know the laws of each state in which they are licensed. National licensure will not happen overnight, but the debate has begun.

LICENSING OF PHARMACIES

State boards of pharmacy issue licenses to business entities that wish to operate a pharmacy at a specified location. The state board will issue a license to operate a pharmacy only to those that meet established standards relating to structural matters (e.g., equipment), library, and assurance of pharmacist supervision. Each location must have a license. States vary in the number of categories under which a pharmacy may license (i.e., hospital, community, nonresident, sterile compounding, limited services) from only one category to as many as 16. These standards are set out in state statutes, regulations, or both. Court cases have exempted some locations from the need to have a pharmacy license to dispense pharmaceuticals, however. For example, in the case of *Love v. Escambia County*, 157 So. 2d 205 (Fla. 1963), the court concluded that a city–county indigent outpatient clinic was not a pharmacy because the nurse dispensed only prefabricated medications under physician supervision.

On the basis of the rationale that pharmacist control is necessary to maintain professional and ethical standards, ensure quality services, and adequately supervise pharmacist employees, some states have laws that restrict the ownership of pharmacies, at least in part, to pharmacists. North Dakota, for example, requires that most of a pharmacy corporation's stock be owned by a pharmacist regularly employed in and responsible for the management, supervision, and operation of the pharmacy. The U.S. Supreme Court upheld this law in *Board of Pharmacy v. Snyder's Drug Stores*, 414 U.S. 156 (1973).

Some states prohibit the ownership of pharmacies by physicians on the theory that, when a prescriber has an interest in the economic success of a pharmacy, the best interest of the patient may not be the primary factor in the selection of the medication to be prescribed. A group of California physicians challenged a law prohibiting physician ownership of pharmacies, arguing that it was unconstitutional because it singled out physicians as the only persons ineligible to obtain a pharmacy permit. The court upheld the law in *Magan Medical Clinic v. Board of Medical Examiners*, 249 Cal. App. 2d 124 (Cal. Ct. App. 1976).

Most states require that the pharmacy owner designate a particular pharmacist as the pharmacist-in-charge or PIC. Generally state laws prevent a person from being the PIC at more than one pharmacy. The PIC has the responsibility, usually together with the pharmacy owner, to ensure that the pharmacy and pharmacy personnel comply with all applicable laws and regulations. A nonpharmacist owner may not subvert or attempt to subvert the PIC's efforts to comply. The pharmacy generally must provide the name of the PIC to the state board, and in some states the board must approve the PIC.

Nonresident (Mail Order) Pharmacies

Licensing of nonresident, primarily mail order pharmacies historically has been challenging for state pharmacy boards. In a relatively few years, mail order pharmacy captured a significant share of the overall prescription drug market. In the 1980s and early 1990s as mail order pharmacy developed, community pharmacy organizations lobbied hard for state laws to regulate the mail order pharmacy industry. Many of the bills introduced, however, were considered by state attorneys general to unduly burden interstate commerce and thus to be unconstitutional. For example, early bills required that nonresident pharmacies be licensed in the same manner as in-state pharmacies. This requirement, however, meant that a mail order pharmacy that mailed prescriptions to 50 states would have to comply with 50 different pharmacy practice acts, and the pharmacists would have to be individually licensed in 50 states. The U.S. Supreme Court has ruled that states can enact laws to evenhandedly serve a legitimate local public interest if the laws only incidentally affect interstate commerce (*Pike v. Bruce Church, Inc.*, 397 U.S. 137 (1970)). Most legal experts, however, believed that state laws requiring nonresident pharmacies to conform to the same requirements expected of in-state pharmacies would be an excessive burden on interstate commerce.

As a result, most states today require that nonresident pharmacies that mail prescriptions into the state must only be registered with the state board. The state boards can require the nonresident pharmacy be licensed in its state of residence and to comply with special recordkeeping requirements and requests for information, and establish other requirements such as a toll-free phone service to communicate with patients. Generally, a state may not require a nonresident pharmacy to meet unduly burdensome requirements such as face-to-face counseling, or require the nonresident pharmacy to comply with more strict regulations than in-state pharmacies.

Technology has created new problems for states regulating nonresident pharmacies. Many mail order pharmacies perform drug use review (DUR) and other cognitive functions in one facility and process the prescriptions in another facility, and these facilities may even be in different states. Boards now have to consider whether to register the nonresident DUR facility, which does no dispensing, as a pharmacy, or instead register the individual pharmacists in the facility, or neither. This is a particular challenge to states that define a pharmacy as a place where dangerous drugs are stored and furnished. This discussion is continued in the following telepharmacy section.

Telepharmacy

Technology now allows pharmacists to provide pharmacy services to remote facilities (such as long-term care facilities and nonprofit clinics) and underserved areas without being physically present. Automated dispensing systems (ADSs) permit pharmacists to remotely dispense a drug to an authorized person (a health care licensee) and provide real-time counseling through audiovisual telecommunication devices to the patient. Telecommunication technology also allows the pharmacist to supervise a technician dispensing the medication at the remote site. Telepharmacy presents boards with questions: Should a pharmacist that is licensed in one state but providing telepharmacy services in another state be licensed in the state where the telepharmacy services are provided? Should an out-of-state pharmacist not licensed in the state (or even an in-state pharmacist) who provides telepharmacy services be licensed as a pharmacy if the pharmacist is not currently working through a pharmacy? Should ADSs be allowed in urban areas where other pharmacies exist? How many ADSs should a pharmacist or pharmacy be allowed to operate? Should only certain drugs be permitted to be dispensed through an ADS? (The Drug Enforcement Agency [DEA] has approved the dispensing of controlled substances through ADSs only in long-term care facilities.) Telepharmacy and the use of ADSs present challenges but offer great opportunities.

Kiosks

Similar in concept to telepharmacy is the "kiosk," resembling an ATM machine for prescription drugs. Located either adjacent to the pharmacy department or nearby, the kiosks allow patients to drop off new prescriptions and pick up refill prescriptions that do not require counseling without having to access the pharmacy department. The patient must consent to the use of the kiosk. Kiosks have been highly controversial, but advocates say they reduce the burden on pharmacists and allow them to spend more time with patients who require their services.

Nonresident (Internet) Pharmacies

The federal Ryan Haight Online Pharmacy Consumer Protection Act of 2008 (discussed in Chapter 5) applies only to controlled substances. Some states have enacted laws prohibiting the dispensing of any prescription via the Internet if the person knows or should know that the prescriptions are not issued pursuant to a good faith prior examination by a prescriber. A good faith medical examination generally is interpreted as including a legitimate patient–physician relationship consisting of a physical examination and documentation on file of the patient's medical records. Internet prescribing pursuant to questionnaires does not qualify. If a state has not passed specific Internet prescribing laws, the board might still be able to discipline pharmacies by establishing that Internet prescriptions are not valid as generally defined under state law, since there is not a legitimate physician–patient relationship. NABP has developed an accreditation process for Internet pharmacies called Verified Internet Pharmacy Practice Sites (VIPPS), and any pharmacy that has been accredited will display the VIPPS seal on its website. The NABP website also lists Internet pharmacies that are "Not Recommended" because they appear not to comply with state or federal law, as well as a midlevel list of Internet pharmacies called "Reviewed Internet Pharmacy Practice Sites," containing sites appearing to comply with the law.

ACTIONS AGAINST A LICENSE

State boards of pharmacy have broad discretion in the discipline of pharmacists and pharmacies. In most states, licenses can be suspended for a period of time or even permanently revoked. Many states allow for monetary civil penalties, public reprimands, or both. Nonetheless, disciplinary actions must be based on specified grounds and must follow administrative procedures outlined in state law.

In 1990, the Office of the Inspector General (OIG) of the Department of Health and Human Services suggested that pharmacy boards focus too much on offenses such as drug or alcohol abuse, Medicaid fraud, and drug diversion and not enough on reviewing the quality of pharmaceutical care in their licensure actions. In essence, the OIG was saying that a pharmacist can be inept and negligent, but as long as the pharmacist is clean and honest, there will be no threat to the pharmacist's license. Only in the past few years have state boards started considering outcomes, as discussed in the last section of this chapter.

State boards of pharmacy are required to follow procedures specified in their state's pharmacy practice and administrative procedures acts. In *Empire State Pharmaceutical Society v. New York State Department of Education*, 469 N.Y.S. 2d 514 (N.Y. Sup. Ct. 1983), the court enjoined a procedure in which penalties were imposed on pharmacists before a hearing. Although the right to notice and an opportunity to be heard before adverse action is taken against a citizen is a fundamental requirement of procedural due process under the U.S. Constitution, the New York board was issuing fines by mail; pharmacists were then allowed to contest a penalty that had already been determined. A pharmacist's options at that point were to

- Pay the penalty.
- Make a statement in mitigation.
- Contest the charges and risk a more severe penalty if found guilty.

In the words of the court, the options were presented in a style intended to encourage the recipient not to contest the charges by making "an offer you cannot refuse." The court held that this procedure was improper because it failed to afford the licensee 15 days' notice before the imposition of the penalty. In effect, the procedure penalized those who opted to contest the charges, and it was for this reason ruled unconstitutional.

Revocation of a pharmacy license by one state may, in and of itself, serve as the basis for revocation in another state. Through centralized communication, boards of pharmacy inform each other of actions taken against licensees, thus making it difficult for a pharmacist who has been disciplined in one state to simply move to another state in which the pharmacist became licensed years earlier and continue, without interruption, the practice of pharmacy within the second state. However, standard procedural requirements apply to disciplinary action taken on the basis of discipline in another state.

A matter of procedure was the issue in *Schram v. Department of Professional Regulation*, 603 So. 2d 1307 (Fla. Dist. Ct. App. 1992). In this case, the pharmacist bringing the lawsuit had lost his license in Michigan, and the Florida board had revoked his Florida license on the basis of the Michigan revocation. The Florida board, having been notified of the Michigan revocation, mailed a registered letter to the pharmacist at the last address the pharmacist had provided to the Florida board. Because the pharmacist had moved from that address years before, the letter was returned as undeliverable. The pharmacist contended that the board had not exercised due diligence in attempting to locate him, particularly because correspondence from the Michigan board to the Florida board had contained the pharmacist's current address. The court agreed that the board had not exercised due diligence, a requirement for notice of an administrative action. Therefore, the board's order revoking the pharmacist's license in Florida was vacated.

Grounds for Discipline

State pharmacy practice acts usually provide several grounds for disciplinary action against a pharmacist or pharmacy. Grounds commonly listed as justification for disciplinary action include such offenses as the provision of false or fraudulent information when applying for a license, violation of any of the statutes or regulations pertaining to the practice of pharmacy, conviction of a felony, conviction of an act involving moral turpitude, unprofessional conduct, immoral conduct or character, gross immorality, habitual intemperance, and incompetence.

If a licensee is a defendant in a criminal case brought in a court of law, the state board of pharmacy often does not bring disciplinary action based on the same incident until the defendant has been adjudicated as guilty. Nonetheless, in most states the board is not required to wait and can take action against a licensee before the judicial outcome in the criminal case. In *Schwartz v. Florida Board of Pharmacy*, 302 So. 2d 423 (Fla. 1974), the state had brought criminal action against a pharmacist for selling narcotics without a prescription. The board then proceeded with disciplinary action. The pharmacist requested that the board wait until the trial was over, but the board refused and ultimately revoked the pharmacist's license. Contending that the board's refusal to postpone the hearing violated due process, the pharmacist appealed; the court, however, found for the board.

In some states, the board may revoke a pharmacist's license because of an act that led to criminal charges, even if the pharmacist was acquitted in court of the charges. This can occur because administrative procedure differs from criminal procedure. For example, the burden of proof is usually not as great in administrative proceedings as it is in criminal proceedings, so the prosecution has a greater chance to succeed. In addition, the rules of evidence permit the person or group making a decision about an administrative case to hear testimony and view documents that would not be admissible in a criminal case.

Nearly all pharmacy practice acts contain catchall phrases that can snare unsuspecting pharmacists who follow the letter, but not the spirit, of the law. Terms such as "unprofessional conduct" and "moral turpitude" can serve as the basis for a successful disciplinary proceeding, even if the pharmacist involved has disobeyed no specific legal requirement. Although these terms have been challenged as unconstitutionally vague because they do not give pharmacists clear guidelines about what they must do or refrain from doing to avoid problems with the board, most courts have upheld the discretionary use of such grounds for discipline by state boards of pharmacy.

Unprofessional Conduct

In *Pennsylvania State Board of Pharmacy v. Cohen*, 292 A.2d 277 (Pa. 1977), the board suspended a pharmacist's license on the grounds of grossly unprofessional conduct. The pharmacist sold large quantities of empty gelatin capsules, along with lactose and quinine hydrochloride, to various customers, even though he knew that these purchases were for the purpose of manufacturing illicit drugs. His actions did not violate any specific law because nothing in the law forbade the sale of these items. Furthermore, although the pharmacy practice act listed 13 specific offenses that constituted unprofessional conduct, none of the 13 described the pharmacist's activity. The court held for the pharmacist, ruling that a pharmacist in Pennsylvania cannot be disciplined for an unlisted act because that would require pharmacists to guess at what is prohibited.

A New Jersey court followed a different approach in *In re Heller*, 374 A.2d 1191 (N.J. 1977). A pharmacist was charged with grossly unprofessional conduct for selling narcotic cough syrups with great frequency to the same people at greatly inflated prices. The pharmacist had complied with all the specific requirements relating to the nonprescription sale of narcotic cough syrups, yet the board disciplined him. The pharmacist's defense was that his conduct was not specifically listed among the acts deemed grossly unprofessional in the practice act. Unlike the Pennsylvania court in *Cohen*, the New Jersey court rejected this argument, ruling that the list is not exclusive because there is no need for the specific identification of conduct that is inherently wrong and obviously dangerous. The New Jersey Supreme Court reasoned that it would be absurd to immunize certain outrageous conduct from disciplinary action simply because it did not happen to be listed in the statute.

Generally, if a state provides that unprofessional conduct includes convictions for violations of the law, there must be a nexus between the convictions and competence to practice. This nexus need not be a strong one, however. In *Griffiths v. Medical Board of California*, 2002 W.L. 307761 (Cal. App. 2 Dist.), the court ruled that the board was justified in determining that three different misdemeanor convictions by a physician for reckless driving involving alcohol over a 5-year period constituted unprofessional conduct.

Moral Turpitude

Determining "moral turpitude" is not an easy task. Many courts have determined that crimes involving fraud constitute moral turpitude because these are intentional acts contrary to honesty and good morals. In *Schaubman v. Blum*, 426 N.Y.S.2d 230 (N.Y. App. Div. 1980), a pharmacist legally dispensed a less expensive generic drug in place of the brand-name drug but illegally billed the state Medicaid agency for the brand-name drug. The excess amount was only $3.39. Nevertheless, the court upheld the board's decision to revoke the pharmacy's license as an effective means to deter Medicaid fraud. Betrayal of the public trust through Medicaid fraud is certain to bring about regulatory action. In *State v. Brown*, 637 So. 2d 669 (La. Ct. App. 1994), the court upheld a sentence of 39 months at hard labor and a $2,500 fine for a pharmacist who was found to have defrauded Medicaid of $3,270.

REINSTATEMENT OF A REVOKED LICENSE

Few things in life can really be said to last "forever," and the revocation of a pharmacist's license is no exception to that rule. Having lost one's pharmacist license, it may be possible to get the license back by making application to the board for reinstatement and showing that the problem that originally led to revocation is no longer operative. In *Schiffman v. Department of Professional Regulation*, 581 So. 2d 1375 (Fla. Dist. Ct. App. 1991), a pharmacist successfully appealed a final order of the Florida Board of Pharmacy denying his application for reinstatement of his previously revoked license. The court noted that it is incompetent, unskilled, and unprofessional pharmacists who are a threat to public safety, not rehabilitated pharmacists. The plaintiff had at one time been found guilty of controlled substance diversion and had his pharmacist license permanently revoked, but he contended that he had been rehabilitated. The court ruled that the board must consider a petition for reinstatement on the basis of rehabilitation. A permanent revocation of a pharmacist's license is not permitted under the law of Florida or of many other states.

Of course, a requirement that a board of pharmacy consider reinstatement of a pharmacist's license does not mean the license will actually be reinstated. The board may not even have to listen to a former pharmacist's arguments as to why a revoked license should be reinstated. In *Jones v. Alabama State Board of Pharmacy*, 624 So.2d 613 (Ala. Civ. App. 1993), a former pharmacist contended that the board of pharmacy was required by due process to afford him a hearing on his motion for reinstatement of his license. The former pharmacist's license had been revoked several years earlier, and the board denied his motion for reinstatement. The pharmacist offered several arguments as to why the board was not legally permitted to deny his motion for reinstatement without a hearing. However, the court ruled that the board of pharmacy had been granted broad discretionary authority, and absent a specific statutory or common law requirement that there be a hearing, the former pharmacist was not entitled to a hearing.

IMPAIRED PHARMACIST PROGRAMS

In the past, boards of pharmacy have had little choice but to revoke or suspend the license of a pharmacist who has been found to be impaired because of alcohol or drug use. Therefore, impaired pharmacists had been hesitant to seek assistance for their problem for fear of public humiliation and board of pharmacy discipline. Two circumstances have exacerbated this situation. First, the pharmacy profession was failing to recognize that alcoholism and drug abuse are diseases that require compassion and treatment rather than aberrant behavior that requires condemnation. Second, the severity of the consequences, should they admit their problem, was forcing impaired practitioners into the closet, and the danger these pharmacists may have posed to the public was unchecked. As a result, state pharmacy associations in many states lobbied for laws to establish programs to assist impaired pharmacists, and most of these laws passed. Most state boards of pharmacy are supportive of such programs, and state laws generally provide impaired pharmacists with two pathways into a rehabilitation program. One pathway allows the pharmacist to voluntarily enter into a rehabilitation program without board of pharmacy involvement or knowledge. The other route would be pursuant to a board of pharmacy disciplinary hearing.

Some state pharmacy laws require pharmacies to have written policies and procedures for taking action to protect the public when a pharmacist is discovered to be impaired. This may involve the pharmacy reporting the individual to the state board within a certain time frame.

ACTIONS AGAINST A PHARMACY LICENSE

License revocations, suspensions, and civil penalties may be assessed against the license of a pharmacy and against the license of a pharmacist. Sometimes a problem develops as the result of actions taken by those who run the pharmacy business, rather than those who practice pharmacy within the business, and the appropriate remedy is to act against the business's pharmacy license and not the pharmacist's professional license. However, in *Sender v. Department of Professional Regulation*, 635 N.E.2d 849 (Ill. App. Ct. 1994), the court reversed disciplinary action taken against a pharmacist "owner" on the basis of the misconduct of an employee in diverting controlled substances. The facts showed that the owner–pharmacist was merely a shareholder in the pharmacy corporation, with no supervisory role and with no authority to control the actions of those who engaged in diversion activities.

An Illinois appellate court reversed disciplinary action taken against a pharmacy for using nonpharmacists to perform tasks that only a pharmacist should perform. In *Walgreen Co. v. Selcke*, 595 N.E.2d 89 (Ill. App. Ct. 1992), the court distinguished between the scientific aspects of the practice of pharmacy and the business aspects of the practice of pharmacy. Describing the actions taken by two pharmacy employees who were not licensed pharmacists, the court concluded that these actions were clerical and supportive in nature. They were not intrusions into the practice of pharmacy. Therefore, disciplinary action against the pharmacy's license was reversed.

Circumstances may warrant disciplinary action against both a pharmacist and a pharmacy. The revocation of a pharmacist's license to practice pharmacy and his or her registration to operate a retail pharmacy were affirmed in *In re 882 East 180th Street Drug Corp.*, 596 N.Y.S.2d 193 (N.Y. App. Div. 1993). An inspection of the pharmacy had disclosed the presence in the back room of large numbers of physician samples, drugs dispensed by other pharmacies, and other large quantities of pharmaceuticals in unlabeled or improperly labeled containers. The board found the pharmacist guilty of gross negligence and unprofessional conduct. The pharmacist claimed that the drugs were all brought to his pharmacy to be destroyed, although he admitted that none had ever been destroyed. He also asserted that none of the drugs so acquired were ever resold to patients. The board found this explanation to be literally "incredible." The court upheld the license revocation for both the pharmacist and pharmacy in view of the threat to the public health posed by the pharmacist's deliberate conduct.

STANDARDS OF PRACTICE

States regulate not only who may practice pharmacy and where it may be practiced but also how pharmacy is practiced. Pharmacists do not dispense drugs in paper envelopes with illegible directions scribbled on them because the standard is to use prescription vials and machine-printed labels. Pharmacists know this to be the standard because it is specified in the law. Standards of practice in many states also stipulate that a pharmacist must be present in a pharmacy when the pharmacy department is open; otherwise there would be access to drugs of abuse, and patients might acquire their medications without the opportunity to discuss them with a pharmacist. Standards of practice specify how pharmacy will be practiced, where it will be practiced, and who will practice it.

Because pharmacy is a self-regulated profession, many laws and regulations merely describe existing standards of practice, rather than establish new standards. For example, checking the work of technicians filling prescriptions is the law, but most pharmacists would do this regardless of the law because checking prescriptions is important to good patient care. Making a standard of practice a law or regulation allows for easier enforcement of the standards against professionals who deviate from the standards. Nonetheless, laws and regulations do not describe all standards of practice. For example, a state law may not specify that the generic drug substituted for the prescribed drug be therapeutically equivalent to the prescribed drug. Yet, this would be an important consideration by a pharmacist for substitution and thus a standard of practice. Laws and regulations do not often set standards of practice related to professional judgment because each situation may require a different judgment. Nonetheless, pharmacists are expected to act appropriately. For example, state law or regulation will require a pharmacist to screen a prescription for a drug–drug interaction but not describe the action a pharmacist should take when detecting the interaction. A pharmacist who detects a potentially serious interaction, yet takes no action because the law does not require it, has not met the standard of practice, or the intent of the law.

Although the states are empowered to regulate the practice of the professions directly, the federal government may indirectly regulate professional practice in two significant ways. First, the federal government regulates the drug product and correspondingly attaches requirements to the product that a practitioner can meet only by behaving in a particular way. Second, the federal government may establish conditions for participation in programs that it funds (or partially funds), requiring states to accept the conditions if they wish to continue receiving federal funds. OBRA '90 establishes such conditions for participation in the Medicaid pharmaceutical program.

The drug use review provisions of OBRA '90 enhance the ability of state enforcement authorities to conduct practice audits of pharmacies to determine whether the quality of practice in the pharmacies meets the standard of care. Claims for payment submitted by pharmacists to Medicaid or another provider of pharmaceutical benefits can serve as a performance database. This database can disclose whether patients who use a particular pharmacy are having drug-related problems despite the fact that the pharmacy has complied with structural requirements. Enforcement activity by the state board of pharmacy can ensure that practice standards are being met. Thus, the OBRA '90 mandate for improved quality of care enables state authorities to enforce practice standards by using data regarding patient outcomes.

Practice of Pharmacy Defined

A state's legal definition of the practice of pharmacy is critical. Historically many states defined the practice of pharmacy in limited terms of dispensing a drug product. Today most states have far broader definitions for the practice of pharmacy, reflecting the clinical roles that pharmacists perform such as drug utilization review, providing clinical consultations to other health care professionals and patients, and administering immunizations. The broader the definition the more latitude provided the state board to implement regulations expanding the practice, as opposed to having to seek legislation. An expansive definition of the practice of pharmacy also establishes professional identity. It becomes instructive to courts and other administrative agencies when making decisions about pharmacy practice. To this end, many states have included a statement in the law that pharmacy is a learned profession, to distinguish it from the perception by some that pharmacy is a commercial business.

The legal definition of the practice of pharmacy is important for several other reasons. It is useful in making distinctions between pharmacists and physicians because a pharmacist may otherwise be accused of practicing medicine without a medical license. In most states, the law prohibits the practice of medicine by anyone who is not licensed as a physician. The law provides that a health care provider who is practicing within the boundaries of another profession is not practicing medicine illegally, however, even though the acts that person is performing may be construed as the practice of medicine. Thus, a pharmacist who is monitoring drug therapy within the definition of pharmacy practice is not illegally practicing medicine, but someone who has no license at all and monitors drug therapy is indeed illegally practicing medicine.

The definition of pharmacy practice also distinguishes between what functions only a pharmacist can perform and what functions a pharmacy technician may be permitted to perform. Technicians may not perform those functions included within the definition of pharmacy practice unless the law specifically permits technicians to do them. Just as pharmacists may now carry out some activities that only physicians have done in the past, so too may pharmacy technicians now perform some functions that only pharmacists have done. The expansion of the pharmacist into medicine and of pharmacy technicians into pharmacy is circumscribed by legal definitions, however.

The legal definition of the practice of pharmacy must distinguish pharmacy not only from other health care professions and ancillary personnel but also from unlicensed persons performing pharmacy-related functions. For example, is someone who makes decisions regarding which drugs will be included on a managed care organization's formulary practicing pharmacy? Is someone who makes drug utilization review decisions about whether a patient can receive a particular drug therapy practicing pharmacy? An even more fundamental question is whether pharmacy can be practiced outside of a facility licensed as a pharmacy. Defining what constitutes the practice of pharmacy and where it may be practiced has quality of care implications that many states must yet address.

ANCILLARY PHARMACY PERSONNEL

For the past several years pharmacy gradually has been shifting its mission from one centered on dispensing to one of providing professional patient care services. In order to allow pharmacists the time to provide professional services, they require assistance in performing routine nonjudgmental dispensing functions. To provide that assistance, states have authorized pharmacy technicians to work in community pharmacy practice, emulating what hospital pharmacies have done for several years prior. Although the duties and tasks that a pharmacy technician may lawfully perform in a community pharmacy are fairly standard among the states, the qualifications, licensure requirements, degree of supervision, and ratio of pharmacist to technician vary between states. Qualifications to become a technician range from no requirements in some states to completion of a board-approved technician program in other states, to national certification in yet other states. To attain national certification, a technician must pass a nationally administered standardized examination. Some states have established two tiers of technicians, certified and noncertified, although NABP announced in 2009 that it has amended its model act to recommend that all technicians be certified by 2015.

Many states have not required that technicians be licensed or registered with the state board. Recently, however, there has been a national trend among the states to license or register technicians. An NABP task force, appointed in 2009 to study this issue, recommended that state boards require that all technicians complete an accredited education and training program, among other requirements. This trend has been accelerated by several factors including recent studies documenting the incidence of dispensing errors; some high-profile injuries resulting from dispensing errors; negligence and even manslaughter lawsuits against pharmacists and pharmacies; and widespread media attention to dispensing errors. A bill was introduced in Congress in 2009 (named Emily's Act for the death of a 2-year old caused by an improperly prepared chemotherapy drug prepared by a pharmacy technician) to mandate education, training, and regulatory standards for all pharmacy technicians. The bill, however, was not passed.

In every state, a supervising pharmacist must check the work of the technician prior to dispensing the prescription to the patient, and that pharmacist is ultimately responsible for the accuracy of the dispensed product. The degree of supervision over ancillary personnel that a pharmacist must provide varies among the states and whether the laws, regulations, and state board combine to formulate a process approach or outcomes approach. Many states specify the supervision requirement as "direct supervision and control." Interpretation of the "direct supervision and control" requirement raises controversies that individual state boards must address such as whether the supervising pharmacist must be in physical proximity of the technician and observe the technician at all times (a process approach). Or, is it acceptable for the pharmacist to perform tasks remote from the technician and just check the technician's prescription before dispensing to the patient (an outcome approach)? Some states even have considered whether it would be appropriate to have a technician check another technician's work, as opposed to a pharmacist checking, a practice that has been authorized by law in some states for hospital pharmacies.

Many states have ratio requirements, generally set at no more than two technicians to one pharmacist, and some states have no ratio requirements. Application of the ratio requirements can cause controversy related to supervision. For example, is the intent of a 1:2 ratio requirement satisfied if a pharmacy has six pharmacists in the facility and 12 technicians, but only three of the pharmacists work with the technicians performing dispensing functions and the other three perform other tasks such as DUR and phoning prescribers? At least one state board has held that the ratio requirement is not satisfied unless one pharmacist is actually supervising two technicians, and this would appear to be the position of most state pharmacy boards.

In addition to technicians, pharmacies may generally employ nonlicensed personnel to assist in a clerk capacity, such as accepting prescriptions from patients, entering information into the pharmacy computer, answering the phone to receive refill requests, and selling the dispensed prescription to the patient. Some states by statute authorize these unlicensed personnel to perform specified clerical functions. In most other states, pharmacy boards tacitly permit these personnel even though the law does not address them.

INTERNS

Most states allow pharmacy students to work as interns starting their first year of pharmacy school and almost all states require that interns be licensed or registered with the board. Generally, interns are allowed to perform any function that a pharmacist may perform under the direct supervision of a pharmacist. As with technicians, some states set ratio requirements for interns, others do not.

AUTOMATION

In addition to the assistance of interns, technicians, and clerks, pharmacists also enjoy the assistance of automation. Automated dispensing equipment and robotics have greatly facilitated the speed, efficiency, and accuracy of dispensing. The issue of whether a pharmacist must check a prescription dispensed by automation (with no technician involvement) arises, however, since most state laws are silent on this issue. Although the state board may not be able to directly cite a pharmacist for a violation if he or she does not check prescriptions, the pharmacist will be legally responsible for any error, both pursuant to a state board action and pursuant to a negligence lawsuit. It would not likely be difficult to establish that a pharmacist must check the dispensed prescription as a standard of practice.

ABSENCE OF A PHARMACIST

One contributing cause of dispensing errors has been identified as long continuous hours worked by pharmacists without breaks. This has led to state laws limiting the number of continuous hours a pharmacist may work in a day. The laws also generally require that employers, depending upon the number of hours of the pharmacist's shift, allow a meal break of usually 30 minutes, together with one or two other breaks of usually 15 minutes. When only one pharmacist is on duty, some states require that the pharmacist must remain in the pharmacy during the break but post a sign that the pharmacist is on break. Some other states allow the pharmacist to take the break away from the pharmacy department. However, the traditional rule of law in nearly all states required that a pharmacist must be present in the pharmacy at all times that the pharmacy is open. Closing a pharmacy for 30 minutes or 15 minutes could cause patients significant inconvenience and disrupt business. As a result, some states have changed their laws to allow the pharmacy to remain open with ancillary personnel during the pharmacist's break and while the pharmacist is absent, provided that the pharmacist agrees. If the pharmacist is not comfortable and does not agree, the pharmacy must close during the break. If the pharmacy remains open, the ancillary personnel may not conduct any activities that require a pharmacist, such as dispensing a new prescription to a patient that requires verification by the pharmacist and counseling. The supervising pharmacist and pharmacist in charge will generally be held responsible and accountable for the diversion of drugs or any pharmacy violations that occur in the pharmacist's absence.

CONTINUING EDUCATION

Pharmacy has recognized the importance of continuing education (CE) or continuing pharmacy education (CPE) for decades, but CE as a legal requirement for relicensure in most states did not occur until the 1970s. Today it is a requirement in every state with most requiring 15 hours, or 1.5 continuing education units (CEU) per year; or 30 hours (3 CEUs) biennially. Some states require that a certain number of those hours be in a specific subject such as law and some states require that a certain number of the hours be from live programs. Some states require that the CE hours or units must be approved by the American Council on Pharmacy Education (ACPE), other states more generally allow for CE hours approved by the board, and the rest of the states specify that either will qualify. Most states allow pharmacists extensions for hardship situations and do not require CE if the pharmacist chooses inactive licensure status.

A collaborative effort among NABP, ACPE, and ACPE providers, called CPE Monitor, provides pharmacists and technicians the opportunity to register on an electronic system so they can easily monitor their completed CPE credits. Licensees can register and receive an e-profile ID number at http://www.nabp.net/programs/cpe-monitor/cpe-monitor-service.

ACPE providers require this ID number together with the licensee's date of birth for the licensee to receive CPE credit. State boards of pharmacy will have access to CPE Monitor, if they desire, to conduct audits to determine whether licensees have completed the required CPEs.

COLLABORATIVE PRACTICE AGREEMENTS

For years, pharmacy has envisioned an expanded scope of practice where the pharmacist prescribes, adjusts, and monitors the patient's drug-therapy regimen, based upon the diagnosis of another health care professional. That vision has advanced a step closer to reality in over 40 states through the enactment of laws authorizing collaborative practice agreements. The requirements vary from state to state, but in general many states now authorize a pharmacist to initiate or adjust a patient's drug therapy pursuant to a written agreement between the physician and pharmacist. That agreement will contain the policies and procedures the pharmacist must follow including any formulary that might be applicable. The scope of authority granted the pharmacist under an agreement can often be as broad or as narrow as the parties agree. The DEA has determined that pharmacists practicing under these arrangements can receive DEA registration if they are authorized by the physician to initiate or adjust controlled substances.

PROSPECTIVE DRUG UTILIZATION REVIEW (DUR)

Because of OBRA '90, every state now requires that pharmacies incorporate prospective drug utilization review into the dispensing process. State regulations requiring counseling, screening, and the maintenance of patient medication records have expanded the scope of practice and most likely the standards of practice. Most states have adopted the same or similar language in their DUR regulations as that of OBRA '90. A few states, however, require that a pharmacist must counsel the patient, rather than permitting the pharmacy to offer to counsel as allowed by OBRA '90. A very few states apply the DUR requirements only to Medicaid patients.

An issue attracting considerable attention in the past few years is whether pharmacists should be required to counsel patients with limited English proficiency in the patient's own language. In 2008, the attorney general of New York announced a settlement agreement with CVS and Rite Aid in which the two chains agreed to counsel all pharmacy customers in their own language and provide written translations in Spanish, Chinese, Italian, Russian, French, and Polish. The requirement to counsel and provide labels in the patient's own language might ultimately be adopted in all states because of federal law. Title VI of the Civil Rights Act of 1964 guarantees equal access to services paid for with federal funds, and applies to providers receiving Medicare or Medicaid payments, including pharmacies. California and New York now require patient-centered standardized labels, including the requirement that the label be interpreted into certain languages other than English when requested by the patient.

REPOSITORY OR TAKE-BACK PROGRAMS

Many states have passed laws establishing some type of drug repository or take-back program. Although a few states include controlled substances in these programs, the DEA does not regard this practice as lawful under federal law. The intent of a repository program is to allow unused drugs to be recycled for use by patients who otherwise could not afford them. In general, a repository program allows a hospital, long-term care facility, pharmacy, manufacturer, or wholesaler to donate sealed, unexpired medications so they can ultimately be distributed to the indigent. Repository programs raise safety concerns. Most notably of course are concerns of adulteration that may affect safety and efficacy since the drugs may have been stored outside the normal course of distribution. An additional concern is drugs, such as thalidomide, which must be distributed by the manufacturer through a restricted distribution program; and some states do specifically exclude drugs that require that the patient must be registered with the manufacturer. Some states allow a pharmacy to dispense the recycled drugs to designated nonprofit clinics provided the county agrees to establish the program and that the pharmacy has a contract with the county to do so.

STATE HOSPITAL PHARMACY LICENSURE ISSUES

The difference between hospital pharmacy and community pharmacy is so great in so many ways that in some states the state board of pharmacy does not have up-to-date laws to regulate hospital pharmacy. Those state pharmacy practice acts that were drafted in the 1950s or earlier may still be relevant to community practice but are unlikely to be relevant to the vastly changed practice of pharmacy in the hospital setting. For this reason, some states have amended their practice acts to include a section specifically covering hospital pharmacy. Other states have passed hospital pharmacy practice acts that stand independently of the pharmacy practice acts. Many states continue to do their best to regulate a type of practice that their enabling legislation does not accurately describe, however.

The court in *Missouri Hospital Association v. Missouri Department of Consumer Affairs*, 731 S.W.2d 262 (Mo. Ct. App. 1987), affirmed a lower court decision in which it was held that the state board of pharmacy had no authority to promulgate rules and regulations relating to in-hospital dispensing of drugs. The court held that the state's pharmacy practice act permitted the board of pharmacy to regulate only pharmacists and community pharmacies and that the authority to regulate hospital pharmacies resided with the state department of health. Although this approach is extreme and may be valid in only a few states, it illustrates the problem that pharmacy boards may face in their efforts to regulate hospital practice. In the absence of specific statutory authority, there is at least some question as to whether state boards may regulate hospital pharmacy practice.

In addition to the issues affecting the licensure of a hospital pharmacy, some issues may arise regarding the licensure of hospital pharmacy personnel. For example, the court in *Sheffield v. State Education Department*, 571 N.Y.S.2d 350 (N.Y. App. Div. 1991), reviewed allegations that a hospital and the hospital's director of pharmacy had illegally permitted persons without pharmacy licenses (in this case, nurses) to compound and dispense medications, including hyperalimentation solutions and intravenous solutions. The hospital, the director of pharmacy, and two nurses were censured, reprimanded, and required to pay a fine.

The hospital pointed out that the nursing practice in question had been going on in the hospital for more than 25 years. In the court's opinion, however, it was permissible for nurses to compound solutions that they themselves administered to patients but not solutions that other nurses administered to patients. The court deemed this latter function to be dispensing, a function that is reserved to the practice of pharmacy. The appellate court affirmed the disciplinary action, emphasizing the distinction between the role of pharmacists and the role of nurses in the institutional setting.

In some hospitals it may not be practical to have a pharmacist in the pharmacy at all times, especially when the pharmacist is performing clinical roles such as making rounds with prescribers; reviewing patient charts; and consulting with prescribers, nurses, and patients. As a result, some states have enacted laws allowing one technician to check another technician's work, rather than a pharmacist. The checking technician generally

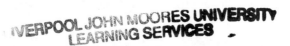

is required to have some type of advanced education or training. Generally, the hospital may only employ a tech-check-tech system if the hospital utilizes its pharmacists in a clinical capacity. Accountability and liability generally fall upon the supervising pharmacist, and because of this, some pharmacists are understandably reluctant to support the practice. Primarily for this reason, tech check tech has not gained approval for community pharmacy practice.

STATE REGULATION OF LONG-TERM CARE

In addition to comprehensive federal regulation, states also extensively regulate long-term care. States may, for example, separately license or issue permits to businesses that wish to operate pharmacies in long-term care facilities. Pharmacists who wish to practice as consultants to long-term care facilities may be required to obtain a specialty license in addition to their pharmacy license. For example, in Florida, a pharmacist who wishes to be employed as a consultant to a long-term care facility must show evidence of special education and experience to become certified as a consultant-pharmacist. Periodic recertification requires continuing education involving specific subjects.

The provision of pharmaceutical care products and services to long-term care facilities has led to legal problems for pharmacists. *Odell v. Axelrod*, 483 N.Y.S.2d 770 (N.Y. App. Div. 1984), affirmed the assessment of a $13,000 fine against a pharmacist who had refilled oral prescriptions without obtaining written authorizations from the prescribing practitioners. Apparently this violation refers to the need to obtain a hard-copy prescription for a schedule II prescription every 60 days. The fact that all but two of the 160 violations involved prescriptions for patients in a nursing home did not permit the conclusion that the violations were insignificant. Although one can understand that a pharmacist would be less concerned with formalities of prescription orders for patients who are essentially institutionalized and for whom drug diversion is probably not as great a problem as it is for patients who present prescriptions at a pharmacy counter, it is easy to understand the court's view that a state's drug abuse prevention program must have the cooperation of pharmacists if it is to be successful. Because of the key role they play in distributing controlled substances, a pharmacist's indifference to legal requirements respecting schedule II controlled substances cannot be tolerated. Rules are not suspended simply because a patient resides in a long-term care facility.

A similar problem arose in Colorado and is described in *Fink v. State Board of Pharmacy*, 515 P.2d 477 (Colo. Ct. App. 1973). A pharmacist's license was suspended for distributing to long-term care facilities a prescription drug without a physician's prescription. The drug was called Virac and was thought to be useful in the treatment of bed sores. For a pharmacist to provide a product of this type is assistance with nursing care, rather than medical care, so it is easy to see how a pharmacist might believe that a nurse could authorize acquisition of the drug. The bottles of the product received by the pharmacist from the manufacturer did not have the federal legend printed on them; thus the pharmacist believed the product to be available without a prescription. Standard pharmacy references available to the pharmacist indicated the prescription-only nature of the product, but the pharmacist did not consult these references. Unfortunately for the pharmacist, evidence revealed that even after he received firm evidence that Virac was not an over-the-counter product, he continued providing it to the long-term care facility without a physician's prescription. The court was unsympathetic with the pharmacist's argument that the status of Virac was confusing. Suspension of the pharmacist's license was affirmed. This case again illustrates the need to avoid becoming too relaxed in dealings with long-term care facilities. Although strong relationships with nursing staff may develop, it is important to remember that the law imposes absolute requirements for a prescription when a legend drug is used on a patient.

STATE REGULATION OF THIRD-PARTY PLANS

Few developments have had as great an economic impact on pharmacy or created more concern among pharmacists as have third-party prescription (managed care) programs. Nationally, the percentage of third-party prescriptions dispensed has rocketed to where the majority of prescriptions dispensed in many areas of the country are third party. A third-party prescription plan is any program in which someone other than the patient receiving the medication pays for all or part of the medication. Today almost all third-party plans are managed care plans, meaning that the plan intervenes in the delivery and reimbursement of services with the intent to reduce costs and unnecessary or inappropriate care. Entities that manage prescription drug services are called prescription benefit managers (PBMs). The patient in a third-party plan is called a beneficiary, an enrollee, or the insured.

Since their inception in the United States in the late 1950s, third-party prescription programs have been the subject of legal and legislative scrutiny. Initially, pharmacists formed and controlled the plans, selling both the insurance and the products and services. The Federal Trade Commission (FTC), however, contended that this relationship could lead to price fixing and threatened legal action unless pharmacists divorced themselves from ownership—which they did. Once nonpharmacists controlled the plans, pharmacy's problems with third-party plans began. These problems have included inadequate professional fees, inadequate reimbursement of product acquisition costs, unequal negotiating power with the plans, unfair audits, insolvent plans that leave pharmacists holding bad debts, exclusive contracts, and slow payments for submitted claims.

Increasing frustration forced pharmacists to take their plight to Congress, first in 1971 and again in 1973. However, even after extensive hearings, investigations, and congressional recommendations, nothing changed. Not enjoying success with litigation, pharmacists pursued state legislation.

STATE LEGISLATIVE EFFORTS TO REGULATE THIRD-PARTY PLANS

In addition to litigation, frustrated pharmacists lobbied for state legislation to regulate third-party insurance plans and pharmacy agreements. The first such law was passed in 1980 in Georgia. This legislation placed several restrictions on third-party prescription plans. It required plans to

- Reimburse pharmacies on a usual and customary basis
- Pay claims within 30 days
- Enroll any pharmacy that wished to participate in the plan
- Conduct audits according to generally accepted accounting principles

Pharmacists hailed the Georgia law as the solution to many of the inequities caused by third-party plans, and pharmacists in several other states rushed to pass similar laws in their states. Within a year, similar laws had been enacted in seven additional states. Pharmacists in approximately 35 other states were either in the process of lobbying for the law in their state or actively considering the introduction of such legislation. The legislative bandwagon came to a halt, however, because of a federal law that most pharmacists had never heard of at the time—the Employee Retirement Income Security Act (ERISA) (29 U.S.C. §§ 1001–1381).

The Legality of State Third-Party Laws Under the Employee Retirement Income Security Act

In 1974, Congress passed ERISA in response to a growing national concern over widespread abuse in the area of employee benefit and pension plans. The act seeks to protect employees from losing the benefits accrued through service to their employers by setting minimum standards for plan reporting and disclosure, vesting, funding, and fiduciary responsibilities. To accomplish its objectives and establish national uniformity, ERISA specifically preempts any and all state laws that relate to any employee benefit plan, except those regulating insurance, banking, or securities. Furthermore, the act prohibits any state law that directly or indirectly regulates the terms and conditions of employee benefit plans.

In Alabama, pharmacists had lobbied successfully for a third-party law modeled after the Georgia law, but the third-party plans ignored the law. Therefore, pharmacists commenced legal action against Blue Cross and Blue Shield of Alabama to force it to comply with the provisions in the law. Before arguments could be heard, however, the U.S. Supreme Court issued an opinion that greatly hurt the plaintiffs' case. In *Shaw v. Delta Airlines*, 463 U.S. 85 (1983), the Court held that ERISA preempted two New York laws: one forbidding employers to discriminate on the basis of pregnancy and the other requiring employers to pay sick leave. In its decision, the Court took an expansive view of the "relate to" phrase in ERISA, finding that a state law "relates to" an employee benefit plan "if it has a connection with or reference to such a plan" (463 U.S. at 96). Until *Shaw*, lower federal courts had varied considerably in their interpretation of "relate to." In fact, many courts had taken the position that a state law would be preempted only if it materially or substantially affected employee benefit plans. The Supreme Court's decision, in contrast, suggested that a state law would be invalidated if it had even the slightest effect on an employee benefit plan.

The *Shaw* decision was the ammunition that Blue Cross needed to challenge the Alabama law. In *Blue Cross and Blue Shield v. Peacock's Apothecary, Inc.*, 567 F. Supp. 1258 (N.D. Ala. 1983), the federal district court relied on *Shaw* to hold that ERISA preempted the Alabama law. The court concluded that, even though the pharmacy agreements regulated by the law are not employee benefit plans in themselves, they are part of an employee benefit plan. Therefore, because the law regulates what employees and employers can do within an employee benefit plan, it "relates to" the plan and must be preempted.

After *Peacock*, several insurance companies and employers in Georgia challenged the legality of the Georgia third-party law in *General Motors Corporation v. Caldwell*, 647 F. Supp. 585 (N.D. Ga. 1986). The Georgia attorney general defended the law on the ground that it only incidentally related to employee benefit plans and certainly could not "relate to" employee benefit plans in the manner that Congress referred to when it enacted ERISA. The court disagreed, however, and found that the Georgia law did "relate to" ERISA and was preempted insofar as the law affected employee benefit programs. The fact that the law indirectly and only incidentally related to employee benefit plans did not save it from preemption. The court also held that the insurance exemption to ERISA would not save the law because of the *Royal Drug* decision. The *Caldwell* case was not appealed, and all attempts to enact legislation of this type ceased.

Freedom-of-Choice Laws

Alarmed by a trend among third-party plans to engage in exclusive contracting, pharmacists have sought legislation allowing any pharmacy the right to participate. These laws have been called freedom-of-choice or any willing provider laws because they require third-party plans to allow their beneficiaries to choose whichever participating pharmacy they wish to patronize for their goods and services. Moreover, third-party plans may not deny any pharmacy the right to participate in the plan, provided that the pharmacy agrees to the terms and conditions of the contract. Third-party plans have vigorously opposed this legislation, arguing that exclusive contracts increase health care costs. There had always been the question that these freedom-of-choice laws may also violate ERISA, but the U.S. Supreme Court determined otherwise in *Kentucky Ass'n of Health Plans, Inc. v. Miller*, 538 U.S. 329 (2003). The Medicare prescription drug plan enacted in December 2003 (Part D) also contains a freedom-of-choice provision.

REGULATION OF MANAGED CARE PLAN FORMULARIES

Managed-care plans often utilize drug formularies. If the prescribed drug is not on the formulary, pharmacies are often required or given incentives to contact the prescriber to authorize a change to the formulary drug. Many health care providers and consumers believe that some of the managed-care formularies are too cost-containment oriented to the detriment of the quality of patient care.

As a result, many states have enacted legislation requiring managed-care plans to provide complete disclosure to consumers of their formulary policies and procedures and provide the list of drugs on their formularies. Some of the laws provide that if a patient is currently taking a medication, the plan cannot exclude coverage of the medication as long as the prescriber continues to prescribe it. Pharmacy was successful in having some formulary provisions included in the Medicare Part D legislation.

In addition to quality issues, pharmacists have been concerned that managed care plans and PBMs include some drugs on their formularies and exclude others based upon discounts, rebates, and special pricing obtained from manufacturers and other suppliers. The plans and PBMs regard this information as proprietary. Pharmacy organizations contend that the PBMs reap the financial gains while insurers and patients pay higher prices and pharmacies suffer lower reimbursements. As a result, there has been legislative activity at both the state and federal levels to require transparency from the plans and PBMs.

REGULATION FOR OUTCOMES

A health services researcher named Avedis Donabedian is usually given primary credit for the categorization of health care quality measures into the three areas of structure, process, and outcomes. An orientation toward this three-part framework has developed into a trend within health care institutions and health care systems, with emphasis being placed on outcomes as the most important factor because outcomes are a direct measure of health care status. Regulatory agencies have generally not followed this trend but instead have continued to focus solely on structure and process. Most regulatory agencies have not yet devised strategies to monitor outcomes, despite widespread recognition in the health care industry that outcomes are more reliable indicators of quality than are structure or process. Thus, the possibility exists that the responsibility to ensure health care quality will shift from government agencies to private health care institutions and health care systems, if government agencies continue to choose regulatory strategies that are not oriented toward health care outcomes.

If they are to continue their prominent role in pharmacy regulation, it is important for state boards of pharmacy to adopt policies aimed toward pharmaceutical care outcomes regulation. This is not to suggest that regulation of structure and process should be abandoned. The importance of outcomes is that they can be linked to particular aspects of structure and process, which can be altered to produce improved outcomes. Correspondingly, the importance of structure and process is that they can be linked with outcomes. The regulator's challenge is to do whatever reasonably can be done to protect the public health. If it is possible to incorporate outcomes into a regulatory approach that already includes structure and process, it would seem necessary to do so as a measure to protect the public health.

STRUCTURE, PROCESS, AND OUTCOMES

When people in the health care industry refer to "outcomes," reference is being made to changes in a patient's health status that result from the provision of health care. The most obvious outcomes are mortality and morbidity. Other important outcomes are disability, discomfort, and dissatisfaction. Sometimes it is not possible to directly measure outcomes, and "proxy" measures are used to indirectly assess outcomes. Examples in pharmacy of directly measured outcomes would be adverse drug reactions, patient dissatisfaction, and diminished quality of life. Proxy outcome measures could include the rate of medication-related emergency department visits or blood pressure readings of hypertensive patients.

"Structure," on the other hand, refers to the characteristics of the setting in which care is provided. The resources (e.g., personnel, computers, equipment) that are available to provide care and the policies in place through which resources are used would be structural measures of quality. In pharmacy, structure would include the ratio of pharmacists to technicians and the completeness of a pharmacy's inventory.

Measurements of "process" would relate to what is actually done with available resources in providing care. The number of patients counseled by a pharmacist or the number of contacts with prescribers regarding potential problems would be process measures. Patient compliance and laboratory values also are usually considered to be process measures, but under some circumstances they might be regarded as proxy outcomes measures.

AN ALTERNATIVE APPROACH TO REGULATION

Pharmacists strive to attain the ability to practice competently, and regulators assess competence (at least initially) to ensure that those who enter the profession are capable of doing it well, yet the potential for doing well is not sufficient for a successful pharmacy practice. One must actually do things well to be considered a success in pharmacy, and regulators have a responsibility to ensure that pharmacists are realizing their potential for success. A pharmacist who is quite capable, but who produces bad results through lack of effort, is not a competent professional. Likewise, the pharmacist who exerts maximal effort, but who simply does not have the requisite ability, can generate unacceptable results. To ensure that the public health is being protected, pharmacy regulators must concentrate on results themselves rather than on the potential for results demonstrated solely by capability or by effort.

The structure-process-outcomes framework relies on the premise that good structure leads to a more appropriate process that promotes better outcomes. A pharmacy that has good structural components and good processes, but produces unsatisfactory outcomes, is inadequate and a threat to the public health. For example, if technicians are properly certified and ointment slabs are readily available if necessary—in fact, if all personnel and equipment requirements are being addressed adequately—this will not be good enough if patients who use the pharmacy are having preventable adverse drug reactions. Regulators may wish to take a hard look at such a pharmacy, despite its apparent compliance with structure and process requirements. Perhaps things are not really as good as they look. On the other hand, if patients at a pharmacy are consistently getting well and are quite satisfied with their care, regulators may wish to be flexible in their evaluation, even if the pharmacy's structure and processes vary somewhat from the standard. Things may not really be so bad. The pharmacy might, for example, be violating a structural rule that requires a pharmacy to be open for business at least 60 hours per week because the pharmacist routinely rounds at the local hospital and makes house calls in the afternoon. The public health may be well served in such a pharmacy.

State boards of pharmacy have many challenges to face in the coming years. One such challenge is the shift to outcomes-oriented health care. Managed care organizations and certification groups have already begun to adopt regulatory measures that are oriented to outcomes and threaten to supersede most activities of the state board of pharmacy.

CONTINUOUS QUALITY IMPROVEMENT PROGRAMS

The shift to outcomes-oriented health care in pharmacy has commenced in some states that have enacted continuous quality improvement (CQI) laws. First Florida, then California, then several other states passed laws mandating that pharmacies must develop and maintain incident reporting systems. Under this system errors must be recorded, investigated, and acted upon. Pharmacies must use the recorded errors to evaluate their dispensing systems in light of determining why the error occurred and how the system can be changed to reduce the probability that this type of error will reoccur. Other states have now passed similar CQI laws. Only North Carolina requires that a pharmacy actually report the error to the state pharmacy board, and then only if the error could have caused or contributed to the death of a patient.

Pharmacies and pharmacists have hesitated to record errors for fear of exposure to negligence liability and fear of disciplinary action by state pharmacy boards. However, states that have enacted CQI laws have included provisions that protect these records from discovery in negligence actions. Moreover, state pharmacy boards have assured pharmacies that they would not use CQI records punitively. Even in states that have not enacted pharmacy CQI laws, pharmacies can still voluntarily engage in a CQI program with protection from discovery by forming a patient safety organization (PSO) pursuant to the Patient Safety and Quality Improvement Act of 2005. It is one thing, however, to legislate that pharmacies have CQI programs and another that pharmacies actually comply. Many state boards of pharmacy do not have the resources to ensure that pharmacies are correctly and effectively utilizing a CQI. As a result, NABP is actively investigating the implementation of a national accreditation program that would establish uniform standards pharmacies must achieve, and provide state boards with resources and a system of measurement to ensure pharmacies are meeting the standards. CQI laws directed at error prevention, however, must only be the beginning. Eventually the focus on outcomes must more broadly include the role of the pharmacy and its pharmacists in improving the health of its patients, not just preventing errors.

STUDY SCENARIOS AND QUESTIONS

1. Ben, a pharmacist in the state of Mordor, set up an office where he provides medication therapy consultations to patients for an hourly fee. Ben neither stocks nor dispenses any drugs. Some on the Mordor Board of Pharmacy feel that Ben should only be able to perform these professional functions through a licensed pharmacy. (The definition of a pharmacy in Mordor is a place where dangerous drugs are stored and furnished at retail.) Some others on the board feel that the definition of a pharmacy must be changed to include places where pharmacy is practiced, such as Ben's office. Others on the board are confident that enough regulatory control exists over Ben's pharmacist license that changing the definition of a pharmacy or requiring Ben to practice out of a traditional licensed pharmacy is not necessary.

   a. Explain the pros and cons of each of the three positions.

   b. What if Ben failed to maintain adequate patient records, kept an unsanitary office, and failed to comply with HIPAA? Explain whether the board has sufficient regulatory authority over Ben if he were not licensed as a pharmacy.

   c. Explain whether Ben is practicing pharmacy pursuant to the definition of pharmacy in your state.

   d. What if Ben, instead of having an office in Mordor, had an Internet consulting practice in another state and provided careless and incompetent advice to a Mordor patient. How would the Mordor Board of Pharmacy be able to discipline Ben if he was not a licensed pharmacist in Mordor? Would the board of pharmacy in your state under its present laws have the authority to discipline Ben? Explain.

2. Billy is a pharmacist at Main Street Pharmacy, and Sue is the pharmacist-in-charge. A routine inspection by a state pharmacy board inspector revealed that Billy had been refilling certain patients' prescriptions without authorization and without Sue's knowledge. State law provides that the pharmacist-in-charge is responsible for any violations of the pharmacy laws and regulations. Therefore, the board of pharmacy found both Sue and Billy in violation of the law, fined each one several hundred dollars, and placed each on probation. Several pharmacists complained to the board that what the board did to Sue was unfair. They argued that the law is unconstitutional because it punishes one for the acts of someone else without having knowledge of the other person's illegal acts. If you were a board of pharmacy member, how would you respond to the pharmacists' complaints? Why have such a law? Is the law unfair?

3. Jim is a pharmacist who works for a chain in a large city. Jim developed a business that illegally solicited bets on sporting events. Jim promoted this to patients, and several patients would place bets with Jim while getting their prescriptions filled. Jim profited handsomely from this business until he was ultimately caught. Because the search by the officers was illegal, however, Jim's criminal case was dismissed. Nonetheless, the state board of pharmacy brought a licensure hearing against Jim and revoked his license based upon unprofessional conduct charges. Jim challenged the board's decision in court, arguing that the state statute does not specify that what he did was unprofessional conduct. Therefore, he argued, his constitutional due process rights were violated because he could not know that what he did was unprofessional conduct.

   Take both sides of this argument. Is it unfair to revoke Jim's license on the basis of a vague charge like unprofessional conduct? Assuming it is not unfair, is Jim's illegal act unprofessional conduct? Why or why not?

BIBLIOGRAPHY

Abood, R. Discretionary justice and state boards of pharmacy. *Contemporary Pharmacy Practice* 5 (1982): 250.

Brushwood, D. Regulating for pharmaceutical care outcomes. *Journal of the American Pharmacy Association* 38 (1998): 524–526.

Duckworth, F. The potential liability of pharmacists arising from announcements of new standards and codes of practice. *Food Drug Cosmetic Law Journal* 43 (1988): 1.

Munger, M., et al. Professional liability for pharmacists: A focus on pharmacy practice acts. *Drug Intelligence and Clinical Pharmacy* 22 (1988): 886.

Murtaugh, P. Unprofessional or immoral conduct: License revocation and professional discipline of pharmacists. *Journal of Legal Medicine* 4 (1983): 525.

National Association of Boards of Pharmacy. Available at: http://www.nabp.net

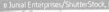

CASE STUDIES

CASE 7-1	*Virginia State Board of Pharmacy v. Virginia Citizens Consumer Council, Inc.,* 425 U.S. 748 (1976)

Issue

Whether a board of pharmacy rule declaring it unprofessional conduct for a pharmacist to advertise the prices of prescription drugs is valid under the "commercial speech" protection provided by the Constitution of the United States of America.

Overview

In any self-regulating profession, there is always a question of whether the regulations enacted by the group to govern itself are really intended to protect the public or are instead intended to protect the profession. This "fox guarding the hen house" issue has plagued pharmacy regulators since boards of pharmacy were first established for the sole purpose of protecting the public health from unsafe pharmacy practices. The history of self-regulation in pharmacy includes several unfortunate episodes of economically driven rules that were intended to protect the finances of pharmacists rather than the health of the public. In this case, one such rule is reviewed. It is a rule from the state of Virginia that forbade pharmacists to advertise price information. As you read this case, make a list of the benefits of such a rule from a public health perspective and also list the ulterior motives for such a rule that may perhaps have been the "hidden agenda" of the profession. Evaluate the entries on the list in terms of their relationship to the public health. Ask yourself whether the list weighs more heavily in favor of the regulation or against the regulation from your perspective within the pharmacy profession. What might you expect to be the public perception of this list? Are there any rules that protect the public health and also promote the profession that would be considered appropriate for a self-regulating group? If so, what are those rules?

The court began its analysis by describing the law that was being challenged as unconstitutional:

> The plaintiffs in this case attack, as violative of the First and Fourteenth Amendments, that portion of [Virginia law] which provides that a pharmacist licensed in Virginia is guilty of unprofessional conduct if he "publishes, advertises, or promotes, directly or indirectly, in any manner whatsoever, any amount, price, fee, premium, discount, rebate, or credit terms . . . for any drugs which may be dispensed only by prescription."

The court then provided a background discussion of the nature of the practice of pharmacy and the role of the board of pharmacy through a review of state laws and other sources of authority.

> The "practice of pharmacy" is statutorily declared to be "a professional practice affecting the public health, safety, and welfare," and to be "subject to regulation and

control in the public interest." Indeed, the practice is subject to extensive regulation aimed at preserving high professional standards. The regulatory body is the appellant Virginia State Board of Pharmacy. The Board is broadly charged by statute with various responsibilities, including the "maintenance of the quality, quantity, integrity, safety, and efficacy of drugs or devices distributed, dispensed, or administered." It also is to concern itself with "maintaining the integrity of, and public confidence in, the profession and improving the delivery of quality pharmaceutical services to the citizens of Virginia." The Board is empowered to "make such bylaws, rules, and regulations . . . as may be necessary for the lawful exercise of its powers."

The Board is also the licensing authority. It may issue a license, necessary for the practice of pharmacy in the State, only upon evidence that the applicant is "of good moral character," is a graduate in pharmacy of a school approved by the Board, and has had "a suitable period of experience [the period required not to exceed 12 months] acceptable to the Board." The applicant must pass the examination prescribed by the Board. One approved school is the School of Pharmacy of the Medical College of Virginia, where the curriculum is for 3 years following 2 years of college. Prescribed prepharmacy courses, such as biology and chemistry, are to be taken in college, and study requirements at the school itself include courses in organic chemistry, biochemistry, comparative anatomy, physiology, and pharmacology. Students are also trained in the ethics of the profession, and there is some clinical experience in the school's hospital pharmacies and in the medical center operated by the Medical College. This is "a rigid, demanding curriculum in terms of what the pharmacy student is expected to know about drugs."

Once licensed, a pharmacist is subject to a civil monetary penalty, or to revocation or suspension of his license, if the Board finds that he "is not of good moral character," or has violated any of a number of stated professional standards (among them that he not be "negligent in the practice of pharmacy" or have engaged in "fraud or deceit upon the consumer . . . in connection with the practice of pharmacy"), or is guilty of "unprofessional conduct." "Unprofessional conduct" is specifically, the third numbered phrase of which relates to advertising of the price for any prescription drug, and is the subject of this litigation.

Inasmuch as only a licensed pharmacist may dispense prescription drugs in Virginia, advertising or other affirmative dissemination of prescription drug price information is effectively forbidden in the State. Some pharmacies refuse even to quote prescription drug prices over the telephone. The Board's position, however, is that this would not constitute an unprofessional publication. It is clear, nonetheless, that all advertising of such prices, in the normal sense, is forbidden. The prohibition does not extend to nonprescription drugs, but neither is it confined to prescriptions that the pharmacist compounds himself. Indeed, about 95% of all prescriptions now are filled with dosage forms prepared by the pharmaceutical manufacturer.

The court reviewed a number of reasons for removing the ban against advertising of pharmaceuticals.

The plaintiffs are an individual Virginia resident who suffers from diseases that require her to take prescription drugs on a daily basis, and two nonprofit organizations. Their claim is that the First Amendment entitles the user of prescription drugs to receive information that pharmacists wish to communicate to them through advertising and other promotional means, concerning the prices of such drugs.

Certainly that information may be of value. Drug prices in Virginia, for both prescription and nonprescription items, strikingly vary from outlet to outlet even within the same locality. It is stipulated, for example, that in Richmond "the cost of 40 Achromycin tablets ranges from $2.59 to $6.00, a difference of 140%," and that in the Newport News-Hampton area the cost of tetracycline ranges from $1.20 to $9.00, a difference of 650%.

Our pharmacist does not wish to editorialize on any subject, cultural, philosophical, or political. He does not wish to report any particularly newsworthy fact, or to make generalized observations even about commercial matters. The "idea" he wishes to communicate is simply this: "I will sell you the X prescription drug at the Y price." Our question, then, is whether this communication is wholly outside the protection of the First Amendment.

As to the particular consumer's interest in the free flow of commercial information, that interest may be as keen, if not keener by far, than his interest in the day's most urgent political debate. Appellees' case in this respect is a convincing one. Those whom the suppression of prescription drug price information hits the hardest are the poor, the sick, and particularly the aged. A disproportionate amount of their income tends to be spent on prescription drugs; yet they are the least able to learn, by shopping from pharmacist to pharmacist, where their scarce dollars are best spent. When drug prices vary as strikingly as they do, information as to who is charging what becomes more than a convenience. It could mean the alleviation of physical pain or the enjoyment of basic necessities.

The court then turned to a description of the reasons justifying a departure from a standard that would forbid advertising by pharmacists.

Arrayed against these substantial individual and societal interests are a number of justifications for the advertising ban. These have to do principally with maintaining a high degree of professionalism on the part of licensed pharmacists. Indisputably, the State has a strong interest in maintaining that professionalism. It is exercised in a number of ways for the consumer's benefit. There is the clinical skill involved in the compounding of drugs, although, as has been noted, these now make up only a small percentage of the prescriptions filled. Yet, even in respect to manufacturer prepared compounds, there is room for the pharmacist to serve his customer well or badly. Drugs kept too long on the shelf may lose their efficacy or become adulterated. They can be packaged for the user in such a way that the same results occur. The expertise of the pharmacist may supplement that of the prescribing physician, if the latter has not specified the amount to be dispensed or the directions that are to appear on the label. The pharmacist, a specialist in the potencies and dangers of drugs, may even be consulted by the physician as to what to prescribe. He may know of a particular antagonism between the prescribed drug and another that the customer is or might be taking, or with an allergy the customer may suffer. The pharmacist himself may have supplied the other drug or treated the allergy. Some pharmacists, concededly not a large number, "monitor" the health problems and drug consumptions of customers who come to them repeatedly. A pharmacist who has a continuous relationship with his customer is in the best position, of course, to exert professional skill for the customer's protection.

The court then provided its final analysis and holding, which favored a change in the rules to permit price advertising by pharmacists.

It appears to be feared that if the pharmacist who wishes to provide low cost, and assertedly low quality, services is permitted to advertise, he will be taken up on his offer by too many unwitting customers. They will choose the low-cost, low-quality service and drive the "professional" pharmacist out of business. They will respond only to costly and excessive advertising, and end up paying the price. They will go from one pharmacist to another, following the discount, and destroy the pharmacist-customer relationship. They will lose respect for the profession because it advertises. All this is not in their best interests, and all this can be avoided if they are not permitted to know who is charging what. There is, of course, an alternative to this highly paternalistic approach. That alternative is to assume that this information is not in itself harmful, that people will perceive their own best interests if only they are well enough informed, and that the best means to that end is to open the channels of communication rather than to close them. If they are truly open, nothing prevents the "professional" pharmacist from marketing his own assertedly superior product, and contrasting it with that of the low-cost, high-volume prescription drug retailer. But the choice among these alternative approaches is not ours to make or the Virginia General Assembly's. It is precisely this kind of choice, between the dangers of suppressing information, and the dangers of its misuse if it is freely available, that the First Amendment makes for us. Virginia is free to require whatever professional standards it wishes of its pharmacists; it may subsidize them or protect them from competition in other ways. But it may not do so by keeping the public in ignorance of the entirely lawful terms that competing pharmacists are offering.

In this sense, the justifications Virginia has offered for suppressing the flow of prescription drug price information, far from persuading us that the flow is not protected by the First Amendment, have reinforced our view that it is. We so hold.

Notes on *Virginia State Board of Pharmacy v. Virginia Consumer Citizens Council, Inc.*

1. This case was the first case from the Supreme Court of the United States to rule on the issue of professional advertising. Before this case, it was virtually unheard of for a professional person to advertise services. Of course, today lawyers, physicians, accountants, and others are all free to advertise. Their advertisements must be truthful, but beyond that relatively basic requirement there is little regulation to limit the advertising done by professionals. Whether the modern view of permitting professional advertising, or the more traditional view of prohibiting professional advertising, is the better view really depends on the preferences of each individual.

2. The court refers to the "highly paternalistic approach" of withholding information from patients on the basis of the fear that patients will misuse that information. In health care, paternalism is benevolent action by a health care provider that either fails to consider the interests of a patient or disregards the expressed interests of a patient. State paternalism is government action that does essentially the same thing. The court obviously, in this case, believed that suppressing the flow of information did more harm than good. It is difficult to argue with this result. One of the cornerstone principles of American democracy is freedom of speech. As long as nobody is being harmed by the speech of an individual, that individual is pretty much free to say what she or he wishes. In this case, the court concluded that the harm done, if there was any at all, was inconsequential when compared with the profound importance of the freedom of speech principle.

3. It was this case in which an early version of the opinion contained language in which it was said that a pharmacist no more performs a true professional service than does a law clerk who retrieves books for a lawyer. That language was removed from the official opinion when it was later published in its permanent form, but memories of the insult linger to this day in the pharmacy profession. A significant issue was made of the Supreme Court's failure to understand the important clinical role of the practicing pharmacist. However, the opinion contains language that does refer to that role, and the overreaction to the language is perhaps a result of "kill the messenger" thinking. Much of what the court had to say as gentle criticism of the pharmacy profession is difficult to refute.

| CASE 7-2 | In the Matter of *CVS Pharmacy Wayne*, 561 A.2d 1160 (NJ. 1989) |

Issue

Whether a New Jersey state law forbidding discounts or rebates by a pharmacist is unconstitutional.

Overview

In this case, the issue was similar to that of the Virginia case previously discussed, but the facts and arguments were sufficiently different to produce a different result. This case reports a challenge to the constitutionality of a New Jersey law that classified as "grossly unprofessional conduct" any offer by a pharmacist to provide discounts or rebates on the sale of drugs or medications. As you read this case, ask yourself how the case differs, if it does, from the preceding Virginia case. What issues in this case differ from the issues in that case? How do the arguments in this case differ from the arguments in that case?

The court began by describing the factual basis of the case:

> In March 1985, Consumer Value Stores (CVS), a chain of retail pharmacies operating in New Jersey, distributed mail circulars for its stores in Wayne, New Jersey, advertising a special one-week $3.00 price for the vast majority of its prescription drugs. The advertisement read: "Prescription Savings. This price valid at both CVS Pharmacy Wayne stores only. All prescriptions $3.00, Saturday, March 23 through Saturday, March 30, 1985." For most drugs, the advertised price was less than the regular price for the drugs; in many instances, the price was less than the cost to CVS.

> The Board subsequently issued a penalty letter to respondent, Timothy Brophy, the resident pharmacist of a CVS drug store in Wayne, charging him with violating [New Jersey law]. The statute provides that it is "grossly unprofessional conduct" for a pharmacist to engage in the distribution of premiums or rebates of any kind whatever in connection with the sale of drugs and medications provided, however, that trading stamps and similar devices shall not be considered to be rebates for the purposes of this chapter and provided further that discounts, premiums, and rebates may be provided in connection with the sale of drugs and medications to any person who is 62 years of age or older.

> Here, the decision to advertise the discounted prices had been made not by respondent but by the CVS corporate management. As the pharmacist in charge, however, respondent was responsible for any advertising by the pharmacy.

The court then described the retail pharmacy marketplace and the conflict that had arisen between the defendant in this case and the board of pharmacy.

> In recent years, as local drug stores and large chains have battled in the marketplace, the Legislature and the Board have sought to maintain the quality of pharmaceutical services. One device for protecting public health is the requirement that pharmacists keep records of drugs purchased by patients through a "patient profile." The underlying thought is that by recourse to the patient profile, a pharmacist can prevent a customer from taking incompatible drugs.

> For several years, CVS and respondent have vigorously challenged the statute on various grounds. In the present case, the Board believes that the legislative purpose behind N.J.S.A. 45:14-12 will be defeated by pricing practices that encourage customers to buy drugs at whatever pharmacy happens to be selling them at the cheapest price that week. CVS, however, believes a 1-week price reduction is in not only its interest but also that of the public. Deprecating the goal of patient monitoring, CVS points to the fact that the statute permits the offer of discount prices to senior citizens.

To this, the Board rejoins that the Legislature may respond to the needs of different segments of the public in various ways. The Board also points out that the Legislature has tried to help people over the age of 62 by providing State funds to limit the cost of prescription drugs through the Pharmaceutical Assistance to the Aged program. According to the Board, the Legislature may recognize, as it has recognized in the PAA program, that for senior citizens, cost is the dispositive concern. For the general population, the Legislature could decide that patient monitoring is the dominant consideration. The Board also maintains that the statute prevents price wars that would reduce the number of pharmacies and adversely affect pharmaceutical services and professional standards. Our analysis proceeds in light of the constant, albeit sometimes conflicting, goals of the Legislature and Board to maintain the quality of pharmaceutical services in a changing market.

The court then proceeded to an analysis of the price control statute it was being asked to examine. The court took care not to challenge the authority of the legislature in this area of regulation but to determine whether the legislature had acted consistent with its authority.

The presumed validity of price-control statutes, such as the present one, can be overcome only "by proofs that preclude the possibility that there could have been any set of facts known to the legislative body or which could reasonably be assumed to have been known which would rationally support a conclusion that the enactment is in the public interest." Even if a court cannot ascertain the actual purpose of the statute, it should sustain the statute if it has any conceivable rational purpose. The judicial task is not to question the wisdom of the legislative decision but to ascertain whether the statute is rationally related to the public health, safety, or welfare. Similarly, courts should approve the means selected by the Legislature to achieve its purposes unless those means are so irrelevant as to be irrational.

For a statute to be rationally related to the public interest, it need not be the best or only method of achieving the legislative purpose. So viewed, we cannot say that N.J.S.A. 45:14-12 is an irrational response to the goal of patient monitoring. Given the deference we are obliged to accord to an act of the Legislature, we likewise conclude that body could have determined that the statute is an effective means of preventing destructive price wars that could adversely affect pharmaceutical services and professional standards.

We also find the exemption for senior citizens to be a reasonable legislative response to economic pressure on the elderly. To some extent, moreover, the effect of the exemption on senior citizens is diluted because of the PAA program, under which those citizens can purchase drugs by making a $2.00 co-payment. According to the Department of Human Services, 246,693 senior citizens were eligible for the program in fiscal year 1988. Because their co-payment is limited to $2.00, discounts for them are unnecessary.

Nor do we find that the statute is an unwarranted exercise in economic protectionism. Nothing in the record suggests that the statute puts any particular group at a competitive disadvantage. Even if the Legislature was moved in part by a desire to accord some degree of economic protection to individual pharmacists, that purpose need not invalidate an otherwise valid statute. As long as the statute has one valid purpose, we are obliged to sustain it.

The court addressed an argument raised by the defendant, in which the defendant had contended it was inconsistent for the law to encourage the use of generic drug products and also to forbid the use of discounts or rebates. The court also responded to the defendant's contention that it was unfair to single out senior citizens as a group to which the prohibition on discounts and rebates was not applied.

We find to be irrelevant respondent's contention that the objectives of N.J.S.A. 45:14-12 are undermined by legislative encouragement to use generic drugs and to advertise prescription drug prices. Nothing in the record would justify the conclusion that the obligation to inform a customer of generic drugs prevents patient monitoring or promotes price wars. The customer who is offered the option of purchasing generic drugs still deals with the same pharmacist. That pharmacist merely offers a lower-priced alternative within his or her drug store. Price advertising simply informs a consumer of the price for prescriptions at a specific pharmacy. Neither practice presents the same threat to the maintenance of a patient profile as short-term price cuts.

We find no merit in respondent's argument that the senior citizen exemption violates the equal protection rights of citizens under age 62. Here, the asserted right is that of a person under age 62 to purchase drugs at a discount. No matter how appealing that right may be to consumers, it does not rise to a constitutional level. Furthermore, the statute restricts the ability to purchase prescriptions only to the extent of preventing discounts, manifested here by sharp reductions for 1 week. According to the Board, the public needs the restriction for pharmacists to monitor the use of prescription drugs by their customers. So viewed, we cannot find that the statute violates the equal protection principles of the State Constitution.

In drawing distinctions, the Legislature need not proceed with mathematical precision. As long as the legislative classification is rational, it is irrelevant that it is not the wisest or the fairest alternative, or one we might choose. So viewed, we find that the Legislature could distinguish between people over and under age 62. The statute not only prevents people under 62 from shifting from pharmacy to pharmacy but also prevents potentially destructive price wars that could erode the integrity of pharmaceutical services.

Notes on In the Matter of *CVS Pharmacy Wayne*

1. One of the most significant differences between this case and the first case is that the issue of freedom of speech was fundamental to the Virginia case but not at all addressed in the New Jersey case. The constitutional issue addressed in this case was "equal protection." Under the Constitution, citizens are entitled to equal protection under the laws. The challengers to the "no rebates" rule contended that the senior citizen exemption violated the equal protection rights of citizens under the age of 62. The court's analysis of this argument required that it first recognize that persons under the age of 62 are not members of a so-called suspect class of persons who are frequently subject to discrimination. The court was required to determine whether there was a "rational basis" for the distinction between those older than and younger than 62. The court concluded that there was such a rational basis because the "no rebates" rule was rationally related to the legislative goals of patient monitoring and the maintenance of pharmaceutical services and professional standards.

2. This case illustrates the possibilities for economically oriented pharmacy regulation that is legitimate because it protects the public health. Even though the rule that was challenged in this case was clearly one that provided an economic advantage to some pharmacies, the overriding benefit of public health protection justified the rule. Profit is not a dirty word. Pharmacists can make money by protecting the public health, and there is nothing shameful in that. In fact, it is hard to provide high-quality pharmaceutical products and services when one is about to go out of business.

3. The facts of this case may have been significant in producing the result of the case. It is quite clear that to offer to fill any prescription for $3.00 for a 1-week period only is an invitation that will result in some people switching their pharmacy

provider for a brief period of time only. This fact may have made it easy for the court to be sympathetic with the argument that the ability to monitor patients' drug therapy would be impaired. Had the offer been more likely to result in a long-term switch of providers, rather than a brief switch, this would perhaps not have been the case. It is not impossible to imagine that pharmacies would take turns being the $3.00 pharmacy of the week, resulting in patients switching each week to take advantage of the weekly special. Such a result would clearly not be consistent with public health protection.

CASE 7-3   In the Matter of *Sobel v. Board of Pharmacy, 882 P.2d 606* (Or. App. 1994)

Issue

Whether a pharmacist may reciprocate a professional license from one state to another, despite a record of disciplinary action in the state from which transfer is being attempted.

Overview

Pharmacists may become licensed in all states by simply transferring their license from another state. This process of license transfer, known as either "reciprocity" or "endorsement" in most states, is designed to remove the burdensome requirement of taking the same board of pharmacy examination (NAPLEX) over again when one moves from one state to another. However, the license transfer methods are not intended as a means to permit pharmacists who are subject to disciplinary action in one state to escape their discipline in that state simply by moving to another state. If that were permitted, discipline would mean little. A pharmacist could break numerous laws in one state, thumb his or her nose at the law, and skip to another state. To stop this, states restrict license transfer to those who have no problems practicing in the state from which they wish to move. In this case, the pharmacist claimed that he had a right to be licensed in Oregon on the basis of his license in Texas. As you read this case, ask yourself whether the pharmacist has been fully truthful with the Oregon Board of Pharmacy. What might the implications be of a pharmacist who is less than truthful in an application for a pharmacy license? Is practicing pharmacy a right or a privilege? Is there a difference between a person who already has a pharmacy license and one who is making application for a license? Does a current licensee have a greater claim to noninterference by government action than does a prospective licensee? In what ways may the public health be protected from license transfer by a pharmacy applicant who would be a bad risk for pharmacy practice in a state?

The court began by describing the process through which one who is licensed in another state would apply for a pharmacy license in the state of Oregon.

To obtain a pharmacist license by reciprocity, an applicant must:

(a) Have submitted a written application in the form prescribed by the board.
(b) Have attained the age of 18 years.
(c) Have good moral character and temperate habits.
(d) Have possessed at the time of initial licensure as a pharmacist such other qualifications necessary to have been eligible for licensure at that time in this state.
(e) Have engaged in the practice of pharmacy for a period of at least 1 year or have met the internship requirements of this state within the 1-year period immediately previous to the date of such application.
(f) Have presented to the board proof of initial licensure by examination and proof that such license and any other license or licenses granted to the applicant by any

other state or states have not been suspended, revoked, canceled, or otherwise restricted for any reason except nonrenewal or the failure to obtain required continuing education credits in any state where the applicant is licensed but not engaged in the practice of pharmacy.

(g) Have successfully passed an examination in jurisprudence given by the board.

(h) Have paid the fees specified by the board for issuance of a license.

[(Oregon law) sets forth the general bases for discipline of a pharmacist, and also provides: "The State Board of Pharmacy may refuse to issue the licenses of any person upon one or more of the following grounds: (f) Fraud or intentional misrepresentation by a licensee or registrant in securing or attempting to secure the issuance or renewal of a license."]

The court then described the facts that were under review for the particular applicant for licensure who brought this lawsuit. The applicant is referred to as the "petitioner" in the language quoted here.

In August 1989, petitioner applied to the Board for licensure by reciprocity. In the section of the application entitled, "Record of Charges, Convictions, and Fines Imposed on Applicant," petitioner stated, "I have not been convicted, fined, disciplined or had my license revoked for violation of pharmacy, liquor, or drug laws, nor am I presently charged with any such violations. I have not been convicted of any felony, nor am I presently charged with the commission of a felony."

A Board investigation revealed that 18 months earlier, on February 23, 1988, the Texas State Board of Pharmacy had entered an "Agreed Board Order," signed by petitioner and his attorney, that disciplined petitioner for violations of the Texas Pharmacy Act and imposed a fine of $1,250. The Board's investigation also revealed a November 7, 1972, report from the Texas Department of Public Safety that documented petitioner's suspensions from pharmaceutical practice for violations of law.

The court then considered the argument by the applicant (the petitioner) that the board of pharmacy should be required to show that he is not competent to practice pharmacy in Oregon. The board had considered it to be the applicant's responsibility to show that he is competent to practice pharmacy in Oregon. The two different perspectives relate to the standard of proof required of the board of pharmacy and the legal significance of a pharmacy license.

We have held that a professional who has been granted a license to practice acquires a right to practice that profession and risks disgrace and loss of livelihood if the license is revoked. Those considerations are absent when the issue is whether to grant a license. In deciding whether to issue a license, the Board of Pharmacy must consider the policy purposes of [Oregon law]: "to promote, preserve, and protect the public health, safety, and welfare by and through the effective control and regulation of the practice of pharmacy," and to ensure "that only qualified persons be permitted to engage in the practice of pharmacy in the State of Oregon." In an application proceeding, it is the applicant who has the burden of establishing eligibility, qualifications, and fitness. Requiring the Board to apply the more rigorous standard of clear and convincing evidence in order to deny a license on the grounds of fraud or misrepresentation would undermine the statutory goal of ensuring that only qualified persons be permitted to practice pharmacy in Oregon.

Notes on In the Matter of *Sobel v. Board of Pharmacy*

1. The process of license transfer known as reciprocity recognizes that the United States is no longer a small group of isolated states, and people no longer live their entire lives where they and their parents were born. We are a mobile society,

and the option of moving from one state to another to practice pharmacy is a realistic possibility for most pharmacists. Because the test that is taken to show competence is NAPLEX in all states, it makes sense that the states would permit reciprocity of license. Some states require that a pharmacist have actively practiced for a period of time before transferring to a state; other states may require that a pharmacist have passed NAPLEX within a certain number of years before making application for licensure by reciprocity.

2. In this case, the pharmacist was almost certainly aware of his disciplinary action in Texas and should have reported that on the application he filed with Oregon. The pharmacist tried the old "I forgot" trick, and it did not work. Discipline by the board of pharmacy is something one cannot, and should not, forget. The pharmacist was denied an Oregon pharmacy license on the basis of his failure to be truthful in his application, not on the basis of the underlying violation that caused his problem in Texas. This is a hard lesson to learn, but it is important for pharmacists to realize that honesty is always the best policy.

3. The law in Oregon permits administrative action against a current pharmacy licensee only when a violation can be shown to be based on "clear and convincing evidence." This standard of proof is a high standard because people base their livelihood on their professional licenses. It would be unfair to permit the government to revoke or suspend a pharmacy license on the basis of anything other than strong proof that a violation had occurred. However, this case says that one who does not yet have a pharmacy license in a state is not subject to that high level of proof in the decision to deny the issuance of an initial license. There is no livelihood yet being earned in a state where one does not yet have a license, and the greater good of protecting the public from threats to health overrides the need to closely scrutinize evidence for board action.

CASE 7-4   *Walgreen Co. v. Selcke*, 595 N.E.2d 89 (III. App. 1992)

Issue

Whether the nonpharmacist personnel being used to support professional pharmacy activities at the pharmacy in question were exceeding the scope of their authority as supportive personnel under the law.

Overview

Technicians are essential to contemporary pharmacy practice. The volume of prescriptions to fill and the expanded practices that pharmacists have available to them make it impossible for pharmacists in today's world to practice in the way pharmacists traditionally have. Supportive personnel can perform some nonprofessional functions for pharmacists, and these activities need not take up the precious time pharmacists must conserve for the more important activities in which they engage. In this case, the Illinois Board of Pharmacy has taken action against a pharmacy company for using technicians in what the board believes are inappropriate ways. As you read this case, ask yourself whether the activities described for the technicians are activities that one must have a pharmacy degree to perform competently. What are the limits on pharmacy technician activities? If a pharmacy is supervised by a pharmacist, and if the pharmacy has a continuous quality improvement program to detect and rectify problems in dispensing, is there really any point in limiting what technicians can do? The distinction often made between what technicians can do and what pharmacists must do is that pharmacists must do the judgmental activities, whereas technicians may engage in nonjudgmental activities. Are there any judgmental activities in which technicians might be able to safely and accurately engage, if properly trained and supervised?

The court began with a description of the pharmacy inspection that led to this court case, and the fallout of that inspection:

> Walgreen was visited by a DPR inspector on February 22, 1987, at its 9503 South Cicero Avenue, Oak Lawn, Illinois store. At that time, Michael Simko, the pharmacist in charge, was not present; another pharmacist was on duty, Thomas Savage. Other employees then working were Brian Gilmartin, a pharmacy technician, and Christine Chrobak. The inspector determined that although these latter two employees were engaged in pharmacy practice, Gilmartin's license had then expired, and Chrobak was unlicensed.

The court then turned to a description of what activities had been done by the unlicensed personnel.

> On the night of the inspection, Chrobak was ringing sales on the cash register. Gilmartin and Savage were present. Her duties, at that time, were to ring sales on the register, clean, and answer the telephone. When someone wanted a refill, she would write the name, prescription number and telephone number on a pad of paper, giving it to a person at the computer terminals, who would put it through. She did not receive new prescriptions, compound prescriptions, package medication in containers, interpret the label directions on prescriptions, or advise about medication or recommend it to customers. When she rang up sales of prescriptions, she handed the sealed package to the customer, in the presence of a registered pharmacist. Simko knew she was not yet licensed.

> Gilmartin testified he had been employed by Walgreen since October 1985 as a pharmacy technician. He described the pharmacy in substantially the same way as did Chrobak. His duties were to put permanent prescription information into the computers; ring sales on the register; and occasionally pull drugs off the shelf for the "pharmacy" to count. He performed these duties on the day of the inspection. When he received a telephone call, he would put the prescription number into the computer. Simko was his supervisor, but Savage performed that function on the night of the inspection. On that night, he did not have a current pharmacy technician license; it had expired on March 31, 1986. He recalled mentioning this to either Simko or his district supervisor. The expired license was posted on the wall at the store. He had applied for a renewal, but it was lost by the Department in Springfield.

The court described in greater detail the circumstances of the technician license that had not been renewed.

> Gilmartin sent in the fee and application for license renewal in January of 1986. Upon inquiry as to non-receipt of the license, he was informed that the Department was backed up and to "keep going." He inquired again in April, but was informed his application was not received. He never received a renewal form as requested. In December of 1986, he was informed that the Department lost his and other licenses and a new renewal form would be sent, which was sent in February. Gilmartin's regular fee and late fee submitted for this period were returned to him. He received his license renewal in March of 1987.

The court then described the disciplinary action that had been recommended by the board of pharmacy to the administrative agency (the DPR) of which it is a part.

The Pharmacy Board (Board), in review of the hearing officer's decision, recommended that Walgreen be found to have allowed persons to engage in the practice of pharmacy when they were not authorized to do so under the Pharmacy Practice Act and, therefore, its license should be put on probation.

The court examined the role of the pharmacy technicians in this particular pharmacy, in light of the arguments that the DPR had made.

The uncontested facts in the present case reveal that Chrobak and Gilmartin each rang up cash register sales of prescription drug products. They took payment for items sealed in packages and handed the packages to customers designated on the packages. They gave no directions, advice, or explanations concerning the products to the customers. At all relevant times, a registered pharmacist was present. In addition, Gilmartin entered refill information into the Walgreen computer. Refill information consists of a customer name, phone number, and prescription number. Gilmartin also retrieved products off the shelves for the pharmacists.

Ringing up a sale on a cash register is no more a dispensing of pharmaceuticals than a delivery boy taking money from a customer at the latter's home, in payment of the package there transferred. It is not in pursuance of study or training in medicine and drugs, their nature, propensities, or traits, but a relatively simple business transaction. Nor does the fact that the cash register is located at or near the pharmacy counter permit the legal conclusion that the salesperson recording the sale is engaged in the practice of pharmacy. It is the straightforward receipt of payment in exchange for a product, under the facts presented here.

Entering refill information by pressing computer keys in order to transcribe the information from a written to an electronic vehicle is no more a practice of pharmacy than allowing an unlicensed employee to write on a pad of paper prescription refill information as received by telephone from a customer; the latter conduct was admitted by DPR to be appropriate under the Act. As the circuit court concluded, this conduct was ministerial, not interpretive.

Nor does merely retrieving a container of a pharmaceutical from the shelf at the request of the pharmacist who is compounding or filling a prescription fall within the exercise of pharmaceutical interpretation, skill, or knowledge of medicine or drugs. The pharmacist chooses and describes the desired ingredient, as prescribed by the physician, and determines from his or her own knowledge, training, and experience whether what has been brought by his employee correctly corresponds with the product requested by him or her. Surely, simply fetching the product requested cannot place the employee within the practice of pharmacy any more than a law clerk bringing law books from a library at a lawyer's request can be deemed tantamount to the practice of law.

DPR insists that the conduct of Walgreen's employees here rises to a "necessary link in the chain of filling prescriptions and delivering them to the ultimate customer." Yet, it concedes that ringing a sale at a cash register and transferring the product to the customer is appropriate if it occurs outside the pharmacy area or at the customer's home. These very acts are as much a "necessary link" at one place as at the other. DPR also admits that the same acts are appropriate when over-the-counter drug products are sold from the pharmacy area register. Why these acts are not as much a "necessary link" at one register for the sale of prescription drug products as for the sale of over-the-counter drug products from the same register is difficult to reconcile.

Last, the court commented on the failure of one technician to timely renew his license in a timely manner.

It should be noted that the case against Walgreen required, in part, that Gilmartin be an unlicensed person. Gilmartin's testimony was that he timely applied for his renewal license, diligently followed-up on its status, was told by the Department to continue working and a new application would be forthcoming. He received that application months later, promptly prepared, and filed it. Through no fault of his own, he received a written certificate from the agency just before its 1-year term expired. He testified that during that entire time, he believed he was licensed. His testimony is uncontroverted. Given the nature of the qualifications for the license—a high school degree, payment of a fee and good moral character—with no examinations or interviews involved, it is unremarkable that the agency would advise one person in Gilmartin's situation to "go on" until the lost application was found or the replacement application processed. Gilmartin's testimony is consistent with the fact that DPR did not give him notice of refused renewal for cause. Absent such notice, renewal cannot be withheld. The absence of notice demonstrates that this was a bureaucratic "foul-up."

The court concluded that neither of the technicians had illegally engaged in the practice of pharmacy.

Notes on *Walgreen Co. v. Selcke*

1. In this case, the court took the pragmatic approach of examining the day-to-day activities of the technicians who were alleged to have practiced pharmacy without authority. The court compared those activities with the legal definition of "the practice of pharmacy" and concluded that the technicians were not practicing pharmacy. The no-nonsense approach of the court opens up the use of technicians in a necessary way for the survival of the pharmacy profession. If pharmacists were relegated to the "ministerial" tasks described by the court (i.e., entering data into the computer, counting dosage units), the profession would be doomed to an insignificant supportive role in health care. The dynamic, expanding profession that we currently have would be brought to a halt.

2. Many of the activities that were subject to scrutiny in this case were activities that seemed similar to activities that were performed by other nonpharmacists in other ways. For example, the handing over of a prescription to a patient in a pharmacy need not necessarily be done by a pharmacist, and this is justified by the fact that often prescriptions are delivered to patients' homes by nonpharmacists. It would be inconsistent to require that pharmacists only give medications to patients in the pharmacy but permit others to deliver medications out to patients' homes.

3. The pharmacy technician's failure to update his certification was deemed to be relatively trivial by the court. The bureaucracy simply did not function as it should have, and the court did not want to punish the technician or his employer for this "foul-up." This is a perspective that has not always been consistently applied. In fact, for pharmacists, it is not the responsibility of the government to get a license renewal to a licensee, it is the responsibility of the licensee to seek out and obtain a renewal. Even if there is a bureaucratic "foul-up," and a pharmacist does not receive an application for license renewal, the requirement is that the pharmacist contact the board to obtain an application for relicensure. Under circumstances similar to those in this case, if a pharmacist were to have not been relicensed, the board and the court would not be so lenient.

CASE 7-5	*Schram v. Department of Professional Regulation* (Fla. App. 1992)

Issue

Whether a pharmacist may be disciplined by a board of pharmacy when the pharmacist has not received notice that disciplinary action is being initiated against the pharmacist.

Overview

The board of pharmacy can take action against a licensee only when the licensee has been given notice of the action and an opportunity to explain the licensee's side of the story at some sort of formal or informal hearing. This due process right is guaranteed to all citizens as a way to prevent unfair government action. As you read this case, ask yourself what the pharmacist could have done to avoid having this problem occur with the Florida Board of Pharmacy. If a pharmacist is required to always keep her or his address up to date with the board of pharmacy, and if the pharmacist fails to do this, whose fault is it if the board of pharmacy cannot find the pharmacist to notify the pharmacist of impending disciplinary action? Should the board of pharmacy be required to hire a private detective to find a pharmacist against whom administrative action is contemplated? On the other hand, if a single telephone call or a brief letter can get the board the information it needs about a pharmacist's whereabouts, is this too much to ask of the board of pharmacy?

The procedure undertaken in this case is important to its disposition. The court described the procedural aspects of the case in detail:

> This is an appeal from a final order of the Florida Board of Pharmacy ("Florida Board") revoking Appellant Schram's license to practice as a pharmacist in the State of Florida. Schram was the respondent in the proceedings below and the Department of Professional Regulation ("DPR") was the petitioner. The Florida Board is the administrative body charged with final agency action in the licensing and regulation of pharmacists pursuant to Florida Statutes. Based on our finding that DPR's action was "impaired by a material error in procedure or a failure to follow prescribed procedure," we vacate the final order and remand the case for further agency action.

The court described the background of the pharmacist having obtained a license in Michigan and Florida, and the action taken against that license in both states.

> In January 1978, Schram was granted a license to practice pharmacy in the State of Florida. From 1978 to the present, he has resided at various addresses in Michigan. As a Florida licensee, Appellant had a duty to apprise the Florida Board as to his current mailing address. The records of the Florida Board showed his last known address as 6209 Ramwyck Court in West Bloomfield, Michigan. In fact, Schram moved to another address in West Bloomfield in February 1988 and moved again in November 1989 to Troy, Michigan. On May 3, 1989, a consent order was issued by the State of Michigan, Department of Licensing and Regulation, Board of Pharmacy, suspending Schram's pharmacist's and controlled substance licenses for 18 months and imposing a fine. The consent order also revoked the pharmacy and controlled substance licenses of Detroit Discount Prescriptions, Inc., of which Schram was a 50% owner.

The Florida agency that at that time regulated the pharmacy profession (DPR) was responsible for ensuring that a pharmacist who is disciplined in another state is subject to discipline in Florida also.

> On September 20, 1989, DPR began investigating the matter for a possible violation of Florida Statutes, which provides for disciplinary action where a pharmacist has

been disciplined by another state's regulatory agency "for any offense that constitutes a violation of this chapter." An administrative complaint was filed on April 3, 1990, based on the DPR panel's memorandum of finding of probable cause.

The Constitutional requirement of due process guarantees all citizens the right to notice and an opportunity to be heard before government action that seriously affects their rights. The court seriously questioned whether the notice requirement had been met in this case.

The applicable notice requirements appear in Florida Statutes, which provides in pertinent part: No revocation, suspension, annulment, or withdrawal of any license is lawful unless, prior to the entry of a final order, the agency has served, by personal service or certified mail, an administrative complaint which affords reasonable notice to the licensee of facts or conduct which warrant the intended action and unless the licensee has been given an adequate opportunity to request a proceeding. When personal service cannot be made and the certified mail notice is returned undelivered, the agency shall cause a short, simple notice to the licensee to be published once each week for 4 consecutive weeks in a newspaper published in the county of the licensee's last known address as it appears on the records of the board. If the address is in some state other than this state, the notice may be published in Leon County.

DPR sent a certified letter, return receipt requested, containing the administrative complaint to the Ramwyck Court address in Michigan. The envelope was returned as "not deliverable as addressed" in April 1990. A notice of action was published weekly over four consecutive weeks in the Leon County News in May 1990.

Because the pharmacist was never personally notified of the pending action (publication in a Tallahassee, Florida, newspaper—Tallahassee is where the Leon County News is located—is hardly likely to be of much use to someone living in Michigan) he defaulted (failed to appear) on the Florida administrative action.

In June 1990, DPR moved for the Florida Board to take final action and to enter an order of default, based on Appellant's failure to respond following service by publication. The motion for default was mailed to the Ramwyck Court address. Schram received actual notice of the hearing for entry of the final order on May 6, 1991, nearly 1 year later. Prior to that, he had received no information concerning the Florida investigation of his license. In a letter dated May 24, 1991, counsel for Appellant apprised DPR of the circumstances and stated further:

Obviously, Mr. Schram is concerned about any licensing action the state of Florida might undertake. Therefore, I would request that any default, if one has been entered by the Board of Pharmacy, be set aside, since Mr. Schram did not have notice sufficient to defend against the instant charges.

Additionally, enclosed please find a signed and notarized copy of Mr. Schram's election of rights: At this point, Mr. Schram is interested in disputing certain allegations of fact contained in the complaint and requests a formal hearing. However, I would be interested in discussing this matter with you since Mr. Schram is presently without a pharmacy license in the State of Michigan. Therefore, he may be willing to enter into a consent order in the state of Florida. However, Mr. Schram is presently in the process of reacquiring his Michigan license and such reacquisition would obviate the state of Florida's need to suspend his license since his Michigan activity is the basis for the state of Florida complaint.

In fact, the Florida Board had already issued a final order on May 13, 1991, finding a default on the Part of Appellant and revoking his license to practice pharmacy in Florida pursuant to Florida Statutes 1989.

The court considered whether the due process right of notice had been met through the efforts of the board of pharmacy.

Clearly, the statutory option of notice by certified mail was unsuccessful. The issue on appeal is whether DPR acted with due diligence to determine whether personal service could be made, pursuant to Florida Statutes, to provide Appellant with reasonable notice of the administrative complaint and licensing investigation.

We hold that the requirements of the statute authorizing service by publication were not met in this case in that there was an absence of diligent inquiry and a conscientious effort to locate appellant reasonably employing knowledge known by or readily available to appellee. As a result, appellant was denied his due process right to request a hearing, and appellee's order was entered without compliance with the requirements of law.

Notes on *Schram v. Department of Professional Regulation*

1. Notice by publication in the newspaper is a vestige of days gone by when most people lived their entire lives in the same community and everyone knew everyone else. Chances were that when someone wanted to officially notify another person of something, publication in the newspaper would do the trick. Obviously those days are long gone—and certainly there is no way a person in Michigan could be expected to read a newspaper in Florida. In contemporary society, this form of notice has to be regarded as a charade and nothing more.

2. In most states, the board of pharmacy is authorized to discipline a pharmacist solely based on disciplinary action in another state and not on the activities that led to the discipline in that other state. If a pharmacist violates a law in a state, the board of pharmacy must prove that the underlying act occurred, and the pharmacist is permitted to defend the allegations of violation by proving that the act did not occur. There is a factual hearing that is much like a trial, with witnesses and testimony and legal arguments. Once that pharmacist is disciplined by a state, any other state in which the pharmacist is licensed may discipline the pharmacist also, if the state laws permit this sort of discipline. The underlying act need not be proved. All that is required is a showing that the discipline occurred in the first state. Pharmacists sometimes try to resist discipline in a second or third state by arguing the facts of the incident in the first state. But it does not matter; discipline in the first state is the only issue, not the acts that led to the discipline.

3. In this case, the pharmacist is likely to be disciplined anyway, even though the board did not provide adequate notice to the pharmacist that the discipline was being undertaken. Apparently the pharmacist has now been found. Although he will be able to set aside the original discipline because of the lack of notice, the board will probably be able to provide notice now, and the allegations will be heard by the board.

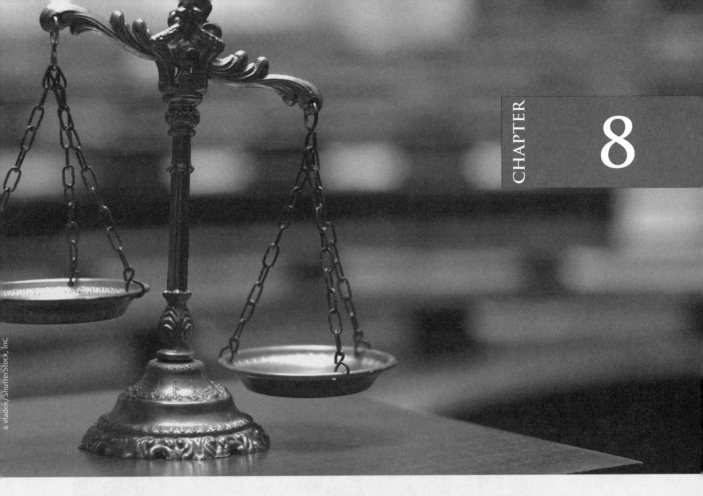

CHAPTER 8

PHARMACIST MALPRACTICE LIABILITY AND RISK MANAGEMENT STRATEGIES

CHAPTER OBJECTIVES

Upon completing this chapter, the reader will be able to:

▸ Identify the elements of a professional malpractice action against a pharmacist.

▸ Describe the legal standard of care for a pharmacist in processing prescriptions and medication orders.

▸ Recognize the types of prescription processing errors that can lead to pharmacist liability.

▸ Discuss the available defenses to a claim of professional negligence.

▸ Describe the purposes of professional malpractice insurance.

▸ Discuss appropriate strategies for risk management.

▸ Describe the expanding liability of pharmacists for the failure to practice pharmaceutical care.

▸ Differentiate professional negligence from drug product liability.

Like other professional people, pharmacists can be held legally accountable for the consequences of their conduct. A pharmacist who unintentionally causes harm to a patient through inattentiveness or carelessness, for example, can be considered legally negligent. Negligence is classified in the law as a "tort," a civil wrong rather than a criminal wrong. It is different from an intentional tort, however, which occurs when one person consciously causes harm to another. Allegations of intentional torts occur infrequently in pharmacy.

Malpractice law serves two purposes: compensation and deterrence. It operates to compensate the victims of a person's negligent conduct by placing them back in the position in which they would have been (as near as possible) had the negligence not occurred. It also operates as a constant reminder that actions have consequences, so the specter of legal liability deters people from acting carelessly and irresponsibly toward one another.

In the case of *Troppi v. Scarf*, 187 N.W.2d 511 (Mich. Ct. App. 1971), the court explained the underlying rationale for malpractice law. The court was asked to rule that a pharmacist could be held liable for dispensing Nardil, a monoamine oxidase inhibitor, to a woman whose prescription had been for Norinyl, an oral contraceptive. The woman gave birth to a healthy child, and the pharmacist argued that no real harm had occurred. The court responded:

> In theory at least, the imposition of civil liability encourages potential tortfeasors to exercise more care in the performance of their duties, and hence, to avoid liability-producing negligent acts. Applying this theory to the case before us, public policy favors a tort scheme which encourages pharmacists to exercise great care in filling prescriptions. To absolve defendant of all liability here would be to remove one deterrent against the negligent dispensing of drugs. Given the great numbers of women who currently use oral contraceptives, such absolution cannot be defended on public policy grounds. (187 N.W.2d at 517)

The pharmacist was held liable for the medical expenses of the pregnancy and for the costs of rearing the child.

LEGAL PROCEDURE

Most pharmacist malpractice cases do not reach a jury verdict. This is not unusual for any type of litigation because out-of-court settlements commonly make it unnecessary to carry the case through to completion. Although law established by a jury verdict that is affirmed on appeal is binding within the same jurisdiction and persuasive outside the jurisdiction, settlements carry no such authority and establish no precedent. Thus, a settlement before the trial of a pharmacist malpractice case, with a payment being made by the defendant pharmacist, does not in any way obligate the same court or another court to decide a similar case in the same way at a later time.

Even though a case may not proceed to trial and appeal, the court may rule on preliminary motions early in the course of proceedings. The most important of these is the motion for summary judgment, in which the defendant says in effect, "Even if everything the plaintiff says is true, I cannot be held legally accountable for what the plaintiff says I did." A ruling granting a defendant-pharmacist's motion for summary judgment legally absolves the pharmacist from liability, no matter what the facts may later show. If the court denies the defendant's motion for summary judgment, the pharmacist may be held liable as a matter of law if the facts support liability, but a jury must consider whether the facts show that the legal requisites for liability have been met.

These early rulings may be appealed, and the decision of the appellate court on a point of law raised on appeal may be binding (on lower courts in the same jurisdiction) or persuasive (on courts outside the jurisdiction). Thus, even though an out-of-court settlement may leave an underlying allegation unresolved, court rulings on preliminary motions in the case make substantive law and reveal the legal expectations of pharmacists.

THE MALPRACTICE ACTION

A legal cause of action for negligence has four elements:

1. Duty owed
2. Breach of duty
3. Causation
4. Damages

The plaintiff must prove each of these elements. If any one element cannot be proved, there will be no legal liability. Once the plaintiff has established all four elements, the defendant tries to show one or more affirmative defenses that should absolve the defendant of liability. The most frequently used affirmative defenses are (1) contributory negligence and (2) statute of limitations. These defenses are called "affirmative defenses" because the defense has responsibility to assert them or the court will not consider them. The plaintiff's challenge is to prove the four elements of negligence and disprove the affirmative defenses. The defendant's response is to disprove the four elements of negligence, prove the affirmative defenses, or both.

ELEMENTS OF NEGLIGENCE

Duty of Care

The well-established rule is that a pharmacist must use the degree of care that a reasonable and prudent person would use under similar circumstances. Recognizing the dangerousness of the products that pharmacists dispense, courts have described the pharmacist's duty of care as "a high degree of care" and "great care." The potential for serious harm that drugs present, combined with the fact that patients usually cannot fully appreciate that harm, creates a special situation in which pharmacists must be particularly cautious. Yet, the duty of care expected of pharmacists is not excessive. A pharmacist is bound simply to exercise the skill generally possessed by well-educated pharmacists who are considered competent in the profession of pharmacy.

As a practical matter, however, pharmacists may be the only health care professionals who are legally required to practice in a completely error-free manner. Pharmacists have traditionally adopted a "no mistakes" approach to practice, and legal standards have reflected this impossible-to-achieve and self-imposed standard.

The case of *DeCordova v. State of Colorado*, 878 P.2d 73 (Colo. App. 1994), affirms this error-free standard. In this case, the hospital pharmacist inadvertently dispensed an overdose of an intravenous antibiotic to an infant patient, resulting in the infant suffering permanent severe hearing loss. The trial court found that the pharmacist's mistake constituted negligence as a matter of law (essentially meaning that the mistake itself amounts to negligence, and whether the pharmacist may have acted reasonably is largely irrelevant). On appeal the pharmacist argued that human error is unavoidable and therefore should not be considered negligence as a matter of law. The court, however, noted that a pharmacist is responsible for accurately filling a prescription and that the error here was avoidable and fell below minimal standards of pharmacy practice. Concluded the judge: "To err is human, to forgive is divine. To be responsible for injuries caused by undisputed negligence is the law of this state."

In contrast to nonjudgmental types of errors, a professional judgment that seems wrong with the benefit of hindsight but was reasonable given the circumstances at the time, is not generally actionable as negligence. Thus, a physician who prescribes two digoxin tablets daily when one tablet is the dosage that most physicians would have chosen, or a physician who prescribes ephedrine when most physicians would have prescribed theophylline is not regarded as a malpractitioner if the prescription was reasonable (albeit somewhat unusual) at the time it was initiated. If harm results to the patient and it becomes obvious in retrospect that the physician made a mistake in prescribing, that mistake will be forgiven as the unavoidable consequence of fallible human judgment.

Pharmacists, on the other hand, would virtually always be held liable if they were to instruct the same patient to take two digoxin tablets daily when one was prescribed or if they were to dispense ephedrine to a patient for whom theophylline had been prescribed. The possibility that two digoxin tablets or ephedrine might have been reasonable for the patient at that time would be considered irrelevant. Unlike prescribing errors, dispensing errors of a nonjudgmental nature are not forgiven. Human fallibility and the inevitability of occasional human error is no defense for a pharmacist in these situations.

Pharmacists have a duty to provide patients with the best care possible. That duty arises out of the relationship between pharmacists and patients, and the extent of the duty is determined by the nature of that relationship. In U.S. law, there is no traditional duty to come to the aid of a stranger. Thus, a passerby who sees a person in a burning building has no duty to help that person, although a firefighter would have such a duty. There is a relationship between people in danger and those whom society trusts to help the endangered. The relationship between pharmacists and the people to whom they dispense medications makes pharmacists something more than casual bystanders when there is a problem with drug therapy.

The key test for the existence of a duty is foreseeability. This point was clearly made in *Docken v. Ciba-Geigy*, 739 P.2d 591 (Or. Ct. App. 1987). In that tragic case, Tofranil had been prescribed for a young boy whose even younger brother took the drug hoping the drug would remedy a problem similar to that for which the drug had been prescribed for the older boy. The younger boy died as a result. The plaintiffs alleged that the dispensing pharmacy should have provided a warning regarding the potentially fatal accumulation of the drug over a short period of time. The pharmacy asserted a "no duty" defense and filed a motion for summary judgment, contending that it only owes a duty to the patient to whom the drug is dispensed. The court noted that a "no duty" defense is only another way of stating that the harm the child suffered by using a drug prescribed for his brother was not a foreseeable risk of the conduct alleged as negligence by the pharmacy. The court felt that it could not say as a matter of law that the harm was not foreseeable and refused to dismiss the case. Rather it remanded the issue to the trial court to determine whether a reasonable pharmacist could foresee this type of harm. On remand, the jury found that the harm was not foreseeable and that the pharmacy was not liable. The plaintiff appealed, but the court affirmed the trial court's ruling (790 P.2d 45 (Or. App. 1990)).

The issue of whether the pharmacist owes a duty to someone other than the patient has also arisen in caregiver situations. In *Huggins v. Longs Drug Stores, Inc.*, 862 P.2d 148 (Cal. 1993), the pharmacy negligently labeled that the drug Ceclor be administered to a 2-month-old child in doses of 2.5 teaspoonfuls every 8 hours rather than 2.5 ccs.

After administering a few doses, the patient's mother noticed that the child was lethargic and unresponsive. The error was ultimately discovered, and the parents sued on the basis of the emotional distress they suffered while observing the harm occur to their child. The California Supreme Court, reversing the court of appeals, found that pharmacists in California owe no duty to the caregiver of the patient. This decision is consistent with the majority of decisions in other states; however, the Utah Supreme Court recently found differently (*B.R. ex rel. Jeffs v. West*, 275 P.3d 228 (Utah 2012)). In this case, the father of the plaintiff children, allegedly under the influence of several prescribed drugs, killed the children's mother, and the plaintiff children sued the prescriber for negligent prescribing. The court reversed the lower court decision and held that health care providers owe a duty to third parties not to prescribe medications that affirmatively cause patients to harm third parties.

In a Nevada case that drew national attention, the patient of several pharmacies, who was an abuser of controlled substances, while driving struck and killed one person and seriously injured another. She was arrested for driving under the influence of controlled substances. One year prior to the accident, a Nevada substance abuse task force had sent a letter to the pharmacies informing them that the patient had obtained approximately 4,500 hydrocodone tablets at 13 different pharmacies over the past year. The plaintiffs (those injured in the accident) sued many of the pharmacies that had continued to dispense the hydrocodone to the patient, alleging that after receiving the task force letter the pharmacies had a duty not to dispense to the patient (*Sanchez ex rel, Sanchez v. Wal-Mart*, 221 P.3d 1276 (Nev. 2009)). The Nevada Supreme Court held that the pharmacies owed no duty to the plaintiffs on the basis that they had no direct relationship with the plaintiffs; and, because the plaintiffs were unknown to the pharmacies, there was no special relationship that would warrant a duty. The court further reasoned that there was nothing in the Nevada Pharmacy Act at the time of the accident that would require the pharmacies to protect third parties from their patients.

Breach of Duty

Dispensing Errors

As noted previously, it is generally accepted that a pharmacist who fills a prescription in a manner other than the way it was ordered by a prescriber has breached a duty of ordinary care owed to the patient. This principle is so well established that, even though the plaintiff technically bears the burden of proof in pharmacist malpractice litigation, evidence of a misfilling error is virtually sufficient for a presumption of negligence.

In most professional malpractice cases, however, proof of breach of duty requires evidence that a standard of professional practice exists and that the defendant did not adhere to the standard. This evidence is frequently offered through the testimony of expert witnesses because a jury of lay people usually must rely on a member of the profession to explain the intricacies of professional practice. When a pharmacist fills a prescription incorrectly, however, the obviousness of the error usually makes expert testimony unnecessary. For example, in *Parker v. Yen*, 823 S.W.2d 359 (Tex. Civ. App. 1991), the defendant pharmacist had improperly filled a prescription for Sinequan with Dalmane. There was no need to establish through expert testimony that standards of practice for pharmacists require accuracy in prescription processing. Law requires this sort of accuracy. The pharmacist must introduce evidence to rebut the presumption created by the fact of error. Unless there is some highly unusual extenuating circumstance (e.g., a natural disaster, an epidemic that has taxed available resources), the pharmacist's rebuttal is likely to be ineffectual.

Courts have clearly established pharmacists' responsibility to dispense the correct medication to patients, and pharmacists accept this responsibility. One of the most common reasons for a wrong drug error by pharmacists is a misunderstanding between the prescriber and the pharmacist, either because of sloppy handwriting or because of slurred speech. In either case, the pharmacist who misfills the prescription has breached a duty because the pharmacist always has the last opportunity to clarify an unclear communication. Attempting to focus blame on physicians who issue unclear orders or manufacturers who use similar drug names does not effectively relieve the pharmacist of responsibility. As the last link in the drug distribution chain, the responsibility for the failure to clarify ambiguity stays with the pharmacist.

Dispensing errors may involve the wrong strength or dosage of the correct drug. In *Lou v. Smith*, 685 S.W.2d 809 (Ark. 1985), the defendant pharmacist changed a prescription for Reglan from the prescribed dosage of 1 mg daily to 10 mg daily because the product was distributed as 10-mg tablets. The higher dosage would have been correct for an adult, but the patient was a 4-month-old child, who had a severe reaction. The pharmacist was held liable.

Dosage errors become particularly important when the drug dispensed is one with a narrow therapeutic index; that is, the toxic dosage is only slightly higher than the therapeutic dosage. Pharmacists have adopted various practice conventions to avoid incorrect dosages. One such convention is an understanding that decimal points are used only when they are absolutely necessary. For example, a dose of one tenth is written *0.1* rather than *.1* because the presence of the zero suggests that a decimal should go before the number one, even if the decimal has become smudged or is otherwise difficult to visualize. Likewise, the convention requires that a dose of one unit be written *1* rather than *1.0* because an illegible decimal point would lead to an overdose. Of course, writing out the dosage by hand, such as 0.1 (one-tenth) mg is the best method of avoiding an overdose because of a disappearing decimal point. The use of such conventions reduces the risk of error even when a pharmacist is rushed or is otherwise momentarily inattentive.

Doctrine of Negligence Per Se

In addition to liability for breach of a professionally recognized standard of care, a pharmacist who violates a statute or regulation concerning the distribution of pharmaceutical products may be liable under the doctrine of negligence per se. Under this doctrine, the court bases its decision on whether the plaintiff is of the class of plaintiffs that the statute or regulation was intended to protect and whether the harm done to the plaintiff was of the type against which the statute or regulation was intended to provide protection. Although not required to do so, a court may choose to adopt the standard expressed within the statute or regulation as the standard for civil liability in a malpractice case. If the defendant has clearly violated the statute or regulation, causation and damages are the only elements left for the plaintiff to prove. Under negligence per se, for example, a court may determine that a pharmacist who substituted a generic drug product for a brand-name product in a way that was not permitted by state law had breached the duty of care if the patient was harmed because the two drugs lacked bioequivalence. Patients are the people whom the law seeks to protect, and harm from bioinequivalence is the type of harm that the drug product selection statute seeks to prevent.

An interesting application of the negligence per se doctrine was presented in *Izzo v. Manhattan Medical Group*, 560 N.Y.S.2d 644 (N.Y. App. Div. 1990). In this case, the widow of an alleged drug addict sued a pharmacy for negligence in filling a forged prescription for the addict. The pharmacy had violated New York law by filling a controlled substance prescription that did not have the prescriber's name imprinted on it.

Although the violation of this law could certainly expose the pharmacist to administrative action, there was some question as to whether it could also expose the pharmacist to civil liability for malpractice. The pharmacist contended that a drug addict who forges a prescription and dies from the effects of the fraudulently obtained drug is not the type of person whom the statute was intended to benefit. The court ruled that this was indeed one type of person whom the statute was intended to protect, however, and allowed the case against the pharmacist to proceed.

Causation

Even if a pharmacist owes a duty of care and that duty is breached, malpractice under the law requires proof that the pharmacist's misconduct caused the alleged damage. Proof of causation is a two-step process. First, the plaintiff must prove that the defendant's conduct was a substantial factor in the harm that occurred (i.e., actual causation). Second, the plaintiff must fix liability with the party or parties whose misconduct most directly caused the damages (i.e., proximate causation). It would be unfair to hold people responsible for every consequence of their conduct, no matter how remote the consequences might be, so proximate causation operates to limit the liability of a person whose conduct was a substantial factor in the harm of another.

Actual Cause

One major problem with proving causation in drug-related cases is that the dispensed drug has often been ingested and eliminated from the body by the time a thorough investigation can be conducted. There may be nothing to do but speculate as to what really happened. When a pharmacist has allegedly dispensed the wrong drug, the identity of the wrong drug may be unknown, and it will be difficult to determine whether the adverse effects are of a kind that the unknown substance can cause. Even when the substance is known, it may not be clear whether the adverse effects are due to the drug or to some other causal factor. This determination is a question of fact that the jury must resolve on the basis of expert testimony. The standard of proof requires an expert's reasonable degree of scientific certainty that the drug dispensed probably caused the adverse effect. The plaintiff does not have to disprove all other possible causal factors, but simply must establish the reasonableness of a causal inference by a preponderance of the evidence.

A pharmacist may have negligently caused some, but not all, of a patient's injuries. In *Cazes v. Raisinger*, 430 So.2d 104 (La. Ct. App. 1983), the pharmacist mislabeled a prescription, and the patient ingested an overdose of digoxin. The patient died 5 months later. The trial court ruled that the pharmacist's error had caused the patient's death. The appellate court limited liability to those damages suffered during the 2 or 3 days after the overdose, however. Even though the pharmacist had made a mistake, and the patient ultimately died, the pharmacist's action was held not to have been the cause of the patient's death.

Proximate Cause

The rules of proximate cause relate primarily to limiting the liability of a defendant whose conduct has been shown to be the actual cause of harm to the plaintiff. Most proximate cause cases address the liability of a defendant who breached a duty of care when the defendant's negligent conduct had an unforeseeable result. For example, assume a pharmacist dispenses the wrong medication to a patient that has a side effect of drowsiness. The patient takes the medication and while driving on a city street, falls asleep, hitting an oncoming car that in turn swerves into a house injuring the occupant. Clearly the pharmacist's negligent act was the cause of the accident. The issue under proximate cause would be the extent to which the pharmacist would be liable. Should the pharmacist be liable for the injuries to the occupants of the other car? To the occupant of the house? The extent of liability often depends upon a determination of foreseeability (although in some jurisdictions the pharmacist could be found liable for all the injury). Because foreseeability is such an important factor in most proximate cause determinations, sometimes the issue is indistinguishable from that of duty. Thus, instead of asking if the pharmacist was the proximate cause of the injury to the occupant of the house, one could also ask whether the pharmacist owed a duty to the occupant of the house.

The rules of proximate cause define the circumstances that break the chain of causation between the defendant's act and the plaintiff's harm. If causation is viewed as a chain of events, with the defendant's conduct at one end of the chain and the plaintiff's harm on the other end, the links in the chain connect the defendant's conduct with the plaintiff's harm. If the defendant is to be liable for the harm, each of the links must be foreseeable to the defendant. Any unforeseeable link in the chain operates as an intervening act between the negligence of the defendant and the harm to the plaintiff; it breaks the chain of causation, so the defendant is no longer responsible for the harm. Called a superseding cause, the intervening act becomes the true causal factor rather than the defendant's conduct. Most cases in which a pharmacist is relieved of liability on the issue of proximate cause involve unforeseeable misuse of the drug by the patient.

In *Speer v. United States*, 512 F. Supp. 670 (N.D. Tex. 1981), the court discussed the superseding cause doctrine. Pursuant to both new prescriptions and refills, Etrafon 4-25 had been dispensed to a patient at frequencies far exceeding what the patient should have needed. The patient was stockpiling an excess quantity of the medication, with which he subsequently committed suicide. The deceased patient's spouse sued the pharmacy, contending that the pharmacists were negligent for refilling the drug in excess of that authorized by the psychiatrist and that the negligence caused the patient's death. In the ensuing lawsuit, the court ruled that although the pharmacists were negligent, the evidence did not establish that they should have foreseen the patient would use the drug to commit suicide. In other words, the ingestion of an overdose by the patient broke the chain between the negligent filling of the Etrafon prescriptions and the patient's death. According to the court, the mere sale of a toxic substance does not give the pharmacists sufficient information to foresee suicide; however, the court left open the possibility that more extensive knowledge would lead to a finding of foreseeability and, thus, to liability.

Causation also was the issue in *Hayes v. Travelers Insurance Co.*, 609 So.2d 1084 (La. Ct. App. 1992). In this case, the pharmacy had erroneously filled a prescription for L-tryptophan with Tofranil; as a result, the patient ingested an overdose of Tofranil. The physician ordered the Tofranil discontinued until the patient's blood level of the drug returned to normal and then restarted the Tofranil therapy. Thereafter, the plaintiff prescribed two other drugs for the patient, which apparently caused an adverse reaction. The plaintiff contended that the two other drugs had been used to treat the Tofranil overdose, which would not have occurred had it not been for the pharmacist's error. Therefore, the plaintiff argued that the pharmacy should be held causally responsible for the adverse reaction. It is well established in the law that if a pharmacist's mistake necessitates medical treatment for an adverse effect, and if the treatment causes harm to the patient, the pharmacist is liable for the harm caused by the medical treatment. In this case, however, the court reasoned that it would have made no sense for the physician to restart Tofranil therapy if the two drugs had really been used to treat the Tofranil overdose. The court concluded that the pharmacy was not the legal cause of the patient's adverse reaction.

Damages

There is no recovery for malpractice if no harm was done. The law does not deal in hypothetical cases. A patient may actually be distressed over a mistake that a pharmacist made, and the distress may actually cause emotional problems. If the mistake was detected and rectified before any physical harm could occur, however, there are unlikely to be any compensable damages.

In malpractice cases, compensable damages are of many types. They can generally be divided into actual damages and punitive damages.

Actual Damages

The purpose of actual damages is compensation. When a patient loses a week of wages, suffers impaired vision, or has severe pain for a month because of a pharmacist's negligence, the legal system seeks to compensate the patient for the harm. The goal is to return the patient to the position in which the patient would have been if the pharmacist had not been negligent.

Reimbursement for lost wages or for medical expenses incurred to treat the problem is relatively easy to determine. A dollar-for-dollar repayment can be arranged to shift the financial burden of the problem from the party who suffered the harm to the party who caused the harm. Compensation for physical injuries, emotional injuries, or pain and suffering are much more difficult to calculate. Usually, it is impossible to correct the injury, remove the pain, and simulate a return to the preinjury status quo. Instead, a second-best approach must be adopted—providing a financial payment to the harmed person. The goal is not to remove the harm (because that cannot be done) but to make the harm more bearable.

Determining the dollar value of harm that has no real value presents a challenge to any court. The jury must decide what dollar figure it believes is reasonable as compensation for essentially noncompensable harm, and the appellate court will uphold any sensible award. Several rules apply to judicial review of this issue. First, the court uses the "eggshell plaintiff" rule, which requires defendants to accept whatever underlying condition the plaintiff had before the defendant's negligent act. A patient who is peculiarly susceptible to harm will not be penalized for that susceptibility. If the patient had a condition that predisposed the patient to harm from the pharmacist's conduct, the plaintiff is still compensated for the harm (even if most other people would not have been harmed in similar circumstances). Second, the plaintiff may be required to mitigate the damages by seeking timely medical assistance or using some other mechanism. If a patient suffered harm and could have done something to lessen the impact of the harm, but did nothing, the avoidable harm is not considered the result of the pharmacist's actions. Finally, reform statutes in a number of states place "caps" or ceilings on liability awards, specifying a maximum dollar amount that can be recovered in a malpractice case. These dollar limits prevent excessive recoveries for the difficult-to-quantify types of harm, and they make it easier for insurance companies to predict what their losses are likely to be during a given time period.

Punitive Damages

Under certain circumstances, the law allows recovery for damages in an amount greater than that necessary to compensate the plaintiff for harm actually suffered. Such damages are known as punitive or exemplary damages because their purpose is to punish or to make an example of the defendant. The plaintiff receives punitive damages only if there is evidence of the defendant's wanton and reckless disregard of the plaintiff's rights or morally culpable conduct. The most likely reasons for punitive damages in a pharmacist malpractice case are a cover-up of a dispensing error; carelessness so significant that an error is almost inevitable; failure to follow a standard procedure in dispensing medications, such as not appropriately supervising technical support personnel; or ignoring the rule that pharmacists observe a compounding machine while a solution is being prepared.

A classic example of willful and wanton conduct that justifies punitive damages appears in *Burke v. Bean*, 363 S.W.2d 366 (Tex. Civ. App. 1962). In this case, the pharmacist discovered that he had mistakenly dispensed Oxsoralen instead of Oxacholin. On the next refill, the pharmacist changed to the correct medication but did not tell the patient about the earlier mix-up. In fact, the pharmacist sold the correct medication at the same price he had charged for the wrong medication so as not to give a clue that a mistake had occurred. The jury found that the pharmacist had affirmatively attempted to conceal his mistake. According to the court, the jury was justified in concluding that the pharmacist had shown a conscious indifference to the rights and welfare of the patient and that he had been grossly negligent. An award of punitive damages was upheld.

DEFENSES TO NEGLIGENCE

Even if the plaintiff can prove the four elements of an action for negligence, the defendant may be able to prove affirmative defenses that will absolve the defendant of liability. Alternatively, of course, the defendant may be able to disprove one of the four initial elements and avoid liability without needing to prove an affirmative defense. The plaintiff bears the burden of proof, and the defendant often chooses to contest every point vehemently.

Contributory and Comparative Negligence

Tort law requires that a plaintiff must act as a reasonable, prudent person in the same or similar circumstance. If the plaintiff could have avoided the consequences of the defendant's negligence by ordinary care, then there is no recovery under the defense of contributory negligence. Until the 1970s, contributory negligence was a complete bar to recovery, even if the plaintiff's fault was slight and the defendant's fault was great. This harsh rule resulted in some unusual verdicts, in which obviously negligent plaintiffs were found not to be at fault because the unfair effect would have been to deny a recovery altogether. If a pharmacist refilled a prescription with the wrong drug, for example, and the physical dissimilarity between the correct drug and the dispensed drug was so obvious that any thoughtful patient should have recognized it as a problem, a court trying to avoid a complete bar to recovery might have pointed out that the patient who did not notice the difference was obviously ill or would not have been taking medication. There could be no contributory negligence, therefore, because people who are ill cannot be expected to think clearly. The unfairness of a complete bar to recovery was a strong bias against finding any contributory negligence whatsoever.

The harshness of the complete bar to recovery for the slightest negligence by the plaintiff, combined with the absurdity of some judicial efforts to contrive explanations of the innocence of plaintiffs who were obviously somewhat at fault, led to a new rule. Comparative negligence has now replaced contributory negligence in most jurisdictions. Although comparative negligence is essentially the same as contributory negligence (i.e., plaintiffs suing a defendant who harmed them are held accountable for the harm that they themselves caused), the complete bar to recovery has been replaced. It is now possible to reduce a plaintiff's recovery by the percentage that corresponds with the percentage of fault attributed to the plaintiff. Thus, assume that a plaintiff was harmed and the dollar value of the harm was determined to be $100,000. If the plaintiff was assigned 20 percent of the fault, and the defendant was assigned 80 percent of the fault, the plaintiff's recovery would be reduced by $20,000.

Most jurisdictions permit recovery under "modified" comparative negligence, in which the plaintiff is permitted to recover whatever percentage of the damages corresponds with the defendant's percentage of fault, provided that the plaintiff is less than 50 percent at fault. In a few jurisdictions, "pure" comparative negligence permits a recovery against a defendant no matter how much at fault the plaintiff was.

Statute of Limitations

A pharmacist who has negligently caused harm to a patient may be able to use the statute of limitations as a defense. Under the statute of limitations, a plaintiff must bring a claim within a specified period of time after the cause of action accrues. The purpose of the statute of limitations is to prevent the litigation of stale claims years after the events that allegedly led to the harm, after memories have faded and witnesses have disappeared.

The public policy favoring the unencumbered practice of the healing arts, without fear of groundless and unjustified malpractice lawsuits, has led to the enactment in many jurisdictions of reform laws that reduce the number of years of a statute of limitations for medical malpractice. For example, if the general negligence statute of limitations is 2 years, the medical malpractice statute of limitations may be 1 year. In many states, pharmacists have specifically been granted this added protection. This approach does nothing to impair the rights of honest and legitimate plaintiffs, but it provides some protection to medical practitioners from the claims-conscious plaintiff whose motives are improper.

Sometimes in drug-related litigation it is difficult to determine when a cause of action accrues. Adverse effects of drugs may not be evident until months or even years after the drug was used, and the time period within which to sue cannot begin until the adverse effects are apparent. A modification of the statute of limitations known as the "discovery rule" specifies that a cause of action does not accrue until the date on which the plaintiff discovers the injury, which could be years after the date the medication was dispensed. In many states, a "statute of repose" limits the length of time after the defendant's alleged negligent action during which the discovery rule can postpone the accrual (and expiration) of the statute of limitations. If this were not the case, drugs that cause latent problems (e.g., diethylstilbestrol [DES]) could give rise to litigation decades after their use despite the statute of limitations.

VICARIOUS LIABILITY

It is well established under tort law that an employer is liable for the negligent acts of its employees. This is vicarious liability under a doctrine called respondeat superior, which places liability upon the employer without regard to any negligence on the part of the employer. Thus, the employer of a pharmacist who commits a negligent act that harms a patient is liable for the act, as is the pharmacist. The justification for respondeat superior arises from the notion that the employer has an obligation to hire and train competent employees.

The plaintiff has the choice of suing either the employer or the pharmacist individually or jointly. Often the plaintiff will sue only the employer on the basis that the employer has greater resources. The employer does have a right to sue the employee for contribution; however, this seldom occurs.

Sometimes the plaintiff will sue both the employer and pharmacist jointly for jurisdictional reasons. For example, in *Crain v. Eckerd Corp.*, 1997 WL 537705, E.D.La.,

Aug. 21, 1997, and *Aucoin v. Vicknair*, 1997 WL 539889, E.D.La., Aug. 29, 1997, the plaintiffs joined the pharmacists as codefendants with the employer, Eckerd, to prevent Eckerd from removing the cases to federal court. Because Eckerd is a Florida corporation and the plaintiffs are Louisiana citizens, the federal courts would have had jurisdiction over the cases on the basis of diversity citizenship. By joining the Louisiana pharmacists who committed the errors, the plaintiffs defeated diversity jurisdiction and were allowed to proceed in state court. Plaintiffs often prefer state court, believing it to be a more sympathetic venue.

© Stockbyte/Thinkstock

STUDY SCENARIOS AND QUESTIONS

1. Pharmacist Dan opened Servemore Pharmacy at 8 a.m., May 3. Shortly thereafter he received phone calls from both of his pharmacy technicians that they would be unable to come to work that day because of illness. On such short notice Dan was unable to find another technician or a pharmacist to assist him. Dan had gotten no sleep the previous night because his 1-year-old daughter became very sick, and she had to be taken to the emergency room in the middle of the night, where she was ultimately admitted into the hospital. Dan was of course very anxious about his daughter. Somehow, Dan made it through the day and was relieved to find out that he could pick up his daughter at the hospital and take her home. About a week later Dan received a call from a physician stating that a patient of Dan's, Mrs. Johnson, had been dispensed Navane on May 3 instead of the prescribed Norvasc and was currently in the hospital with serious injuries. A few weeks later Mrs. Johnson filed a negligence lawsuit against Dan.

   a. Explain what Mrs. Johnson must prove in order to establish that Dan is negligent and liable for her injuries.

   b. Based upon the scenario, did Dan breach his standard of care? Does it matter to his case that the technicians did not come to work and that his daughter was ill? Explain.

2. Pharmacist Mary managed Compoundit Pharmacy and employed an intern, Jim, who impressed her with his intelligence and maturity. Mary never needed to show Jim how to do anything more than once. One day Mary showed Jim how to compound a prescription for a topical product for a facial skin disorder. A few weeks later the patient requested a refill, and Mary told Jim to prepare it while she tended to other business. After Jim compounded the drug, he asked Mary if she would like to check it. Mary looked at the label and told Jim it was fine. A couple of days later the patient called saying that his skin was burning up. Mary told him to go to the emergency room immediately. The hospital determined that the compound contained 46 percent of the active ingredient as opposed to the required 0.46 percent and that the error caused the patient to suffer third-degree burns and permanent facial scarring. The patient sued Jim, Mary, and Compoundit.

   a. Who is the cause in fact of this injury? Why? Who is the proximate cause of the injury? Why? What is the difference? Should Jim be liable?

   b. Explain why Compoundit might be liable.

3. Pharmacist Sue worked as a relief pharmacist at Philmore Pharmacy and dispensed two prescriptions for a patient, Ralph. One prescription was a refill for digoxin and the other was a new prescription for erythromycin. Sue was very busy and inadvertently switched the labels on the vials. Ralph is legally blind and normally his daughter serves as his caregiver and picks up his prescriptions. That day, however, she was out of town and would be for the whole week, and Ralph's son assumed the role of caregiver. The son picked up the prescriptions and administered them to Ralph as directed: digoxin four times daily and erythromycin once daily. After a few days Ralph suffered digitalis toxicity and his bacterial infection worsened. He was hospitalized and later sued Sue and Philmore.

   a. What procedures could Sue have followed that would have prevented this unfortunate incident?

   b. What procedures should Sue follow after discovering the error? Does your state require pharmacies to maintain an incident reporting system?

c. Explain how the defense of contributory or comparative negligence could be used in this case. Explain whether it would be a good defense here.
d. Explain whether punitive damages should be applicable in this case.

LIABILITY FOR FAILURE TO PERFORM EXPANDED RESPONSIBILITIES

Pharmacists have always been charged with the legal responsibility to process prescriptions and drug orders accurately, and this responsibility will continue for the foreseeable future. Times are changing, however, and pharmacists are increasingly being given the legal responsibility to improve the outcomes of drug therapy. Ironically, the law has traditionally placed limits on pharmacists that would prevent the type of expanded practice that it is now demanding.

The pharmacist's exercise of professional discretion has been limited primarily because of the omnipotent position that physicians occupy in health care. Until recently, generic substitution was the only discretionary function that pharmacists have been permitted to perform (in many states it is now actually required), and they received legislative authority to perform that function only after repeatedly expressed consumer demand overcame opposition from physicians and the pharmaceutical industry. The opposition was because of fear of interference with physician autonomy and the reduction of revenue from the sale of trade name drug products. Because of the limiting effect of the law on pharmacy practice, pharmacists have come to think of the law as a set of mandates and prohibitions rather than as an opportunity to serve the public. To survive the transformations in health care that will occur in the next decade, that view of pharmacy law will have to change. The law should be viewed as enabling rather than restricting because expanded legal expectations provide pharmacists with the authority to grow professionally.

One of the first judicial opinions to recognize an expanded role for pharmacists was in the case of *Riff v. Morgan Pharmacy*, 508 A.2d 1247 (Pa. Super. Ct. 1986). The plaintiff was a woman who had been given Cafergot suppositories for the treatment of migraine headaches without being told to limit her use to two suppositories per headache or five suppositories per week. The directions were to use one suppository every 4 hours. The pharmacist filled the prescription exactly as written. Unfortunately, the patient used too many suppositories (always one every 4 hours as she had been directed, but for 3 or 4 days), and she had a toxic reaction to ergotamine. In her subsequent lawsuit against the pharmacy and the physician, the pharmacy argued that the limits of a pharmacist's responsibility to a patient are to process medication orders accurately, which was done in this case. The court disagreed with the pharmacy, specifically noting that each member of the health care team "has a duty to be, to a limited extent, his brother's keeper" (508 A.2d at 1253). The court in *Riff* eloquently justified this position.

Fallibility is a condition of the human existence. Doctors, like other mortals, will from time to time err through ignorance or inadvertence. An error in the practice of medicine can be fatal; and so it is reasonable that the medical community, including physicians, pharmacists, anesthesiologists, nurses, and support staff, have established professional standards which require vigilance not only with respect to primary functions, but also regarding the acts and omissions of the other professionals and support personnel in the health care team. (508 A.2d at 1253)

The duty that Morgan Pharmacy was found to have breached was a duty to warn the patient or to notify the prescribing physician of the obvious inadequacies on the face of the prescription that created a substantial risk of serious harm to the patient. The duty is one of notification only. The pharmacist has no duty to assume complete control of the patient's drug therapy. The *Riff* opinion opened the door to expanded legal responsibility for pharmacists, but it did not open the door widely. Subsequent legal developments have, however, built on the foundation established by *Riff*.

EXPANDED RESPONSIBILITIES IN PERSPECTIVE

The history of pharmacy practice reflects the limitations put in place by pharmacy laws, with their clear distinction between the practice of medicine and the practice of pharmacy. For example, before the 1950s, pharmacists were often taught not to tell patients about prescribed medications. In 1951, the Durham-Humphrey Amendment to the Food, Drug, and Cosmetic Act listed for the first time the information that federal law required a pharmacist to place on the label of a dispensed medication, and the name of the drug was not on the list. Although patient counseling and other patient-oriented facets of practice have played a significant role in pharmacy since the middle of the 20th century, the promise that patient-oriented practice brings with it has not yet fully materialized. Many pharmacists today still practice within the technical model. They believe that it is their responsibility to tell the patient several important facts about a drug but not to elaborate further by providing clinical information.

The clinical pharmacist does more than provide warnings. Clinical practitioners interview patients and explain the importance of drug therapy. They collaborate with physicians on decisions about therapeutic alternatives. Historically, a significant component of clinical pharmacy has been assuring patients that the physician knows what is best and admonishing patients about problems that can arise if the physician's orders are not followed. This historic approach to clinical pharmacy, however, is yielding to one of pharmaceutical care.

The pharmaceutical care model empowers a pharmacist to encourage patients to assume responsibility for drug therapy within the framework of their own lifestyle, values, and environmental factors. Pharmaceutical care is the responsible provision of drug therapy for the purpose of achieving definite outcomes that improve the patient's quality of life. A pharmacist who practices pharmaceutical care is not as concerned with the objective correctness of therapy from a medical viewpoint as with the subjective appropriateness of therapy from a patient viewpoint. Pharmaceutical care is patient oriented rather than physician oriented. In recent years, courts of law have come to understand the significant role that pharmacists can play in the care of patients, but this recent understanding did not develop without a struggle, and in fact has not been completely realized yet today.

Historically, the courts have taken a narrow view of the role of pharmacists, a role that certainly does not include pharmaceutical care. The case of *Ingram v. Hook's Drug*, 476 N.E.2d 881 (Ind. Ct. App. 1985) typifies this view. In *Ingram*, the pharmacist dispensed Valium to the plaintiff, providing no warnings of possible adverse effects or side effects. A few days later the plaintiff fell off a ladder and fractured his leg, allegedly due to the dizziness and drowsiness caused by the Valium. He sued the pharmacy contending that the pharmacist had a duty to warn him of the drug's dangers. The trial court granted the pharmacy's motion for summary judgment and the plaintiff appealed. On appeal the court held that the duty to warn of a drug's dangers rests with the physician and that the pharmacist has no duty to warn.

Court decisions such as *Ingram* that have rejected the pharmacist's duty-to-warn argument have articulated similar rationale in support for their decisions. That rationale is that the pharmacist has no duty to advise a patient about a drug's risks, or to monitor a patient's drug use because the physician is the primary health care provider and the one upon whom the patients place their reliance (this rationale often is called the learned intermediary doctrine as discussed later in the product liability section); that pharmacists do not have access to sufficient medical information about the patient in order to advise the patient properly; that pharmacists would interfere with the physician–patient relationship; and that to require pharmacists to warn would place an undue burden upon them because they would have to question every prescription and warn of every danger. (For a detailed analysis of these rationale, see *McKee v. American Home Products, Inc.*, 782 P.2d 1045 (Wash. 1989).) These rationale seem specious when applied to today's practice of pharmacy yet are still persuasive today to courts in many jurisdictions, even in the face of state regulations requiring the maintenance of patient medication records, the screening of prescriptions for potential problems, and counseling of common and severe adverse risks.

AN EXPANDED VIEW OF PHARMACIST DUTY

One of the first cases to describe pharmacist duty consistently with the precepts of pharmaceutical care was *Hooks SuperX, Inc. v. McLaughlin*, 642 N.E.2d 514 (Ind. 1994), in which the Indiana Supreme Court reversed an earlier ruling of the Indiana Court of Appeals. Filed in late 1994, the opinion in this case thoroughly analyzed the concept of duty, based on three factors:

1. Relationship
2. Foreseeability
3. Public policy

The *Hooks SuperX* decision warrants discussion because the rationale the court used to find duty was the basis for recent court decisions finding that pharmacists owe a patient a duty beyond simply dispensing prescriptions correctly and accurately.

Factual Background of the *Hooks SuperX* Case

The plaintiff in this case injured his back while working as a lumberjack. In the course of treatment for that injury, he became addicted to propoxyphene. He was treated for the addiction in 1982, 1983, and 1987, but he did not stop using the drug. In 1988, because he was still having pain from the injury, he began treatment under a new physician. Over a period of months in 1988, the plaintiff obtained from the physician numerous prescriptions for drugs containing propoxyphene. Most of these prescriptions were filled at the defendant pharmacy. The propoxyphene was dispensed on the basis of valid written prescriptions, telephoned prescriptions, or authorized refills.

The plaintiff ingested propoxyphene at a much greater rate than prescribed. The records of the defendant pharmacy showed that dozens of prescriptions for propoxyphene were filled for the plaintiff between May 1987 and December 1988. For example, during one 60-day period in 1988, the plaintiff received 24 separate refills of propoxyphene compounds totaling 1,072 tablets. If consumed according to the prescription, the dosage units dispensed would have lasted 138 days, yet the plaintiff consumed the tablets in 62 days. In 1 month alone, propoxyphene prescriptions were filled 12 times, which meant that the plaintiff or his wife appeared in the defendant pharmacy every 2 or 3 days.

In late 1988 the physician, apparently aware that the plaintiff was consuming propoxyphene tablets at the increased rate, refused to furnish any more prescriptions. Shortly thereafter, the plaintiff's wife found her husband holding a shotgun to his head during an acute episode of depression. He did not pull the trigger. After treatment for drug addiction in early 1989, the plaintiff stopped taking all prescription medication.

The plaintiff sued the pharmacy under the theory that the pharmacy had breached its duty of care by failing to stop filling the prescriptions because the pharmacist knew that the plaintiff was consuming the drugs so quickly that they posed a threat to his health. The defendant moved for dismissal of the case on the grounds that it owed no such duty. The trial court denied the motion and the defendant appealed. The Indiana Court of Appeals concluded that no duty existed and that imposition of a duty for pharmacists to monitor drug therapy and intervene to prevent potential problems would be contrary to public policy because it would undermine the physician–patient relationship.

On appeal to the Indiana Supreme Court, the most important issue was whether pharmacists have any duty to refuse to fill validly issued prescriptions that pose a threat to the welfare of the patient. As indicated earlier, the opinion in this case analyzes the concept of duty on the basis of three factors. In essence, the court reasoned that it would make good legal precedent to expand pharmacist duties to include the duty to monitor and intervene if:

1. The relationship between pharmacist and patient is of the kind that should give rise to an expanded duty.
2. Harm to the patient is reasonably foreseeable to a pharmacist.
3. Public policy concerns (such as increased health care costs and diminished patient confidence in physicians) favor recognizing such an expanded duty.

The Relationship Factor

The court in *Hooks SuperX* reaffirmed that the law recognizes the relationship between pharmacist and patient as one that creates a duty under traditional order-processing circumstances. Pharmacists are clearly liable for dispensing the wrong medicine or for failing to inform the patient of warnings included in the prescription. The court noted that the relationship between the pharmacist and the patient is a direct one, independent of the physician–patient relationship. The court recognized that pharmacists possess expertise in the dispensing of prescription drugs and that patients rely on them for that expertise. All these factors combined led the court to conclude that "the relationship between the pharmacist and customer is sufficiently close to justify imposing a duty" (642 N.E.2d at 517) to monitor drug use and intervene when a problem becomes evident.

The court apparently recognized that in evaluating the relationship of one party to another, it is necessary to first identify the characteristics of the two parties. A relationship is forged from the identities of the individuals in the relationship; thus people relate to each other only in ways that reflect their own personal, or professional, characteristics. The *Hooks SuperX* opinion noted that a pharmacist is a person who knows about drugs and that a patient is a person who needs information about drugs. Given these individual characteristics, it is logical to conclude that the pharmacist–patient relationship is one in which the pharmacist has a duty to provide information. Under this analysis, the duty of a pharmacist expands and contracts on the basis of the pharmacist's knowledge. A knowledge-based duty would serve as the foundation for requiring some action by pharmacists but not for requiring unlimited action. Pharmacists would have a duty to warn patients of known risks, but there would be no duty to warn of risks that are not known. Thus, the answer to a question of pharmacist duty would begin with a determination of pharmacist knowledge. The availability of knowledge would define the minimum that could be expected of a pharmacist, and the unavailability of knowledge would set limits on what could be expected of a pharmacist.

Knowledge, by itself, however, is not a sufficient foundation for a duty from pharmacists to patients. For there to be a duty to intervene to protect patients from known adverse effects, it is also necessary that pharmacists foresee harm to patients.

The Foreseeability Factor

Turning to the factor of foreseeability, the court found it undisputed that an individual who consumes sufficient quantities of addictive substances may become addicted to them, and that such an addiction carries with it certain foreseeable consequences. The court was satisfied that, for the purpose of determining whether a duty exists, the risk of the plaintiff's addiction was foreseeable from the events that took place. Under the court's analysis, it would be good legal precedent to require that one who can anticipate harm to another intervene to prevent that harm. Simply knowing of a potential adverse effect would not be sufficient to require that a pharmacist provide a warning to a patient; it would also be necessary for the pharmacist to foresee harm to the patient.

The foreseeability requirement takes the pharmacist's duty from the realm of the hypothetical into the realm of the practical. A known but relatively unlikely adverse effect would not require a warning because it would not be foreseeable. Under this approach, a pharmacist's duty to warn requires first that the adverse effect be known and second that there be foreseeable negative consequences for the patient if a warning about the adverse effect is not given. Many adverse effects are known because they have occurred at some time in the past, and at that time they were associated with the use of a medication. However, the incidence of the adverse effect may be so low that it is not realistically foreseeable. Although McLaughlin's addiction to propoxyphene was foreseeable under the circumstances, many adverse effects would not be foreseeable.

Public Policy Considerations

The final factor considered in determining the existence of the duty for pharmacists was that of public policy. The court deemed three public policy considerations to be at stake:

1. Preventing intentional and unintentional drug abuse
2. Not jeopardizing the physician–patient relationship
3. Avoiding unnecessary health costs

The court's purpose in identifying these considerations was to determine whether public policy should or should not favor recognition of the duty.

On the first issue, the court recognized that there are a variety of reasons why a patient might try to have a prescription for a potentially harmful drug refilled at a rate higher than that prescribed, of which an addiction to the drug and diversion of the drug for an illicit purpose were two. Both of these explanations for too-frequent refills give rise to a strong public policy interest in preventing intentional and unintentional drug abuse. This public policy interest is reflected in the enactments of the state legislature. For example, the Indiana Code empowers a pharmacist to exercise professional judgment and refuse to honor a prescription when the pharmacist believes in good faith that honoring the prescription might aid or abet an addiction or habit. This statute demonstrates that public policy concerns about proper dispensing of prescription drugs and preventing drug addiction are paramount to policy concerns about interfering with the physician–patient relationship. A physician–patient relationship that is causing drug addiction or diversion needs to be interfered with. As a matter of policy, pharmacists should be required to act to prevent intentional and unintentional drug abuse.

Next, the court reasoned that, as a matter of public policy, the imposition of a duty to cease filling prescriptions in certain circumstances would not lead to the development of an adverse relationship between pharmacists and physicians. The court offered three separate reasons for this conclusion:

1. Pharmacists already have authority to intervene through statute.
2. Physicians remain ultimately responsible for the proper prescription of medications, and recognition of a duty on the part of pharmacists would not replace the physician's obligation to evaluate a patient's needs.
3. The recognition of a legal duty would encourage pharmacists and physicians to work together in considering the best interests of their patients. Public policy should encourage collaboration to protect the public.

The last public policy concern reviewed by the court related to the possibility of an increase in health care costs if the duty in question were to be imposed on pharmacists. The court implied that if health care costs were to rise as the result of recognizing the expanded duty, public policy might not favor the recognition. The defendant had argued that recognition of the expanded duty would require pharmacies to buy expensive new technologies, thus driving up the cost of health care. However, the defendant pharmacy already had a computer-based information system that showed the plaintiff's entire prescription history on the screen at the time of each fill or refill. The cost of computerizing the pharmacy had already been incurred and would not increase with recognition of the expanded pharmacist duty. Thus the public policy of holding down health care costs was not at odds with recognition of the duty.

The court concluded that all three relevant factors (relationship, foreseeability, and public policy) supported imposition of the expanded duty on pharmacists. Although any of the three factors could individually have justified the decision, the collective force of the three was compelling.

RATIONALE FOR EXPANDED PHARMACIST DUTIES

Consistent with the rationale of the *Hooks SuperX* opinion, some courts across the country have begun to recognize expanded responsibilities for pharmacists. To escape liability for negligence, it is still necessary for pharmacists to process orders accurately, but it is no longer sufficient to be technically accurate. Pharmacists must competently monitor drug therapy and thoroughly discuss drug therapy with patients if they wish to avoid exposure to legal liability.

The emerging judicial view of the pharmacist–patient relationship was summarized by Judge Pittman in his opinion in *Griffin v. Phar-Mor, Inc.*, 790 F. Supp. 1115 (S.D. Ala. 1992). Judge Pittman stated:

> The relationship between a pharmacist and a client is one in which the client puts extreme trust in the pharmacist. Pharmacists possess important specialized knowledge that is possessed by few, if any, non-pharmacists, and it is this specialized knowledge that puts patients in the position of having to put complete trust and confidence in a pharmacist's skill. (790 F. Supp. at 1118)

Judge Pittman then described the specific responsibility of pharmacists to educate patients about their medications.

> The importance of the particular facts does not need to be explained in any great detail. In general, it is important that a person know the type of medicine the person

is taking. For example, a person may be allergic to a particular medicine, or a person may need to inform another doctor of what medications the person is taking. Also, and this is another thing that patients depend on pharmacists to provide, a person needs to know the type of medicine he or she is taking so the person can know what activities (i.e., drinking alcohol or dairy products) to avoid while taking the medications. (790 F. Supp. at 1118)

The responsibility of pharmacists to convey such information is important; in fact it is potentially lifesaving, and the cost of providing this information is not great.

The Tennessee Supreme Court has described the drug information responsibility of pharmacists using similar language. In the opinion from *Pittman v. The Upjohn Co.*, 890 S.W.2d 425 (Tenn. 1994), the court quoted with approval rules of the Tennessee Board of Pharmacy, which state:

A pharmacist should, on dispensing a new prescription, explain to the patient or the patient's agent the directions for the use and a warning of all effects of the medication or device that are significant and/or potentially harmful. (890 S.W.2d at 435)

The disclosure standard recognized by this language relates to both the content of the information to be given by a pharmacist to a patient and the process through which the information is to be provided. Accurate and complete information must be provided in a way that will promote appropriate medication use.

A Florida appellate court took a similar position to *Pittman* in a 2005 decision, diverting from prior Florida court decisions. In *Powers v. Thobhani*, 903 So.2d 275 (Fla. App. 2005), the defendant pharmacy filled numerous lawful controlled substance prescriptions issued by the prescriber too closely in time to previously issued prescriptions. The patient ultimately overdosed and died, and her husband brought a wrongful death action against the pharmacy for failure to exercise due and proper care by not notifying the prescriber or the patient of the risks associated with frequently prescribed multiple controlled substance prescriptions. The trial court followed prior Florida court decisions and held that pharmacists have no duty other than to properly dispense a lawful prescription. The appellate court, however, reversed the trial court, noting that "There is a strong policy basis to support a pharmacy's duty to warn customers of the risks inherent in filling certain repeated prescriptions" (at 279). The court found the social policy was reflected in Florida laws and regulations requiring that pharmacists interpret and assess prescriptions and counsel patients. (For more discussion of this issue see Case 8-1: *Happel v. Wal-Mart Stores, Inc.* and the notes following the case.)

The *Baker* Case: Assumption of a Duty

An interesting case regarding the pharmacist's expanded duty is *Baker v. Arbor Drugs, Inc.*, 544 N.W.2d 727 (Mich. App. Ct. 1996). Decided by the Michigan Court of Appeals, *Baker* departed from a clear line of precedent in the Michigan appellate courts. Before *Baker*, courts in Michigan had been reluctant to recognize expanded responsibilities for pharmacists. Although the pharmacist's duty to process prescriptions correctly was clear, Michigan courts had held that pharmacists had no duty to warn the patient of possible side effects of a medication or to monitor drug use. The *Baker* opinion adopted a different perspective on the issue in part on the basis of the compelling facts of the case.

The plaintiff in *Baker* was a patient who suffered from depression and was prescribed the drug tranylcypromine after an attempted suicide in October 1989. The patient was well aware of the dangers of adverse reactions with tranylcypromine, and he had strictly followed instructions given by his physician and the drug's manufacturer. On February 26, 1992, the patient developed a cold and went to see a different physician.

This physician's records indicated that the patient was taking tranylcypromine. In addition, the patient later told his wife that he had twice told the physician that he was taking this drug. The physician prescribed two products for the patient. One product contained the drug phenylpropanolamine.

The patient took his prescriptions to the pharmacy where he normally had his prescriptions for tranylcypromine filled. A prescription for that drug had been filled for him at this pharmacy 11 days earlier. A computer at the pharmacy detected a potential interaction between the previously prescribed tranylcypromine and the newly prescribed phenylpropanolamine. However, a pharmacy technician overrode the computer prompt, and a pharmacist filled the prescription without becoming aware that the patient was also using a drug with which the prescribed drug could interact.

The patient ingested his prescribed cold remedy. Later that evening he complained to his wife that he was not feeling well. The two of them referred to literature that had been provided to them with tranylcypromine and concluded that the patient was suffering from a hypertensive attack. The patient was taken to the hospital, where he was diagnosed as having suffered a stroke. The stroke was a result of having ingested both the monoamine oxidase inhibitor and phenylpropanolamine. The patient eventually died.

The defendant pharmacy had advertised that its computer system was designed in part to detect harmful drug interactions such as the one that led to Baker's death. For example, one advertisement said:

> Do you know what happens when you bring your prescription to Arbor Drugs? First, it's checked for insurance coverage and screened for possible drug interactions and therapeutic duplication. That's done very quickly by the Arbortech Plus computer. Then your prescription is filled and labeled. That's done very carefully, by your Arbor pharmacist. The bottom line? Your prescription is not just filled quickly, it's filled safely. Only at the Arbor Pharmacies. You can't get any better. (544 N.W.2d at 731)

Despite providing this assurance in its advertising, the defendant did not prevent the plaintiff's drug interaction. The available technology was not used correctly because the pharmacy technician overrode the interaction indicated on the computer.

In reversing summary judgment granted in favor of the defendant pharmacy by the trial court, the Michigan Court of Appeals held that the pharmacy "voluntarily assumed a duty to utilize the Arbortech Plus computer technology with due care" (544 N.W.2d at 731). Citing prior case law for the precedent that a defendant can be held liable when it voluntarily assumes a function that it was under no legal obligation to assume, the court expanded pharmacist responsibilities in Michigan beyond technical accuracy to include drug therapy monitoring with the assistance of computer systems.

Representations, Reliance, and Duty

The ubiquitous nature of computers in contemporary pharmacy practice turns what could have been a narrow exception to a general rule of "no duty" into a new and opposite general rule. Computers are hardly voluntary in pharmacy practice of the 21st century. They are as necessary as prescription vials (which replaced paper envelopes) and machine-printed instructions for patients (a vast improvement over pen and ink scribbling by a pharmacist or physician). Escaping liability such as that imposed by *Baker* is hardly possible by opting not to use computers. Technology has enabled pharmacists to provide greater value to patients, and the pharmacist who fails to use available technology has failed in a duty owed to patients.

Pharmacists have the ability to define the relationship they have with patients. The opinion in *Baker* recognized that the "defendant's advertisements were made to induce customers to utilize its pharmacy" (544 N.W.2d at 733). If patients are told to expect nothing more than technical accuracy from pharmacists, then they are likely to expect only that they will receive the right drug, in the right strength, with the right directions for use. "Rightness" would be determined only by the physician's prescription, not the patient's needs. However, a pharmacy that advertises, "We accept responsibility for accurately filling your prescription with the drug ordered by your physician" is not likely to see an increase in business. Patients expect pharmacists to be accurate, and such an advertisement does not distinguish the advertising pharmacy from any other pharmacy.

If patients are told to expect more than technical accuracy from pharmacists, they likely will elevate their expectations. The *Baker* opinion noted that the "decedent reasonably relied on the allegedly false representation" (544 N.W.2d at 732). This finding served as the basis for the court's ruling that the pharmacy could be liable for fraud or deception. Pharmacist duties expand with patient expectations. Representations by a pharmacist that are relied on by a patient create a covenantal relationship between pharmacist and patient. A pharmacist's promise to perform, in exchange for a patient placing himself or herself in the care of the pharmacist, obligates the pharmacist to keep the promise and meet a duty to the patient.

EXPANDED RESPONSIBILITIES: A JUDICIAL COMPROMISE

Many recent court decisions have been reluctant to find that pharmacists have a general duty to warn, but instead have held that pharmacists have a duty to warn only in certain circumstances. In essence, these courts have fashioned a middle ground. The case of *Happel v. Wal-Mart Stores, Inc.* (see Case 8-1) is one example. Another example is *Morgan v. Wal-Mart Stores, Inc.*, 30 S.W.3d 455 (Tex. Ct. App. 2000), which was cited favorably in *Happel*. In *Morgan*, the plaintiffs sued the pharmacy, alleging that the death of their son was caused by an adverse reaction to Desipramine. The plaintiffs contended that the pharmacy was negligent for failing to warn of the possibility of the adverse reaction. The court held that pharmacists do not have a generalized duty to warn absent "special circumstances." The court interpreted special circumstances as: (1) when the manufacturer gives special instructions to warn patients, (2) contraindications, and (3) when the pharmacist has special knowledge of the patient's medical condition. In *Morgan*, the court found against the plaintiff because these special circumstances did not exist. In contrast, *Happel* found that special circumstances did exist.

© Stockbyte/Thinkstock

STUDY SCENARIOS AND QUESTIONS

1. Joe, who is a pharmacist and the owner of Pillum Pharmacy, dispensed codeine and glutethimide prescriptions to George for over 10 years. The prescriber authorized all the prescriptions dispensed by Pillum. As a result of taking the two drugs in combination for such an extended period of time, George required in-patient hospitalization for glutethimide detoxification and psychiatric treatment for addiction. He also suffered from major clinical depression and related disorders. Subsequently, George sued Joe, Pillum, and the prescriber. Joe and Pillum filed a motion to dismiss for failure to state a claim upon which relief could be granted. The defendants argued that, as a matter of law, a pharmacist has neither a duty to warn of a prescribed drug's dangerous propensities nor a duty to control or keep track of a customer's reliance on drugs prescribed by a licensed treating physician.
   a. Discuss who should prevail in this case. Should a pharmacist have a duty to warn a patient of a drug's adverse effects and monitor a patient's drug therapy? (Contrast the traditional approach of the courts on this issue with the emerging trend.) What arguments can be made either way?

  b. Assuming that the court concludes that pharmacists have a duty to warn and monitor, would a reasonable pharmacist have warned a patient of the potential dangers of long-term treatment with these two drugs?

2. Mary took a prescription for Indocin to Sauter Pharmacy. She had never traded at Sauter's previously and did not know Bill, who was a licensed pharmacist there. Mary presented the prescription to Bill, and a discussion followed concerning her drug allergies. Mary told Bill she was allergic to Percodan and described an earlier brush with death. On Mary's prescription, Bill wrote, "Allergic to Percodan." Mary asked Bill if Percodan and Indocin were related. Bill replied that the two drugs were in different classes. The next morning, Mary suffered a severe attack of bronchial asthma, apparently triggered by an anaphylactic reaction, and died in the emergency room. Mary's estate sued Sauter and Bill contending that the pharmacist had a duty to advise Mary that since she was allergic to Percodan she also might be allergic to Indocin.

  a. Explain whether Bill should have a legal duty to warn Mary of the possible allergic reaction. Would a reasonable pharmacist know that Percodan contains aspirin and that Mary might be allergic to the aspirin and also the Indocin?

  b. How is this case different from the previous case? Is this a stronger case for duty than the previous case? Why or why not?

RISK MANAGEMENT STRATEGIES

Failures of quality not only produce human suffering, but also produce lawsuits that are financially and emotionally costly. Pharmacy errors may also lead to state board of pharmacy disciplinary activities and uncomplimentary media coverage. Risk management activities are designed to reduce the incidence of errors, so as to prevent the negative fallout that adversely affects a business at which errors have occurred. Primarily a business activity, risk management has the additional benefit of protecting patient welfare; thus, it is entirely consistent with good patient care. Managing the risk of legal liability requires an effective system to reduce error and a commitment to remediation when error does occur.

  It is important to remember that pharmacy risk management is not risk elimination. In health care, some risk is necessary in order to benefit patients. In pharmacy, one way to eliminate the risk of litigation caused by error is to practice so conservatively that patient welfare is compromised. For example, a pharmacy could refuse to fill any prescription with a dose that is out of the ordinary or refuse to stock drugs that have a narrow therapeutic index and are inclined to cause problems for patients. Assuming a pharmacy could stay in business with such a restrictive approach to practice, the risk of litigation would be reduced because patients would be less likely to be harmed. However, patients would also be less likely to derive benefit from their medications because some patients need doses that are out of the ordinary, or they need drugs with a narrow therapeutic index, or they need both.

  This overly restrictive approach to risk management would conflict with the goal of good patient care. Effective risk management requires the development of systems to reduce the incidence of preventable error and lessen the consequences of error that cannot be prevented. Risk management is the responsibility of the institutions in which pharmacists work and of pharmacists themselves, who must be effective risk managers every minute of every day.

INSTITUTIONAL CONTROLS

The importance of developing and maintaining appropriate systems for order processing, and to detect and "absorb" errors by pharmacists before a patient is harmed, has been judicially recognized. The Alabama Supreme Court affirmed a jury verdict against a pharmacy, awarding $100,000 in compensatory damages and $150,000 in punitive damages on the basis of the plaintiff's allegation that the pharmacy had failed to initiate sufficient institutional controls over the manner in which prescriptions were filled. In *Harco Drugs, Inc. v. Holloway*, 669 So. 2d 878 (Ala. 1995), the court ruled that the jury could properly have concluded that in failing to conduct quality assurance activities, the pharmacy had acted with reckless disregard for the safety of others. In effect, this case is a call for more substantial quality assurance systems in retail pharmacy chains, so as to recognize circumstances that give rise to error and modify those circumstances to prevent error.

The facts of the case, as described in the majority opinion, disclosed that a pharmacist employed by the defendant–pharmacy had incorrectly processed a prescription order for the plaintiff. The pharmacist, in attempting to fill a prescription for Tamoxifen, incorrectly entered into the computer information relating to Tambocor. As a result, the plaintiff's prescription was misfilled on three separate occasions. According to the court, the pharmacist knew that the patient's physician was an oncologist, and that the medication she was dispensing was a heart medication. Although the pharmacist recognized what the court refers to as an "obvious conflict," the pharmacist did not telephone the oncologist to confirm the prescription.

Another pharmacist, who was on duty when the plaintiff came in to question the misfilled prescription, testified that the prescription written by the oncologist was not legible and that he would have had trouble reading it if he had been busy. He agreed that being busy is no excuse for misfilling a prescription. He admitted that the responsibility for correctly filling a prescription rests with the pharmacist, and that if a pharmacist has any questions whatsoever with regard to a prescription, it is the pharmacist's responsibility to telephone the physician and to take whatever steps are necessary to see that the prescription is filled correctly.

One of the pharmacy's district managers testified that misfilling a prescription could have serious consequences and that the pharmacy had a responsibility to support its pharmacists to ensure that misfillings did not happen. The district manager testified that it is the pharmacy's job to make certain that prescriptions are not misfilled.

The jury was informed of 233 incident reports that had been prepared by the pharmacy's employees during the 3 years preceding the incident involving the plaintiff in this case. These reports dealt in some way or another with customer complaints of errors on the part of pharmacy employees in filling prescriptions, and most of them indicated that the pharmacy's employees had committed errors in filling prescriptions.

Punitive Damages for "Wantonness"

On appeal, the key issue was the appropriateness of punitive damages and the legal conclusion that the defendant pharmacy had acted "wantonly" toward the plaintiff. "Wantonness" is defined in Alabama as "conduct which is carried on with a recklessness or conscious disregard of the rights or safety of others." With this standard in mind, the Alabama Supreme Court noted that the pharmacy's management had evidence of numerous incidents of incorrectly filled prescriptions; however, it failed to share this information with the stores in the chain. The jury could have inferred, said the court, that although the incident reports were in the possession of the pharmacy, the pharmacy did not see fit to disseminate the information to all of its pharmacists as a matter of course, despite undisputed testimony that a misfilled prescription could be fatal. Instead of providing this information to all of its stores once a year, a company representative merely encouraged the pharmacists to "be careful." The court noted that given knowledge on the company's part that misfilling a prescription could be fatal, the jury could have found that there was a reckless disregard on the company's part for the safety of its customers in not disseminating the information to all the pharmacists in the chain.

In addition, the court pointed to the failure of the company to use nonprofessional personnel to look at prescriptions to make sure that the prescriptions were being filled correctly by pharmacists. The company had conceded that having two people, a pharmacist and a clerk, look at a prescription would reduce the chances of making a mistake in filling that prescription. The company believed, however, that it would cost too much to adopt such a policy. On the basis of this review of the evidence, the court concluded that the jury could have properly determined that the company had acted wantonly in connection with its handling of its pharmacies. The jury verdict for punitive, as well as compensatory, damages was upheld in a majority opinion agreed to by five of eight justices.

In a vigorous dissenting opinion, three of the eight justices explained why they would have overruled the punitive damages judgment. This minority view disclosed a version of the facts of the case that was distinct from the facts as described in the majority opinion. According to the minority opinion, the incident reports on which the plaintiff relied in support of her argument had all been sent to the company's director of pharmacy operations for review. The director of pharmacy operations testified that he reviewed each report and counseled any pharmacist who misfilled a prescription as reflected in an incident report. Occasionally, a pharmacist would be transferred to a store with less volume if the company believed that the pharmacist could perform better in a low-volume store. The company had terminated the employment of some pharmacists that it believed could not perform their duties.

In addition, the dissenters pointed out that the plaintiff had relied heavily on the fact that the company management had considered the implementation of a policy of having clerical workers verify prescriptions but had rejected the idea. However, the director of pharmacy operations had testified that the use of supportive personnel for this purpose was discretionary with the pharmacists. Although the use of supportive personnel to check the accuracy of pharmacists was not expressly required, it was not forbidden. The dissenters disagreed with the majority's view that the company's decision not to require a clerical worker to inspect the work of a professionally trained and licensed pharmacist could constitute wantonness. Nevertheless, although the minority dissenting opinion did not support the award of punitive damages, the rationale of the majority opinion resulted in affirmation of the punitive damages verdict.

On reconsideration, the Alabama Supreme Court endorsed all of its previous holdings regarding the failure to maintain institutional controls. However, the new opinion clarified the responsibility of an individual pharmacist when the pharmacist is presented a prescription that is difficult to interpret. The court said:

> We believe that a prescription from an oncologist that a pharmacist believes to call for Tambocor, a heart medication used by cardiologists to treat arrhythmias or serious heart ailments, should cause her grave concern and necessarily prompt further inquiry. The extreme unusualness of a prescription from a cancer specialist supposedly calling for a dangerous heart medication, combined with the alleged illegibility of the prescription, is sufficient evidence of a reckless disregard of the safety of others to create a jury question as to whether Harco acted wantonly. A jury could infer that Harco's actions under those circumstances rose to the level of a conscious disregard for the safety of Ms. Holloway. (669 So. 2d at 880–881)

Interpreting Unclear Prescriptions

According to this interpretation of the law, pharmacists who are asked to dispense a medication pursuant to an unclear order should make sure they consider the therapeutic context of the order—particularly the prescriber's area of practice and the patient's condition. The shapes of letters on paper may suggest one drug, whereas the circumstances of therapy indicate an altogether different drug. A pharmacist focusing on pharmaceutical care, rather than on technical activities, can prevent error and reduce the risk of resulting liability.

Corporate Responsibility (Corporate Negligence)

The essence of *Harco Drugs* is the allegation that a corporate pharmacy with many community-based outlets has a responsibility to develop and maintain a comprehensive quality assurance program to ensure "institutional control" over the system of prescription processing. This type of negligence is called "corporate negligence," meaning that the corporation is itself responsible for its own actions, apart from those of its employees. This is a novel claim of primary responsibility of the corporate pharmacy. This sort of claim is distinct from the traditional approach of alleging that an employer is responsible only secondarily for the acts of its employees. In the past, when corporate pharmacies have been sued as the result of a misfilled prescription, the legal theory has almost always been that under the principle of vicarious liability the employer must answer for the wrongs done by the employee. The focus has been on the improper conduct of a single person, the pharmacist who misfilled the prescription, and the company has been held liable on the basis of a legal theory connecting it with the wrongful act of its employee rather than for its own wrongful act. This case changes that approach because the focus is on the acts of management and the system itself within which the pharmacist works, rather than the acts of the practitioner. The idea that a pharmacist's error might be caused by a system failure, rather than by an individual failure, has until recently not been considered in litigation based on community pharmacy practice.

Harco Drugs departs from precedent because it considers the possibility that a pharmacist may be given circumstances that are predisposed to error (e.g., inadequate supportive personnel, outdated technologies, or inadequate lighting or other deficiency in the physical layout), so a pharmacy can fairly be characterized as an accident that is waiting to happen. Despite the conscientious activities of a pharmacist under such circumstances, an error is likely to occur—not because of a pharmacist's inattentiveness, but despite a pharmacist's attentiveness. It is the provision of such an environment within which a company's pharmacists are required to practice that could expose the pharmacy company to punitive damages. Punitive damages punish wrongdoers. They deter future wrongdoing. They are intended to force people to think about the consequences of their actions for other people and to act responsibly to prevent harm to others.

Whether the jury was justified in awarding punitive damages in this case and whether the Alabama Supreme Court was justified in affirming the award are interesting questions on which it is possible to disagree. The disagreement among the justices of the Alabama Supreme Court illustrates the difficulty of resolving such questions.

CONTINUOUS QUALITY IMPROVEMENT (CQI) PROGRAMS AS RISK MANAGEMENT

The implications of *Harco Drugs* and corporate negligence lawsuits go beyond the wrongness or rightness of the result and are of greater significance to pharmacies as practices rather than pharmacists as practitioners. This case shows that courts have begun to consider the implications for public safety of the order-processing systems developed and used by community pharmacies. In the face of this evolving body of law, community pharmacies must seriously consider not only developing effective CQI programs but also using them.

As *Harco Drugs* suggests, the generation and use of incident reports is an essential component of CQI. To anticipate problems that may occur in the future and to implement systems to detect and prevent those problems is a daunting task. A flaw in a system is difficult to see without the benefit of hindsight. By using incident reports, a quality assurance manager can identify flaws within the system and implement strategies to address those flaws. Incident reports should be generated at any time a patient might have been harmed by a misfilled prescription. Each report should be investigated to determine whether a particular cause of the problem can be identified and if so, whether the cause can be eliminated or mitigated. Reports should be evaluated in the aggregate to determine whether collectively it is possible to see a problem that is not evident from the investigation of a single incident. Many states have mandated that pharmacies develop a CQI program that includes an incident reporting system.

Periodic evaluation of employees is also an essential element of institutional control to meet legal requirements. Pharmacists or technicians who seem to be particularly error prone may simply be practicing in situations that create error, or they may be hampered by a knowledge deficit or misunderstanding of procedures. Practice situations that create error should be resolved, and personnel problems should be addressed to reduce the rate of error. This latter problem may require that a pharmacist work under the supervision of an experienced and more capable pharmacist, or it may even require a period of retraining. The *Hundley v. Rite Aid* case discussed in the case studies section of this chapter provides an excellent example of the consequences to a corporation that fails to monitor and supervise a pharmacist properly.

Perhaps the most important aspect of *Harco Drugs* and similar corporate negligence decisions is that they place the responsibility for the quality of distributive systems squarely on the shoulders of the pharmacy company. The responsibility for working competently within the system is the individual pharmacist's responsibility. This includes the responsibility to think about the context of a medication order, not just about the appearance of ink on paper—yet the overall responsibility for assessing and improving quality rests with the pharmacy company. To meet this newly recognized legal responsibility, community pharmacies must conduct CQI activities. This does not mean that the law requires elimination of all error. It means that aggressive efforts must be undertaken to reduce error to the greatest extent possible. To fail in this effort is to increase a pharmacy company's exposure to liability for punitive damages.

THE PHARMACIST AS RISK MANAGER

No matter how good a pharmacy's system of quality assurance may be, and no matter how hard a pharmacist may try to adhere to policies within the system, failures of quality will continue to occur. Patients will receive inaccurately filled prescriptions, they will be inadequately counseled, and obvious problems with drug therapy will be undetected by prospective drug-use review. When problems of this sort do occur, patients will understandably become upset, and the person who will be confronted by the patient, or a representative of the patient, will be the pharmacist. This initial confrontation is the best opportunity to avoid litigation by means of an appropriate response by the pharmacist, and it is the time at which the pharmacist can guarantee litigation through an inappropriate response. It is the defining moment in risk management.

Pharmacists should always do whatever they can to assist in resolving a pharmacy error and minimizing its impact. This includes notification to anyone whom the pharmacist suspects may have been the object of an error and absolute openness with information necessary to ensure a good outcome for the patient. The patient's physician should be contacted any time there is reason to believe that a pharmacy error may have affected the patient's health. Patients should be made to know that their safety and welfare are the most important concern. Many times patients have said, "I understand that anyone can make a mistake, but what upsets me is that the pharmacist didn't seem to care when I asked him to talk with me about the mistake he made." A patient who feels this way may file a lawsuit for malpractice or a complaint with the board of pharmacy, simply to get the pharmacist's attention. Reacting to patient concerns in a way that does not show respect and caring is poor professional judgment and a poor risk management technique.

Pharmacists must ensure that, when they react to a problem with drug therapy, the things they say and the things they write are done in ways that are sensitive to risk management issues. Otherwise, the words spoken and written will come back to haunt them in a lawsuit.

PROBLEMS AND PITFALLS OF RISK MANAGEMENT

Verbal communication and written documentation by pharmacists can be a cause of problems for risk managers. The things pharmacists say and the things they write have a way of coming up in lawsuits, and they can be difficult to explain. There is no question that some problems, which would have gone undetected otherwise, are made obvious through careless comments, and suspicions are cast on previously unidentified health care providers through a carelessly drafted written record. However, the advantages of verbal communication and written documentation clearly outweigh the disadvantages. It would not be good risk management advice, and certainly not good patient care advice, to instruct pharmacists, "Don't ever say anything or write anything." Verbal communication is necessary to ensure that patients make good decisions about drug therapy, and documentation by pharmacists can prevent harm to patients. Both of these activities are positive from a risk management perspective because they prevent litigation. Nobody sues when harm does not occur. Even if harm does occur, documentation may show that a pharmacist did everything that could reasonably have been done for a patient and that the bad outcome was unavoidable. Litigation will be unsuccessful if it is based on harm that could not have been prevented, and a pharmacist's written record can refute the patient's contention that a medication error was preventable.

RULES FOR EFFECTIVE RISK MANAGEMENT

Every pharmacist is a risk manager, and it is important to remember that there are certain approaches to verbal discussions and written notes that can reduce exposure to liability. No set of rules can absolutely produce good risk management outcomes, but the following suggestions serve as the basis for an approach to patient care that is sensitive to the concerns of risk management.

1. *Be correct.* The admonition to "be correct" reflects the fact that most errors in verbal communication or recordkeeping result from a failure to accurately convey information. Word use is important. Consider the following statements that do not really say what was intended:
   - "Patient has difficulty walking on diazepam."
   - "Patient experiences difficulty swallowing tires easily."
   - "She moves her bowels roughly, three times a day."

Sometimes the placement of punctuation or voice tone can alter the meaning of a statement. Being correct also includes the notion that when things go wrong, one should tell it like it is. Cover-ups are never to be tolerated. The facts will speak for themselves eventually, so honesty is always the best policy.

2. *Be complete.* That conversations and written documents should "be complete" means that they should include all information that is necessary to provide a continuing high level of care for the patient. Everything necessary to promote a good outcome for a patient should be spoken of and appear in the patient's record. A pharmacist who is wondering whether a particular piece of information should be mentioned in a conversation or included in a patient care record should ask whether the information is necessary to promote the patient's welfare. If the answer to that question is yes, then the information should be included.

3. *Be concise.* Being complete does not mean saying whatever comes to mind or putting every known tidbit of information in the patient care record because that would conflict with the rule to "be concise." Nothing that is not necessary for patient care should be spoken or appear in the patient care record. Some pharmacists confuse consults with other health care providers and notes entered in the patient care record with an in-service or pharmacy grand rounds. They photocopy articles from journals and staple them to the patient care record. Their chart entries are lengthy treatises designed to demonstrate their proficiency with pharmacotherapy. They overdo the job of information provision just to prove a point that does not need to be made.

   When the attending physician has not followed pharmacy advice and a bad result has occurred, these pharmacists write "Told Ya So" notes in the chart referencing back to a previous note containing what now (with the benefit of hindsight) looks like golden information. This is a real problem because notes in the patient care record are fully available to the patient's lawyer if the patient decides to sue. It is better to put information that is not necessary for patient care in an incident report. Under some circumstances, it is possible to refuse disclosure of an incident report. However, the fact of having filed an incident report should not be referred to in the patient care record.

4. *Be consistent.* To urge that pharmacists "be consistent" reflects the fact that once a pattern of verbal comments or documented remarks develops, a break from that pattern can be interpreted in a way that was not intended. Pharmacists should develop patterns of verbal observation and written documentation and adhere to them. If a pharmacist has a habit of recording a particular finding, and that information is not recorded, then the record overall will lead to the conclusion that the pharmacist did not observe something that should have been observed or that the pharmacist did not do something that should have been done. The pharmacist may in fact have acted appropriately, but to have omitted from the record a type of notation that is habitually made will be compelling evidence of inaction. Remember the saying: "If it isn't documented, then it didn't happen."

5. *Be cautious.* A pharmacist's verbal statements and documentation must "be cautious" to avoid misinterpretation of even the most innocuous comments. In particular, pharmacists should be cautious enough to avoid beginning a conversation or written note with a word or phrase that "handcuffs" the attending physician. For example, to begin a note with "Recommend . . ." or "Strongly recommend . . ." has the effect of saying "You are committing malpractice if you don't do. . . ." This is obviously a risk management nightmare.

   Of course, there are some circumstances when strong language needs to be used and attending physicians need to be handcuffed, yet caution dictates using softer beginnings for most pharmacy notes. The best approach for a pharmacist is to use a less-demanding beginning to a note, such as "Suggest . . ." or "Consider . . ." or even "Possibly consider . . ." Using this more cautious language makes it easier for an attending physician to explain why a decision was made not to do what the pharmacist thought was best after things had not gone well (e.g., "It was only a suggestion, and I gave it careful consideration"). This language also enables a pharmacist to provide attending physicians with information about an idea that the pharmacist may have, even if the pharmacist is less than absolutely certain that the idea is a good one. Patients deserve to have pharmacists make suggestions that pharmacists will not have to defend and justify later because a pharmacist's suggestion may be just what is needed to improve the possibility of a good outcome for the patient. Pharmacists will have to defend and justify a recommendation, so there may be a disincentive to making a recommendation under situations of uncertainty, thus potentially depriving the patient of the full benefit of a pharmacist's expertise. Use of the words "consider" and "suggest" can relieve the pharmacist of concerns about accountability that may accompany use of the word "recommend."

MALPRACTICE INSURANCE

Professional malpractice insurance is a necessity in modern pharmacy practice, just as it is in the practice of virtually every other profession. If a pharmacist who carries malpractice insurance is sued, the insurance company will both assume the costs of the defense (e.g., fees for attorneys and expert witnesses) and pay a claim if recovery is permitted.

Employee-pharmacists often wonder whether it is advisable for them to purchase their own individual insurance policy. One view is that having separate insurance invites litigation because the assets of an insurance company are obviously greater than are those of a pharmacist. On the other hand, an individual insurance policy provides added protection just in case a claim against a pharmacist is based on an occurrence that is not related to the pharmacist's employment. The current low cost of individual pharmacist malpractice policies makes it difficult to argue against their purchase.

Most pharmacist malpractice insurance policies contain a provision that expressly excludes coverage for personal injury or property damage caused by the willful violation of a penal statute. These "illegal act" exclusions are narrowly interpreted in favor of the insured pharmacist. A minor violation of a technical requirement will probably not permit an insurance company to deny coverage of a pharmacist who has diligently paid premiums for many years. When there is evidence of intentional illegal conduct, however, a pharmacist should not expect the malpractice policy to cover claims of harm made by those who were victimized by the conduct. Pharmacists should carefully read their insurance policy for scope of coverage and make certain it covers all activities in which they might be engaged including compounding, blood testing, immunizations, and initiating or adjusting drug therapies pursuant to a collaborative practice agreement.

© Stockbyte/Thinkstock

STUDY SCENARIOS AND QUESTIONS

1. The plaintiffs, parents of an infant who died at birth, sued K-Rite Pharmacy, allegedly because the pharmacist mistakenly filled a prescription for the mother for Ritalin instead of Ritodrine when the mother was 25 weeks pregnant. The plaintiffs contend negligence against K-Rite on two separate grounds: that the pharmacist was negligent in furnishing the wrong drug, and that K-Rite was

corporately negligent in failing to establish and maintain proper protocol and procedures to ensure that appropriate drugs were dispensed to consumers. Plaintiffs sought by interrogatories, by requests for the production of documents, and by oral depositions to discover from K-Rite information about other, earlier lawsuits involving allegations of professional liability relating to dispensing errors. Plaintiffs also requested information about training of K-Rite's pharmacy staff, as well as information relating to prior incidents involving negligence in the filling or dispensing of prescriptions in K-Rite's pharmacies. Plaintiffs also requested all incidence reports kept as a result of dispensing errors.

   a. Regarding the second allegation that K-Rite Pharmacy was negligent, should the court allow the plaintiffs' requests for information? Is there any specific information that the court should not allow the plaintiffs to discover?
   b. What is the social policy on both sides of the issue of whether the employer should furnish all this information to the plaintiffs?
   c. What do the plaintiffs hope to gain by reviewing all of this information? What might the plaintiffs find that would be most damaging to the defendant?
   d. How could K-Rite reduce its risk of liability?

2. The plaintiff appeals a jury verdict in favor of the defendant pharmacy. The plaintiff charged the pharmacy with corporate negligence on the basis that the pharmacy lacked a quality control dispensing system that caused errors to occur. The plaintiff alleged that the pharmacy erroneously switched labels for two prescription medications, Prozac and Restoril, and that as a result, she consumed an overdose of Prozac for over a week, and that she became increasingly disturbed and ultimately was hospitalized in a psychiatric facility for 5 weeks. She asked for damages in compensation for her pain and suffering as well as for medical expenses, and also for punitive damages. The pharmacy employed three full-time pharmacists and a part-time pharmacist, dispensing about 800 prescriptions per day. Based on the average 8-hour day, counsel for plaintiff figured that the average number of prescriptions filled per hour was 28.5, or one prescription every 2.1 minutes. The pharmacist who dispensed the prescription stated that this took a great deal of concentration, and if interrupted during the process, he would have to start over again. He often was interrupted to answer questions or to answer the telephone. When filling a prescription, he would first receive a computer-generated three-part label; he would then read the prescription to check for accuracy of the information. The first portion of the label is attached to the prescription; the second part of the label contains refill information and the pharmacist's name along with the name of the medication, directions, and the like. The pharmacist would then get the medicine, bring it to the counter and check it against the prescription, check it against the computer-generated document, count the pills, and put them in the bottles. After stamping his name on the bottle, the contents would then be checked again to make sure that the medication was correctly dispensed. According to the pharmacist, "There is a rule about the whole thing that if there is any doubt about what you're doing then you don't do it." When filling more than one prescription for the same patient, both medications are pulled at the same time, and each one is filled separately, as outlined earlier. After so doing, the bottles are again opened and checked before handing the prescriptions down. Each pharmacist is responsible for checking his or her own work. The pharmacist admitted that he has made errors in the past of miscounting pills; he also has erred in putting the wrong pills in the wrong bottle, but due to his checking procedures, this did not result in giving the patient the wrong medication.

   During the trial, an expert witness testified that dispensing a prescription every 2.1 minutes "could be considered safe" depending on other circumstances of the business. To fill prescriptions at that rate for 8 hours requires intense concentration, and there is a high likelihood of making a mistake, especially if there are other interruptions. However, he had no personal information about the plaintiff herself and gave no opinion as to the negligence of the defendants. The testimony of the plaintiff conflicted with other witnesses, and she was not able to clearly explain what had happened. Although the pharmacist who dispensed the prescription did not have specific recollection of this particular event, his testimony as to his usual practices was consistent. The plaintiff presented no evidence to contradict the pharmacist.

   a. If you were the appellate court, how would you decide this corporate negligence case, and why? Should punitive damages be applicable?
   b. Can workload be the cause of error and result in corporate negligence? Why? How could the risk of liability be reduced?

DRUG PRODUCT LIABILITY

If a physician, a pharmacist, or a hospital is sued after harm occurs from drug use, the argument is usually that the drug was improperly prescribed, improperly dispensed, or improperly administered, resulting in harm to the patient. In other words, that professional negligence or malpractice occurred. Whereas professional malpractice litigation focuses on a problem with the way in which the product was used, drug product liability litigation focuses on the product itself. Drug product liability law deals with claims that a drug was so inherently dangerous that harm to someone was inevitable, no matter how carefully the drug was used, and that the risk of harm was unreasonable. Professional malpractice law deals with claims that a drug could have been used safely, but was not, because the professional who was responsible for the outcomes of drug therapy did not meet the requisite standard of care.

DRUG PRODUCT DEFECT

A central principle in all product liability cases is that for there to be exposure to liability, the product itself must be proved defective. Because perfect safety is neither technologically possible nor economically feasible, the basis of the liability analysis is a reasonableness test that balances the benefits of having a drug marketed in a particular way against the detriments of having the drug marketed in that way. If the manufacturer is to be held liable, the product must be both defective and unreasonably dangerous.

There are three categories of defect:

1. Design defect
2. Manufacturing defect
3. Warning defect

Most drug products cannot be designed any differently and are manufactured in strict accordance with exacting specifications; therefore, the discussion of defectiveness in drug product liability is concerned primarily with the adequacy of the warning, that is, whether the warning was defective.

GROUNDS FOR LIABILITY ACTIONS

Most product liability actions are based on three seemingly separate grounds: (1) negligence, (2) breach of warranty, and (3) strict liability.

The theoretical basis for each of these actions is different. Negligence, as has been extensively discussed, is fault based, and to prevail on such a claim, the plaintiff must show that the defendant did not act reasonably to prevent foreseeable harm. A breach-of-warranty claim is based on an allegation that a seller violated either an express or an implied agreement that the goods would not be harmful to the buyer. The theory of strict liability holds the seller of a product responsible for an injury caused by its defective product, even if the seller was not negligent in any manner and exercised all possible care in the design, manufacture, and distribution of the product. Reasonableness of conduct is irrelevant to an action for strict liability. Needless to say, strict liability is the action of choice for plaintiffs in a product liability action because they have no burden of proving that the defendant acted substandardly. This does not necessarily mean, however, that the plaintiff will obtain a favorable judgment.

For example, in *Brown v. Superior Court*, 751 P.2d 470 (Cal. 1988), one of many cases relating to DES litigation, the plaintiff brought a strict liability action against the manufacturer, alleging that the drug was defective because it caused injury to the daughters of women who used it in the 1950s to prevent miscarriages. Although it is now known that there is a relationship between maternal use of DES and cervical adenocarcinoma in female offspring, that fact was not known when the drug was widely distributed for maternal use. The lower court ruled that the defendant manufacturers could not be held strictly liable for the alleged defect in DES. The court stated:

> Public policy favors the development and marketing of beneficial new drugs, even though some risks, perhaps serious ones, might accompany their introduction, because drugs can save lives and reduce pain and suffering. If manufacturers were subject to strict liability, they might be reluctant to undertake research programs to develop some pharmaceuticals that would prove beneficial or to distribute others that are available to be marketed, because of the fear of large adverse monetary judgments. Further, the additional expense of insuring against such liability—assuming insurance would be available—and of research programs to reveal possible dangers not detectable by available scientific methods could place the cost of medication beyond the reach of those who need it most. (751 P.2d at 477)

The court also rejected the plaintiff's assertion that a drug manufacturer should be held strictly liable for failure to warn of the risks inherent in a drug, even if it did not know nor could have known by the application of scientific knowledge that the drug could produce the undesirable side effects suffered by the patient.

Duty to Warn Under Strict Liability

In virtually every drug product liability case, the court cites section 402A of the Restatement (Second) of Torts. The Restatement is a compilation of rules established by decades of litigation. It is written by a group of legal experts and is considered authoritative by most courts. Section 402A deals with strict liability and states:

> **(1)** One who sells any product in a defective condition unreasonably dangerous to the user or consumer or to his property is subject to liability for physical harm thereby caused to the ultimate user or consumer, or to his property, if
>   **(a)** the seller is engaged in the business of selling such a product, and
>   **(b)** it is expected to and does reach the user or consumer without substantial change in the condition in which it is sold.
> **(2)** The rule stated in Subsection (1) applies although
>   **(a)** the seller has exercised all possible care in the preparation and sale of his product, and
>   **(b)** the user or consumer has not bought the product from or entered into any contractual relation with the seller.

Section 402A makes the manufacturer of a product the guarantor of the product's safety. Pharmaceutical products, however, are unique from most other products because all are necessarily unsafe to some degree. A drug cannot be manufactured to be any safer. As noted in the *Brown* decision previously discussed, if the law were to impose a guarantee of safety for these products, the only way for a drug manufacturer to avoid liability simply would be not to market any drugs, an outcome that would have serious ramifications for health care. Recognizing this potential problem, the writers of the Restatement included a comment to address the special circumstances posed by pharmaceutical products. Comment k to section 402A reads:

> Unavoidably unsafe products. There are some products which, in the present state of human knowledge, are quite incapable of being made safe for their intended and ordinary use. These are especially common in the field of drugs. An outstanding example is the vaccine for the Pasteur treatment of rabies, which not uncommonly leads to very serious and damaging consequences when it is injected. Since the disease itself

invariably leads to a dreadful death, both the marketing and the use of the vaccine are fully justified, notwithstanding the unavoidable high degree of risk which they involve. Such a product, properly prepared, and accompanied by proper directions and warning, is not defective, nor is it unreasonably dangerous. The same is true of many other drugs, vaccines, and the like, many of which for this very reason cannot legally be sold except to physicians, or under the prescription of a physician. It is also true in particular of many new or experimental drugs as to which, because of lack of time and opportunity for sufficient medical experience, there can be no assurance of safety, or perhaps even of purity of ingredients, but such experience as there is justifies the marketing and use of the drug notwithstanding a medically recognizable risk. The seller of such products, again with the qualification that they are properly prepared and marketed, and proper warning is given, where the situation calls for it, is not to be held to strict liability for unfortunate consequences attending their use, merely because he has undertaken to supply the public with an apparently useful and desirable product, attended with a known but apparently reasonable risk.

Comment k is directed toward drugs and other products that are highly regulated in their design and manufacture and have a high utility in spite of a known risk. These products are deemed to be free of defects as long as they are accompanied by proper directions and warnings. An unavoidably unsafe drug product that is marketed without an adequate warning of its known dangers does not fall within the comment k exception to section 402A, and strict liability will be imposed for damages caused by the drug. Because the reasonableness standard for a warning established by comment k is virtually the same as the standard that would be applied under either negligence or breach of warranty, the three legal grounds for liability are indistinguishable when the alleged defect is a warning defect.

It is usually less costly (and theoretically just as effective) to warn the user of a product about potential adverse effects than to redesign the product in such a manner as to eliminate the problem. Moreover, the duty to warn is premised on the superior knowledge of the manufacturer concerning its own product. Manufacturers cannot make all decisions about risk for product consumers, but they can provide the information necessary for a consumer to make a fully informed decision. Perhaps the most frequently occurring question in warning-defect cases is whether the information supplied was adequate, given the nature of the particular circumstances of product use.

An adequate drug warning presents a reasonably balanced picture of the effectiveness, hazards, and safety of the drug. A drug cannot be promoted in such a way that the net effect is to nullify an otherwise adequate warning. In addition to being adequate, a warning must also be timely. If a serious and unanticipated adverse effect is discovered, a warning must be made promptly, even though a causal relationship between the adverse effect and the drug has not yet been clearly established.

DUTY TO WARN UNDER THE LEARNED INTERMEDIARY DOCTRINE

A somewhat unusual aspect of drug product liability is that the manufacturer owes a duty to the patient to warn the physician, but not the patient. For prescription drugs, the ordinary user of the product has traditionally been considered the physician, who acts as a learned intermediary between the manufacturer and the patient, evaluating the patient's needs, assessing the benefits and detriments of available drugs, prescribing a drug, and supervising its use. A patient who is harmed by drug use most often has no right of action against the manufacturer if the physician received an adequate warning, even if the patient did not. If the basis of a patient's lawsuit is that the manufacturer's warning was inadequate, then the learned intermediary doctrine is not applicable because the patient is alleging harm as a result of the prescriber being denied adequate information.

The learned intermediary doctrine rests on the fact that the physician is trained to assess risks and to select the appropriate mode of therapy for an individual person. A manufacturer's warning directly to an unsophisticated or uneducated patient may not give the patient adequate protection from the specified risks because the patient is not trained to evaluate risks. Included in the learned intermediary doctrine is the presumption that a physician will be mindful of a manufacturer's warning and, when the physician deems it appropriate, will transmit the warning to the patient. A physician who fails to convey an appropriate warning may be civilly liable if the omission breaches the standard of care. In this event, however, physician liability would fall under the law of professional malpractice, not product liability.

Although the challenge to the learned intermediary doctrine in *Ferrara v. Berlex Laboratories, Inc.*, 732 F. Supp. 552 (E.D. Pa. 1990), was particularly creative, it fared no better than did most of those that preceded it. The plaintiff in this case suffered from chronic sinusitis. She advised her physician that she was taking a monoamine oxidase (MAO) inhibitor, but the physician prescribed a sympathomimetic amine—despite an explicit warning in the product labeling that MAO inhibitors may interact negatively with sympathomimetic substances. The combination of the two drugs caused the plaintiff to suffer a hypertensive reaction, culminating in a stroke. She brought a lawsuit against the manufacturers of both drugs for failure to warn her directly of their products' dangerous side effects when taken together.

The novelty of the argument lay in the claim that the learned intermediary doctrine was inapplicable because of the especially dangerous nature of MAO inhibitors. The patient contended that because more than 40 types of foods and beverages can cause hypertensive crises if consumed with an MAO inhibitor, too much responsibility for advising the patient is placed on the prescribing physician. Therefore, the patient argued, drug manufacturers must be required to warn patients directly of the risks associated with a particular drug. The patient suggested that a wallet-sized insert should have been required to provide an adequate warning. She argued that an informational card is the only effective means of protecting patients, who may forget the long complicated list of prohibited foods and drugs given by their physician.

This argument has a certain appeal because it recognizes that not all potential risks can be identified at the time a drug is prescribed. A risk may materialize weeks or months later because of a patient's altered behavior (e.g., beginning to drive a car, drinking alcohol, eating particular foods). The physician is not present at that time to help patients make decisions about risk. Therefore, the information should be provided in an enduring form at the time of prescribing so patients can refer to it later. Despite the novelty of this approach and the obvious reality that it reflects, the court did not consider it persuasive, and the learned intermediary doctrine was left in place. The adequate warning to the physician was sufficient to absolve the manufacturers of liability for harm to this patient.

The learned intermediary doctrine was successfully challenged, however, in *Perez v. Wyeth Laboratories, Inc.*, 734 A.2d 1245 (N.J. 1999). In *Perez*, a group of women sued Wyeth for injuries suffered while using the contraceptive Norplant, contending that the manufacturer failed to adequately warn them of the drug's side effects. Wyeth contended that it owed no duty to warn patients, only physicians under the learned intermediary doctrine. The trial court agreed with Wyeth, but the New Jersey Supreme Court reversed, finding for the plaintiffs. The court found that Wyeth engaged in a nationwide direct-to-consumer advertising campaign directed at women, not physicians. Because Wyeth marketed directly to consumers, held the court, Wyeth had an obligation to properly warn consumers of the drug's adverse effects. Considering the extent of direct-to-consumer advertising occurring today, *Perez* may signal a significant weakening of the learned intermediary doctrine as a defense for drug manufacturers. However, many state courts have ruled since *Perez* that the learned intermediary doctrine applies even though the manufacturer has engaged in direct-to-consumer advertising (See, for example, *Centocor, Inc. v. Hamilton et al.*, ___S.W.3d___, 2012 WL 2052783 (June 2012)).

WHETHER FDA-APPROVED LABELING PREEMPTS STATE PRODUCT LIABILITY ACTIONS

For years a debate waged over whether FDA approval of a drug's labeling preempts a plaintiff's product liability claim in state court alleging that the manufacturer's labeling inadequately warned of risks. The Supreme Court decided this issue in *Wyeth v. Levine*, 129 S.Ct. 1187 (March 4, 2009). In this case, a physician's assistant injected the plaintiff with Phenergan by the IV-push method, where the drug is injected directly into the vein. Unfortunately, the drug entered the plaintiff's artery resulting in gangrene and the amputation of her forearm. The plaintiff, a professional musician, sued Wyeth under strict liability contending that the labeling failed to adequately warn of the risks of administering the drug by IV-push. Finding for the plaintiff, a Vermont jury determined that the injury would not have occurred had the warning in the labeling been adequate, and the Vermont Supreme Court affirmed.

Wyeth appealed in federal court, contending that FDA approval of the label is a complete defense to state tort claims. The U.S. Supreme Court rejected Wyeth's argument on the basis that it was not the intent of Congress that federal labeling requirements preempt state tort claims. Although Wyeth contended it had no authority to revise the labeling without FDA approval, the court found otherwise, noting the "changes being effected" (CBE) regulation. This regulation permits manufacturers to make certain changes to its labeling without waiting for agency approval. *Levine* does leave the door open for a manufacturer to assert a preemption defense by proving that the FDA would have rejected a proposed labeling change under the CBE regulation.

The court's ruling contrasts with its decision about one year earlier that the Medical Device Amendments Act of 1976 preempts state product liability actions over device safety or efficacy (*Riegel v. Medtronic, Inc.*, 128 S.Ct. 999 (Feb. 20, 2008)). The court in that case found convincing language in the device law that Congress intended to preempt state actions.

Two years later the Supreme Court was faced with the issue of whether its holding in *Wyeth v. Levine* applied to generic drug manufacturers. In *Pliva, Inc. v. Mensing*, 131 S.Ct. 2567 (2011), the plaintiffs had received a generic version of Reglan (metoclopramide) and had taken the drug as prescribed for several years. They developed tardive dyskinesia and contended that despite growing evidence of this adverse effect in long-term use, the manufacturers did not change their labeling to adequately warn of the risk. In a 5-to-4 decision, the court found that the FDCA regulations preempt state law failure to warn claims, reversing three Courts of Appeals decisions to the contrary. Unlike with brand-name drug manufacturers as in *Levine*, found the majority, generic manufacturers cannot change their labeling under the CBE regulation because regulations require them to carry the exact same labeling information as the brand-name drug. The majority recognized that it made little sense that had the plaintiffs taken Reglan they could have brought a lawsuit, but because they took a generic, they cannot. Nonetheless, said the court, it was bound by the FDCA and the regulations and it was up to the FDA or Congress to change the law. In response, bills were introduced into both the House and Senate in 2012 to allow generic drug manufacturers to be liable under state law for failing to warn adequately. In the meantime, the *Pliva* decision may mean that plaintiffs will attempt to bring failure to warn lawsuits against brand-name manufacturers for injuries caused by the generic drug.

PHARMACISTS AND PRODUCT LIABILITY

Simple logic seems to suggest that, in a legitimate drug product liability case against a pharmaceutical manufacturer, the pharmacist who dispensed the drug should not be joined as a codefendant. If a manufacturer should be held liable because a drug is defective, the pharmacist's dispensing of that drug does not increase its defective character. If a drug is not defective, the dispensing of that drug does not make it defective. Thus, logically, the bodies of law known as pharmacist malpractice and drug product liability are mutually exclusive. Either a pharmacist should be held liable for causing unsafe and/or ineffective use of a safe and effective drug, or a manufacturer should be held liable for marketing an unsafe and/or ineffective drug. One cannot be held liable for what the other did.

Nevertheless, there is a significant body of case law in which the pharmaceutical manufacturer appears to be the target defendant, and the dispensing pharmacist (perhaps along with the prescribing physician) is joined as an additional party defendant. Such cases must include some rationale to explain why the pharmacist should remain in the case. It is usually asserted that pharmacists are much more than product sellers and that they owe some sort of duty to the patient to prevent harm from defective drugs. The pharmacist who defends such claims by arguing that the pharmacist's role goes no farther than the proper filling of prescriptions risks running afoul of a developing body of pharmacist malpractice law. Pharmacists do have responsibilities to ensure that drugs are used safely and effectively, but they cannot take an inherently unsafe and/or ineffective drug and make it safe and effective. Therefore, a pharmacist should not be liable for having failed to do so.

Strict Liability and Pharmacists

Under professional malpractice litigation, a pharmacist has no duty to warn a patient of a risk that the pharmacist could not know. Plaintiffs attempting to circumvent certain defeat in a negligence action for this reason will sometimes allege strict liability against a pharmacist because strict liability is not fault based.

The question of whether the doctrine of strict liability should apply to cases in which the sellers are pharmacists and the goods are pharmaceuticals is as significant today as it was more than 140 years ago when the first reported case on this issue was considered. The case of *Fleet and Semple v. Hollenkemp*, 52 Ky. (1B Mon.) 219 (Ky. Ct. App. 1852), stemmed from the dispensing by defendant pharmacists of a compounded medication that was contaminated with a toxic impurity. A drug-compounding machine had not been properly cleaned following its use to prepare a medication that included a certain toxic substance; as a result, the substance was improperly included in the medication dispensed to the plaintiff.

The defendant pharmacists asked the judge to instruct the jury that, if the pharmacists used due and reasonable skill, care, and diligence, the jury must find in favor of the pharmacists. The judge refused to do this, and the refusal was affirmed on appeal. The court said that pharmacists are absolutely responsible for a consequence that their knowledge enabled them to avoid. When asked by attorneys for the defendants whether pharmacists were to be regarded as insurers of their products, the court responded that a vendor of drugs is not entitled to a relaxation of the rule that applies to vendors of all products, which is that a vendor undertakes and ensures that the article is wholesome.

During the 20th century, this approach was modified significantly. Pharmacists, as professional retailers, have been afforded special exempt status from the general rule of retailer liability under a strict liability theory. Although retailers of most consumer products can be held strictly liable for product defects, pharmacists have not been held to such a standard of liability when dispensing prescription drugs, as the following cases demonstrate.

The first modern court to consider this issue seriously was the court in *McLeod v. W. S. Merrell Co.*, 174 So.2d 736 (Fla. 1965). The court noted that application of strict liability to pharmacists under the facts presented in this case would convert retail pharmacists into insurers of the safety of premanufactured drugs. As the pharmacist in *McLeod* had done nothing more than correctly dispense an unmodified medication obtained from the manufacturer, the court was unwilling to apply strict liability principles. The distinguishing feature of *McLeod*, and several cases that followed, is that the pharmacist was in no position to take any action to prevent harm to the patient. This presents a factually distinct situation from the scenario in *Fleet and Semple*.

The court in *Batiste v. American Home Products*, 231 S.E.2d 269 (N.C. Ct. App. 1977), also rejected a strict liability claim against a pharmacist, citing *McLeod* as authority. Both *Batiste* and *McLeod* were relied upon by the court in *Bichler v. Willing*, 397 N.Y.S.2d 57 (N.Y. App. Div. 1977), another case in which strict liability against a pharmacist was rejected. In this case, the court noted that a retail pharmacist should not be put under an obligation to test a drug's chemical structure for side effects or other possible risks, which is precisely what the imposition of strict liability would do.

Not all courts easily find a distinction between commercial retailers and retail pharmacy and the distinction is critical under strict liability. Strict liability applies to products, not services. Courts have generally acknowledged the principle that strict liability is not applicable when a product is merely incidental to the performance of a professional service. Thus, courts have denied actions for strict liability against a dentist when a defective drill used by a dentist broke in the patient's mouth (*Magrine v. Krasnica*, 227 A.2d 539 (N.J. 1971), aff'd 241 A.2d 637 and 250 A.2d 129); and against a physician for implementation of a defective device (*Cafazzo v. Central Medical Health Services, Inc.*, 668 A.2d 521 (Pa. 1995)). The important issue in pharmacy is whether the dispensing of a prescription is primarily the sale of a product, or whether it is provided incidental to a professional service. The California Supreme Court conducted a thorough review of this issue in *Murphy v. E.R. Squibb and Sons, Inc.*, 221 Cal. Rptr. 447 (Cal. 1985). In affirming the earlier opinion of the appellate court in the same case, the state supreme court reached a judgment in favor of the pharmacy but for various reasons. The court of appeals had made several flattering statements about professionalism in pharmacy before unanimously holding that pharmacists function as service-performing professionals, in contrast to product sellers, and can be held liable only for negligence or intentional misconduct. The state supreme court, however, was far less flattering in its 4-to-3 split opinion (four justices against holding the pharmacy liable and three in favor of holding the pharmacy liable). All three dissenters advocated the application of strict liability principles in describing pharmacists as product sellers, not professionals. Two majority justices felt that pharmacists are professionals to whom strict liability should not apply. The other two majority justices felt that the pharmacist is not a professional but is an extension of the physician, who is a professional, and that strict liability should not apply because of the widely recognized physician exemption. Thus, the pharmacy in *Murphy* was not held strictly liable, but a majority of the court expressed the view that pharmacy is not a profession.

Pharmacist Malpractice vs. Drug Product Liability

Current litigation involving pharmacists as defendants in drug product liability cases usually confuses the idea of a warning defect created by a manufacturer with a pharmacist's failure to warn patients of adverse drug effects. The arguments presented by the plaintiff assert that the manufacturer distributed a defective product without a warning of an adverse effect on its label and that the pharmacist failed to warn the patient about the adverse effect. These two contentions are factually inconsistent, except under exceedingly rare circumstances where the pharmacist may know of a problem that has not been included in the lengthy list of possible adverse effects noted in the product labeling.

In *Makripodis v. Merrell-Dow Pharmaceuticals*, 523 A.2d 374 (Pa. Super. Ct. 1987), the plaintiffs were parents who brought a product liability action against both the pharmaceutical manufacturer and the dispensing pharmacist, alleging that their child was born with certain congenital abnormalities as a result of the mother's ingestion of Bendectin during her pregnancy. The two relevant allegations against the pharmacist were (1) breach of an implied warranty of merchantability, because Bendectin was alleged to be unsafe for its ordinary use, the treatment of nausea in pregnant women, and (2) strict liability, because Bendectin was alleged to be an unsafe product, unreasonably dangerous because of the absence of proper warnings concerning its teratogenic potential. The trial court dismissed the complaint against the pharmacist, concluding that the complaint failed to state a cause of action against the pharmacist.

The appellate court affirmed this decision, holding that the very nature of prescription drugs precludes the imposition of an implied warranty of merchantability. The appellate court held also that the pharmacist could not be held strictly liable as the retailer of a defective product. The plaintiffs contended that the failure of the pharmacist to warn the mother concerning the teratogenic potential of Bendectin caused the drug to be unreasonably dangerous. In evaluating this argument, the court reasoned that the benefits and detriments have been weighed and the drug selected by the time the patient presents the pharmacist with a prescription for a certain drug. The court concluded that the absence of adequate warnings from the manufacturer at the time the drug was dispensed by the pharmacist does not have an impact on the safe use of the drug as sold by the pharmacy. Therefore, the court could not see any benefit to be derived from the imposition of strict liability upon the pharmacist who properly dispensed the prescription drug upon the prescription of a duly licensed physician.

Allegations of a different sort were brought in *Leesley v. West*, 518 N.E.2d 758 (Ill. App. Ct. 1988), a case in which the plaintiff's primary thrust was a challenge to the learned intermediary doctrine. As a corollary argument, the plaintiff asserted that both negligence and strict liability principles require the pharmacist to warn the patient of two known, although infrequent, side effects of the drug Feldene—peptic ulceration and gastrointestinal bleeding. Evaluating this argument, the court concluded that when the manufacturer gives the required warnings to the prescribing physician and the pharmacist distributes the drug in the usual manner, the drug is not an unreasonably dangerous product. In fact, the court characterized as "unreasonable" the contrary conclusion that a product can become unreasonably dangerous while it is in the pharmacist's hands. Furthermore, the court reasoned that placing a burden on pharmacists to warn patients under these circumstances is inconsistent with the exemption afforded manufacturers by the learned intermediary doctrine. In the court's opinion, a manufacturer's adequate warning to a physician that is sufficient to protect the manufacturer from liability is also sufficient to protect the pharmacist from liability.

In true product liability cases, such as *Makripodis* or *Leesley*, the focus is on the quality of the product as it arrived in the pharmacy, not on the pharmacist's dispensing of the product. Pharmacists have no control over the product prior to its arrival in the pharmacy, just as manufacturers have no control over the product after its arrival. Although the likelihood is remote, it is theoretically possible that a product was defective on arrival and was also improperly dispensed by the pharmacist. It is far more likely, however, that one or the other occurred. If the product is nondefective when it arrives, an action based on adverse drug effects is not an action for product liability; it is an action for professional malpractice. If the product is defective when it arrives, the action is for product liability against the manufacturer and no one else.

Fortunately, the courts have recognized the implausibility of arguments asserting that pharmacists should be liable along with manufacturers in cases alleging defective product. Although pharmacists may be held liable for malpractice, manufacturers must be responsible for product defects.

© Stockbyte/Thinkstock

STUDY SCENARIOS AND QUESTIONS

1. Syrup of ipecac is a commonly used product to induce emesis after the ingestion of some toxic substances. The active ingredient in syrup of ipecac is emetine, which is toxic itself in high doses, but is safe if ingested in the doses necessary to produce emesis after the ingestion of poisons. Emetine is directly cardiotoxic. Unfortunately, some people who suffer from bulimia have used syrup of ipecac to induce emesis after binge eating. There have been deaths of bulimics due to the toxic effects of emetine. Psychiatrists who treat patients suffering from anorexia nervosa and bulimia believe that the availability of syrup of ipecac should be restricted. Poison control center representatives believe that additional restrictions would be dangerous to their efforts. Jane B., suffering from bulimia, purchased 15 bottles of ipecac at a single time from a convenience store. She used all 15 bottles over a 2-day period to purge her body of food after binge eating. She died from cardiac arrest due to emetine toxicity. The labels on the bottles of ipecac syrup that she bought did not have a warning concerning misuse or overdosage. Jane B.'s relatives have filed a products liability lawsuit against the manufacturer of the ipecac syrup that they claim was inadequately labeled.
    a. Assume that the medical profession had been adequately warned of the hazards of ipecac overuse. Would that warning enable the manufacturer to successfully use the learned intermediary rule in this case? Why or why not?
    b. What are the arguments for and against holding the manufacturer of syrup of ipecac liable to the plaintiffs in this case?
    c. If the place where Jane B. purchased 15 bottles of ipecac all at once had been a pharmacy rather than a convenience store, would that change the manufacturer's exposure to liability?
2. The plaintiff received a prescription from LessPay Drug Store for Pediotic Otic Suspension as treatment for acute severe left otitis media with bullous myringitis. The plaintiff claims that he carefully took all the drugs as directed on the labeling but contends that the Pediotic Otic Suspension was not properly labeled in that it did not contain a warning that the use or administration of the suspension should be discontinued and the prescribing physician promptly contacted in case of symptoms of tympanic membrane rupture. The manufacturer does package the drug product in a box that contains this warning and the manufacturer intends that the patient receive the product in this box. The pharmacist, however, allegedly dispensed the drug without the box. The plaintiff contends that due to the defective and unreasonably dangerous manner in which the drug was dispensed (without appropriate labeling and/warning), he suffers from severe and permanent injuries, including brain damage. Plaintiff sued on the basis of strict liability and negligence and defendant moved for summary judgment.

a. Should the summary judgment motion be denied? In other words, should the pharmacy be subject to strict liability in this case?
b. How does this case differ from one where a patient suffers an adverse effect from a drug and sues under strict liability? Should a pharmacy be subject to strict liability in these cases?
c. What are the social policy consequences if the court finds the pharmacy in this case liable for strict liability?

BIBLIOGRAPHY

Brushwood, D., and R. Abood. Strict liability in tort: Appropriateness of the theory for retail pharmacists. *Food, Drug, Cosmetic Law Journal* 42 (1987): 269.

Fleischer, L. From pill counting to patient care: Pharmacist's standard of care in negligence law. *Fordham Law Review* 68 (1999): 165–187.

King, G. Liability for negligence of pharmacists. *Vanderbilt Law Review* 12 (1959): 695.

Nelson, L., and S. Susina. The case against applying strict liability to pharmacists: A reply to Professor Vandall. *Toledo Law Review* 19 (1988): 783.

Sveska, K. Pharmacist liability. *American Journal of Hospital Pharmacy* 50 (1993): 1429.

Termini, R. B. The pharmacist duty to warn revisited: The changing role of pharmacy in health care and the resultant impact on the obligation of a pharmacist to warn. *Ohio Northern Law Review* 24 (1998): 551–565.

Vandall, F. Applying strict liability to pharmacists. *Toledo Law Review* 18 (1986): 1.

Willig, S. Physicians, pharmacists, pharmaceutical manufacturers: Partners in patient care, partners in litigation? *Mercer Law Review* 37 (1986): 755.

CASE STUDIES

CASE 8-1 | *Happel v. Wal-Mart Stores, Inc.*, 766 N.E.2d 1118 (Ill. 2002)

Issue

Whether a pharmacy has a duty to warn a patient about a known drug contraindication where the pharmacy is aware of a customer's drug allergies and knows that the medication prescribed by the customer's physician is contraindicated for a person with those allergies.

Overview

As discussed in this chapter, courts have historically ruled that the duty of a pharmacist does not include warning a patient of a drug's dangers unless directed by the prescriber. This perspective is changing in many jurisdictions as courts take notice of the knowledge and education of pharmacists and the technology available to them in pharmacies. As you read this case consider: Should pharmacists have a legal obligation to warn patients of a drug's dangers? If so, should that obligation exist only in special circumstances, such as in this case? If pharmacists have an obligation to warn, what risks and burdens does this create for pharmacists? If pharmacies take the position they have no duty to warn, as Wal-Mart did in this case, what message does this send to the public?

The Illinois Supreme Court began its analysis by reviewing the facts of the case.

A physician phoned the defendant, Wal-Mart Pharmacy, ordering a prescription for Toradol for the plaintiff. The plaintiff had been to the pharmacy six times previously, and each time the pharmacy personnel would ask the patient if she was allergic to any medications. Each time she told them she was allergic to aspirin, acetaminophen, and ibuprofen. This information was entered in the pharmacy's computer and available to the pharmacists. When the plaintiff's husband went to the pharmacy to pick up the prescription, an employee of the pharmacy again asked him if the patient had any known allergies to which he responded, aspirin, acetaminophen, and ibuprofen. The pharmacy dispensed the drug supplying no warnings, either written or oral, of any contraindications.

After the plaintiff took the first dose of the drug, she suffered a severe reaction experiencing respiratory problems. She called the pharmacy and was told there should be no drug reaction problem. She then called a pharmacist friend who told her to go to the emergency room where she was found to be experiencing anaphylactic shock. The Wal-Mart pharmacists acknowledged that Toradol is contraindicated in patients allergic to aspirin and ibuprofen. They stated that the computer system should have alerted them of the contraindication, which would have required an override only after contacting the physician. The physician testified he would not have prescribed Toradol had he known of the contraindication. The pharmacists did not remember whether there was a computer warning or whether the physician was ever contacted. They admitted that a pharmacist is required to know a patient's allergies and to know whether a particular drug would be contraindicated in the patient's condition. They also testified that overriding a computer warning without first contacting the physician would deviate from a pharmacist's standard of care.

The plaintiff filed a negligence action against Wal-Mart, and Wal-Mart moved for a summary judgment. The trial court granted the summary judgment motion and the plaintiff appealed. The court of appeals reversed the summary judgment motion, concluding that Wal-Mart did owe the plaintiff a duty to warn but that the duty was a narrow one. The Illinois Supreme Court then rendered its decision as described here.

The supreme court noted that the critical issue involves whether a duty exists between Wal-Mart and the plaintiff such that Wal-Mart owes the plaintiff an obligation of reasonable conduct. The court stated that four factors are important to determining the existence of a duty and they include: (1) the reasonable foreseeability that the defendant's conduct may injure another, (2) the likelihood of an injury occurring, (3) the magnitude of the burden of guarding against such injury, and (4) the consequences of placing that burden on the defendant.

As to the first three factors, the court stated:

> It is undisputed that, at the time Heidi's prescription was filled on August 4, 1993, Wal-Mart was aware not only of Heidi's drug allergies but also that the drug prescribed by Dr. Lorenc, Toradol, was contraindicated for persons such as Heidi who are allergic to aspirin. Given this superior knowledge on the part of Wal-Mart, and particularly given the nature of the knowledge, i.e., that Toradol was contraindicated, it was reasonably foreseeable that a failure to convey this knowledge might result in injury to Heidi. Both the likelihood and the reasonable foreseeability of injury here were great. These factors thus favor the imposition of a duty on Wal-Mart.

> The burden on defendant of imposing this duty is minimal. All that is required is that the pharmacist telephone the physician and inform him or her of the contraindication. Alternatively, the pharmacist could provide the same information to the patient. Since this burden of warning about a contraindication is extremely small, this factor also favors the imposition of a duty here.

As to the fourth factor, Wal-Mart argued that the consequences of imposing a duty to warn on pharmacies would be so substantial as to have a "chilling effect." Because duty is premised on knowledge, pharmacies therefore would not gather patient medical information or record it and thus patients would be deprived of potentially beneficial warnings. The court responded:

> The consequence of accepting Wal-Mart's "chilling effect" argument would be to sanction the status quo, where pharmacies solicit allergy information from their customers but are under no obligation to follow through with a warning, even where the pharmacy knows that the drug being prescribed is contraindicated for the individual customer. The difficulty with this approach is that the status quo is unacceptable. By asking customers about their drug allergies, the pharmacy is engendering reliance in the customer that the pharmacy will take steps to ensure that the customer does not receive a drug to which the customer is allergic. There can be no other reason for a pharmacy's seeking this information regarding drug allergies. Where the pharmacy fails to warn the customer, then the customer is placed at risk of serious injury or death. . . . We therefore conclude that any negative consequences of recognizing a duty to warn here are far outweighed by the substantial reasons favoring such a duty.

Wal-Mart argued one final point; that in spite of this analysis, the learned intermediary doctrine exempts pharmacists and pharmacies from warning patients by placing the responsibility upon the physician. The court noted that Illinois courts have interpreted the learned intermediary doctrine in this manner on the rationale that the physician is in the best position to know the medical history of the patient and that it would require too much of the pharmacist to learn the patient's medical condition. However, continued the court, the reasons for justifying application of the learned intermediary doctrine do not apply to this case.

> Here, Wal-Mart was aware not only of Heidi's drug allergies, but also that Toradol was contraindicated for persons such as Heidi with allergies to aspirin. Imposing a duty to warn of this contraindication would not require the pharmacist to "learn the customer's condition and monitor his drug usage." On the contrary, Wal-Mart already had the knowledge it needed in order to give an effective warning, and this warning required Wal-Mart only to notify Dr. Lorenc or Heidi of the Toradol contraindication, not to monitor Heidi's drug usage.

The court concluded that a pharmacy has a duty to warn when it has patient-specific information about drug allergies, and knows that the drug being prescribed is contraindicated. In these instances, the pharmacy has a duty to warn either the physician or the patient of the potential danger.

Notes on *Happel v. Wal-Mart Stores*

1. As discussed in the chapter, courts have historically taken the position that pharmacists do not owe patients a general duty to warn them of a drug's adverse effects. Even relatively recent Illinois court decisions prior to *Happel* have followed this position. *Happel* may not be inconsistent with prior decisions in Illinois because the duty established here is a narrow one, requiring that the pharmacy or pharmacist have specific knowledge of the patient's condition. *Happel* raises the issue that if pharmacists owe patients a duty to warn, just how broad should that duty be? This case is an example of where the court rejects that pharmacists owe a general duty and instead has determined that pharmacists owe a duty to warn in only certain situations.

   Happel, *Morgan*, and most duty-to-warn decisions center on whether the pharmacist owed a duty as a question of law, meaning that if a judge determines that as a matter of law a pharmacist does not owe a duty to warn, the case is dismissed. One could argue that courts should not approach the issue as one of duty, but rather as a question of fact from the perspective of the pharmacists' standard of care. For example, in *Lasley v. Shrake's Country Club Pharmacy, Inc.*, 880 P.2d 1120 (Ariz. App. 1994), the court held that pharmacists owe patients a general legal duty to conform to a standard of reasonable conduct. What a pharmacist should or should not do is a question of fact for the jury to determine. Under this approach, the court would not deliberate whether a duty exists or not, but rather would rely upon expert witnesses to establish to a jury whether a reasonable pharmacist would have acted in a similar manner.

2. Wal-Mart contended that it was exempt from a duty to warn under the learned intermediary doctrine. This doctrine holds that the prescriber is the person responsible for providing warnings and risk information to the patient, not the pharmacist. Defendant pharmacies often assert the doctrine in this manner, and this argument persuades many courts to rule for the defendants. (See *Springhill Hospitals, Inc. v. Larrimore*, 5 So.3d 513 (Ala. 2008), where the court held that the doctrine severs the liability of a pharmacist who provided dosing information to a physician.) The learned intermediary doctrine, however, was never conceived as a defense for pharmacists in a negligence suit. For the reasons articulated in the chapter, the doctrine materialized as a defense for manufacturers in strict product liability actions. It is difficult for many to understand how courts can continue to apply this doctrine given the education, knowledge, and role of the pharmacist in today's health care system, and given the regulatory obligation of pharmacists to conduct prospective drug utilization review. Nonetheless, courts even today seem to favor the doctrine. In *Klasch v. Walgreen Co.*, 264 P.3d 1155 (Nev. 2011), the court accepted the learned intermediary doctrine as sound policy but rejected the notion that it insulates a pharmacist from liability when the pharmacist has knowledge of a customer-specific risk.

3. Interestingly in this case, the National Association of Chain Drug Stores (NACDS) filed an amicus (friend of the court) brief in support of Wal-Mart's position. The National Association of Boards of Pharmacy (NABP) filed an amicus brief for the plaintiff. It is unusual that two national pharmacy organizations would take contrary positions in a case where neither is a party. It demonstrates the importance of the social policy involved in this type of case and the polarization of views. Needless to say, NACDS, as an organization representing pharmacy employers, felt obligated to support the position that would minimize its members' exposure to liability. NABP, on the other hand, has historically articulated and supported an expanded scope of practice for pharmacists. Wal-Mart and NACDS's position to defend rather than settle the case is somewhat troubling in light of the particular facts of this case and considering that even the Wal-Mart pharmacists acknowledged that they acted below the standard of care.

CASE 8-2   *Hundley v. Rite Aid*, 529 S.E.2d 45 (S.C. App. 2000)

Issue

Whether a pharmacy may be liable for punitive damages based on allegations of negligent retention and supervision of a pharmacist.

Overview

The liability of pharmacies increasingly depends on not simply an error by a pharmacist but also perhaps the alleged failure to provide appropriate supervision of pharmacists.

This is primary liability of a pharmacy company for its own failure, rather than secondary liability as the employer of a pharmacist who has erred. To complicate the picture, courts have begun to entertain the notion that the failure to use systems to prevent error, or the failure to learn from the past and improve in the future, may subject a pharmacy company to punitive damages. This case that follows resulted in a verdict for a huge amount of money. As you read this case, ask yourself what the solution might be to the workload problem in pharmacy and how pharmacies might be able to address the dilemma of a public that demands cheaper prices and highest quality. How can pharmacists and the pharmacies they work for find solutions to this dilemma by working together? Are we condemned in pharmacy to unrealistic public expectations of perfection and huge jury verdicts for failure to attain unrealistic expectations? Can the threat of liability force pharmacists and pharmacies to develop new quality improvement systems to learn from the past and improve in the future? Is coercion of new system development the role of litigation, or would other avenues be better suited to this activity?

The court began by outlining the misfilling of the prescription by the pharmacist who worked for the defendant pharmacy:

> On February 20, 1995, Dr. Jan Shaw diagnosed 7-year-old Gabrielle Hundley with attention deficit hyperactivity disorder ("ADHD") and prescribed Ritalin. Dr. Shaw is a pediatric neurologist. Peggie Hundley, Gabrielle's mother, took the prescription to a Rite Aid pharmacy in Rock Hill, South Carolina, where it was filled that evening.
>
> The next morning, Mrs. Hundley gave Gabrielle one tablet from the prescription bottle as directed. She then took several tablets to Gabrielle's school with appropriate instructions to give Gabrielle one tablet each day at 11:30 A.M. School officials administered a second dose at 11:30 as instructed. Unfortunately, the Rite Aid prescription did not contain Ritalin, but instead contained six-milligram tablets of Glynase, an adult medication used to treat diabetes.
>
> Shortly before 2:30 P.M., Gabrielle had a seizure. She lost consciousness and was taken by emergency service personnel to the hospital. She was in a hypoglycemic coma. She stayed in a coma for several hours and remained in the hospital overnight.
>
> Gabrielle's doctors determined her coma was induced by her ingestion of Glynase. Glynase is a medication designed to lower blood sugar levels in adult diabetics. It is not prescribed for children at any dose, and a six-milligram tablet is a high dosage, even for an adult.
>
> According to doctors, while Gabrielle was in a hypoglycemic coma her blood sugar fell to a level at which her brain cells, particularly the gray cells of the cerebral cortex, began using their own proteins and lipids as fuel to avoid necrosis. As a result, Gabrielle suffered permanent brain damage.
>
> Experts opined at trial that Gabrielle's ability to learn has decreased since the incident, and she has not progressed academically or behaviorally at her previous rate of progress. She has fallen behind her peers despite extra help from her parents, tutors, and summer school. Evidence indicated that Gabrielle's ability to care for herself has also decreased. According to Gabrielle's parents, she can no longer manage personal hygiene without assistance. She cannot fully dress herself, and she is unable to manage clothing fasteners. She makes poor choices, endangering herself further.
>
> In addition to her brain injury, Gabrielle was described as suffering mental trauma, including major depression, post traumatic stress disorder, and separation anxiety disorder. At trial, Gabrielle was categorized for the first time as mentally retarded because of her brain injury.

The jury held in favor of the plaintiff and awarded damages to the plaintiff.

A jury trial resulted in a verdict for Gabrielle Hundley (Gabrielle) against Howard Jones, the pharmacist, and Rite Aid of South Carolina (Rite Aid) (collectively "defendants") in the sum of $5,000,000 actual damages, and against Rite Aid in the sum of $10,000,000 punitive damages. The jury returned a verdict in the parents' companion case against both defendants for actual damages in the sum of $20,000, and against Rite Aid for punitive damages in the sum of $1,000,000. Both defendants appeal.

One of the most significant issues in the case was the award of punitive damages. This award was challenged by the defendant. The defendant first argued that the evidence did not support an award of punitive damages, but the court disagreed, noting that the jury could have based the award on the claims of negligent retention and supervision of the pharmacist.

Jones and Rite Aid argue that because there is no clear and convincing evidence of gross negligence in the misfilling of Gabrielle's prescription, the punitive damages against Rite Aid should be reversed. We disagree.

The power to assess punitive damages is within the discretion of the jury, as reviewed by the trial judge. In order to receive an award of punitive damages, the plaintiff has the burden of proving by clear and convincing evidence the defendant's misconduct was willful, wanton, or in reckless disregard of the plaintiff's rights.

We need not determine whether the jury was presented with sufficient evidence of gross negligence in the misfilling of Gabrielle's prescription, because the jury may have awarded punitive damages against Rite Aid solely on the negligent retention and supervision claims, a possibility Rite Aid does not address in this issue.

The defendant next argued that it was inconsistent to hold the pharmacy liable for punitive damages and not to hold the pharmacist liable for punitive damages.

The court disagreed with this argument also.

Next, Jones and Rite Aid argue that the award of $11,000,000 against Rite Aid with no punitive damage award against Jones constitutes an inconsistent verdict.

Rite Aid argues that because the jury apparently did not find Jones guilty of willful, wanton, or reckless conduct, that level of conduct may not be imputed against Rite Aid by respondent superior or by way of the supervision and retention claim.

The Hundleys presented evidence that at the time of the mis-fill, Jones was nearing the end of one of his 12-hour work shifts. Jones was 65 years old, and his wife had died less than 1 month before the mis-filled prescription. He worked these shifts 5 days per week without another pharmacist present to relieve him. Rite Aid permitted him to work these shifts despite his age and personal trauma, and despite the fact that he had a history of mis-filling prescriptions, did not keep his paperwork up to date, and had been cited for failing to keep the pharmacy up to regulations. A memo in his personnel file recounted that his supervisor once took 14 hours to clean up the pharmacy and found violations such as multiple bottles of the same drug open and pill bottles on the counters without their caps.

The evidence also reflects that Rite Aid has no policies or procedures designed to ensure the competence of its pharmacists. Rite Aid considers its pharmacists fit to work as long as they maintain their state licenses. Rite Aid also has no policies, procedures, manuals, or directives dealing with the storage or handling of medications or the filling and labeling of prescriptions, leaving all such matters to the judgment of its pharmacists.

Considering the evidence of Rite Aid's conduct in retaining and supervising Jones, we conclude the trial court properly submitted the issue of punitive damages to the jury, and there is ample evidence from which the jury could have concluded that Rite Aid alone was reckless. Consequently, this verdict is not inconsistent.

The verdict against the defendant was affirmed.

Notes on *Hundley v. Rite Aid*

1. Pharmacies have a tradition of permitting their employee pharmacists significant leeway in determining how they are to practice their profession. As licensed health care providers, pharmacists differ from bakers or florists or cosmeticians because the employers do not set standards for what they do, the profession sets standards. Cases such as this one may change that tradition and force pharmacy companies to be more involved in the development and enforcement of standards that affect the profession. If this is to occur, it would be important for pharmacists to work with management to ensure that the standards represent realistic expectations of the profession, and that they promote the public health.

2. The award of punitive damages in this case is based, apparently, on the alleged failure of the pharmacy employer to supervise the pharmacist thoroughly. There is no litmus test for appropriate supervision. Each pharmacist requires supervision of a different kind. To meet the challenge of providing appropriate supervision, pharmacy managers will probably have to develop systems that adjust to individual and specific needs. There will perhaps be some aspects of the systems that will be standardized, but the use of them must be flexible. At a minimum, such systems probably would include periodic performance evaluation, periodic inquiries of pharmacists by management to determine what resources and support might be necessary to assist in the competent provision of pharmaceutical care, and periodic review of failures of quality to learn from the past and improve in the future.

3. This case obliquely raises the issue of continuing competency assessment in the pharmacy profession. To some in the profession, it makes little sense to simply assume that merely because one is competent to practice at age 25, one will continue to be competent to practice for the next 50 years. Those who challenge this assumption have suggested that there is a need to periodically assess the competence of pharmacists and not just require that they attend continuing education programs that may, or may not, maintain competence. There are no clear answers to the concerns some have expressed on this issue. Clearly the issue of continuing competency is a matter for further discussion, and it should be addressed by the profession before those outside the profession decide to find a solution to it.

CASE 8-3   *Cackowski v. Wal-Mart Stores, Inc.*, 2000 Ala. LEXIS 22 (Ala. 2000)

Issue

Whether a patient is held to the same standard of proof in establishing contributory negligence as the pharmacist is in establishing negligence in dispensing.

Overview

Patients who sue pharmacists bear the burden of proving their negligence case, and pharmacists who are sued by patients bear the burden of proving their defenses to negligence. As a practical matter, what this generally means is that the patient must prove breach of duty, causation, and damages. If the patient is successful in this proof, then the pharmacist may still defend successfully by proving that the patient was contributorily negligent and thus not deserving of an award. In Alabama, as in many other states, health care providers have been granted a reprieve from the burdensomeness of defending numerous lawsuits that might lead to defensive practice or even close down some sorts of health care practice. This reprieve is part of what has been called by some "tort reform" in response to a perceived "malpractice crisis." Whether there was really a malpractice crisis is an issue on which it is possible to disagree—but there is little disagreement that tort reform has made it more difficult (perhaps appropriately so, perhaps not) to sue health care providers in some states.

This case reviews an interpretation of Alabama's malpractice reform law, specifically the law that requires a patient to show negligence of a health care provider consistent with the high standard of proof known as "substantial evidence." In this case, the patient was required to meet that high standard of proof in the lawsuit against the defendant pharmacy. However, the lower court ruled that the pharmacy was required to show the contributory negligence of the patient only through the lower standard of "reasonable satisfaction." It is less difficult to meet the "reasonable satisfaction" standard than it is to meet a "substantial evidence" standard. The lower court's ruling resulted in a non-level playing field favoring the pharmacy. The patient appealed that ruling, contending that the playing field should be leveled by applying the same standard of proof to both parties—the plaintiff and the defendant.

The court began its analysis of the case by reviewing the factual basis of the litigation:

> On October 11, 1995, Brenda Cackowski enrolled in a physician-supervised weight-loss program and was prescribed a number of medications: Verelan, Profast, and Pondimin. Verelan is a medication commonly prescribed for high blood pressure. Profast and Pondimin are diet medications. The next day, Mrs. Cackowski went to the Wal-Mart pharmacy in Arab and had the prescriptions filled. The clerk on duty at the pharmacy counter asked Mrs. Cackowski if she wanted to have her prescriptions filled with generic medication, rather than the brand-name medication. Mrs. Cackowski stated that she did. Gavin Gilleland, the pharmacist on duty that day, correctly filled the Profast prescription. However, Gilleland misread the word "Pondimin," thinking the prescription was for Prednisone, a steroid. Instead of giving Mrs. Cackowski Pondimin or its generic equivalent, he gave her Deltasone, the generic equivalent of Prednisone. Because it was the cold and flu season, Gilleland did not think it unusual that a physician would prescribe a diet drug and a steroid (which causes weight gain) for the same person and to be taken at the same time.

> Although Mrs. Cackowski left the prescription with the pharmacist, her physician had also given her a list of the drugs he was prescribing for her. This list stated that he was prescribing Profast, Pondimin, and Verelan for her. Mrs. Cackowski knew that Gilleland gave her Deltasone rather than Pondimin, but she did not ask Gilleland the difference. Mrs. Cackowski took the Deltasone for 30 days, in accordance with the directions on the prescription. When Mrs. Cackowski finished the prescription, she went back to Wal-Mart to have it refilled. When the prescription was refilled, it was correctly filled and she received Pondimin. However, several days after she began taking the Pondimin, Mrs. Cackowski began to experience blurred vision and lethargy. Her husband became concerned and contacted her physician. Further investigation revealed Gilleland's error.

The court then described the legal proceedings that occurred at the trial court after the patient's lawsuit was filed.

> The trial court ruled that a pharmacist fell within the definition of "other health care provider" set out in [Alabama law]. Therefore, the court determined, the Cackowskis'

claims against Gilleland and Wal-Mart were governed by the Alabama Medical Liability Act ("AMLA"), and that those statutes required them to prove their case by "substantial evidence." At the close of the Cackowskis' case, the trial court granted Wal-Mart's motion for a directed verdict as to the Cackowskis' wantonness claim, but denied its motion for a directed verdict on the negligence and loss-of-consortium claims. At the close of all the evidence, the Cackowskis dismissed their claims against Gilleland, leaving only their claims against Wal-Mart. The case was submitted to the jury, which returned a verdict in favor of Wal-Mart. The court entered a judgment on that verdict, and the Cackowskis appeal.

The court described the main issue on appeal, which was that the differing standards of proof were unfair to the plaintiff in that they created a nonlevel playing field. The court then addressed the question of whether the "substantial evidence" standard was appropriate for the pharmacy. Only if a pharmacy is considered to be a "health care provider" would that standard be an appropriate one.

The Cackowskis first argue that the trial court erred by requiring them to prove their case by "substantial evidence," as mandated by the AMLA, while Wal-Mart, they say, was required to prove its defense of contributory negligence only to the jury's "reasonable satisfaction." In order to answer this argument, we must determine whether a pharmacist is a "health care provider," as that term is defined in [Alabama law]. That statute defines "health care provider" as "[a] medical practitioner, dental practitioner, medical institution, physician, dentist, hospital, or other health care provider as those terms are defined in § 6-5-481." Section 6-5-481(8) defines "other health care providers" as "any professional corporation or any person employed by physicians, dentists, or hospitals who are directly involved in the delivery of health care services."

The question whether a pharmacist is a health care provider for purposes of the AMLA is a question of first impression. This is not, however, the first time this Court has been called upon to determine whether an individual fell within the definition of "other health care providers" for purposes of the AMLA.

After careful consideration, we conclude that the pharmacist who filled Mrs. Cackowski's prescription was included within the AMLA definition of "other health care provider." To hold otherwise would be inconsistent with our prior decisions. Based on the foregoing, we conclude that the trial court correctly determined that claims against a pharmacist and/or a pharmacy must be proven by substantial evidence.

The court then turned to the appropriateness of applying the less challenging "reasonable satisfaction" standard to the proof required of the pharmacy in showing contributory negligence of the patient.

The Cackowskis also contend that the trial court erred in charging the jury that the Cackowskis had to prove their case by "substantial evidence," while, they say, the court required Wal-Mart to prove its affirmative defense of contributory negligence only to the jury's reasonable satisfaction.

In an effort to ensure the continued availability of quality medical services, the AMLA altered the standard of proof in a medical-malpractice case, to require that a plaintiff prove his or her case by "substantial evidence." Thus, Wal-Mart was also required to prove its affirmative defense of contributory negligence by substantial evidence.

The court reversed the verdict, which had been in favor of the defense, and remanded the case to the trial court with instructions to proceed based on the ruling that both parties must prove their case (the defendant's negligence must be proven by the plaintiff and the plaintiff's contributory negligence must be proven by the defense) under the same standard, that being "substantial evidence."

Notes on *Cackowski v. Wal-Mart Stores, Inc.*

1. Contributory negligence is an issue that is ever-present in pharmacy malpractice litigation. In this case, the patient received medication that was labeled with a name that she knew to be different from the name that she expected. Why didn't she raise the issue with the pharmacist? Apparently she had been asked whether she wanted a generic product, and she had replied that she did. This interaction with the pharmacist may have led her to believe that the prednisone she received (labeled as Deltasone) was the generic form of Pondimin. Although it is clear to any pharmacist that this assumption is a mistaken one, it is not clear to patients. The jury will have to decide whether the patient's failure to alert the pharmacist to this potential mistake rises to the level of contributory negligence. If it does, there is the possibility that the patient will recover nothing as compensation for her damages.

2. The decision by the court that the pharmacist and the patient are held to the same standard of proof serves as a reminder that pharmacists and patients are partners in health care. They share responsibility for outcomes from drug therapy, and it would be unfair to apply a higher burden of proof to one as opposed to the other. Of course, the standard of care is different for the two, even though the burden of proof may be the same. The patient's standard of care is that of a reasonable and prudent patient, the pharmacist's standard of care is defined by the profession, and it assumes that a significant level of expertise has been acquired by the pharmacist through education, training, and experience.

3. Tort reform measures have been adopted in many states, but pharmacists have not always been included within the coverage of tort reform directed to medical malpractice. In some states, pharmacists have been granted the protection of tort reform, but pharmacies have not. Tort reform efforts have imposed shorter statutes of limitation for health care malpractice, requirements that lawsuits against health care providers be accompanied by expert affidavits, and limitations on the credential of experts who may testify as to malpractice. Whether these measures have reduced frivolous malpractice litigation is an open question.

CASE 8-4   *Nelms v. Walgreen Co.,* 1999 Tenn. App. LEXIS 437 (Tenn. App. 1999)

Issue

Whether a slight deviation from state pharmacy rules justifies an award of punitive damages against a pharmacy.

Overview

Pharmacists are subject to numerous regulations that prescribe how they are to practice. No pharmacy adheres to these regulations at all times. It is a simple fact that any pharmacy may be found in violation of some rule at some time, although most pharmacies are in compliance with most rules most of the time. Requirements relating to the number of spatulas and stirring rods that must be owned by a pharmacy seem only distantly related to patient outcomes in a contemporary world. In this case, the question is asked whether it is willful disregard to exceed the allowed ratio for technicians to pharmacists during a brief time when a pharmacist takes a meal break. The plaintiff contends that the pharmacist is liable for punitive damages caused by the violation of the technician ratio rule. As you read this case, ask yourself whether there is really any purpose to limits on technicians. If a pharmacy is conducting a meaningful continuous quality improvement program (perhaps a big if), then does it really matter whether the pharmacy limits the technicians to a 2:1 ratio with pharmacists? Should a pharmacist be permitted to take a meal break if this means that an arbitrary technician/pharmacist ratio will be violated during the meal break? If technicians are not used more extensively in the future than they have been in the past, who will fill the prescriptions that are expected to almost double in volume during the next 5 years?

The court began its summary by describing the events that led to the lawsuit:

> In the fall of 1995, Inez Nelms suffered from depression that was associated with other health problems she had experienced over the years. Nelms' physician, Kirby Smith, prescribed the drug Paxil to treat Nelms' depression. On October 2, 1995, Plaintiff Jerry Nelms took a written prescription for Paxil to Walgreen Company's pharmacy on Knight Arnold Road in Memphis. The Plaintiff returned later that evening to pick up the filled prescription.
>
> Approximately 2 weeks later, the Plaintiff returned to the same Walgreen Company pharmacy to pick up a refill of his wife's Paxil prescription. Upon his return home, the Plaintiff noticed that the pills were smaller than the ones Inez Nelms had been taking. The Plaintiff returned to the pharmacy and learned that the first prescription had contained Tagamet pills instead of Paxil pills. While Paxil is a drug commonly used to treat depression, Tagamet generally is prescribed to treat stomach ailments, such as indigestion and ulcers. Paxil pills and Tagamet pills are not similar in appearance; they are different sizes and colors. The Walgreen Company pharmacist on duty informed the Plaintiff that the pharmacy had made a mistake in filling Inez Nelms' Paxil prescription on October 2, 1995.
>
> In November 1995, Inez Nelms was hospitalized for thrombocytopenia, or a low platelet count, the symptoms of which included bruising and mouth sores. Nelms blamed this condition on the Tagamet that she had taken as a result of the mistake of Walgreen Company's pharmacy. Consequently, Nelms filed this lawsuit against Walgreen Company for the negligent filling of her Paxil prescription. Nelms' complaint sought both compensatory and punitive damages. After Inez Nelms' death in October 1997, Jerry Nelms was substituted as the Plaintiff in this action as Inez Nelms' next of kin and as executor of her estate.

The court then described the basic controversy that related to alleged violations of state pharmacy laws by the defendants. The crux of the allegations was that a pharmacy technician had misfilled the plaintiff's prescription and that the technician had been illegally practicing pharmacy at the time.

> At trial, the evidence initially suggested that Walgreen Company pharmacist Ed Daniel had filled Inez Nelms' Paxil prescription on October 2, 1995.
>
> The computer-generated prescription label contained Daniel's initials, indicating that Daniel was the pharmacist who filled the prescription at 7:19 P.M.; however, Walgreen Company's schedules, which were introduced at trial, indicated that Daniel's shift was scheduled to end at 5:00 P.M. on that day. The original written prescription contained no pharmacist's initials, although the Tennessee Board of Pharmacy's regulations and Walgreen Company's policies required the pharmacist who filled the prescription to initial the original prescription form.
>
> As a result of this discrepancy in Walgreen Company's records, the Plaintiff sought to show that a pharmacy technician, rather than a licensed pharmacist, filled Inez Nelms' Paxil prescription in violation of both the Board of Pharmacy's regulations and Walgreen Company's policies. Walgreen Company employed pharmacy technicians

to assist its pharmacists in filling prescriptions. In filling the typical prescription, pharmacy technicians were permitted to obtain customer information, generate a computer prescription label, pull and count the medication, place the medication in the correct vial or bottle, and affix thereto the computer-generated label. The pharmacist on duty then was required to verify the prescription's accuracy before approving it for the customer's purchase. According to the Plaintiff's theory, a pharmacy technician filled and dispensed Inez Nelms' Paxil prescription without obtaining the approval of the pharmacist on duty.

Another Walgreen Company pharmacist, Steve Presson, testified that he had spoken with Ed Daniel two or three times during the last 6 months of 1995 about concerns Presson had with Daniel's performance. Specifically, Presson was concerned because Daniel would become distracted by other job duties and he would allow prescriptions to stack up waiting for his verification. Presson could not say for sure, however, if Daniel was the pharmacist on duty at 7:19 P.M. on October 2, 1995, when Inez Nelms' Paxil prescription was filled. Presson himself might have been the pharmacist on duty at that time because, according to Walgreen Company's records, Presson was scheduled to work from 1:00 P.M. to 10:00 P.M. on that day.

The Plaintiff argues that, from this evidence, a jury could have inferred that Walgreen Company's representatives engaged in fraudulent conduct in an attempt to conceal the fact that a pharmacy technician, and not Daniel, filled Inez Nelms' prescription.

The court evaluated the claim brought by the plaintiff, adopting a more forgiving and realistic perspective than one might have expected in a lawsuit involving serious injury to a patient.

We conclude that this argument is without merit. Although a jury could have found from the foregoing evidence that Ed Daniel was not the pharmacist who filled Inez Nelms' prescription, such a finding would not necessarily lead to the inference that a pharmacy technician rather than a pharmacist filled the prescription. Steve Presson, the pharmacist who was scheduled to work from 1:00 P.M. to 10:00 P.M. on October 2, 1995, testified that either he or Daniel was the pharmacist on duty when the prescription was filled. Thus, the Plaintiff's proof presented two equally probable scenarios: that a pharmacy technician filled the prescription in Ed Daniel's absence and, alternatively, that Steve Presson filled the prescription. Inasmuch as the proof failed to establish that one of these conclusions was more probable than the other, we hold that this proof cannot constitute clear and convincing evidence that Walgreen Company's representatives fraudulently concealed the fact that a pharmacy technician filled Inez Nelms' prescription.

The court then turned to the argument by the plaintiff that the pharmacy had permitted technicians to fill prescriptions without their being checked by a pharmacist.

In the present case, the Plaintiff contended that the following evidence demonstrated recklessness by Walgreen Company's representatives: Walgreen Company permitted medications to be dispensed without verification by a pharmacist; Walgreen Company allowed Ed Daniel to be responsible for filling prescriptions despite the fact that Daniel had been counseled for failing to stay at his workstation to verify prescriptions; Walgreen Company permitted its pharmacy technicians to bag medications; and Walgreen Company scheduled three pharmacy technicians to work with one pharmacist when the Board of Pharmacy's regulations permitted a ratio of only two to one.

The court disagreed with the plaintiff's contention that this evidence proved a violation of state law by the defendant.

The evidence failed to establish with a high degree of probability that Walgreen Company permitted medications to be dispensed without verification by a pharmacist.

Instead, the evidence indicated that, if a pharmacist was unavailable to verify prescriptions, the prescriptions simply accumulated until the pharmacist's return to his workstation. The record contains no evidence that Walgreen Company's pharmacy technicians ever bypassed the Company's verification procedures by dispensing medications without a pharmacist's approval. Similarly, although the evidence was undisputed that Steve Presson counseled Ed Daniel a few times regarding his absence from his workstation, the record contains no evidence that any unverified prescriptions were dispensed during Daniel's shifts. Rather, the evidence showed that the prescriptions accumulated until Daniel returned to his workstation. As for the Plaintiff's complaint that Walgreen Company permitted its pharmacy technicians to bag medications, we note that the Board of Pharmacy's regulations specifically allowed this practice: the Board authorized pharmacy technicians to "retrieve medication from stock, count or measure medication, and place the medication in its final container."

We also reject the Plaintiff's contention that Walgreen Company's violation of the Board of Pharmacy's regulation governing the ratio of pharmacy technicians to pharmacists constituted clear and convincing evidence of recklessness. As we previously stated, in order to be considered reckless, the challenged conduct must demonstrate a conscious disregard of a substantial and unjustifiable risk of such a nature that its disregard constitutes a gross deviation from the required standard of care. In the present case, the evidence showed that Walgreen Company usually scheduled three pharmacy technicians and two pharmacists to work during various shifts on each weekday. For as long as thirty minutes to one hour of the typical weekday, three pharmacy technicians remained on duty while only one pharmacist worked. Although this 3:1 ratio technically violated the applicable Board regulation permitting only a 2:1 ratio of pharmacy technicians to pharmacists, the evidence failed to show that this scheduling violation constituted a gross deviation from the required standard of care. Any violation occurred during only a thirty-minute to one-hour period of the fourteen-hour workday, and the evidence failed to suggest that Walgreen Company's representatives were aware that this scheduling violated a Board regulation or deviated from the required standard of care. Moreover, the rules and regulations promulgated by the Tennessee Board of Pharmacy do not necessarily establish the duty of care owed by a pharmacist, although they may provide guidance in determining if there is a duty of care under the circumstances. In any event, we note that Walgreen Company was not violating this regulation at the time Inez Nelms' prescription was filled.

The appellate court affirmed a ruling of the lower court, which had supported an award of compensatory damages but did not support an award of punitive damages.

Notes on *Nelms v. Walgreen Co.*

1. Pharmacy technicians are an absolute necessity in any modern pharmacy practice. It is just not possible for pharmacists to perform the necessary judgmental functions and for them also to conduct the order-processing activities that nonpharmacists are capable of doing. Pharmacists must supervise pharmacy technicians, but the requirement for supervision does not mean that pharmacists must look over the shoulder of technicians at every minute of every working day. It would be pointless to require this high level of supervision because pharmacists might as well do the order-processing tasks themselves if they are required to be at the technicians' side at all times. Rather, the approach usually taken is to require that the pharmacists check the work of technicians. In this case, the court was satisfied with an arrangement that required checking of pharmacy technicians' work and not constant supervision by a pharmacist. This is a sensible approach that permits the efficient use of pharmacists and at the same time provides reasonable protection of the public.

2. The court in this case was respectful of the state board of pharmacy rule regarding technician ratios, but the court was also careful to point out that board of pharmacy rules do not necessarily establish the standard of care. Although state board of pharmacy rules may be of some relevance in determining the standard of care for pharmacists, they are not the beginning and ending of pharmacist duties. The court was willing to be flexible in its interpretation of the board of pharmacy rules, resulting in a tolerant attitude toward the defendant that apparently had committed a relatively minor infraction of state law.

3. Pharmacists deserve to have breaks during their work day, just as all workers deserve breaks. When there are two or more pharmacists working at a pharmacy, as was described in this case, breaks can be taken by pharmacists in shifts through the day, and the relaxation of state laws regarding technician supervision, and other matters, is relatively minor. However, when pharmacists work by themselves and need a break, laws that require a pharmacist to be "present and on duty," or laws that require "direct and immediate personal supervision" of pharmacy technicians may have to be interpreted flexibly. Of course, it is always possible to close the pharmacy department down during a pharmacist break. However, no work gets done when the pharmacy department is shut down, and the saved-up work that greets the pharmacist after the break makes it almost not worth taking a break at all. In some states, boards of pharmacy have begun to lighten up on the rule that requires pharmacists to be present in the pharmacy at all times that the pharmacy is open, permitting the pharmacy to continue to be open during brief breaks by the pharmacist on duty. During these breaks, no prescription that has not been checked by a pharmacist may be delivered to a patient, but checked prescriptions may be delivered to patients and work can continue by technicians, subject to its being checked when the pharmacist returns. The posture of the court in this case suggests a tolerance of such an approach, as long as the pharmacist remains responsible for the quality of what is done in the pharmacy.

CASE 8-5   *Van Hattem v. Kmart Corporation*, 719 N.E.2d 212 (Ill. App. 1999)

Issue

Whether a mistrial should be granted to a pharmacy on the basis of possible prejudice from a television news investigative story about pharmacy misfills that aired during the trial of the pharmacy malpractice case.

Overview

The media have discovered pharmacy as a profession to criticize. A decade ago it was rare to have any criticism of the pharmacy profession in the media, but newspapers, magazines, and television shows are now filled with horror stories of "Danger and the Drugstore" and "Death by Prescription." In these stories, sad tales are told of patients who were dispensed incorrect medications and suffered terrible adverse effects as a consequence. Some pharmacists have met this criticism with a "kill the messenger" response, refusing to believe that there could be any truth to it. However, most in pharmacy are willing to confess that problems exist with quality in order processing and that the stories ring true at least to a certain degree. In this case, the court reviewed a claim by a pharmacy that publicity regarding pharmacy errors, during a trial for malpractice caused by an alleged pharmacy error, was prejudicial and led to a verdict against the pharmacy. As you read this case, ask yourself what the public's general impression of pharmacy tends to be and how that general impression may be altered by media coverage of pharmacy error. How can the pharmacy profession best respond to such media coverage of pharmacy error? Is there validity to the claim that media coverage may bias a jury? To what sort of bias is a pharmacist subjected anyway, even if there is no negative media coverage, if the evidence shows that an error occurred?

The court began by describing actions that led to the filing of a lawsuit against the pharmacy:

> The evidence adduced at trial established that, on June 15, 1995, 76-year-old Ernest died at St. James Hospital following an intracerebral hemorrhage, or massive brain bleed. At the time of his death, Ernest was taking several prescription medications, including Coumadin, a drug for reducing clotting factors and thinning the blood.
>
> Dr. Habib, Ernest's physician, had first prescribed Coumadin for him during a 3-month period in 1991 to prevent phlebitis, for which he had been hospitalized. Thereafter, in June 1994, after being hospitalized for acute thrombophlebitis, Ernest again was prescribed a 2-milligram dosage (one pill) of Coumadin once per day by Dr. Habib. On July 15, 1994, Dr. Habib increased Ernest's dosage from 6 milligrams every 3 days to 8 milligrams every 3 days. His specific instructions were for Ernest to take one pill on the first day, one pill on the second day and two pills on the third day, repeating that dosage, or a 1-1-2 regimen.
>
> On October 14, 1994, Dr. Habib again prescribed a 1-1-2 regimen of 2-milligram-strength Coumadin for Ernest. The prescription was filled at Kmart's Steger pharmacy, as it had been by the pharmacy previous times: on June 17, 1994; on July 29, 1994; and on September 7, 1994. Refills of the October 1994 Coumadin prescription also were filled by the Kmart pharmacy on December 29, 1994, March 10, 1995, and May 30, 1995.
>
> Each time Dr. Habib prescribed Coumadin, he warned Ernest about the dangers associated with that drug, specifically abnormal bleeding. Upon his discharges from the hospital, Ernest also was warned about Coumadin and was told to report any unusual symptoms or bleeding to his doctor. In addition, each time the Kmart pharmacy filled Ernest's Coumadin prescription, written warnings were provided and stapled to the bag containing the prescription bottle.
>
> According to Hazel, who picked up all Ernest's prescriptions at Kmart's Steger pharmacy, warnings were attached to each prescription bag, but she regularly removed those warnings before she gave Ernest the medication. Although she could not specifically remember picking up the May 30, 1995, Coumadin refill, Hazel testified that it was her custom to telephone a refill request to the Steger pharmacy whenever Ernest placed his pill bottle by the telephone. She then brought the prescription home, removed the warning labels and receipt and gave the bag containing the prescription bottle to Ernest. She believed she had done this for the May 30, 1995, prescription, but could not remember specifically. After giving her husband his prescription, she did not monitor the manner in which he took his medication. Ernest took his own medicine and kept a "drug diary," entering a check mark each time he took medication.
>
> While Ernest was on Coumadin, Dr. Habib checked his prothrombin time (the number of seconds it takes for a plasma sample to clot) monthly. From June 1994 until June 1995, Ernest's prothrombin time remained therapeutic. On June 14, 1995, after he was brought to the hospital, however, Ernest's prothrombin time was abnormally high and more than twice the previous result from a test taken on May 24, 1995.

Unfortunately, the use of Coumadin by this patient led to problems that were later attributed to the use of a wrong strength of Coumadin.

On the afternoon of June 13, 1995, Hazel and Ernest were vacationing in Dowagiac, Michigan. There, Ernest remarked to a friend that he might have passed blood in his urine. Ernest's friend advised him to see his doctor. That evening, after returning to their home in Crete, Illinois, Hazel noticed spatters of blood in front of their toilet; Ernest told her he would see his doctor in the morning about his "prostate." Ernest, who suffered from migraines, also complained of a headache. The next morning, Hazel found her husband unconscious and bleeding from his mouth and nose. Paramedics were called and Ernest was transported to St. James Hospital.

On June 15, 1995, while Ernest was in the hospital, Hazel remembered the warnings about Coumadin and bleeding. At home, she removed the Coumadin prescription bottle from the drawer in their home where her husband kept it, looked at its contents, and noticed the number "5" on the 79 pills remaining in the bottle, although the prescription label indicated that the dosage was 2 milligrams. While at the hospital, the Van Hattems' daughter Marilyn Neumeyer, a registered nurse since 1968, overheard her mother express concern that the Coumadin prescription bottle contained pills imprinted with a "5." Neumeyer then requested a *Physician's Desk Reference* and saw that the number "5" on the pills meant that they were 5-milligram strength. On September 6, 1995, plaintiffs filed the present suit.

It was impossible to know exactly how the 5-mg Coumadin tablets could have been dispensed instead of the 2-mg tablets that were prescribed. To discern how perhaps this error occurred, the court reviewed testimony regarding the procedures followed by the pharmacy in filling prescriptions.

At trial, further evidence was presented as to Kmart's custom and practice in filling prescriptions. According to a Kmart pharmacist, when a new prescription is brought into Kmart, a review is done to establish that all the pertinent information is legible. Then, the pharmacist enters onto a computer the patient's name, the name of the medication, its quantity, its directions, the number of refills and the doctor's name. A second check is done by comparing the computer screen to the written prescription. The computer then generates a label, patient information, warnings and a receipt. To fill the prescription, a member of the pharmacy staff removes the indicated drug, which is labeled with a National Drug Code (NDC) number, from the shelf. The pharmacy staff consists of pharmacists and technicians.

A member of the pharmacy staff then matches the NDC, the name and the strength of the drug on the stock bottle to that on the prescription label. Thereafter, the pills from the stock bottle are poured into a tray, counted out, and then poured from the tray into the prescription bottle, which is capped and labeled. If the prescription is completed by a technician, the bottle is left to be checked by a pharmacist. Similar procedures are used for refills. None of the pharmacists or technicians on duty the day Ernest's May 30, 1995, refill was prepared remembered refilling that prescription.

As bad luck would have it, during the trial the local television station decided to run an investigative news story on the subject of pharmacy error. The plaintiff was, at least to some degree, involved with the story.

After presentation of testimony was concluded, but before argument, Kmart's attorney moved for a mistrial based upon a news segment which appeared on television concerning misfilled prescriptions. The Channel 5 News program aired during the trial and featured interviews of Hazel in which she discussed how Ernest's death was caused by a misfilled prescription. After polling the jury and questioning the jurors who had seen the program, the circuit court denied Kmart's motion.

Kmart asserts that the circuit court erred in denying its motion for a mistrial based on the Channel 5 News broadcast, "Prescription for Error?" which aired during trial.

Plaintiffs respond that the court polled the jury and properly determined the news report did not prejudice or affect the fairness of trial.

During jury selection, plaintiffs' attorney reported to the circuit court that Hazel had spoken to the local news media about the case, but that he, himself, had "not made any comments for publication at this time." Attorneys for Kmart asked the court to explore plaintiffs' attorney's involvement. The court declined, but ordered all the attorneys, parties and their agents to refrain from speaking to the media during the pendency of the case.

On January 12, 1998, in the midst of trial, Kmart's attorney noted to the circuit court that a Channel 5 News reporter had been present in the courtroom. The attorney asked that the court "revisit" the question concerning media coverage and suggested that "before something comes up on the 10:00 o'clock news," the court instruct the jurors not to watch it. The court declined, stating "the minute I do, all 12 of them are going to watch it."

On January 14, 1998, plaintiffs' attorney advised the circuit court that the investigative story would be televised the next night and suggested that the court admonish the jurors "not to watch Channel 5 tomorrow." The court again declined to do so.

After the testimony had concluded, but before argument in the case, Channel 5 News broadcast a story on its 10 P.M. program about prescription misfills entitled, "Prescription for Trouble?" The report began by stating that the use of prescription drugs had dramatically increased in recent years and posed the question, "but can your pharmacy meet that demand without jeopardizing your health and safety?" The report also questioned whether enough trained workers were available to fill the increasing number of prescriptions.

Intermittently, throughout the Channel 5 News report, Hazel was interviewed. She discussed her belief that "somebody" had made a "mistake" with respect to Ernest's prescription. The newscast then reported that other prescription misfills had occurred: one at a Chicago-area Walgreen's pharmacy and one each in Florida and South Carolina at unnamed pharmacies.

The Channel 5 News report also discussed the prevalence of pharmacy technicians and the National Association Board of Pharmacies' concern that no testing was required to become a technician in Illinois. Channel 5 News also acknowledged Kmart's contention that its workers "double-checked" all prescriptions prepared by technicians. The report then showed Hazel again, stating that "something" had to be done which, although it could not help "Ernie," might help someone else. The report then noted that there were "good" technicians, but that the Pharmacy Board wanted better regulations and a task force of pharmacists was meeting the following week to discuss the use of technicians and work schedules.

After the news story was carried on the local television station, the defendant filed a motion for a mistrial on the basis of the potential bias of the jury as a result of exposure to the prejudicial information contained within the news story.

On January 16, 1998, Kmart moved for a mistrial, citing the Channel 5 News report. The circuit court reviewed the video tape and, on January 20, 1998, polled the jurors to determine whether the news program would influence their verdict. Four jurors had seen the program; one juror had seen the commercial preceding the program, but had not seen the program itself; six jurors had heard the program was broadcast, but had not watched it; and one juror knew nothing about the report. The court then questioned individually the jurors who had seen the program and its commercial to determine its effect, if any, upon their ability "to render a fair and impartial verdict, especially as it relates to Kmart." The first juror saw only the commercial, which he stated would not cause him to be unfair to Kmart. The second juror saw the entire report, but understood that the information was not evidence; he answered "yes" to the court's question of whether he would be "fair" and return a verdict based only on the evidence heard in the case. The third juror, who also saw the program, described the program as "so incidental" that he "couldn't even tell what he saw in that program" and also answered "yes" to the court's question as to whether he would be fair and impartial to Kmart. The fourth juror, who also had seen the program, denied that it would cause her to be partial, and answered "right" to the court's question as to whether she would base her verdict on the evidence and not on the program's contents. The fifth juror, who had seen the program, also indicated that she would be fair and impartial and base her verdict only on the evidence heard at trial.

After hearing the jurors' responses, Kmart's attorney argued that a mistrial should be granted. "Based on the responses of the jurors," the circuit court denied Kmart's motion for a mistrial.

In reviewing the trial court's ruling to deny the motion for mistrial, the appellate court first described the basic rules applicable to the appellate review of a decision by a trial court regarding a mistrial.

Whether to grant or deny a mistrial rests within the sound discretion of the circuit court and that decision will not be reversed unless a clear abuse of discretion is apparent. Only when there is an occurrence of such character and magnitude as to deprive one party of a fair trial and actual prejudice results will a mistrial be granted. Where publicity occurs during trial which may be prejudicial, a court must determine whether any of the jurors have been influenced to the extent that they could not be fair or impartial. The determination of whether the publicity has impacted upon the fairness of trial rests within the sound discretion of the court; "each case must be determined on its own peculiar facts and circumstances, with due consideration to the nature and character of the statements themselves."

In the instant case, the jurors who had seen the program answered the circuit court's question of whether they would remain fair to all parties, and would base their verdict only on the evidence presented at trial in the affirmative. The determination as to the effect of the broadcast, however, does not rest solely upon the jurors' responses.

A determination of this question involves the court's consideration of all the facts and circumstances and conjecturing upon the effect that the incompetent information has had upon the minds of the jurors, a determination incapable of absolute accuracy of a very high degree of reliability. It has been held that jurors themselves are incapable of knowing the effect which prejudicial matters might have upon their unconscious minds.

In any event the statement of a juror that reading a prejudicial newspaper article has not influenced him should not be considered conclusive. Basing the determination solely upon the statements of the jurors ignores and evades the real issue. The determination of that issue must, therefore, rest in the sound judicial discretion of the court to reach an inference, from all the facts and circumstances, that a fair trial has, or has not, been interfered with.

The court then applied the general rules for appellate review of trial court decisions to the facts of the present case.

A review of the Channel 5 News tape "Prescription for Trouble?" and of the evidence presented at trial, reveals that the content of the program was palpably prejudicial, particularly its timing, and was of such character and magnitude as to deprive Kmart of a fair trial. Although the investigative piece purported to report upon the general problem in the pharmaceutical industry, specific references to Hazel and Ernest's "tragedy" were replete and repeated throughout its content. Further, the implication of Hazel's appearance on the news report was that she was seeking to protect others by publicizing her own "ordeal."

The circuit court questioned those jurors who actually had seen the Channel 5 News report; however, it did not question those jurors who merely had "heard" about the program. Six jurors responded affirmatively when asked by the court whether they had heard from some "third-party source" about that particular broadcast. One juror volunteered that he had seen the commercial but intentionally missed the program, explaining that he did not want to become prejudiced against Kmart. Nevertheless, the court failed to determine how those other jurors had heard about the program or what they had heard. The court further failed to inquire whether any of the six jurors heard about the investigative report from any of the jurors who had seen it and, if so, what conversation or information was exchanged.

Given that the commercial itself was highly prejudicial in its portrayal of the pharmaceutical industry—declaiming the need for better regulations "behind the counter"—the court should have questioned those six jurors more specifically, as indicated above.

The circuit court further erred in basing its determination to deny a mistrial solely upon the jurors' responses which, for the most part, merely involved raising their hands, and answering the court's question by saying "the same," "yes, I did," "no, I didn't," or simply "yes" or "no." In refusing to grant a mistrial, the court stated, "a mistrial will be denied based upon the responses of the jurors." Although the determination of this issue rests within the sound discretion of the court, "basing the determination solely upon the statements of the jurors ignores and evades the real issue." Here, the court questioned only those jurors who had seen the program, accepted their responses with scant inquiry, and failed to question more closely those six jurors who had heard about the manifestly prejudicial program. The effect (upon eleven jurors) of such a prejudicial newscast, timed so as to be aired during trial just before jury deliberations, cannot be underestimated and certainly cannot be gauged by the limited inquiry pursued here by the court. Clearly, the court abused its discretion in failing to grant a mistrial where the program and its commercial indicted the entire pharmaceutical industry as lax in safety precautions, which would have included Kmart, and portrayed the Van Hattems as crusaders for the public benefit. The verdict that might have been rendered had no jurors seen the commercial or the report, or had not "heard" of them, is purely speculative.

Kmart also asserts that actual prejudice resulted because the jurors who had seen the broadcast were apprised of other pharmacy errors or misfills. In the newscast, the discussion of other misfills concerned a Chicago Walgreen's pharmacy and two other out-of-state pharmacies; Kmart was not mentioned. The impact of a supposedly unbiased newscast, however, cannot be underestimated, where that report articulated, bolstered and supported plaintiffs' theory of the case. The news report implied that pharmacies in general were understaffed and overworked allowing viewers to infer that prescriptions were filled by "untrained" technicians across the industry, which could, of course, include Kmart.

Moreover, the commercial for the program, standing alone, was prejudicial. The commercial for the news report promised a program about "one family's painful ordeal in their fight for better regulations behind the counter," but did not provide any information as to what better regulations were needed, who was responsible for providing them, how they might have affected Kmart's procedures, or how they could have alleviated the cause of the "ordeal."

For the forgoing reasons, the circuit court should have granted Kmart's motion for a mistrial. We reverse, based upon the foregoing ground.

Notes on *Van Hattem v. Kmart Corporation*

1. There have been many news stories about pharmacy error in the past 5 years. Although no pharmacist welcomes any discussion of error that casts aspersions on the profession, there is the possibility that the negative media coverage may be a blessing in disguise. If the issue of quality in pharmacy is put squarely on the table, perhaps price will no longer be the only factor when decisions are made about the acquisition of pharmaceutical products and services. In a society that views all pharmacy services as being of equal quality, price is the only factor that distinguishes one provider from another. Media coverage of pharmacy quality may persuade purchasers to think differently about pharmacy, and it may provide an incentive to pay a bit more money for a bit higher quality service.

2. In the American legal system, juries are supposed to be unbiased. In the selection of juries for trials, questions about beliefs and attitudes are asked of each potential juror, and great care is taken to ensure that any possible bias is removed from jury decisions. In this case, the court was concerned that jurors might have been biased by the television show that many of them saw and about which most of them had heard. Realistically, it is difficult to remove all bias from a jury's deliberations. It is difficult to look back on any situation and evaluate that situation without bias. So-called hindsight bias makes it difficult to fairly evaluate anything that happened in the past, because it is not possible to know everything that happened in the past. Hindsight bias causes evaluators to digitize an otherwise analogue situation, oversimplifying what happened and leading to a conclusion that there was clear error when things at the time were probably not nearly so clear.

3. In any situation of pharmacy error it is important to determine whether a system problem may have caused the error. In this case, an obvious potential source of error is the difficult dosing schedule that the physician prescribed. According to the court, the patient was directed to "take one pill on the first day, one pill on the second day and two pills on the third day, repeating that dosage, or a 1-1-2 regimen." Whether this difficult-to-understand dosing regimen had anything to do with the dispensing of 5-mg Coumadin is impossible to know. It is obvious, however, that directions for use in this way would be difficult to communicate and that patients would be likely to misunderstand them. Confusion of any kind can lead to the failure by the patient to detect a pharmacy error, and the pharmacist loses the patient as an important quality improvement ally.

TABLE OF CASES

GLOSSARY

Note: Words defined within the text are generally not included in the glossary.

A

acquit   The act of freeing a person by judicial determination.
adjudicate   To hear or try and determine judicially.
adversary   Opponent. Plaintiffs and defendants are adversaries.
affirmed   Upheld, agreed with.
allege   To declare or claim.
amendment   A change in an existing law, bill, or regulation made by modifying it, adding to it, or deleting part of it.
amicus curiae   Latin for a "friend of the court." A nonparty to a proceeding that the court permits to present its views through a brief.
appeal   A proceeding to have a case examined by an appropriate higher court to see if a lower court's decision was made correctly according to law.
appellant   The party who appeals a losing decision to a higher court to have the lower court decision reversed or modified.
appellate court   A court with the power to review the judgment of another court.
appellee   The party to an appealed lawsuit who wins in the lower court only to have the other party (called the appellant) file for the appeal.
arbitrary and capricious decision   A decision not based upon substantial evidence.

B

beyond a reasonable doubt   The burden of proof the prosecution needs to obtain a guilty verdict.
bill   A proposed bill presented to a legislature.
bona fide   In good faith.
breach   Violation of a law or legal duty.
brief   A written document prepared by attorneys on each side of a lawsuit presented to the court setting forth their legal arguments.
burden of proof   The obligation of a party in convincing the court as to why it should win.

C

certiorari   A writ from a higher court to a lower court to produce records.
common law   The body of law that originated in England and upon which present day U.S. court decisions are based.
compensatory damages   Damages awarded for actual injury or loss, in contrast to punitive damages.

concurring opinion   An opinion of a justice agreeing with the majority of other justices but for reasons different from the majority.

consent order   An order from a court or administrative agency based upon the voluntary consent of the party or parties involved.

contempt of court   Disobedience of a court order.

contingency fee   A legal arrangement where the attorney usually receives a percentage of the damages awarded, as opposed to an hourly fee.

counterclaim   A claim filed by the defendant against the plaintiff.

cross-examination   Questioning by a party of an adverse party or witness called by the adverse party.

D

damages   Monetary compensation for wrong or injury caused by the violation of a legal right.

declaratory judgment   A court decision informing the parties of their rights and responsibilities without awarding them damages or ordering them to do anything.

de facto   In fact or actuality.

default judgment   A decision by a trial court awarded to the plaintiff when the defendant fails to contest the case.

dissenting opinion   An opinion of a justice that disagrees with the majority.

diversity jurisdiction   The authority of federal courts to decide cases between two citizens of different states.

due process of law   Following legal procedures according to established rules and principles. Providing judicial fairness.

E

elements of a case   The component parts of a legal claim. The plaintiff must prove every element.

enabling law or clause   A statute upon which an administrative regulation must be based.

enjoin   *See* injunction.

et al   Abbreviation of *et alia*, meaning "and others."

et seq   Abbreviation for *et sequentia*, meaning "and the following."

F

federal question   A legal issue involving the U.S. Constitution or a federal law.

felony   A serious crime, as defined by statute, that is punishable by imprisonment or death.

fraud   Intentional deception for the purpose of causing another to suffer loss.

G

grandfather clause   A provision in a new law creating an exemption for previous circumstances.

grand jury   A group that decides whether enough evidence exists to justify a criminal indictment and a trial.

H

hearing   A preliminary proceeding where evidence and arguments are presented in order to reach a decision.

holding   The ruling by the court.

I

incarcerate   To imprison.

injunction   A court order requiring a person to stop doing or start doing a particular act.

in re   In the matter of.

intentional tort   A deliberate act causing harm to another for which the victim may sue the wrongdoer for damages.

ipso facto   Latin for "by the fact itself." When something is so obvious no further explanation is necessary.

J

joint stipulation of facts   A document stating that both parties agree to the facts.

judgment   The decision of the court.

judgment notwithstanding the verdict (NOV)   Reversal of a jury verdict by a judge when the judge believes the decision was based on insufficient facts or that the jury did not properly apply the law.

jurisdiction   The authority of a court to hear and decide a case.

jury   A group of people selected to find the facts, apply the law to the facts, and render a decision.

L

liability   Being legally responsible for an act or omission.

libel   To defame in writing.

litigation   A lawsuit.

M

malpractice   Provision of substandard care or services by a professional (negligence).

may   When used in statutes, it generally means not mandatory (in contrast to *shall*).

misdemeanor   A crime less serious than a felony and punishable by no more than 1 year imprisonment, a fine, or both.

mitigate   Reduce, abate, or diminish.

moot   Unsettled, undecided. Not requiring a decision.

motion   An oral or written request to a judge for a decision.

N

negligence   Failure to use the care a reasonably prudent person would have used under similar circumstances.

nolo contendere   A plea in a criminal case meaning the defendant will not contest the case. The defendant is neither admitting nor denying guilt but agrees to a punishment.

nominal damages   Conclusion by a court that no real harm was committed and thus the award of a small sum of money.

O

ordinance   A law adopted by a city council, county board of supervisors, or other municipal governing board.

original jurisdiction   Authority of a court to hear a case for the first time (as opposed to on appeal).

P

partnership   A form of business owned by two or more people.

party   The person either filing the lawsuit (plaintiff) or defending the lawsuit (defendant).

patent   A legal monopoly of 20 years granted by the federal government for the use, manufacture, and sale of an invention.

per se   In or by itself.

petitioner   The party who initiates the lawsuit. Usually a synonym to *plaintiff*.

police power   Authority of a state government to enact laws related to the public health, safety, and welfare of its people.

power of attorney   A document giving one person legal authority to act on behalf of another.

precedent   A legal principle or rule formed by one or more appellate court decisions that serve as authority in similar later cases.

prima facie case   "On its face." A case that presents sufficient evidence on its face for the plaintiff to win.

probable cause   The amount and quality of information police must have before they can arrest or search without a warrant, or that a judge must have before he or she will sign a warrant allowing a search or arrest.

promulgate   To proclaim or declare something officially; to publicize that a law or regulation is in effect.

R

relief   Legal remedy.

remand   To send back.

repeal   To annul or abolish a previous law by enacting another law.

respondent   Synonymous to *defendant* or *appellee*.

ruling   A decision by a judge.

S

sanction   A punishment or penalty.

service   The delivery of a notice, such as a subpoena.

settlement   Agreement reached between the two parties in a civil case prior to a judicial decision.

shall   When used in a statute, it means that something must be done or somebody must do something.

sole proprietorship   A business owned by one person.

standards of practice   Either written or unwritten rules followed by professionals in the course of professional practice.

statute   A written law enacted by a legislature.

stipulation   An agreement to settle a controversy.

suit   A legal action.

summary judgment   A final decision by a judge in favor of one of the parties. A motion for summary judgment is made after discovery but before trial and is granted if one side convinces a judge that, based upon the evidence, the case could only be decided in favor of the moving party.

T

testimony   An oral declaration made by a witness or party under oath.

tort   An injury or wrong to one person for which the person who caused the injury is legally responsible.

transcript   The official record of a trial or hearing.

U

ultra vires   "Beyond powers." Exceeding the authority granted to an entity such as a corporation or a board of pharmacy.

unprofessional conduct   Conduct below the ethical standards of a professional.

V

vacate   To set aside a previous action.

venue   A geographical place where the case can be heard by the appropriate court.

verdict   The determination by a jury based on the facts.

W

waiver   An intentional and voluntary relinquishment of a right.

wantonly   Reckless disregard for the health and safety of others.

witness   A person who gives testimony.

writ   A written order from a court requiring the performance of a specified act or giving authority to have it done.

wrongful death   Death caused by the fault of another.

INDEX